Chronic Pelvic Pain and Dysfunction

Chronic Pelvic Pain and Dysfunction

Practical Physical Medicine

Leon Chaitow ND DO
Osteopathic Practitioner and Honorary Fellow, University of Westminster, London, UK

Ruth Lovegrove Jones PhD MCSP
Specialist Physiotherapist and External Lecturer University of Southampton UK

Foreword by

Magnus Fall MD, PhD

ELSEVIER
CHURCHILL
LIVINGSTONE

ELSEVIER
CHURCHILL
LIVINGSTONE

ISBN 9780702035326

British Library Cataloguing in Publication Data
A catalogue record for this book is available from the British Library

Library of Congress Cataloging in Publication Data
A catalog record for this book is available from the Library of Congress

Notices

Knowledge and best practice in this field are constantly changing. As new research and experience broaden our understanding, changes in research methods, professional practices, or medical treatment may become necessary.

Practitioners and researchers must always rely on their own experience and knowledge in evaluating and using any information, methods, compounds, or experiments described herein. In using such information or methods they should be mindful of their own safety and the safety of others, including parties for whom they have a professional responsibility.

With respect to any drug or pharmaceutical products identified, readers are advised to check the most current information provided (i) on procedures featured or (ii) by the manufacturer of each product to be administered, to verify the recommended dose or formula, the method and duration of administration, and contraindications. It is the responsibility of practitioners, relying on their own experience and knowledge of their patients, to make diagnoses, to determine dosages and the best treatment for each individual patient, and to take all appropriate safety precautions.

To the fullest extent of the law, neither the Publisher nor the authors, contributors, or editors, assume any liability for any injury and/or damage to persons or property as a matter of products liability, negligence or otherwise, or from any use or operation of any methods, products, instructions, or ideas contained in the material herein.

Commissioning Editor: Alison Taylor
Development Editor: Carole McMurray
Project Manager: Kerrie-Anne McKinlay
Designer/Design Direction: Kirsteen Wright
Illustration Manager: Merlyn Harvey

The Publisher's policy is to use paper manufactured from sustainable forests

Printed in China

Contents

Contributors

Tracey Adler DPT
Physical Therapist, Orthopedic Physical Therapy Inc., Richmond, Virginia, USA

Giannapia Affaitati MD
University of Chieti, Italy

Rodney Anderson MD
Professor of Urology, Stanford University School of Medicine, Stanford, California, USA

Andrew Baranowski MB BS BSc FRCA MD FFPMRCA
Consultant in Urogenital Pain Medicine, The National Hospital for Neurology and Neurosurgery, London, UK

Eric Blake ND, MSOM
Adjunct Faculty, National College of Natural Medicine, Portland, Oregon USA

Raffaele Costantini MD, PhD
University of Chieti, Italy

Jan Dommerholt PT, DPT, MPS, DAAPM
President & Physical Therapist, Bethesda Physiocare, Inc., Bethesda, Maryland, USA

César Fernández de las Peñas PT, PhD
Doctor of Physiotherapy, Department of Physiotherapy, University Rey Juan Carlos, Madrid, Spain

Maria Adele Giamberardino MD
University of Chieti, Italy

Christopher Gilbert PhD
Psychologist, Chronic Pain Management Program, Kaiser Permanente Medical Center, San Francisco, California, USA

Howard I. Glazer Ph.D.
Clinical Associate Professor, Weill College of Medicine, Cornell University; Associate Attending, New York Presbyterian Hospital of Columbia and Cornell Medical Colleges, New York, USA

Diane Lee BSR, FCAMT, CGIMS
Owner, Director and Physiotherapist, Diane Lee & Associates, Surrey, British Columbia, Canada

Linda-Joy (LJ) Lee BSC, BSC(PT), FCAMPT, CGIMS, PhD Candidate
Owner, Director and Physiotherapist, Synergy Physio, North Vancouver, British Columbia, Canada
Co-Founder, Discover Physio

Andrzej Pilat PT
Professor, School of Physiotherapy, San Lorenzo de El Escorial, Madrid, Spain

Stephanie Prendergast MPT
Physiotherapist, Pelvic Health and Rehab Center, San Francisco California, USA

Hallie J. Robbins DO
Osteopathic Physician, Integral Rehabilitation, Salt Lake City, Utah, USA

Elizabeth Rummer MSPT
Physiotherapist, Pelvic Health and Rehabilitation Center, San Francisco, California, USA

Michael A. Seffinger DO
Associate Professor and Chair, Department of Neuromusculoskeletal Medicine/Osteopathic Manipulative Medicine, College of Osteopathic Medicine of the Pacific, Western University of Health Sciences, Pomona, California, USA

William Taylor PT
Owner and Director, Taylor Physiotherapy, Edinburgh, UK

Melicien Tettambel DO, FAAO, FACOOG
Doctor of Osteopathy, Pacific Northwest University of Health Sciences, College of Osteopathic Medicine, Yakima, Washington, USA

Andry Vleeming PT, PhD
Department of Rehabilitation and Kinesiotherapy, Medical University Ghent, Belgium Medical University of New England, Department of Anatomy, Maine, USA

Maeve Whelan PT
Chartered Physiotherapist, Milltown Physiotherapy Clinic, Dublin, Ireland

Foreword

The treatment of pelvic pain and dysfunction spans a very wide field of knowledge, expertise and practice. Accurate diagnosis and successful treatment can be very tricky; to get to the root of the problem within this area can be extremely difficult, and many specialists in related fields may well find this a very challenging an area into which to venture.

In this book, various aspects of chronic pelvic pain are brought together. Although some may be well known to experts in a particular field of knowledge, they may be unknown to experts in other fields, so this book is a very welcome addition for any practitioner whose work may routinely include treating patients with pelvic pain of any kind. In making an informed diagnosis, the anatomy of joints, ligaments, fasciae, muscles and viscera, biomechanics, and structural properties are just some of the factors that have to be taken into account, and these are all widely discussed and examined here. What this book further recognises is that the nature of pelvic pain is often complicated, and although pain may be diagnosed and treated as a strictly physiological symptom, it is often the case that this underpins a constellation of symptoms, necessitating the consideration, in diagnosis, of all anatomical and pelvic structures, and including the essential role the nervous system plays.

This book provides a wide-reaching and extremely comprehensive range of practical solutions to the treatment and diagnosis of patients presenting with chronic pelvic pain and dysfunction. Approaches including breath work and chronic pelvic pain, biofeedback techniques, and soft tissue manipulations are discussed. The result is a very practical, generously illustrated guide to the treatment and diagnosis of chronic pelvic pain, and one that is innovative in its approach to dealing with pelvic pain and dysfunction. In a difficult and challenging subject area, this is a coherent volume that helpfully gathers together the variety of regimens and techniques that are often required in effectively diagnosing these all too common conditions with which so many patients present. This will be a welcome edition to the library of many a practitioner for years to come!

Magnus Fall, MD, PhD
Göteborg
Sweden
May 2011

Acknowledgements

As co-editors we wish to express our thanks to the editorial team at Elsevier, whose friendly support has helped to bring this text to the point of publication. There are too many to mention, but a special vote of thanks goes to Alison Taylor, whose steadying advice helped us through difficult periods.

Our sincere gratitude also goes to the wonderful team of chapter authors, without whose knowledge and skills the breadth and depth of the pelvic pain story could not have been adequately told. We are hopeful that the contents of this book will shine some light and ease the journey of those patients with chronic pelvic pain.

LC: I wish to offer particular praise and thanks to my co-editor, Ruth Lovegrove Jones, who I believe agreed to participate in this project without realising just how much time and effort it would demand. Her intellectual focus, innate skills and natural enthusiasm helped to make the almost three years of collaboration both harmonious and productive.

My personal thanks go to my wife, Alkmini, for creating and maintaining the peaceful and loving environment in which the arduous hours of writing and editing passed peacefully.

RLJ: It's true, I had no idea how much time and effort co-editing this, my first book, would take, yet I am delighted that Leon Chaitow asked me, even if times I have thought "what was I thinking?!" It has been a privilege and honour to work with this wonderful teacher and his dedication to his path shone through, even at our most difficult times. Finally, as is always the way; my personal thanks to Stevie Steve and our magnificent daughter Hannah Morgan, for all their love and support. Namaste.

Leon Chaitow, *Corfu, Greece*
Ruth Lovegrove Jones, *Hampshire, UK*

An introduction to chronic pelvic pain and associated symptoms

1

Leon Chaitow Ruth Lovegrove Jones

CHAPTER CONTENTS

Introduction

This book has a single primary aim – to offer a one-stop source of relevant information for clinicians – specialists, practitioners and therapists – on the subject of non-malignant chronic pelvic pain (CPP), with particular emphasis on current trends in physical medicine approaches to assessment, treatment, management and care.

The purpose of this chapter is to:

1. Highlight the current classifications of chronic pelvic pain syndromes (CPPS) and define the terms used within this book;
2. Summarize the layout of the book and the topics covered in individual chapters;
3. Inform the reader of how little is known about the aetiology of CPP;
4. Remind the reader that as most treatment options are currently empirical, there is a great requirement for careful clinical reasoning when approaching the management of a patient with CPP.

Definitions of chronic pelvic pain syndromes

It is suggested that approximately 15–20% of women, aged 18–50 years, have experienced CPP lasting for more than one year (Howard 2000) and a prevalence of 8% CPPS is estimated in the US male population (Anderson 2008). However, overall prevalence rates of CPP are likely to be underdiagnosed, in part due to the lack of agreed-upon definitions and subsequent difficulty in categorizing CPP (Clemens et al. 2005, Fall et al. 2010).

Pain is defined as 'an unpleasant sensory and emotional experience, associated with actual or potential tissue damage, or is described in terms of such damage' (Merskey & Bogduk 2002) and central neurological mechanisms will play a major role in the aetiology and pathophysiology of CPP. To emphasize that pathology would not always be found where the pain was perceived and that there would most likely be overlapping mechanisms and symptoms between different CPP conditions, the updated European Association of Urology (EAU) classification of CPP (Fall et al. 2010) reflected a shift from definitions based on assumptions of pathophysiological causes, to one based on recommendations of the International Association for the Study of Pain (IASP) (Merskey & Bogduk 2002) and the International Continence Society (ICS) (Abrams et al. 2003).

Chronic pelvic pain is non-malignant pain perceived in structures related to the pelvis of either men or women. In the case of documented nociceptive pain that becomes chronic, pain must have been continuous or recurrent for at least 6 months. If non-acute and central sensitization pain mechanisms are well documented, then the pain may be

> regarded as chronic, irrespective of the time period. In all cases, there often are associated negative cognitive, behavioural, sexual and emotional consequences
>
> (Fall et al. 2010)

Chronic pelvic pain is then subdivided into those conditions with well-defined classical pathology, such as infection and cancer, and those where no obvious pathology is found. Chronic pelvic pain syndrome (CPPS) is therefore defined as:

> The occurrence of chronic pelvic pain where there is no proven infection or other obvious local pathology that may account for the pain. It is often associated with negative cognitive, behavioural, sexual and emotional consequences as well as with symptoms suggestive of lower urinary tract, sexual, bowel or gynaecological dysfunction.

Therefore in most examples of CPP-related syndromes, and those listed in Box 1.1, marked with an asterisk, it is important to note that they are not the result of infection or pathology, and are characterized by persistent, recurrent or episodic pain (Abrams et al. 2002, Fall et al. 2010).

This shift in definition is important to avoid incorrect diagnostic terms and descriptors as erroneous diagnostic terms are frequently associated with

Box 1.1

Common chronic pelvic pain syndromes (Fall et al. 2010, Abrams et al. 2003)

Note: The selection of CPP-associated syndromes on this list does not include acute variants, and the word *chronic* implies the presence of the symptom for not less than 6 months.

Note: Syndromes marked * have no proven infection or other obvious pathology and are characterized by persistent, recurrent or episodic pain.

- **Anorectal pain syndrome:** * Persistent or recurrent, episodic rectal pain with associated rectal trigger points/tenderness related to symptoms of bowel dysfunction.
- **Bladder pain syndrome:** * Suprapubic pain related to bladder filling, accompanied by other symptoms such as increased daytime and night-time frequency, with no proven urinary infection or other obvious pathology. The European Society for the Study of IC/PBS (ESSIC) publication places greater emphasis on the pain being perceived in the bladder (Van de Merwe et al. 2008).
- **Clitoral pain syndrome:** * Pain localized by point-pressure mapping to the clitoris.
- **Endometriosis-associated pain syndrome**: Chronic or recurrent pelvic pain where endometriosis is present but does not fully explain all the symptoms (Fall et al. 2010).
- **Epididymal pain syndrome:** * Persistent or recurrent episodic pain localized to the epididymis on examination. Associated with symptoms suggestive of urinary tract or sexual dysfunction. No proven epididymo-orchitis or other obvious pathology (a more specific definition than scrotal pain syndrome (Fall et al. 2010).
- **Interstitial cystitis (IC):** Within the EUA guidelines, IC is included within painful bladder pain syndromes. It is frequently diagnosed by exclusion. Positive factors leading to a diagnosis of IC include: bladder pain (suprapubic, pelvic, urethral, vaginal or perineal) on bladder filling, relieved by emptying, and characterized by urgency, and (commonly) the finding of submucosal haemorrhage (glomerulations) on endoscopy. IC is immediately ruled out in the presence of a variety of pathological conditions, including bacterial infection (Hanno et al. 1999, Peeker & Fall 2002).
- **Pelvic floor muscle pain:** * Persistent or recurrent, episodic, pelvic floor pain with associated trigger points, which is either related to the micturition cycle or associated with symptoms suggestive of urinary tract, bowel or sexual dysfunction.
- **Pelvic pain syndrome:** Persistent or recurrent episodic pelvic pain associated with symptoms suggesting lower urinary tract, sexual, bowel or gynaecological dysfunction. No proven infection or other obvious pathology (Abrams et al. 2002).
- **Penile pain syndrome:** * Pain within the penis that is not primarily in the urethra. Absence of proven infection or other obvious pathology (Fall et al. 2010).
- **Perineal pain syndrome:** * Persistent or recurrent, episodic, perineal pain either related to the micturition cycle or associated with symptoms suggestive of urinary tract or sexual dysfunction.
- **Post-vasectomy pain syndrome**: Scrotal pain syndrome that follows vasectomy.
- **Prostate pain syndrome**: Persistent or recurrent episodic prostate pain, associated with symptoms suggestive of urinary tract and/or sexual dysfunction (Fall et al. 2010). This definition is adapted from the National Institutes of Health (NIH) consensus definition and classification of prostatitis (Krieger et al. 1999) and includes conditions described as 'chronic pelvic pain syndrome'. Using the NIH classification system, prostate pain syndrome may be subdivided into type A (inflammatory) and type B (non-inflammatory).
- **Pudendal pain syndrome:** A neuropathic-type pain arising in the distribution of the pudendal nerve with symptoms and signs of rectal, urinary tract or sexual

Box 1.1

Common chronic pelvic pain syndromes (Fall et al. 2010, Abrams et al. 2003)—cont'd

dysfunction. (This is not the same as the well-defined pudendal neuralgia.)

- **Scrotal pain syndrome:** * Persistent or recurrent episodic scrotal pain associated with symptoms suggestive of urinary tract or sexual dysfunction. No proven epididymo-orchitis or other obvious pathology (Abrams et al. 2003). This may be unilateral or bilateral, and is a common complaint in urology clinics.
- **Testicular pain syndrome:** * Persistent or recurrent episodic pain localized to the testis on examination, which is associated with symptoms suggestive of urinary tract or sexual dysfunction. No proven epididymo-orchitis or other obvious pathology. This is a more specific definition than scrotal pain syndrome (Abrams et al. 2002).
- **Urethral pain syndrome:** * Recurrent episodic urethral pain, usually on voiding, with daytime frequency and nocturia (Abrams et al. 2003).
- **Vaginal pain syndrome:** * Persistent or recurrent episodic vaginal pain associated with symptoms suggestive of urinary tract or sexual dysfunction.
- **Vestibular pain syndrome** (formerly *vulval vestibulitis*): Refers to pain that can be localized by point-pressure mapping to one or more portions of the vulval vestibule.
- **Vulvar pain syndrome:** Subdivided into generalized and localized syndromes:
  - **Generalized** (formerly *dysaesthetic vulvodynia*): Refers to vulval burning or pain that cannot be consistently and tightly localized by point-pressure 'mapping' by probing with a cotton-tipped applicator or similar instrument. The vulval vestibule may be involved but the discomfort is not limited to the vestibule. Clinically, the pain may occur with or without provocation (touch, pressure or friction) (Abrams et al. 2002).
  - **Localized:** Refers to pain that can be consistently and tightly localized by point-pressure mapping to one or more portions of the vulva. Clinically, the pain usually occurs as a result of provocation (touch, pressure or friction) (Abrams et al. 2002).

inappropriate investigations, treatments, patient expectations and potentially a worse prognostic outlook (Fall et al. 2010).

Terms that imply infection or inflammation should be avoided unless these are known to exist. For example, treatment choices for chronic prostate pain are often based on anecdotal evidence, with most patients requiring multimodal treatment aimed at their symptoms and comorbidities. Only between 5% and 7% of all chronic prostatitis complaints yield evidence of bacterial involvement (Anderson 2008), and the concept of chronic pain deriving from inflammatory conditions of the prostate is questionable (Nickel et al. 2003). Similarly, a diagnosis of interstitial cystitis (IC) suggests that the bladder interstitium is inflamed, despite evidence to the contrary in most cases.

Additional confusion results from the presence of lesions necessary for diagnosis of type 1 IC in healthy women following bladder distension (Waxman et al. 1998). It appears that urologic chronic pelvic pain syndromes (UCPPS) frequently evolve in otherwise healthy men and women, with no obvious pathogenic aetiological evidence, or objective biological markers of disease (Anderson 2008). EAU guidelines have therefore moved away from using 'prostatitis' and 'interstitial cystitis' in the absence of proven inflammation or infection.

Baranowski (2009) suggests that where pain is a major feature of a condition it is appropriate to name the region/area/organ where the individual perceives the pain – for example *painful bladder syndrome*. Such a label does not imply any mechanism, merely a location, while inclusion of the word *syndrome* takes account of any 'emotional, cognitive, behavioural and sexual [associations or] consequences of the chronic pain'. The mechanisms involved may be associated with local, peripheral or central neural behaviour, and may involve psychological and/or functional influences, reaction and effects. None of these aspects are however implied by the name '*bladder pain syndrome*', although all are subsumed into its potential aetiology and presentation.

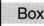

In general management of CPP Fall et al. (2010) suggest a sequence in which initial consideration is given to the organ system in which the symptoms appear to be primarily perceived. Where a recognized pathological process exists (infection, neuropathy, inflammation, etc.), this should be diagnosed and treated according to national or international guidelines. However, when such treatment is ineffectual in relation to the pain, additional tests, such as cystoscopy or ultrasound, should be performed. If such tests reveal pathology this should be treated appropriately; however, if such treatment has no effect, or no pathology is found by additional tests, investigation via a multidisciplinary approach is called for (see Chapters 6, 7 and 8).

Chronic pain

As practitioners working with people in chronic pain, we therefore need to remind ourselves that the structural–pathology model for explaining chronic pain is outdated, particularly as the relationship between pain and the state of the tissues becomes weaker as pain persists (Moseley 2007). A summary of the sensitization processes involved in CPP (Fall et al. 2010) suggests that persistent pain is associated with changes in the central nervous system (CNS) that may maintain the perception of pain in the absence of acute injury. The CNS changes may also magnify non-painful stimuli that are subsequently perceived as painful (allodynia), with painful stimuli being perceived as more painful than expected (hyperalgesia). For example, pelvic floor muscles may become hyperalgesic, and may contain multiple trigger points. This process may lead to organs becoming sensitive, for example the uterus with dyspareunia and dysmenorrhoea, or the bowel with irritable bowel syndrome (IBS). Berger et al. (2007) have indicated that men with chronic prostatitis have more generalized pain sensitivity, and current thinking suggests that if there has been an inciting event, such as infection or trauma, it results in neurogenic inflammation in peripheral tissues *and* the CNS (Pontari & Ruggieri 2008). Later chapters – particularly Chapter 3 – will consider both the local and the general influences on, as well as the nature of, pain, occurring in pelvic structures.

The following chapters include pain-oriented discussion:

- Chapter 3: Chronic pain mechanisms;
- Chapter 8: Multispeciality and multidisciplinary practice; Chronic pelvic pain and nutrition;
- Chapter 10: Biofeedback in the diagnosis and treatment of chronic essential pelvic pain disorders;
- Chapter 11.1: Soft tissue manipulation approaches to chronic pelvic pain (external);
- Chapter 11.2: Connective tissue and the pudendal nerve in chronic pelvic pain
- Chapter 13: Practical anatomy, examination, palpation and manual therapy release techniques for the pelvic floor;
- Chapter 15: Intramuscular manual therapy: Dry needling.

Pelvic girdle pain and CPP: To separate or combine?

The American College of Gynecologists (ACOG) has proposed the following definition of CPP (limited to females):

> Noncyclical pain of at least six months' duration, involving the pelvis, anterior abdominal wall, lower back, and/or buttocks, serious enough to cause disability or to necessitate medical care.
>
> (ACOG 2004)

The definitions from ACOG and EUA, include phrases such as '*structures related to the pelvis*' and '*involving the pelvis*' which suggests inclusion in such definitions of the structural supporting features of the region – and not only the pelvic organs and soft tissues.

However, many researchers and clinicians make a distinction between pelvic pain and dysfunction that relates to the organs and soft tissues of the region, and those chronic pain problems that involve the structural, osseous and ligamentous structures that frame the pelvis – the *pelvic girdle*. Pelvic girdle pain (PGP) therefore has its own definition, which *specifically excludes* gynaecological and/or urological disorders:

> PGP generally arises in relation to pregnancy, trauma, osteo-arthrosis and arthritis. Pelvic girdle pain is experienced between the posterior iliac crest and the gluteal fold, particularly in the vicinity of the sacroiliac joints. The pain may radiate in the posterior thigh, and can also occur in conjunction with/or separately in the symphysis. The endurance capacity for standing, walking, and sitting is diminished. The diagnosis of PGP can be reached after exclusion of lumbar causes. The pain or functional disturbances in relation to PGP must be reproducible by specific clinical tests.
>
> (Vleeming et al. 2008)

A reading of this definition of PGP can be seen to *specifically exclude* the pelvic organs and soft tissues, while the definition of CPP as provided in Table 1 in Fall et al. (2004, 2010) appears to allow for the consideration of *all pelvic structures*, including the pelvic framework.

So whilst simultaneously reminding the reader of 'no brain, no pain' (Butler & Moseley 2003), one of the aims of this book is to avoid what can be considered to be an artificial separation of the functions and structures of the entire pelvic region.

The *urological* and *gynaecological*, as well as the *biomechanical* (and other), features and functions of the pelvis are therefore considered, throughout this text, as having the potential to mutually influence each other.

Whenever the term *chronic pelvic pain* (or CPP) is used in this text, unless specifically stated to the contrary, this will refer to *pain anywhere in the pelvis*, arising from, or being referred to part, or all, of the region that lies inferior to the lumbar spine (although this will be involved at times) and superior to the gluteal folds – whether involving osseous, neurological, ligamentous, or other soft tissues, including the viscera.

Connecting PGP with CPP

O'Sullivan & Beales (2007) suggest that the motor control system can become dysfunctional in a variety of ways, and that such changes may represent a response to a pain disorder (i.e. it may be adaptive), or might promote abnormal tissue strain, and therefore be seen to be 'mal-adaptive', or provocative of subsequent pain disorders (see Figure 1.1).

Maladaptive changes might in turn lead to reduced force closure (involving a deficit in motor control of, for example, the sacroiliac joint) or excessive force closure (involving increased motor activation) resulting in a mechanism for ongoing peripheral pain sensitization, leading to chronic pain involving the sacroiliac and/or other pelvic structures.

Additionally the pelvic floor itself may be involved in such adaptations – with the possibility of CPP symptoms emerging (O'Sullivan 2005).

Consideration of the biomechanical aspects of CPP and PGP will be found in:

- Chapter 2: The anatomy of pelvic pain;
- Chapter 9: Breathing and chronic pelvic pain: Connections and rehabilitation features;
- Chapter 11.1: Soft tissue manipulation approaches to chronic pelvic pain (external);
- Chapter 11.2: Connective tissue and the pudendal nerve in chronic pelvic pain;
- Chapter 12: Evaluation and pelvic floor management of urologic chronic pelvic pain syndromes;
- Chapter 14: Patients with pelvic girdle pain – An osteopathic perspective.

Aetiological features of CPP

Some identifiable aetiological features commonly associated with CPP often involve one or more of the following factors summarized in Box 1.2.

However, in most cases the aetiology of CPP remains unknown, with no identifiable organic cause (Gomel 2007). Susceptibility to ill-health – in general – and to particular conditions such as those involving CPP, usually has multiple causes, since all manner of features, factors and events can compromise the individual's ability to self-regulate.

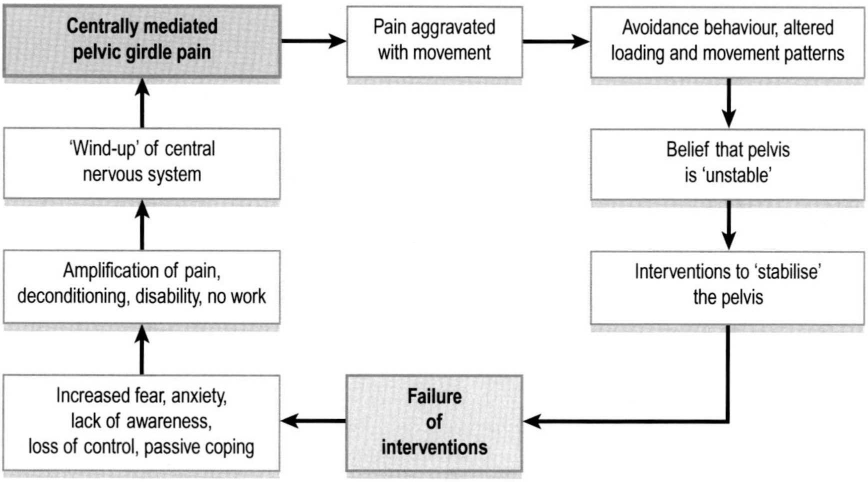

Figure 1.1 • The vicious cycle of pain for centrally mediated pelvic girdle pain. Adapted from O'Sullivan P, Beales D (2007) Diagnosis and classification of pelvic girdle pain disorders, Part 2: Illustration of the utility of a classification system via case studies. Manual Therapy 12 with permission

Box 1.2

Aetiological aspects of CPP

- **Abuse** (see also Trauma, below): Studies designed to evaluate factors predisposing to CPP and recurrent pelvic pain have demonstrated that several psychological factors, including sexual abuse and alcohol and drug abuse, are strongly associated with CPP and with dysmenorrhoea and dyspareunia (Raphael et al. 2001, Latthe et al. 2006).
- **Adhesions:** Found in 25% of women with CPP, but a direct causal link with associated pain has not been established (Stones & Mountfield 2000).
- **Autoimmune conditions** (Tomaskovic et al. 2009, Twiss et al. 2009).
- **Biomechanical:** Levator ani spasm, piriformis syndrome, and other musculoskeletal conditions have been associated with CPP in many instances (Tu et al. 2006) as have trigger points (Carter 2000, Fitzgerald et al. 2009).
- **Circulatory:** In one study presence of pelvic varicose veins was noted in 30 of 100 women with CPP of undetermined origin (Gargiulo et al. 2003).
- **Gender:** Females predominate – with studies showing prevalence ranging from 10 per 100 000 to 60 per 100 000 (Bade & Rijcken 1995, Curhan & Speizer 1999), with significantly higher rates in young women (Parsons & Tatsis 2004).
- **Hormonal:** Dysmenorrhoea and endometriosis may benefit from hormonal therapy (Howard 2000).
- **Infection:** Previous or concealed – for example involving the periurethral glands or ducts (see note at start of Box 1.1) (Parsons et al. 2001).
- **Inflammation** (though not always) (Bedaiwy et al. 2006, Twiss et al. 2009).
- **Neurological:** A recent study suggested that 'denervation that is caused by injuries to uterine neuromuscular bundles and myofascial supports is succeeded by re-innervation that may provide an explanation for some forms of chronic pain that is associated with endometriosis' (Atwal et al. 2005). Pontari & Ruggieri (2008) note that 'Pelvic pain also correlates with the neurotrophin nerve growth factor implicated in neurogenic inflammation and central sensitization'.
- **Psychiatric:** The rate of major depression among patients with CPP has been found to be in the order of 30–45% (Gomel 2006, Latthe et al. 2006). In a different study depression was present in 86% of women with both endometriosis *and* CPP, and only in 38% of the women with endometriosis *and no* CPP (Lorencatto et al. 2006).
- **Trauma** (see also Abuse, above): 40–50% of women with chronic pelvic pain have a history of physical or sexual abuse, which could explain psychological or neurological components of pain. Research also suggests that trauma may heighten physical sensitivity to pain (Howard 2000).

Beyond single causes

A linking of genetic susceptibility with some instances of CPP (discussed further below) suggests an interaction between lifestyle and environmental factors, and the unique genetic make-up of the individual (Dimitrakov & Guthrie 2009).

As to what such environmental factors might be, Tak & Rosmalan (2010) discuss the role of the body's 'stress responsive systems' in what have been termed functional somatic syndromes, for example IBS (Lane et al. 2009), as involving a 'multifactorial interplay between psychological, biological, and social factors'. They conclude that *stress responsive system dysfunction* may be involved in the aetiology of such conditions. There is therefore a need to move beyond a search for single causes of most conditions involving CPP, since, like many other complex and difficult-to-treat conditions, CPP commonly has multifactorial aetiological features – possibly interacting with predispositions and altered stress-coping functions.

Beales (2004) has described a scenario that highlights multiple contributory factors to functional somatic syndromes:

> Too much sustained, unhealthy, down slope arousal (see Figure 1.2) leads to the loss of internal balance, and results in reduced performance and a mind–body system in overdrive. In this state, the metabolism is struggling and cholesterol, blood sugar and blood pressure are often raised, resulting in ill-health. The more aroused we become, the more sleep, which would be to some degree restorative, decreases. Signals of mind–body protest multiply. For instance, sufferers from irritable bowel syndrome may also commonly experience back pain, fatigue and loss of libido. Negative emotions, such as frustration and despair, can trigger exhaustion, which in turn can trigger breathing pattern disorders, as a consequence of the perceived threat to survival eliciting fight, flight or freeze reactions.

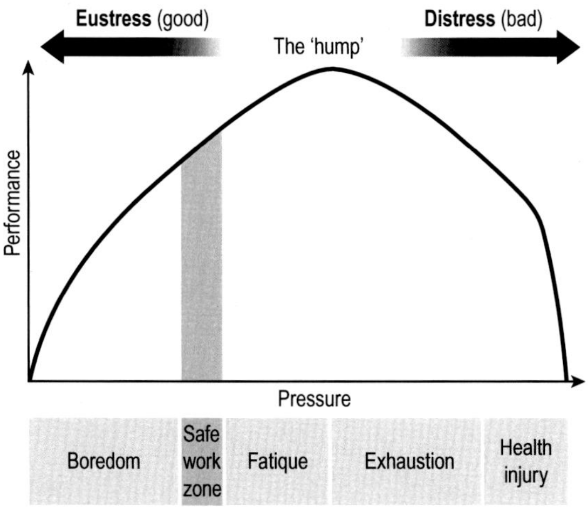

Figure 1.2 • Human function curve. Healthy tension is represented by the up slope of the curve, where performance tends to improve in proportion to arousal. In this state of mind and body, activity can be balanced by restoration, and so homeostasis is maintained. On the down slope, effort continues despite fatigue; arousal increases but performance deteriorates, and eventually exhaustion worsens and health breaks down. Adapted from Beales (2004) "I've got this pain . . ." Human Givens Journal 11(4):16–18 with permission

Recent research has indicated that there may be a genetic tendency operating in some people with CPP. Dimitrakov & Guthrie (2009) note that:

> An increasing body of evidence showing familial clustering of urological chronic pelvic pain syndrome (UCPPS) supports the notion of it being a genetic disease. Indeed, familial clustering appears to apply to IC in families with other comorbidities such as panic disorder, social anxiety disorder and thyroid problems. The well established prevalence of comorbidities of interstitial cystitis, such as fibromyalgia, allergies and Sjogren's, irritable bowel and chronic fatigue syndromes, present an enticing picture of UCPPS as a set of conditions with significant pathophysiological overlap with many other diseases due to central, genetically defined risk factors.

Interesting as such considerations might be to researchers, a finding of a genetic link to CPP is unlikely to offer solutions to a patient's current CPP problem. Yet phenotypes result from the expression of an organism's genes, as well as the influence of environmental factors and the interactions between the two. Understanding the classifications, and possible aetiological features of a particular manifestation of CPP, should help determine a successful therapeutic plan. For example, Baranowski (2009) explains:

> A chronic bladder pain condition may be associated with the presence of Hunner's ulcers and glomerulations on cystoscopy, whereas another condition may have a normal appearance on cystoscopy. There will be two different phenotypes. The same is true for the irritable bowel syndrome (IBS) that may be subdivided into those with primarily diarrhoea or those with primarily constipation or both.

Making sense of the multiple clinical features in any individual with CPP and arriving at a therapeutic plan therefore calls for careful evaluation of the evidence. In Chapter 7 the question of the role of clinical reasoning, in the differential diagnosis and management of chronic pelvic pain, is explored in depth. How individuals and organizations set about combining clinical assessment and therapeutic expertise, experience and evidence is clearly of major importance when handling complex problems such as CPP and its multiple associated symptoms.

Treatment aimed at pathology is only part of the answer

There would be little need for this book were current treatment strategies that focus on CPP proving successful. Anderson (2006) notes that traditional medical therapy to treat CPP conditions has failed, 'whether involving antibiotics, anti-androgens, anti-inflammatories, α-blockers, thermal or surgical therapies, and virtually all phytoceutical approaches'. Shoskes & Katz (2005) concur – demonstrating that a series of monotherapies, used to treat hundreds of men with prostatitis, resulted in only 19% reporting any relief of symptoms. However a randomized clinical trial designed to assess the feasibility of conducting a full-scale trial of physical therapy methods in 48 patients with urological CPPS has shown promise (Fitzgerald et al. 2009). It compared two methods of manual therapy: myofascial physical therapy and global therapeutic massage. The global response rate of 57% in the myofascial physical therapy group was significantly higher than the rate of 21% in the global therapeutic massage treatment group ($P = 0.03$) suggesting a beneficial effect of myofascial physical therapy.

However, Pontari & Ruggieri (2008) note that the symptoms of CP/CPPS appear to result from interplay between psychological factors and dysfunction in the immune, neurological and endocrine systems. It therefore seems unarguable that therapeutic approaches should adopt strategies that take account of these multiple interacting factors. And this is precisely the approach that this book takes.

For example psychological issues are considered in:

- Chapter 4: Psychophysiology and pelvic pain;
- Chapter 6: Musculoskeletal causes and the contribution of sport to the evolution of chronic lumbopelvic pain;
- Chapter 8: Multispeciality and multidisciplinary practice;
- Chapter 9: Breathing and chronic pelvic pain: Connections and rehabilitation features;
- Chapter 10: Biofeedback in the diagnosis and treatment of chronic essential pelvic pain disorders;
- Chapter 12: Evaluation and pelvic floor management of urologic chronic pelvic pain syndromes.

As expressed throughout this book, a background of different influences will be found to accompany the evolution of CPP, and its associated symptoms. Identifying the *particular* influences that have caused, maintained and/or exacerbated a CPP patient's condition is therefore an appropriate clinical ambition. In the context of this book, a further ambition is the identification of those influences that may be amenable to therapeutic attention involving physical medicine. However, as pain involves many thoughts and emotional contributions, how we treat, talk, listen to and educate our patients about 'their' pain requires great skill. Reminiscent of the Indian parable regarding the elephant and a group of six blind men, many clinicians would agree that if there were six therapists examining one chronic pain patient, the most likely outcome would be six different diagnoses and six different treatment approaches. Further resembling the wise man's explanation, all could be correct but no-one would know the whole truth. The patient may have all the features the therapist individually described, but it would be influenced by the therapist's perspective and different belief systems. Further complicating matters, any dysfunction observed may not even be relevant to the presenting condition.

So how can the therapist explain CPP to their patient and what makes one patient more susceptible to chronic pain than another? As outlined previously, the aetiology is unclear but it is apparent that multiple factors somehow contribute to the pain experience. With this belief system in mind, a '10 points for pain' model is one concept that a number of patients and clinicians have found useful (Jones 2003) (Figure 1.3). It is an easy way to demonstrate that pain can develop through many different reasons

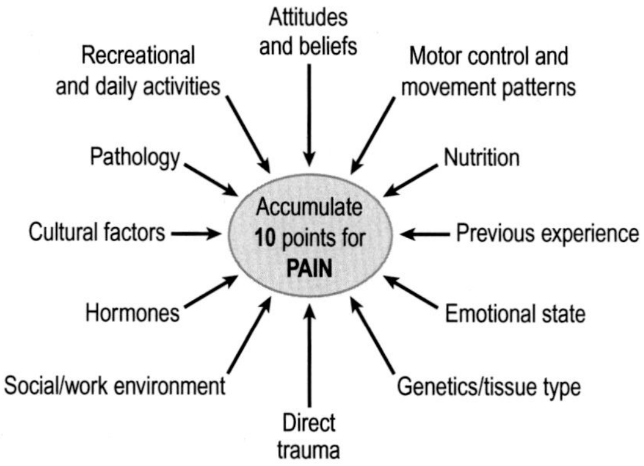

Figure 1.3 • Accumulate 10 points for pain; some factors that appear to influence the accumulation of a pain experience. Reproduced, with permission, from Jones (2003)

and works on the premise that pain is rarely the result of one single incident, but normally stems from a range of different issues or *a whole lifestyle* that contribute to the 10 points and painful state.

In this way, the patient and therapist can move away from the solely structural pathological model, to one that considers, for example, the brain in pain, their beliefs about their pain, nutritional issues, in addition to any pathology or motor control issues. For example, there is evidence that understanding pain reduces the threat of it, altering patients' attitudes and beliefs, increasing pain thresholds and, when combined with physiotherapy, reduces pain and disability (Moseley 2007). It is therefore important to understand what the patient believes the pain means and help explain modern pain biology, thereby reducing the patient's attitude and beliefs points. For example the patient may have a belief that:

- All pain is harmful;
- Pain only occurs when they have damaged or injured themselves;
- Chronic pain means that an injury has not healed properly;
- Worse injuries always result in worse pain;
- All pain must go before they can resume work or their hobbies;
- Exercise will hurt;
- Something is terribly wrong with their back/pelvis/pelvic organs, it is just that no-one has performed the right tests;
- They are unable to help themselves overcome their pain, and think that someone else has to fix it.

One consequence of these beliefs is that the patient may be afraid to do an activity just in case it hurts or avoid it completely. For example, patients who have been diagnosed with pudendal neuralgia typically are afraid to sit, as they have read that prolonged sitting causes compression to their nerve so if they sit for too long (or at all) they will develop greater compression and more pain. In this way, they avoid sitting at all costs, which can severely affect their work, recreation and quality of life. Similarly sex can be painful, so if the patient equates pain with damage, not only does the patient avoid an activity that can provide great pleasure, cessation of sexual intimacy can produce immense strain on their relationship.

The 10 points for pain is not an exhaustive list, and the patient is encouraged to fill out their own chart, adding in any factor that they believe may contribute to their pain. Furthermore, it is important to emphasize that this is not an absolute scoring system that says that diagnosed pathology is 4 points, having negative beliefs and attitudes is 2 points, having poor motor control is 3 points, being angry or fearful is 2 points. Some patients will accumulate more points in one area than another, or those same factors will have a higher (or lower) weighting in different patients. The task of the therapist and patient is to start piecing the different parts of the puzzle together in order to understand the unique accumulation of factors that tip the patient over the threshold from a pain-free (below 10 points) to a painful (above 10 points) state. Over time the patient then can reduce their points by choosing to change the areas in their life that they believe are contributing to their pain experience and let go of the things that they cannot. The therapist assists by reducing the patient's accumulated pain points in areas amenable to the therapist's particular discipline.

It is our hope that some of the ideas contained within this book may be of use in the clinic, either in their current form, or with additional creative input from the reader. However, as stated at the beginning of the chapter, currently most treatment options for CPP are empirical, so there is a great requirement for careful clinical reasoning when approaching the management of a patient with CPP, if indeed we are to do no harm.

The next chapter describes the anatomy of structures that may need to be examined and treated in patients with pelvic pain.

References

Abrams, P., Cardozo, L., Fall, M., et al., 2002. The standardisation of terminology of lower urinary tract function: report from the Standardisation Subcommittee of the International Continence Society. Am. J. Obstet. Gynecol. 187, 116–126.

Abrams, P., Cardozo, L., Fall, M., et al., 2003. The standardisation of terminology of lower urinary tract function: report from the Standardisation Subcommittee of the International Continence Society. Urology 61 (1), 37–49. http://www.ncbi.nlm.nih.gov/pubmed/12559262.

ACOG, 2004. Practice Bulletin No. 51. Chronic pelvic pain. Obstet. Gynecol. 103 (3), 589–605.

Anderson, R., 2006. Traditional therapy for chronic pelvic pain does not work: What do we do now? Nat. Clin. Pract. Urol. 3 (3), 145–156.

Anderson, R., 2008. The role of pelvic floor therapies in chronic pelvic pain syndromes. Current Prostate Reports 6, 139–144.

Atwal, G., du Plessis, D., Armstrong, G., Slade, R., Quinn, M., 2005. Uterine innervation after hysterectomy for chronic pelvic pain with, and without endometriosis. Am. J. Obstet. Gynecol. 193, 1650–1655.

Bade, J.J., Rijcken, B., 1995. Interstitial cystitis in the Netherlands: prevalence, diagnostic criteria and therapeutic preferences. J. Urol. 154, 2035–2037.

Baranowski, A., 2009. Chronic pelvic pain. Best Pract. Res. Clin. Gastroenterol. 23, 593–610.

Beales, D., 2004. "I've got this pain ..." Human Givens Journal 11 (4), 16–18.

Bedaiwy, M.A., Falcone, T., Goldberg, J.M., et al., 2006. Peritoneal fluid leptin is associated with chronic pelvic pain but not infertility in endometriosis patients. Hum. Reprod. 21, 788–791.

Berger, R., Ciol, M., Rothman, I., Turner, J., 2007. Pelvic tenderness is not limited to the prostate in chronic prostatitis/chronic pelvic pain syndrome (CPPS) type IIIA and IIIB: comparison of men with and without CP/CPPS. BMC Urol. 7, 17.

Butler, D., Moseley, G.L., 2003. Explain pain. NOI Group Publishing, Adelaide.

Carter, J., 2000. Abdominal wall and pelvic myofascial trigger points. In: Howard, F.M. (Ed.), Pelvic pain. Diagnosis and management. Lippincott Williams & Wilkins, Philadelphia, PA, pp. 314–358.

Clemens, J.Q., Meenan, R.T., Richard, T., et al., 2005. Prevalence of interstitial cystitis symptoms in a managed care population. J. Urol. 174 (2), 576–580.

Curhan, G.C., Speizer, F.E., 1999. Epidemiology of interstitial cystitis: a population based study. J. Urol. 161, 549–552.

Dimitrakov, J., Guthrie, D., 2009. Genetics and phenotyping of urological chronic pelvic pain syndrome. J. Urol. 181 (4), 1550–1557.

Fall, M., Baranowski, A., Fowler, C., et al., 2004. EAU guidelines on chronic pelvic pain. Eur. Urol. 46 (6), 681–689.

Fall, M., Baranowski, A., Elneil, S., et al., 2008. EAU guidelines on chronic pelvic pain. European Association of Urology web site. http://www.uroweb.org/fileadmin/tx_eauguidelines/2009/Full/CPP.pdf.

Fall, M., Baranowski, A., Elneil, S., et al., 2010. EAU guidelines on chronic pelvic pain. Eur. Urol. 57 (1), 35–48.

Fitzgerald, M.P., Anderson, R., Potts, J., et al., 2009. Randomized multicenter feasibility trial of myofascial physical therapy for the treatment of urological chronic pelvic pain syndromes. J. Urol. 182 (2), 570–580.

Gargiulo, T., Mais, V., Brokaj, L., et al., 2003. Bilateral laparoscopic transperitoneal ligation of ovarian veins for treatment of pelvic congestion syndrome. J. Am. Assoc. Gynecol. Laparosc. 10, 501–504.

Gomel, V., 2006. Foreword. In: Li, T.C., Ledger, W.L. (Eds.), Chronic Pelvic Pain. Taylor and Francis, London, UK.

Gomel, V., 2007. Chronic pelvic pain: A challenge. J. Minim. Invasive Gynecol. 14, 521–526.

Hanno, P., Landis, J., Matthews-Cook, Y., 1999. The diagnosis of interstitial cystitis revisited: lessons learned from the National Institutes of Health Interstitial Cystitis Database study. J. Urol. 161 (2), 553–557.

Howard, F., 2000. The role of laparoscopy as a diagnostic tool in chronic pelvic pain. Baillieres Best Pract. Res. Clin. Obstet. Gynaecol. 14, 467–494.

Jones, R.C., 2003–2010. The Back Detective: Course notes and book in preparation.

Krieger, J., Nyberg, L., Nickel, J., 1999. NIH consensus definition and classification of prostatitis. JAMA 282, 236–237.

Lane, R., Waldstein, S., Critchley, H., et al., 2009. The rebirth of neuroscience in psychosomatic medicine, Part II: clinical applications and implications for research. Psychosom. Med. 71, 135–151.

Latthe, P., Mignini, L., Gray, R., et al., 2006. Factors predisposing women to chronic pelvic pain: systematic review. BMJ 332, 749–755.

Lorencatto, C., Petta, C., Navarro, M., et al., 2006. Depression in women with endometriosis with and without pelvic pain. Acta Obstet. Gynecol. Scand. 85, 88–92.

Merskey, H., Bogduk, N., 2002. Classification of Chronic Pain. Descriptions of Chronic Pain Syndromes and Definitions of Pain Terms. IASP Press.

Moseley, G.L., 2007. Reconceptualising pain according to modern pain science. Phys. Ther. Rev. 12 (3), 169–178.

Nickel, J., Alexander, R., Schaeffer, A., et al., 2003. Leukocytes and bacteria in men with chronic prostatitis/chronic pelvic pain syndrome compared to asymptomatic controls. J. Urol. 170 (3), 818–822.

O'Sullivan, P.B., 2005. Clinical instability of the lumbar spine: its pathological basis, diagnosis and conservative management. In: Jull, G.A., Boyling, J.D. (Eds.), Grieve's modern manual therapy, third ed. Churchill Livingstone, Edinburgh, pp. 311–331 [Chapter 22].

O'Sullivan, P., Beales, D., 2007. Diagnosis and classification of pelvic girdle pain disorders, Part 2: Illustration of the utility of a classification system via case studies. Man. Ther. 12, e1–e12.

Parsons, C., Zupkas, P., Parsons, J., 2001. Intravesical potassium sensitivity in patients with interstitial cystitis and urethral syndrome. Urology 57, 428–432.

Parsons, C.L., Tatsis, V., 2004. Prevalence of interstitial cystitis in young women. Urology 64, 866–870.

Peeker, R., Fall, M., 2002. Toward a precise definition of interstitial cystitis: further evidence of differences in classic and nonulcer disease. J. Urol. 167 (6), 2470–2472.

Pontari, M., Ruggieri, M., 2008. Mechanisms in prostatitis/chronic pelvic pain syndrome. Urology 179, S61–S67.

Raphael, K., Widom, C., Lange, G., 2001. Childhood victimization and pain in adulthood: a prospective investigation. Pain 92, 283–293.

Shoskes, D., Katz, E., 2005. Multimodal therapy for chronic prostatitis/chronic pelvic pain syndrome. Curr. Urol. Rep. 6 (4), 296–299.

Stones, R.W., Mountfield, J., 2000. Interventions for treating chronic pelvic pain in women. Cochrane Database Syst. Rev. (4), CD000387.

Tak, L., Rosmalan, J., 2010. Dysfunction of stress responsive systems as a risk factor for functional somatic syndromes. J. Psychosom. Res. 68 (5), 461–468.

Tomaskovic, I., Ruzica, B., Trnskia, D., et al., 2009. Chronic prostatitis/chronic pelvic pain syndrome in males may be an autoimmune disease, potentially responsive to corticosteroid therapy. Med. Hypotheses 72 (3), 261–262.

Tu, F.F., As-Sanie, S., Steege, J.F., 2006. Prevalence of musculoskeletal disorders in a chronic pain clinic. J. Reprod. Med. 51, 185–189.

Twiss, C., Kilpatrick, L., Triaca, V., et al., 2009. Evidence for central hyperexitability in patients with interstitial cystitis. J. Urol. 177, 49.

van der Merwe, J.P., Nordling, J., Bouchelouche, P., et al., 2008. Diagnostic criteria, classification, and nomenclature for painful bladder syndrome/interstitial cystitis: an ESSIC proposal. Eur. Urol. 53, 60–67.

Vleeming, A., Albert, H., Östgaard, H., et al., 2008. European guidelines for the diagnosis and treatment of pelvic girdle pain. Eur. Spine J. 17 (6), 794–819.

Waxman, J.A., Sulak, P.J., Kuehl, T.J., 1998. Cystoscopic findings consistent with interstitial cystitis in normal women undergoing tubal ligation. J. Urol. 160, 1663–1667.

An introduction to the anatomy of pelvic pain

2.1

Ruth Lovegrove Jones

The anatomy of pelvic pain can conveniently be divided into the clinical anatomy and biomechanics of the pelvis (see Chapter 2.2) and the anatomy of the pelvic floor (Chapter 2.3). However, the human body operates as a system (Ahn et al. 2006, Reeves et al. 2007) and cannot be divided quite so simplistically. Each component of the movement system is likely to influence distal and proximal regions, it is modulated by many factors from across somatic, psychological and social domains (Moseley 2007, Fall et al. 2010) and ultimately it is controlled by the central nervous system (CNS). It is therefore important always to remind ourselves not to focus solely on the end organ that we may perceive to be 'at fault', particularly as the relationship between pain and the state of the tissues becomes weaker as pain persists (Moseley 2007).

The lumbopelvic spine is encompassed by a dense ligamentous connective tissue stocking (Willard 2007) containing five lumbar vertebrae, sacrum, coccyx and two innominates, which are joined by strong ligamentous attachments posteriorly at the sacroiliac joints and anteriorly at the symphysis pubis. Furthermore, the thoracolumbar junction (T10–L2) can, when stimulated, result in pain perceived in the pelvis, and will also need to be evaluated in patients with chronic pelvic pain (CPP). The stiffness of the spine will be the result of reaction forces acting across it, and is modified by gravity, the shape of the articular surfaces, the actual joint position, proprioceptive muscle reflexes, the level of muscle (co)contractions and increased ligament tension.

European guidelines proposed the following functional definition of joint stability:

> The effective accommodation of the joints to each specific load demand through an adequately tailored joint compression, as a function of gravity, coordinated muscle and ligament forces, to produce effective joint reaction forces under changing conditions.
>
> (Vleeming et al. 2008)

To emphasize the importance of muscle and neural control when the muscles of the spine are removed, the spine can buckle with compressive loads of just 90 N (Crisco et al. 1992). The nervous system is therefore likely to coordinate muscle activity to match the internal and external forces placed on the spine in order to meet the demands for stable movement (for a review see Hodges & Cholewicki 2007). Simultaneous co-activation of many muscle groups will increase the stiffness of the spine, but the relative contribution will vary with the task, posture, movement direction and potentially the high real or perceived risk of injury (Cholewicki et al. 1997, 2000, Reeves & Cholewicki 2003). In situations of high real or perceived risk, the CNS may opt to limit the possibility of error and utilize a strategy to stiffen the spine, thus increasing the safety margin; conversely if the threat is low, the CNS could opt to use a more versatile strategy (Hodges & Cholewicki 2007). The lumbopelvic spine therefore forms a key role in the transfer of load from the upper body to the lower limbs, and the stability of the spine and pelvis is a complex, dynamic system with feedback control involving the bony architecture, muscles, connective tissue and the CNS. All anatomical structures that influence the thoracolumbar junction, the lumbopelvic spine and lower limbs may therefore need to be evaluated in patients with CPP. Further details can be found in Chapters 11.1 and 11.2.

References

Ahn, A.C., Tewari, M., Poon, C.S., Phillips, R.S., 2006. The limits of reductionism in medicine: could systems biology offer an alternative? PLoS Med. 3 (6), e208.

Cholewicki, J., Panjabi, M.M., Khachatryan, A., 1997. Stabilizing function of trunk flexor-extensor muscles around a neutral spine posture. Spine 22 (19), 2207–2212.

Cholewicki, J., Simons, A.P., Radebold, A., 2000. Effects of external trunk loads on lumbar spine stability. J. Biomech. 33 (11), 1377–1385.

Hodges, P.W., Cholewicki, J., 2007. Functional control of the spine. In: Vleeming, A., Mooney, V., Stoeckart, R. (Eds.), Movement, Stability and Lumbopelvic Pain. Elsevier, pp. 489–512.

Moseley, G.L., 2007. Reconceptualising pain according to modern pain science. Phys. Ther. Rev. 12 (3), 169–178.

Reeves, N.P., Cholewicki, J., 2003. Modeling the human lumbar spine for assessing spinal loads, stability, and risk of injury. [Review] [238 refs]. Crit. Rev. Biomed. Eng. 31 (1–2), 73–139.

Reeves, N.P., Narendra, K.S., Cholewicki, J., 2007. Spine stability: the six blind men and the elephant. [Review] [58 refs]Clin. Biomech. 22 (3), 266–274.

Vleeming, A., Albert, H.B., Ostgaard, H.C., Sturesson, B., Stuge, B., 2008. European guidlines for the diagnosis and treatment of pelvic girdle pain. Eur. Spine J. 17 (6), 794 –819.

Anatomy and biomechanics of the pelvis

2.2

Andry Vleeming

Authors' note: This chapter is adapted from Chapter 9 of Movement, Stability & Lumbopelvic Pain: Integration of research and therapy 2nd edition by Andry Vleeming Vert Mooney Rob Stoeckart (Hardcover - 9 Mar 2007) Churchill Livingstone, Edinburgh.

CHAPTER CONTENTS

(Adapted from Chapter 8 of Movement, Stability and Lumbopelvic Pain (Vleeming & Stoeckart 2007).)

This chapter presents the clinical anatomy and biomechanics of the pelvis and lumbar spine. Primarily the goal of this chapter is to present research that enhances knowledge about the anatomy of the pelvis, how it needs to be actively stabilized, and how this knowledge can assist in more effective treatment for patients with chronic pelvic pain (CPP).

In all quadrupeds and bipeds, the pelvic girdle forms a firm connection between the spine and the lower extremities. In bipeds, the pelvis has to serve as a basic platform with three large levers acting on it (the spine and the legs). To allow bipedal gait in humans, evolutionary adaptations of the pelvis have been necessary, i.e. changing the shape of the ilia, flaring out into the sagittal plane, providing a more optimal lateral attachment site for the gluteus medius as an important muscle for hip pelvic stability. In particular, a dramatically increased attachment site for the gluteus maximus muscle has changed this muscle – a relatively minor muscle in the chimpanzee – into one of the largest muscles of the human body (Lovejoy 1988).

Additional evolutionary changes in humans are the muscular and ligamentous connections between the sacrum and ilia: (1) muscles, like the lower lumbar multifidi, that insert into the sacrum and also into the medial cranial aspects of the ilium; (2) changes in the position of the coccygeus and the piriform muscles, and of the gluteus maximus muscle originating from the sacrum and sacrotuberous ligaments; (3) extensive fibrous connections adapted to the typical anatomy of the sacroiliac joints (SIJs), like the interosseous ligaments, surrounding an iliac protrusion fitting in a dorsal sacral cavity, called the axial joint just behind the auricular surfaces of the SIJ (Bakland & Hansen 1984); (4) ventral and dorsal SIJ ligaments, sacrotuberous and sacrospinous ligaments between sacrum and lumbar spine (anterior longitudinal ligaments). In addition, direct fibrous connections exist between the iliac bone and L4 and L5, the iliolumbar ligaments.

A recent study has described the influence of the iliolumbar ligaments on SIJ stability (Pool-Goudzwaard et al. 2003). Due to the above-mentioned muscular and ligamentous connections, movement of the sacrum with respect to the iliac bones, or vice versa, affects the joints between L5–S1 and between the higher lumbar levels. Anatomical and functional disturbances of the pelvis or lumbar region influence each other. Due to the tightness of the fibrous connections and the specific architecture of the SIJ, mobility in the SIJ is normally very limited, but movement does occur and has not been scientifically challenged (Weisl 1955, Solonen 1957, Egund et al. 1978, Lavignolle et al. 1983, Miller et al. 1987, Sturesson et al. 1989, 2000a, 2000b, Vleeming et al. 1990a, 1990b, 1996) (Figure 2.2.1).

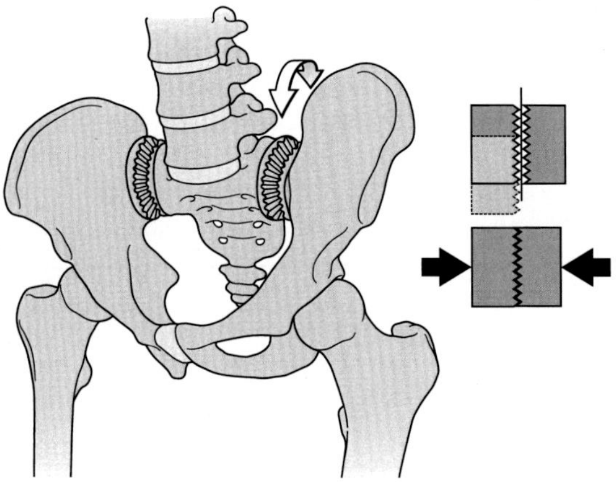

Figure 2.2.1 • Whimsical depiction of sacroiliac joints with friction device

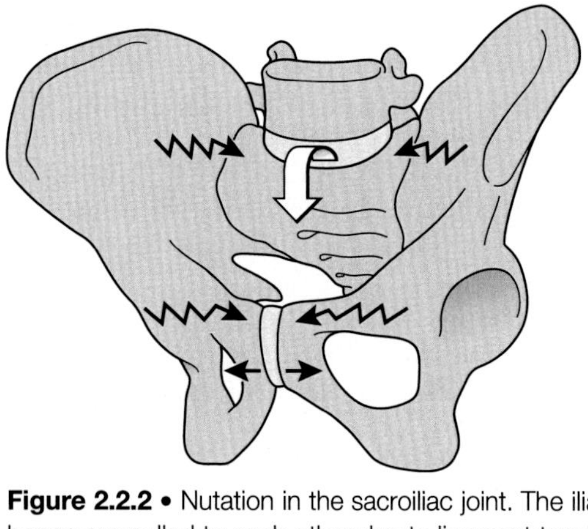

Figure 2.2.2 • Nutation in the sacroiliac joint. The iliac bones are pulled to each other due to ligament tension (among others) and compress the sacroiliac joints (upper black arrows). It can be expected that especially the upper (anterior) part of the pubic symphysis is compressed

The main movements in the SIJ are forward rotation of the sacrum relative to the iliac bones (nutation) and backward rotation of the sacrum relative to the ilia (counternutation) (Figure 2.2.2). It was shown that even at advanced age (>72 years) the combined movement of nutation and counternutation can amount to 4°; normally movements are less than 2° (Vleeming et al. 1992a). In the latter study, the SIJ with the lowest mobility showed radiologically marked arthrosis. Ankylosis of the SIJ was found to be an exception, even at advanced age. This finding is in agreement with the studies of Stewart (1984) and Miller et al. (1987).

Nutation is increased in load-bearing situations, e.g. standing and sitting. In lying prone, nutation is also increased compared to supine positions (Weisl 1955, Egund et al. 1978, Sturesson et al. 1989, 2000a, 2000b). Counternutation normally occurs in unloaded situations like lying down (supine). Counternutation in supine positions can be altered to nutation by maximal flexion in the hips, using the legs as levers to posteriorly rotate the iliac bones relative to the sacrum, as in a labour position, creating space for the head of the baby during delivery.

The anatomy of the sacroiliac joint

The SIJs are relatively flat, unlike ball and socket joints such as the hip. Generally speaking, flat articular surfaces are less resistant to shear forces and therefore the presence of flat surfaces in the pelvis seems surprising. This anatomical configuration gives rise to three questions:

1. Why did nature create a seemingly flat SIJ?
2. What specific adaptations are available to prevent shear in the SIJs?
3. Why is the SIJ not perpendicularly orientated to the forces of gravitation?

Why did nature create a seemingly flat SIJ?

A large transfer of forces is required in the human SIJ, and indeed flat joints are theoretically well-suited to transfer large forces (Snijders et al. 1993a, 1993b). An alternative for effective load transfer by these flat joints would be a fixed connection between sacrum and iliac bones, for instance by ankylosis of the SIJ. The SIJs in humans serve a purpose: to economize gait, to allow shock and shear absorption, and to alleviate birth of (in the evolutionary sense) abnormally large babies. The principal function of the SIJs is to act as stress relievers, ensuring that the pelvic girdle is not a solid ring of bone that could easily crack under the stresses to which it is subjected (Adams et al. 2002).

What specific adaptations are available to prevent shear in the SIJs?

The SIJs are abnormal compared to other joints because of cartilage changes that are present already before birth. These occur especially at the iliac side of the joint and were misinterpreted as degenerative arthrosis (Sashin 1930, Bowen & Cassidy 1981). These cartilage changes are more prominent in men than in women and, according to Salsabili et al. (1995), the sacral cartilage is relatively thick in females. This gender difference might be related to childbearing and possibly to a different localization of the centre of gravity in relation to the SIJ (Dijkstra et al. 1989, Vleeming et al. 1990a, 1990b). Vleeming et al. (1990a, 1990b) considered these changes to reflect a functional adaptation. The features seem to be promoted by the increase in body weight during the pubertal growth spurt and concern a coarse cartilage texture and a wedge and propeller-like form of the joint surfaces.

Studies of frontal slides of intact joints of embalmed specimens show the presence of cartilage-covered bone extensions protruding into the joint. These protrusions seemed irregular but are in fact complementary ridges and grooves. Joint samples taken from normal SIJ with both coarse texture and complementary ridges and grooves were characterized by high-friction coefficients (Vleeming et al. 1990b). All these features are expected to reflect adaptation to human bipedality, contributing to a high coefficient of friction and enhancing the stability of the joint against shear (Vleeming et al. 1990a). As a consequence, less muscle and ligament force is required to bear the upper part of the body (Figure 2.2.3).

The 'keystone-like' bony architecture of the sacrum further contributes to its stability within the pelvic ring. The bone is wider cranially than caudally, and wider anteriorly than posteriorly. Such a configuration permits the sacrum to become 'wedged' cranially and dorsally into the ilia within the pelvic ring (Vleeming et al. 1990a, 1990b). The SIJ has evolved from a relatively flat joint into a much more stable construction (Figure 2.2.4).

To illustrate the importance of friction in the SIJ, the principles of form and force closure were introduced (Vleeming et al. 1990a, 1990b). Form closure refers to a theoretical stable situation with closely fitting joint surfaces, where no extra forces are needed to maintain the state of the system, given the actual load situation. If the sacrum would fit in the pelvis with perfect form closure, no lateral forces would be needed. However, such a construction would make mobility practically impossible. With force closure (leading to joint compression) both a lateral force and friction are needed to withstand vertical load. Shear in the SIJ is prevented by the combination of the specific anatomical features (form closure; see Figure 2.2.5) and the compression generated by muscles and ligaments that can be accommodated to the specific loading situation (force closure). Force closure is the effect of changing joint reaction forces generated by tension in ligaments, fasciae and muscles and ground reaction forces (Figure 2.2.5).

Why is the SIJ not perpendicularly orientated to the forces of gravitation?

Force closure ideally generates a perpendicular reaction force to the SIJ to overcome the forces of gravity (Vleeming et al. 1990b). This shear prevention system was named the self-bracing mechanism and such a mechanism is present elsewhere in the body, e.g. in the knee, foot and shoulder. When a larger lever is applied and/or coordination time becomes less, the general effect in the locomotor system will be closure or reduction of the degrees of freedom of the kinematic chain, leading to a reduction in the chain's mobility or a gain of stability by increasing force closure (Huson 1997).

In self-bracing of the pelvis, nutation of the sacrum is crucial. This movement can be seen as an anticipation for joint loading. Hodges et al. (2003) use the terminology 'preparatory motion' for a comparable phenomenon in the lumbar spine. So, nutation is seen as a movement to prepare the pelvis for increased loading by tightening most of the SIJ ligaments, among which are the vast interosseous and short dorsal sacroiliac ligaments. As a consequence the posterior parts of the iliac bones are pressed together, enlarging compression of the SIJ.

Ligaments and their role in self-bracing the pelvis

In self-bracing the pelvis, nutation in the SIJ is crucial (see above); this involves several ligaments. To further explain self-bracing of the pelvis we will

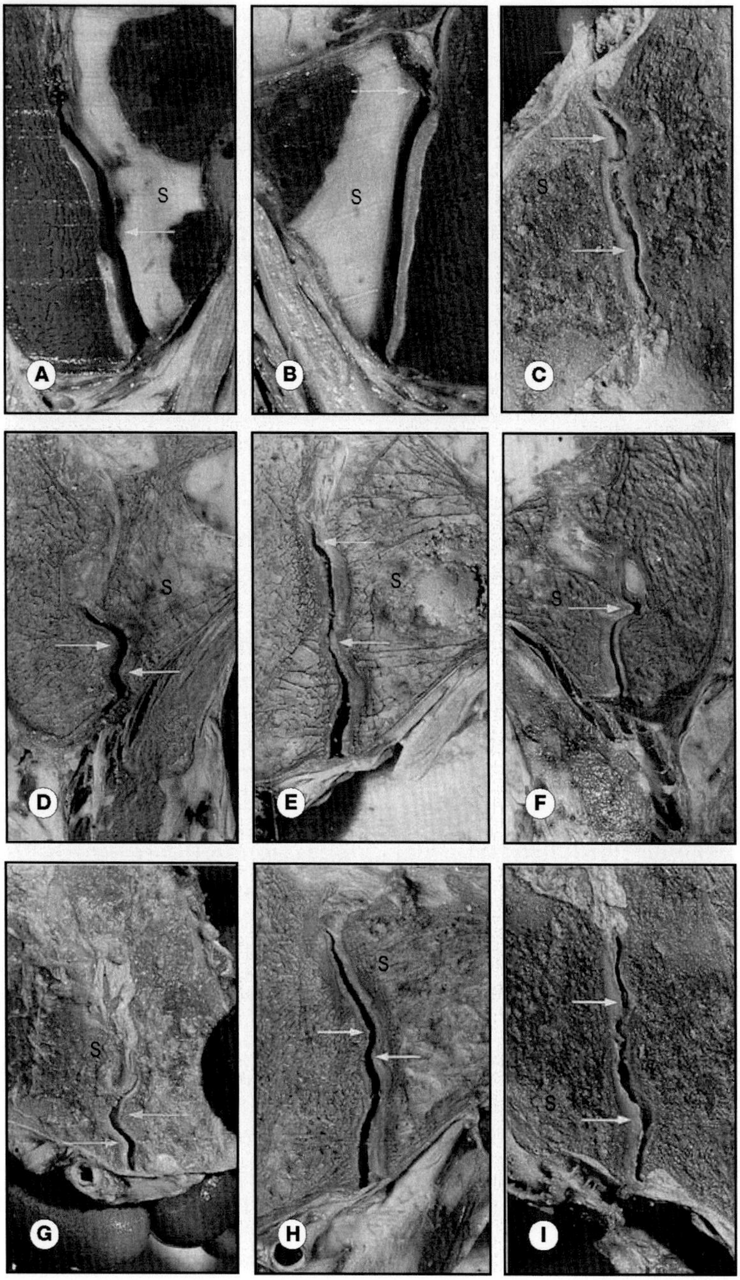

Figure 2.2.3 • Frontal sections of the sacroiliac joint (SIJ) of embalmed male specimen. S indicates the sacral side of the SIJ. (A) and (B) concern a 12-year-old boy; (C)–(I) concern specimen older than 60 years. Arrows are directed at complementary ridges and depressions. They are covered by intact cartilage, as was confirmed by opening the joints afterwards

discuss two sets of ligaments (Figure 2.2.6): the sacrotuberous ligaments (Vleeming et al. 1989a, 1989b, van Wingerden et al. 1993) and the long dorsal SI ligaments (Vleeming et al. 1996, 2002). In the literature, specific data on the functional and clinical relevance of the long ligaments are not available. In several anatomical atlases and textbooks, the long ligament and the sacrotuberous ligament are portrayed as fully continuous ligaments. The drawings generally convey the impression that the ligaments have identical functions. As shown by the contrasting effects of nutation and contranutation on these ligaments (see below), this is not the case. Essentially, the long ligament connects the sacrum and posterior superior iliac spine (PSIS), whereas the main part of the sacrotuberous ligament

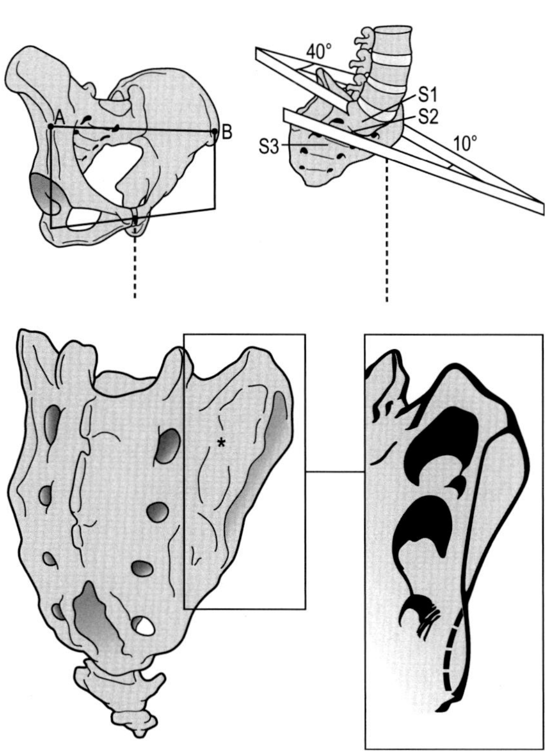

Figure 2.2.4 • (Top left) Pelvis in erect posture. (Top right) View of the sacrum from ventrolateral side, showing the different angles between left and right sacral articular surface. (Bottom left) Dorsolateral view of the sacrum. The * indicates a cavity in the sacrum in which an iliac tubercle fits. (Bottom right) Sacral articular surface at the right side. The different angles reflect the propeller-like shape of an adult sacroiliac joint

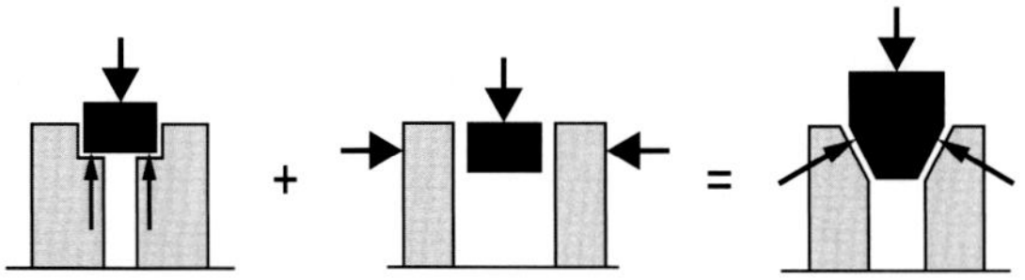

Figure 2.2.5 • Model of the self-locking mechanism. The combination of form closure and force closure establishes stability in the sacroiliac joint

connects the sacrum and ischial tuberosity. However, some of the fibres derived from the ischial tuberosity pass to the iliac bone. Generally, they are denoted as part of the sacrotuberous ligament, although 'tuberoiliac ligament' would be more appropriate. In the *terminologia anatomica* such a ligament does not exist. In fact, this also holds for the long (dorsal SI) ligament, reflecting one of the problems of topographical anatomy.

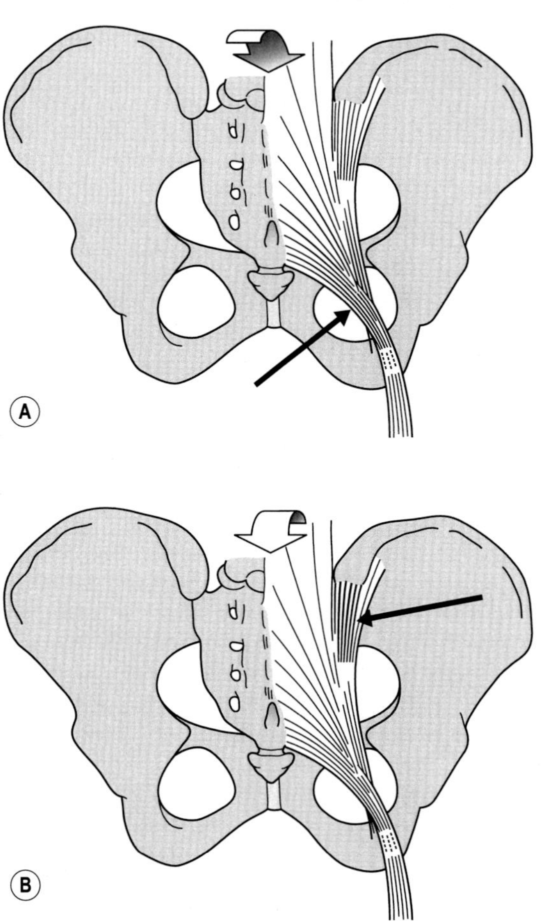

Figure 2.2.6 • (A) Nutation winds up the sacrotuberous ligament. (B) Counternutation winds up the long dorsal sacroiliac ligament

Sacrotuberous ligaments

In embalmed human specimens, we could demonstrate a direct relation between nutation and tension of the sacrotuberous ligament (Figure 2.2.6A). By straining this ligament, we found a decrease of nutation (Vleeming et al. 1989a, 1989b), indicating that these ligaments are well-suited to restrict nutation. It can be expected that the opposite (diminished ligament tension) will increase nutation.

Long dorsal sacroiliac ligaments

In view of the capability of the sacrotuberous ligaments to restrict nutation, we wondered which ligament(s) could restrict counternutation. Because of its connection to the PSIS and to the lateral part of the sacrum (Figure 2.2.6B), we expected that the long dorsal SI ligament could fulfil this function. The ligament can be easily palpated in the area directly caudal to the PSIS and is of special interest since women complaining of lumbopelvic back pain during pregnancy frequently experience pain within the boundaries of this ligament (Mens et al. 1992, Njoo 1996, Vleeming et al. 1996). Pain in this area is also not uncommon in men. The ligament is the most superficially located SIJ ligament and therefore well-suited to mirror asymmetric stress in the SIJ. As this ligament is not well known in medical practice, we will summarize data from an anatomical and biomechanical study (Vleeming et al. 1996) that assessed the function of the ligament by measuring its tension during incremental loading of biomechanically relevant structures.

For that purpose, the tension of the long ligament ($n = 12$) was tested under loading. Tension was measured with a buckle transducer. Several structures, including the erector spinae muscle and the sacrum itself, were incrementally loaded (with forces of 0–50 N). The sacrum was loaded in two directions (nutation and counternutation).

Anatomical aspects

At the cranial side, the long ligament is attached to the PSIS and the adjacent part of the iliac bone, at the caudal side to the lateral crest of the third and fourth sacral segments. In some specimens, fibres also pass to the fifth sacral segment. From the sites of attachment on the sacrum, fibres pass to the coccyx. These are not considered to be part of the long ligament.

The lateral expansion of the long ligament directly caudal to the PSIS varies between 15 and 30 mm. The length, measured between the PSIS and the third and fourth sacral segments, varies between 42 and 75 mm. The lateral part of the long ligament is continuous with fibres of the sacrotuberous ligament, passing between the ischial tuberosity and the iliac bone. The variation is wide. Fibres of the long ligament are connected to the deep lamina of the posterior layer of the thoracolumbar fascia, to the aponeurosis of the erector spinae muscle and to the multifidus muscle.

Biomechanical aspects

Forced incremental nutation in the SIJ diminished the tension in the long ligament, whereas forced counternutation increased the tension. Tension increased also during loading of the ipsilateral sacrotuberous ligament and erector spinae muscle. Tension decreased during traction on the gluteus maximus muscle. Tension also decreased during traction on the ipsilateral and contralateral posterior layer of the thoracolumbar fascia in a direction simulating contraction of the latissimus dorsi muscle.

Obviously, the long dorsal SI ligament has close anatomical relations with the erector spinae/multifidus muscle, the posterior layer of the thoracolumbar fascia, and a specific part of the sacrotuberous ligament (tuberoiliac ligament). Functionally, it is an important link between legs, spine and arms. The ligament is tensed when the SIJs are counternutated and slackened when nutated. Slackening of the long dorsal SI ligament can be counterbalanced by both the sacrotuberous ligament and the erector spinae muscle.

Pain localized within the boundaries of the long ligament could indicate, among others, a spinal condition with sustained counternutation of the SIJ. In diagnosing patients with a specific low back pain (LBP) or pelvic girdle pain (PGP), the long dorsal SI ligament should not be neglected. Even in cases of arthrodesis of the SIJ, tension in the long ligament can still be altered by different structures.

This observation implies that the tension of the long ligament can be altered by displacement in the SIJ as well as by action of various muscles. Obviously, nutation in the SIJ induces relaxation of the long ligament, whereas counternutation increases tension. This is in contrast to the effect on the sacrotuberous ligament (see Figure 2.2.5). Increased tension in the sacrotuberous ligament during nutation can be due to SIJ movement itself as well as to increased tension of the biceps femoris and/or gluteus maximus muscle. This mechanism can help to control nutation. As counternutation increases tension in the long ligament, this ligament can assist in controlling counternutation (see Figure 2.2.6).

Ligaments with opposite functions, such as the long and sacrotuberous ligaments, apparently do not interact in a simple way. After all, loading of the sacrotuberous ligament also leads to a small increased tension of the long ligament. This effect will be due to the connections between long ligament and tuberoiliac (part of the sacrotuberous ligament) ligament, and possibly also to a counternutating moment generated by the loading of the sacrotuberous ligament.

A comparable complex relation might hold for the long ligament and the erector spinae, or more specifically the multifidus muscle. As the multifidus is connected to the sacrum (MacIntosh & Bogduk 1986, 1991; see Chapter 1), its action induces nutation. As a result, the long ligament will slacken. However, the present study shows an increase in tension in the long ligament after traction to the erector spinae muscle. This counterbalancing effect is due to the connections between the erector spinae muscle and the long ligament, and opposes the slackening. In vivo, this effect might be smaller because the moment of force acting on the sacrum is raised by the pull of the erector spinae muscle and the resulting compression force on the spine (Snijders et al. 1993b). This spinal compression was not applied in this study. Both antagonistic mechanisms – between long and sacrotuberous ligaments and between the long ligament and the erector spinae muscle – might serve to preclude extensive slackening of the long ligament. Such mechanisms could be essential for a relatively flat joint such as the SIJ, which is susceptible to shear forces (Snijders et al. 1993a, 1993b). It can be safely assumed that impairment of a part of this interconnected ligament system will have serious implications for the joint as load transfer from spine to hips and vice versa is primarily transferred via the SIJ (Snijders et al. 1993a, 1993b).

As shown earlier (Vleeming et al. 1996), traction to the biceps femoris tendon hardly influences tension of the long ligament. This is in contrast to the effect of the biceps on the sacrotuberous ligament (Vleeming et al. 1989a, 1989b, van Wingerden et al. 1993). The observations might well be related to the spiralling of the sacrotuberous ligament. Most medial fibres of the ligament tend to attach to the cranial part of the sacrum, whereas most fibres arising from a lateral part of the ischial tuberosity tend to attach to the caudal part of the sacrum (see Figure 2.2.6A). The fibres of the biceps tendon, which approach a relatively lateral part of the ischial tuberosity, pass mainly to the caudal part of the sacrum. As a consequence, the effect of traction to the biceps femoris on the tension of the long ligament can only be limited.

The effect on the long ligament of loading the posterior layer of the thoracolumbar fascia depends on the direction of the forces applied. Artificial traction to the fascia mimicking the action of the transverse abdominal muscle has no effect. Traction in a craniolateral direction, mimicking the action of the latissimus dorsi muscle, results in a significant decrease in tension in the ipsilateral and contralateral long ligaments. As shown in another study (Vleeming et al. 1995), traction to the latissimus dorsi influences the tension in the posterior layer of the thoracolumbar fascia, ipsilaterally as well as contralaterally, especially below the level of L4. Thus slackening of the long ligament could be the result of increased tension in the posterior layer by the latissimus dorsi. This might itself lead to a slight nutation, leading to more compression and force closure of the SIJ. As shown in this study, slackening of the long ligament can also occur due to action of the gluteus maximus muscle, which is ideally suited to compress the SIJ.

It is inviting to draw conclusions when palpation, directly caudal to the PSIS, is painful. However, pain in this area might be due to pain referred from the SIJ itself (Fortin et al. 1994a, 1994b), but also due to counternutation in the SIJ. Counternutation is part of a pattern of flattening the lumbar spine (Egund et al. 1978, Lavignolle et al. 1983, Sturesson et al. 1989) that occurs in particular late in pregnancy when women counterbalance the weight of the fetus (Snijders et al. 1976). However, such a posture combined with counternutation could also result from a pain-withdrawal reaction to impairment elsewhere in the system. Hence, only specific pain within the boundaries of the long ligament can be used as a diagnostic criterion (Vleeming et al. 2002). An example of a pain-withdrawal reaction could be the following: pain of the pubic symphysis following delivery (Mens et al. 1992) could preclude normal lumbar lordosis and hence nutation owing to pain of an irritated symphysis. After all, lumbar lordosis leads to nutation in the SIJ (Weisl 1955, Egund et al. 1978, Lavignolle et al. 1983, Sturesson et al. 1989). Nutation implies that the left and right PSISs approach each other slightly while the pubic symphysis is caudally extended and cranially compressed (Lavignolle et al. 1983, Walheim & Selvik 1984). In this example the patient will avoid nutation and flattens the lower spine, leading to sustained tension and pain in the long ligament. In a study by Mens et al. (1999), it was shown that a positive active straight leg raise test coincides with a counternutated position of the SIJ in many patients.

In conclusion: functionally, the long dorsal SI ligament is an important link between legs, spine and arms. In women with lumbopelvic back pain frequently pain is experienced within the boundaries of this ligament, which is tensed with counternutation and slackened with nutation. The erector muscle and the sacrotuberous ligament can counterbalance this slackening. The connections between ligaments and muscles with opposing functions could serve as a mechanism to preclude excessive slackening of ligaments.

Before focusing on the role of the muscles, we will draw attention to the thoracolumbar fascia.

The role of the thoracolumbar fascia in stabilizing the lumbopelvic area

To deepen our knowledge of the role of the thoracolumbar fascia the posterior layer of the thoracolumbar fascia was loaded by simulating the action of various muscles (Vleeming et al. 1995).

Anatomical aspects

The posterior layer of the thoracolumbar fascia covers the back muscles from the sacral region, through the thoracic region as far as the fascia nuchae. At the level of L4–L5 and the sacrum, strong connections exist between the superficial and deep lamina. The transverse abdominal and internal oblique muscles are indirectly attached to the thoracolumbar fascia through a dense raphe formed by fusion of the middle layer (Bogduk & MacIntosh 1984) of the thoracolumbar fascia and both laminae of the posterior layer. This 'lateral raphe' (Bogduk & MacIntosh 1984, Bogduk & Twomey 1987) is localized laterally to the erector spinae and cranial to the iliac crest.

Superficial lamina (Figure 2.2.7)

The superficial lamina of the posterior layer of the thoracolumbar fascia is continuous with the latissimus dorsi, gluteus maximus, and part of the external oblique muscle of the abdomen and the trapezius muscle. Cranial to the iliac crest, the lateral border of the superficial lamina is marked by its junction with the latissimus dorsi muscle. The fibres of the superficial lamina are orientated from craniolateral to caudomedial. Only a few fibres of the superficial lamina are continuous with the aponeurosis of the external oblique and the trapezius. Most of the fibres of the superficial lamina derive from the aponeurosis of the latissimus dorsi and attach to the supraspinal ligaments and spinous processes cranial to L4. Caudal to L4–L5, the superficial lamina is generally loosely (or not at all) attached to midline structures, such as supraspinal ligaments, spinous processes and median sacral crest. In fact, they cross to the contralateral side, where they attach to sacrum, PSIS and iliac crest. The level at which this phenomenon occurs varies; it is generally caudal to L4 but in some preparations already occurs at L2–L3.

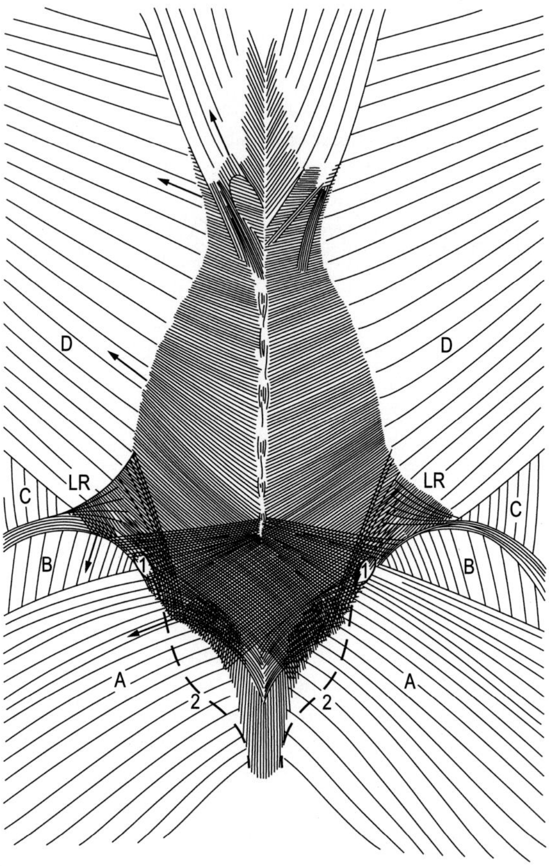

Figure 2.2.7 • The superficial lamina. A, Fascia of the gluteus maximus; B, fascia of the gluteus medius; C, fascia of external oblique; D, fascia of latissimus dorsi. 1, posterior superior iliac spine (PSIS); 2, sacral crest; LR, part of lateral raphe. Arrows (at left) indicate, from cranial to caudal, the site and direction of the traction (50 N) given to trapezius, cranial and caudal part of the latissimus dorsi, gluteus medius and gluteus maximus muscles, respectively. Reproduced from Vleeming et al. (1995), *Spine*, with permission.

Barker & Briggs (1999) showed that the superficial lamina is also continuous superiorly with the rhomboids. They could not confirm the findings of Bogduk et al. (1998) in relation to thickening of the fascia and the presence of posterior accessory ligaments. This is in agreement with the findings of Vleeming et al. (1995).

At sacral levels, the superficial lamina is continuous with the fascia of the gluteus maximus. These fibres are orientated from craniomedial to caudolateral. Most of these fibres attach to the median sacral crest. However, at the level of L4–L5, and in some specimens even as caudally as S1–S2, fibres *partly or completely* cross the midline, attaching to the contralateral PSIS and iliac crest. Some of these fibres fuse with the lateral raphe and with fibres derived from the fascia of the latissimus dorsi. Owing to the different fibre directions of the latissimus dorsi and the gluteus maximus, the superficial lamina has a cross-hatched appearance at the level of L4–L5, and in some preparations also at L5–S2. The lamina becomes thicker and stronger especially over the lower lumbar spine and SIJ.

Barker & Briggs (1999) showed that the *deep lamina* (Figure 2.2.8) is continuous cranially with the tendons of the splenius cervicis and capitis muscles. At lower lumbar and sacral levels, the fibres of the deep lamina are orientated from craniomedial to caudolateral. At sacral levels, these fibres are fused with those of the superficial lamina. As, in this region, fibres of the deep lamina are continuous with the sacrotuberous ligament, an indirect link exists between this ligament and the superficial lamina. There is also a direct connection with some fibres of the deep lamina. In the pelvic region, the deep lamina is connected to the PSIS, iliac crests and long dorsal SI ligament. This ligament originates from the sacrum and attaches to the PSIS. In the lumbar region, fibres of the deep lamina derive from the interspinous ligaments. They attach to the iliac crest and more cranially to the lateral raphe, to which the internal oblique is attached. In some specimens, fibres of the deep lamina cross to the contralateral side between L5 and S1. In the depression between the median sacral crest and the posterior superior and inferior iliac spines, fibres of the deep lamina fuse with the fascia of the erector. More cranially, in the lumbar region, the deep lamina becomes thinner and freely mobile over the back muscles. In the lower thoracic region, fibres of the serratus posterior inferior muscle and its fascia fuse with fibres of the deep lamina.

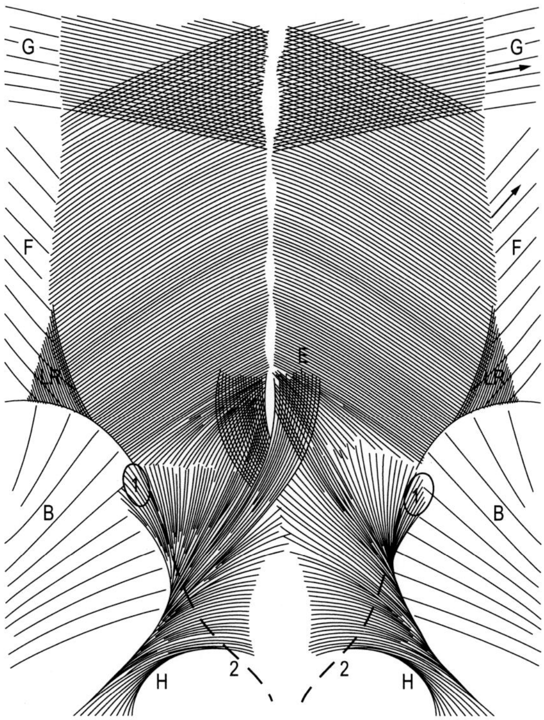

Figure 2.2.8 • The deep lamina. B, Fascia of the gluteus medius; E, connections between the deep lamina and the fascia of the erector spinae; F, fascia of the internal oblique; G, fascia of the serratus posterior inferior; H, sacrotuberous ligament; 1, the posterior superior iliac spine (PSIS); 2, sacral crest; LR, part of lateral raphe. Arrows (right) indicate, from cranial to caudal, traction to serratus posterior inferior and internal oblique muscles, respectively. Reproduced from Vleeming et al. (1995) *Spine*, with permission.

Biomechanical aspects

Traction to the superficial lamina

Depending on the site of the traction, quite different results were obtained (Vleeming et al. 1995). Traction to the cranial fascia and muscle fibres of the latissimus dorsi muscle showed limited displacement of the superficial lamina (homolaterally up to 2–4 cm). Traction to the caudal part of the latissimus dorsi caused displacement up to the midline. This midline area is 8–10 cm removed from the site of traction. Between L4–L5 and S1–S2, displacement of the superficial lamina occurred even contralaterally. Traction to the gluteus maximus also caused displacement up to the contralateral side. The distance between the site of traction and visible displacement varied from 4 to 7 cm. The effect of traction to the external oblique muscle varied markedly between the different preparations. In all preparations, traction to the trapezius muscle resulted in a relatively small effect (up to 2 cm).

Traction to the deep lamina

Traction to the biceps femoris tendon, applied in a lateral direction, resulted in displacement of the deep lamina up to the level L5–S1. Obviously, this load transfer is conducted by the sacrotuberous ligament. In two specimens, displacement occurred at the contralateral side, 1–2 cm away from the midline. Traction to the biceps tendon directed medially showed homolateral displacement in the deep lamina, up to the median sacral crest.

As shown by the traction tests, the tension of the posterior layer of the thoracolumbar fascia can be influenced by contraction or stretch of a variety of muscles. It is noteworthy that especially muscles such as the latissimus dorsi and gluteus maximus are capable of exerting a contralateral effect especially to the lower lumbar spine and pelvis. This implies that the ipsilateral gluteus maximus muscle and contralateral latissimus dorsi muscle both can tension the posterior layer.

Hence, parts of these muscles provide a pathway for mechanical transmission between pelvis and trunk. One could argue that the lack of connection between the *superficial* lamina of the posterior layer and the supraspinous ligaments in the lumbar region is a disadvantage for stability. However, it would be disadvantageous only in case strength, coordination and effective coupling of the gluteus maximus muscle and the caudal part of the contralateral latissimus dorsi muscle are diminished. It can be expected that increased strength of these mentioned muscles accomplished by torsional training could influence the quality of the posterior layer. Following this line of thinking, the posterior layer of the thoracolumbar fascia could play an integrating role in rotation of the trunk and in load transfer, and hence instability of the lower lumbar spine and pelvis.

Barker & Briggs (1999) make the interesting comment that the posterior layer is ideally positioned to receive feedback from multiple structures involved in lumbar movements and may regulate ligamentous tension via its extensive muscular attachments to both deep stabilizing and more superficial muscles. They also report that the fascia displays viscoelastic properties and thus is capable of altering its structure to adapt to the stresses placed on it. The posterior layer has been reported to stiffen with successive loading and adaptive fascial thickening is possible.

Barker & Briggs (1999) also comment that when adaptive strengthening of the posterior layer takes place, one might expect to facilitate this by using exercises that strengthen its attaching muscles, both deep and superficial. Adaptive strengthening therefore would be expected to occur with exercises using contralateral limbs such as swimming and walking and torsional training. It also might occur with recovery of muscle bulk and function (erector spinae/multifidus) during lumbopelvic stabilization exercises.

Bogduk et al. (1998) do not agree with the concept that the latissimus dorsi has a role in rotating the spine and comment that the muscle is designed to move the upper limb and its possible contribution to bracing the SIJ via the thoracolumbal fascia is trivial. In contrast to this, Kumar et al. (1996) showed that axial rotation of the trunk involves agonistic activity of the contralateral external obliques, and ipsilateral erector spinae and latissimus dorsi as agonistic muscles to rotate the trunk.

Mooney et al. (2001) used the anatomical relation of the latissimus dorsi and the contralateral gluteus maximus muscles to study their coupled effect during axial rotation exercises and walking. They concluded that in normal individuals, walking a treadmill, the functional relationship between the mentioned muscles could be confirmed. It was apparent that the right gluteus maximus muscle had on average a lower signal amplitude compared to the left ($n = 15$; 12 right-handed). This reciprocal relationship of muscles correlates with normal reverse rotation of shoulders versus the pelvis in normal gait. They showed that during right rotation of the trunk the right latissimus dorsi muscle is significantly more active than the left, but that the left gluteus maximus muscle is more active than the right. In patients with SIJ problems a strikingly different pattern was noticed. On the symptomatic side the gluteus maximus was far more active compared with the healthy subjects. The reciprocal relation between latissimus and gluteus maximus muscles, however, was still present. After an intense rotational strengthening training programme, the patients showed a marked increase in latissimus dorsi muscle strength and diminished activity of the gluteus muscle on the symptomatic side.

The importance of these findings could be that rotational trunk muscle training is important, particularly for stabilizing the SIJ and lower spine. These findings contradict the conclusion of Bogduk et al. (1998) that the latissimus dorsi muscle has no function besides upper limb movement.

Pelvic girdle pain can be partially relieved by application of a pelvic belt, a device that 'self-braces' the SIJ (Vleeming et al. 1992b). By exerting compression on the lower lumbar spine and pelvis, the posterior layer of the thoracolumbar fascia and its attached muscles can accomplish self-bracing physiologically. It is noteworthy that, as shown in this study, the coupled function of the gluteus maximus and the contralateral latissimus dorsi muscles creates a force perpendicular to the SIJ.

Attention is drawn to a possible role of the erector muscle and multifidus in load transfer. Between the lateral raphe and the interspinous ligaments, the deep lamina encloses the erector muscle and multifidus. It can be expected that contraction of the erector/multifidus will longitudinally increase the tension in the deep lamina. In addition, the whole posterior layer of the thoracolumbar fascia will be 'inflated' by contraction of the erector spinae/multifidus (Vleeming et al. 1995), comparable to pumping up a ball. Consequently, it can be assumed that the training of muscles such as the gluteus maximus, latissimus dorsi and erector spinae, and the multifidus can assist in increasing force closure also by strengthening the posterior layer of the thoracolumbar fascia.

In conclusion: the posterior layer of the thoracolumbar fascia could play an important role in transferring forces between spine, pelvis and legs, especially in rotation of the trunk and stabilization of lower lumbar spine and SIJ. The gluteus maximus and the latissimus dorsi merit special attention because they can conduct forces contralaterally via the posterior layer. Because of the coupling between the gluteus maximus and the contralateral latissimus dorsi via the posterior layer of the thoracolumbar fascia, one must be very cautious when categorizing certain muscles as arm, spine or leg muscles. Rotation of the trunk is mainly a function of the oblique abdominals. However, a counter muscle sling in the back helps to preclude deformation of the spine. Rotation against increased resistance will activate the posterior oblique sling of latissimus and gluteus maximus.

Muscles and self-bracing

Various muscles are involved in force closure of the SIJ. With respect to SIJ function, we focus here on four muscles: the erector spinae/multifidus, gluteus maximus, latissimus dorsi and biceps femoris (Figure 2.2.9).

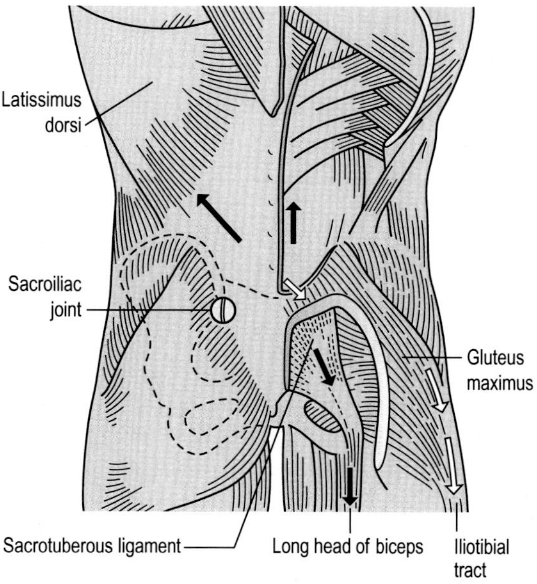

Figure 2.2.9 • Schematic dorsal view of the low back. The right side shows a part of the longitudinal muscle–tendon–fascia sling. Below this is the continuation between biceps femoris tendon and sacrotuberous ligament, above this is the continuation of the erector spinae. To show the right erector spinae, a part of the thoracolumbar fascia has been removed. The left side shows the sacroiliac joint and the cranial part of the oblique dorsal muscle–fascia–tendon sling, latissimus dorsi muscle and thoracolumbar fascia. In this drawing the left part of the thoracolumbar fascia is tensed by the left latissimus dorsi and the right gluteus maximus muscle

The erector spinae/multifidus is the pivotal muscle that loads and extends spine and pelvis. The sacral connections of the erector/multifidus induce nutation in the SIJ, tensing ligaments such as the interosseous, sacrotuberous and sacrospinal. Nutation is anticipatory for preloading the SIJ (preparatory movement; Hodges et al. 2003 and see above). These muscles have a double function because their iliac connections pull the posterior sides of the iliac bones towards each other, constraining nutation. This implies that during nutation, due to action of the erector spinae/multifidus, the cranial side of the SIJ tends to be compressed whereas the caudal side has a tendency to widen. The latter is restricted by the sacrotuberous ligament, tensed by nutation, which has direct fascial connections with the erector spinae. A comparable process will occur in the pubic symphysis where the largest symphyseal ligament passes caudally to the joint (see Figure 2.2.2).

Owing to its perpendicular orientation to the SIJ, the gluteus maximus can compress the joints directly and also indirectly by its vast muscular connections with the sacrotuberous ligament. Gibbons (2004) speculates that the caudal part of the gluteus maximus, originating from the sacrotuberous ligament, can function in conjunction with the pelvic floor. Vleeming et al. (1995) noted in a study on the SIJ that compression, among others, also can be established by coupling of the gluteus maximus with the contralateral latissimus dorsi muscle via the thoracolumbar fascia (Figure 2.2.9).

Tension in the sacrotuberous ligament is increased by caudal traction to the long head of the biceps femoris. This is possible because not all fibres of the long head of the biceps attach to the ischial tuberosity; partly, and occasionally completely, its proximal tendon is continuous with the sacrotuberous ligament (Figure 2.2.9). This tension mechanism of the biceps femoris depends on body position (van Wingerden et al. 1993). In most specimens, a higher percentage of force was transferred from the biceps to the sacrotuberous ligament in a flexed, stooped position than in an erect stance. This could be expected because the flexion torque on the lumbar spine increases when changing from an erect to a flexed stance. Consequently, in stooped positions, larger compression forces are needed to prevent the sacrum from tilting forward. This force can be derived in part from the biceps femoris but also from other muscles attached to the sacrotuberous ligament (the sacral part of the aponeurosis of the erector spinae and gluteus maximus). Barker (2005) showed that besides the biceps muscle also part of the semimembranosus muscle regularly is connected to the sacrotuberous ligament. In her studies, Barker confirmed the biceps connection with the sacrotuberous ligament.

Comparable to the erector muscle, a double function of the hamstrings (including the biceps femoris muscle) can be described. Particularly in stooped positions and in sitting with straight legs, sitting upright, the hamstrings are well positioned to rotate the iliac bones posteriorly relative to the sacrum. This nutating effect (Sturesson et al. 1989) can be constrained by the biceps femoris with its connections to the sacrotuberous ligament. Nutation in stooped positions can help to avoid excessive loading of the posterior part of the lumbar discs.

This polyarticular coupling effect of muscles can also be seen in the arm where the long tendon of the biceps brachii, forming an integrated part of the glenohumeral joint, is one of the key structures for shoulder stabilization.

Self-bracing during forward bending

When stooped, the sacrum assumes a more or less horizontal position. When lifting objects in this posture, the vertical force from the upper part of the body and the object acts almost perpendicularly to the longitudinal axis of the sacrum. In this situation, the joint also becomes loaded in the transverse plane and stability will depend on effective compression of the SIJ in a transverse plane. The transverse diameter is small in comparison with the longitudinal diameter, so additional forces are needed to protect the SIJ. An electromyography (EMG) study found that, during lifting, the activity of the gluteus maximus muscle paralleled that of latissimus dorsi and erector spinae muscles (Noe et al. 1992). These observations indicate that, in this position, self-bracing of the pelvis can be established by contraction of the mentioned muscles and core muscles like the transversus, multifidus, the pelvic floor and the diaphragm (Hodges et al. 2003).

Self-bracing in unconstrained positions

The question of how the SIJ can be stabilized in unconstrained sitting and standing led to the following experiment: we expected that during unconstrained sitting, especially the oblique abdominals would be active to self-brace the pelvis, to deliver the necessary compression force. Using electromyography (EMG) the abdominal muscle activity was recorded in different positions (supine, unconstrained standing, and sitting with and without crossed legs on an office chair with the use of a backrest and armrests). For both the external and internal obliques, the activity was significantly higher in standing than in sitting. The activity of particularly the internal obliques turned out to be significantly higher in sitting than in a supine position (Figure 2.2.10). Surprisingly, the activity of the oblique abdominals was lowered by crossing the legs (Snijders et al. 1995; cross-legged or ankle on knee as preferred by the individual; Figure 2.2.10). By contrast, the activity of the rectus abdominis was not altered by leg-crossing. We concluded that to stabilize the pelvis: (1) unconstrained sitting and standing initiates an oblique ventral muscle–tendon sling; and (2) leg-crossing is a functional habit. Crossing the legs causes rotation

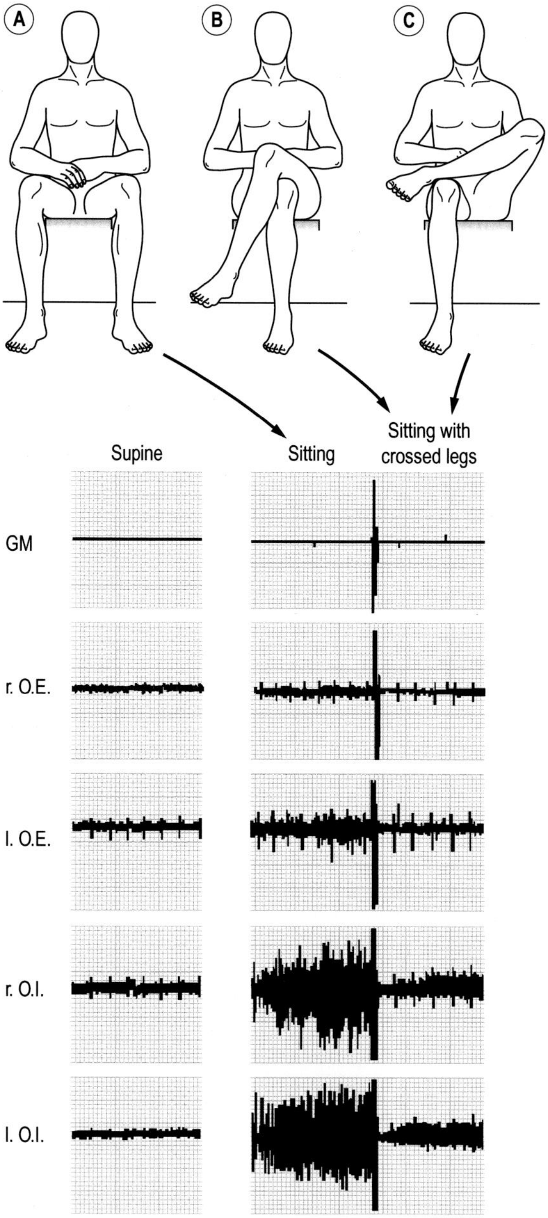

Figure 2.2.10 • Normal sitting (A) and sitting with crossed legs (B and C). The electromyographic data show a remarkable increase of the internal obliques during sitting with uncrossed legs (A). The activity diminishes when the legs are crossed (B and C). GM, gluteus maximus; lOE, left external oblique; lOl, left internal oblique; rOE, right external oblique; rOl, right internal oblique

in the pelvis and possibly tenses the thoracolumbar fascia. Due to creep of tissues (elongation), leg-crossing is only temporarily functional; as a consequence the legs are crossed to the other side (Snijders et al. 1995).

Failed self-bracing

The different mechanisms that warrant stability of the SIJ can become less effective as a result of a decline in muscle performance and/or increased laxity of ligaments. This could occur in people withdrawing from sports or undertaking sedentary work. A characteristic case could be a young girl performing top-level gymnastics. Through excessive training, the mobility of spine and pelvis is markedly enhanced and the girl will develop extremely strong muscles. Thus the mobile pelvis can be adequately constrained with force closure. If such an athlete abruptly terminates high-level training, the muscles rapidly decline. The muscles are not up to their task and form closure will be limited because of enlarged mobility and laxity.

Laxity of pelvic ligaments especially occurs during pregnancy, due to relaxin. In addition, patients with a painful pubic symphysis will avoid nutation because this strains the symphysis. Consequently, these women will 'choose' a counternutated position.

One method to facilitate pelvic stability and reduce pain is the use of a pelvic belt (Mens et al. 1996). In a loading experiment on embalmed human preparations, nutation of the sacrum decreased by about 20% when applying a belt force of only 50 N. Based on the biomechanical model presented here, such a belt must be applied with a small force, like the laces of a shoe. This will be sufficient to generate a self-bracing effect in the SIJ under heavy load (Vleeming et al. 1992a, 1992b, Snijders et al. 1993a, 1993b). The model indicates that the belt must be positioned just cranial to the greater trochanters; it crosses the SIJ caudally, and can assist in preventing gapping of the caudal part of the SIJ. However, this is not what we propose to our patients. Only in very severe cases do patients wear belts for a short period in the beginning and during training.

We like to emphasize that, according to the model presented here, weakening of the erector spinae/multifidus (insufficient nutation) and the gluteus maximus muscles (insufficient ligament pull and SIJ compression) will lead to diminished straining of the sacrotuberous ligament. Weakness of these muscles has in addition implications for the strength of the thoracolumbar fascia, especially if combined with a weak latissimus dorsi muscle. Weakening or inadequate use of the transversus abdominis muscle precludes, among others, sufficient tension of the thoracolumbar fascia. This leads to diminished self-bracing of the SIJ. With insufficient bracing, the body can be expected to use other strategies, for example tensing the sacrotuberous ligament through activation of the biceps femoris or exaggerated contraction of parts of the gluteus maximus. Although definitive experimental data are lacking, we presume that tension of the biceps and other hamstring muscles can be increased over an extended period. Hungerford et al. (2003) showed altered firing patterns of these muscles in SIJ patients. Higher tension of the hamstrings will force the pelvis to rotate backwards, leading to flattening of the lumbar spine. The biceps femoris muscle, in particular, will strain the sacrotuberous ligament, diminishing nutation. Both processes will be harmful if hamstring tension is continuously increased because, in this relatively counternutated position, load will be unnaturally distributed to the lower lumbar discs. In our opinion, it is important to realize that counternutation of the SIJ seems to be a pain-withdrawal reaction that disengages the normal self-bracing of the pelvis. The patient seeks to compress the SIJ in a new joint position, with less adequate and strong ligaments to be tensed. Hence, the lower spine can become unstable and prone to infringement, leading to LBP.

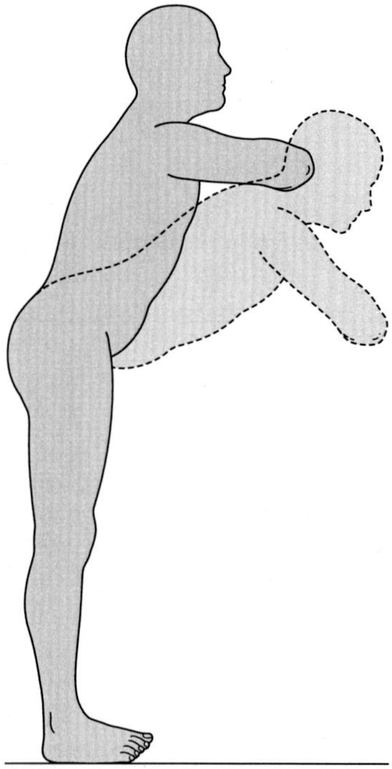

Figure 2.2.11 • A suggested exercise with lordosis of the lumbar spine and nutation of the sacroiliac joint. The biceps femoris, gluteus maximus and erector muscle are simultaneously activated

We tried to define a simple exercise that could assist in preventing LBP and counteract the detrimental effects of modern life. The exercise shown in Figure 2.2.11 facilitates nutation of the SIJ and couples the action of biceps femoris, erector spinae and gluteus maximus. We suppose this to be an effective and natural way to stretch the hamstring. To evaluate its effectiveness, the exercise needs further practical study. This is an exercise that has to be demonstrated carefully to patients with the main movement occurring in the hip joints with a relaxed spine. In case of lumbar impairments, of course, care has to be taken with this exercise.

Optimal and non-optimal pelvic girdle stability

Since the mid-1990s, several clinicians and researchers have studied PGP and its causes. In the past, PGP research focused on the functional and clinical analysis, mainly in women; this was a consequence of former publications emphasizing relaxation of the pelvic girdle as a primary cause for instability of the pelvic ring. By the 1870s, Snelling was of the impression that relaxation of the pelvic articulations becomes apparent either suddenly after parturition or gradually during pregnancy, permitting mobility which hinders locomotion and gives rise to distressing and alarming sensations (in Svensson et al. 1990).

Abramson et al. (1934) described pelvic pain and instability and made the distinction between symptoms related to the pubic joint, to the SIJ, or to a combination. They also described pain in the symphyseal region with radiation to the thighs. The SIJ symptoms are presented as low (lowest) backache and localized pain in the SIJ. Furthermore, they noted a waddling gait and a positive Trendelenburg sign (during walking the patient shows inability to hold the pelvis in the horizontal plane). The authors used, among others, screening techniques like X-rays of the pubic symphysis, even in women who were 8 months pregnant (Abramson et al. 1934). So before the hazards of X-rays were realized, increased mobility and widening of the symphysis in relation to PGP were well-documented. Postmortem studies in former days, when mortality during pregnancy and labor was not exceptional, showed increased mobility of the SIJ and an increased amount of synovial SIJ and symphyseal fluid in pregnant women (Brooke 1924).

After these studies on pelvic instability in the nineteenth and twentieth centuries, analysis of pelvic pain shifted towards a more functional approach. By contrast, the study of lumbar pain after Mixter and Barr's (1934) study (which explained that radiating pain in the leg is the consequence of a rupture of the intervertebral disc) has been particularly addressed to the study of pain generators that could generate the symptoms. Since the 1980s there have been increasing efforts to study the lumbar and pelvic area as an integrated part of a complex kinematic system.

More recent functional pelvic studies have stated that PGP can be related to non-optimal stability, which is underpinned by the fact that a pelvic belt reduces pain symptoms and influences the laxity of the pelvic ring. Vleeming et al. (1992b) conclude that pelvic belts enhance pelvic stability because they reduce SIJ laxity. Mens et al. (1999) suggested that, after initial provocative pelvic tests, these tests should be repeated with application of a pelvic belt to assess possible differences. In these studies, only a small amount of tension (50 N) is applied to the belt, just above the greater trochanter. Larger forces did not yield better results, as predicted in a biomechanical study (Vleeming et al. 1990a, 1990b). The efficacy of the pelvic belt was primarily determined by the location of the belt and the effects were explained by increased compression of the SIJ.

Buyruk et al. (1995a, 1995b, 1999) applied unilateral oscillations to the anterior-superior iliac spine to assess laxity of the pelvic joints. With sonoelasticity, using Doppler imaging of vibrations (DIV), they measured the stiffness/laxity ratio of artificially unstabilized SIJ in comparison with stabilized pelvices. The new method was objective and repeatable. In vivo studies have used the same technology in healthy subjects (Damen et al. 2002a, 2002b). It was shown that pelvic belts are effective to alter the laxity of the SIJ with an applied force of the pelvic belt of maximally 50 N. Subsequently, they showed that the laxity values of the SIJ decreased after application of a pelvic belt in patients with pelvic pain (Damen et al. 2002a). In another study (Damen et al. 2002b), patients with asymmetric SIJ laxity reported significantly more pain during pregnancy when compared with patients with symmetric laxity. According to the authors, increased general laxity is not associated with pelvic pain. Pregnant women with moderate or severe pelvic pain have the same laxity of the SIJ as pregnant women with no or mild pain. According to these studies, the *asymmetry* of laxity correlates with the symptomatic individual. In keeping with these data, perhaps manual motion testing should focus more on the (a)symmetry of SIJ motion. However, up to now, there has been no evidence that manual motion tests have a sufficient level of intra- and inter-tester reliability.

In 1999, Mens et al. developed a new diagnostic test. They studied the relation between impaired active straight leg raising (ASLR) and the mobility of pelvic joints with and without the application of a pelvic belt (testing the hypothesis that the pelvis is the basic bony platform that has to be stabilized before levers, like the legs and spine, can be used effectively). They conclude that impairment of the ASLR test correlates highly with the level of laxity of the pelvis, because application of a pelvic belt generally reduces the impairment of the ASLR test. The sensitivity and specificity of the test is high for PGP and the test is suitable to discriminate between PGP patients and healthy individuals (Mens et al. 1999).

The same authors (Mens et al. 1999) showed – by means of X-rays taken after pregnancy – that the pubic bone on the symptomatic side shifts caudally relative to the other side when the symptomatic leg is freely hanging down in a standing position. This procedure differs from the classical Chamberlain X-ray method, which screens the symptomatic loaded side. The authors conclude that this symphyseal shift is the result of an anterior rotation of the iliac bone relative to the sacrum on the symptomatic side (counternutation in the SIJ).

Hungerford et al. (2001) came to the same conclusion. Using an external motion analysis system, they studied (three-dimensionally) the angular and translational displacements in patients with SIJ problems and in healthy persons. They concluded that posterior rotation of the iliac bones relative to the sacrum (nutation) occurs in normals on the weightbearing side. By contrast, the iliac bones rotated anteriorly relative to the sacrum (counternutation; see Figure 2.2.6B) in the patient group. They found the same in the standing flexion test. Only on the loaded (standing) symptomatic side did an anterior rotation of the iliac bone occur.

The conclusion of these recent studies is that a relation exists between pelvic asymmetric laxity and the severity of complaints (Buyruk et al. 1999, Damen et al. 2002b). Damen et al. state that subjects with asymmetric laxity of the SIJ during pregnancy have a threefold higher risk of moderate to severe pelvic pain persisting into the postpartum period, compared to subjects with symmetric laxity during pregnancy. They also conclude that pelvic belt application can diminish the laxity and stiffen the pelvis and influence an impaired ASLR test with application of the DIV method. Based on the studies mentioned here, a dysfunctional SIJ is normally not related to a subluxated position of the joint, but to an altered position within the normal range of motion due to asymmetric forces acting on the joint.

The focus in this section has been to clarify the anatomy and biomechanics of the pelvic girdle and SIJ. However, spinal function and pelvic function are fully coupled. Any SIJ movement has consequences for the lumbar spine and vice versa. Nutation of the SIJ is coupled to extension of the lumbar spine. The spine and pelvis cannot be studied in isolation.

Nutation of the sacrum generally is the result of load-bearing and a functional adaptation to stabilize the pelvic girdle.

The intervertebral discs are loaded by compression, bending and torsion. As a result of body weight and force moments, the largest force acts perpendicularly to the discs. By contrast, this force is almost parallel to the surfaces of the practically flat SIJ. As a result, there is considerable shear loading in the SIJ and a risk of damaging the ligaments. In general, the ligamentous structures surrounding the SIJ are assumed to be sufficient to prevent shear and stabilize the joints. We do not agree with this view. We put forward evidence that the ligaments alone are not capable of transferring lumbosacral load effectively to the iliac bones. This holds especially for heavy loading situations and for conditions with sustained load resulting in creep, such as standing and sitting.

According to the self-bracing mechanism, resistance against shear results from the specific properties of the articular surfaces of the SIJ (form closure) and from the compression produced by body weight, muscle action and ligament force (force closure). Different aspects of this mechanism are operating in standing, sitting and walking and during actions such as forceful rotation and lifting in a stooped posture. The study reveals a functional relation between the biceps femoris, gluteus maximus, latissimus dorsi and erector spinae/multifidus muscles. Also, a relation exists with core muscles like the transversus abdominis and internal obliquus abdominis muscles, pelvic floor and diaphragm. In understanding their coupled function, the SIJ plays a central role.

We state that knowledge of the coupling mechanisms between spine, pelvis, legs and arms is essential to understand dysfunction of the human locomotor system, particularly the lower back. It has led us to describe three muscle slings (one longitudinal and two oblique) that can be energized (Figure 2.2.12).

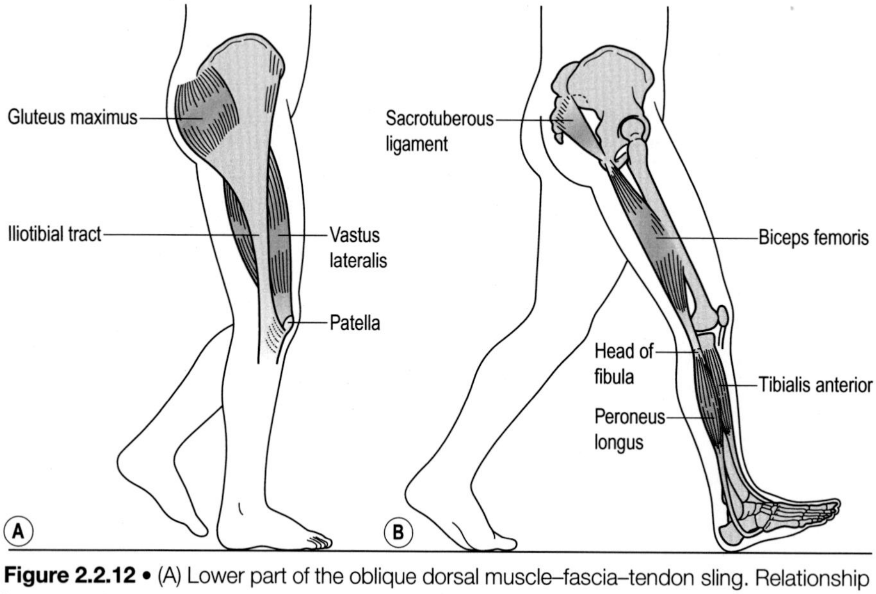

Figure 2.2.12 • (A) Lower part of the oblique dorsal muscle–fascia–tendon sling. Relationship between gluteus maximus muscle, iliotibial tract, vastus lateralis muscle and knee in the single support phase. The iliotibial tract can be tensed by action of the dorsally located gluteus maximus and ventrolaterally located tensor fascia latae muscle. The tract can also be tensed by contraction of the vastus lateralis muscle. (B) The longitudinal muscle–tendon–fascia sling. Relations at the end of the swing phase

We have provided evidence that non-optimal pelvic connections can be a main cause of complaints in patients with LBP. Diminished and/or unbalanced muscle function can lead to sustained counternutation in the SIJ. According to the model, the SIJ becomes especially prone to shear forces if loaded in a counternutation position. Counternutation, which is coupled to a supine position and to flattening of the spine in standing and sitting, could lead to abnormal loading of the lumbar discs and, in the end, herniation. Based on the data presented, disc herniation is not necessarily a separate syndrome but could be the result of failed stabilization of the pelvis and lower spine.

As a consequence, 'non-specific LBP' can be prevented and treated by modifying posture and by specific training methods. On the basis of the model presented above, advice is to treat and prevent LBP by appropriately strengthening and coordinating trunk and leg muscles to reach core stability. Initially, big levers like the legs and spine in the case of sub/non-optimal stability should not be used and only trained when core stability is sufficiently established.

Acknowledgement

We would like to extend our gratitude to Frans van der Helm, Cees de Vries, Annemarie van Randen, Jan-Paul van Wingerden, Annelies Pool, Ria van Kruining, Eddy Dalm, Jan Velkers and Cees Entius.

References

Abramson, D., Roberts, S.M., Wilson, P.D., 1934. Relaxation of the pelvic joints in pregnancy. Surg. Gynecol. Obstet. 58, 595–613.

Adams, M.A., Dolan, P., Burton, K., Bodguk, N., 2002. The biomechanics of back pain. Churchill Livingstone, Edinburgh.

Ahn, A.C., Tewari, M., Poon, C.S., Phillips, R.S., 2006. The limits of reductionism in medicine: could systems biology offer an alternative? PLoS Med. 3 (6), e208.

Bakland, O., Hansen, J.H., 1984. The axial sacroiliac joint. Anat. Clin. 6, 29–36.

Barker, J., 2005. The thoralumbar fascia. Thesis. University of Melbourne, Australia.

Barker, J., Briggs, C.A., 1999. Attachments of the posterior layer of the lumbar fascia. Spine 24 (17), 1757–1764.

Bogduk, N., MacIntosh, J.E., 1984. The applied anatomy of the thoracolumbar fascia. Spine 9 (2), 164–170.

Bogduk, N., Twomey, L.T., 1987. Clinical anatomy of the lumbar spine. Churchill Livingstone, Melbourne.

Bogduk, N., Johnson, G., Spalding, D., 1998. The morphology and biomechanics of the latissimus dorsi. Clin. Biomech. 13, 377–385.

Bowen, V., Cassidy, J.D., 1981. Macroscopic and microscopic anatomy of the sacroiliac joints from embryonic life until the eighth decade. Spine 6, 620.

Brooke, R., 1924. The sacroiliac joint. J. Anat. 58, 299–305.

Buyruk, H.M., Stam, H.J., Snijders, C.J., et al., 1995a. The use of colour Doppler imaging for the assessment of sacroiliac joint stiffness: a study on embalmed human pelvises. Eur. J. Radiol. 21, 112–116.

Buyruk, H.M., Snijders, C.J., Vleeming, A., et al., 1995b. The measurements of sacroiliac joint stiffness with colour Doppler imaging: a study on healthy subjects. Eur. J. Radiol. 21, 117–121.

Buyruk, H.M., Stam, H.J., Snijders, C.J., et al., 1999. Measurement of sacroiliac joint stiffness in peripartum pelvic pain patients with Doppler imaging of vibrations (DIV). Eur. J. Obstet. Gynecol. Reprod. Biol. 83 (2), 159–163.

Cholewicki, J., Panjabi, M.M., Khachatryan, A., 1997. Stabilizing function of trunk flexor-extensor muscles around a neutral spine posture. Spine 22 (19), 2207–2212.

Cholewicki, J., Simons, A.P., Radebold, A., 2000. Effects of external trunk loads on lumbar spine stability. J. Biomech. 33 (11), 1377–1385.

Crisco, J.J., Panjabi, M.M., Yamamoto, I., Oxland, T.R., 1992. Euler stability of the human ligamentous lumbar spine. Part II: experiment. Clin. Biomech. 7 (1), 27–32.

Damen, L., Spoor, C.W., Snijders, C.J., Stam, H.J., 2002a. Does a pelvic belt influence sacroiliac laxity? Clin. Biomech. 17 (7), 495–498.

Damen, L., Buyruk, H.M., Guler Uysal, F., et al., 2002b. The prognostic value of asymmetric laxity of the sacroiliac joint in pregnancy related pelvic pain. Spine 27 (24), 2820–2824.

Dijkstra, P.F., Vleeming, A., Stoeckart, R., 1989. Complex motion tomography of the sacroiliac joint: an anatomical and ro entgenological study. Fortschr. Geb. Rontgenstr. Nuklearmed. 150, 635–642.

Egund, N., Ollson, T.H., Schmid, H., Selvik, G., 1978. Movements in the sacroiliac joints demonstrated with roentgen stereophotogrammetry. Acta Radiol. Diagn. 19, 833.

Fortin, J.D., Dwyer, A.P., West, S., Pier, J., 1994a. Sacroiliac joint: pain referral maps upon applying a new injection/arthrography technique. 1: Asymptomatic volunteers. Spine 19, 1475–1482.

Fortin, J.D., Aprill, C.N., Ponthieux, B., Pier, J., 1994b. Sacroiliac joint: pain referral maps upon applying a new injection/arthrography technique. 2: Clinical evaluation. Spine 19, 1483–1489.

Gibbons, S., 2004. The caudomedial part of the gluteus maximus and its relation to the sacrotuberous ligament. In: Fifth Interdisciplinary World Congress on Low Back Pain, Melbourne, Australia.

Hodges, P.W., Cholewicki, J., 2007. Functional Control of the Spine. In: Vleeming, A., Mooney, V., Stoeckart, R. (Eds.), Movement, Stability and Lumbopelvic Pain. Elsevier, pp. 489–512.

Hodges, P.W., Kaigle, A., Holm, S., et al., 2003. Intervertebral stiffness of the spine is increased by evoked contraction of transversus abdominus and the diaphragm: in vivo porcine studies. Spine 28 (23), 2594–2601.

Hungerford, B., Gilleard, W., Lee, D., 2001. Alteration of sacroiliac joint motion patterns in subjects with pelvic motion asymmetry. In: Proceedings from the Fourth World Interdisciplinary Congress on Low Back and Pelvic Pain. Montreal, Canada.

Hungerford, B., Gilleard, W., Hodges, P.W., 2003. Evidence of altered lumbo–pelvic muscle recruitment in the presence of sacroiliac joint pain. Spine 28 (14), 1593–1600.

Huson, A., 1997. Kinematic models and the human pelvis. In: Vleeming, A. et al., (Eds.), Movement stability and low back pain. Churchill Livingstone, Edinburgh, pp. 123–131.

Kumar, S., Narayan, B.S., Zedka, M., 1996. An electromyographic study of unresisted trunk rotation with normal velocity among healthy subjects. Spine 21 (13), 1500–1512.

Lavignolle, B., Vital, J.M., Senegas, J., et al., 1983. An approach to the functional anatomy of the sacroiliac joints in vivo. Anat. Clin. 5, 169.

Lovejoy, C.O., 1988. Evolution of human walking. Sci. Am. 259, 118–125.

MacIntosh, J.E., Bogduk, N., 1986. The biomechanics of the lumbar multifidus. Clin. Biomech. 1, 205–213.

MacIntosh, J.E., Bogduk, N., 1991. The attachments of the lumbar erector. Spine 16, 783–792.

Mens, J.M.A., Stam, H.J., Stoeckart, R., et al., 1992. Peripartum pelvic pain: a report of the analysis of an inquiry among patients of a Dutch patient society. In: Vleeming, A. et al., (Eds.), First Interdisciplinary World Congress on Low Back Pain and its Relation to the Sacroiliac Joint, San Diego, CA, 5–6 November, pp. 521–533.

Mens, J.M.A., Vleeming, A., Stoeckart, R., et al., 1996. Understanding peripartum pelvic pain: implications of a patient survey. Spine 21 (11), 1303–1369.

Mens, J.M.A., Vleeming, A., Snijders, C.J., et al., 1999. The active straight leg raising test and mobility of the pelvic joints. Eur. Spine J. 8, 468–473.

Miller, J.A., Schultz, A.B., Andersson, G.B., 1987. Load displacement behavior of sacroiliac joint. J. Orthop. Res. 5, 92.

Mixter, W.J., Barr, J.S., 1934. Rupture of the intervertebral disc with involvement of the spinal canal. N. Engl. J. Med. 211, 210–215.

Mooney, V., Pozos, R., Vleeming, A., et al., 2001. Exercise treatment for sacroiliac joint pain. Orthopedics 24 (1), 29–32.

Moseley, G.L., 2007. Reconceptualising pain according to modern pain science. Phys. Ther. Rev. 12 (3), 169–178.

Njoo, K.H., 1996. Nonspecific LBP in general practice: a delicate point. Thesis, Erasmus University, Rotterdam.

Noe, D.A., Mostardi, R.A., Jackson, M.E., et al., 1992. Myoelectric activity and sequencing of selected trunk muscles during isokinetic lifting. Spine 17 (2), 225.

Pool-Goudzwaard, A., Hoek van Dijke, G., Mulder, P., et al., 2003. The iliolumbar ligament: its influence on stability of the sacroiliac joint. Clin. Biomech. 18 (2), 99–105.

Reeves, N.P., Cholewicki, J., 2003. Modeling the human lumbar spine for assessing spinal loads, stability, and risk of injury. [Review] [238 refs]. Crit. Rev. Biomed. Eng. 31 (1–2), 73–139.

Reeves, N.P., Narendra, K.S., Cholewicki, J., 2007. Spine stability: the six blind men and the elephant. [Review] [58 refs]. Clin. Biomech. 22 (3), 266–274.

Salsabili, N., Valojerdy, M.R., Hogg, D.A., 1995. Variations in thickness of articular cartilage in the human sacroiliac joint. Clin. Anat. 8, 388–390.

Sashin, D., 1930. A critical analysis of the anatomy and the pathological changes of the sacroiliac joints. J. Bone Joint Surg. 12, 891.

Solonen, K.A., 1957. The sacroiliac joint in the light of anatomical, roentgenological and clinical studies. Acta Orthop. Scand. 27, 1–127.

Snijders, C.J., Seroo, J.M., Snijder, J.G.N., Hoedt, H.T., 1976. Change in form of the spine as a consequence of pregnancy. In: Digest of the Eleventh International Conference on Medical and Biological Engineering, May 1976, Ottawa, Canada, pp. 670–671.

Snijders, C.J., Vleeming, A., Stoeckart, R., 1993a. Transfer of lumbosacral load to iliac bones and legs. 1: Biomechanics of self-bracing of the sacroiliac joints and its significance for treatment and exercise. Clin. Biomech. 8, 285–294.

Snijders, C.J., Vleeming, A., Stoeckart, R., 1993b. Transfer of lumbosacral load to iliac bones and legs. 2: Loading of the sacroiliac joints when lifting in a stooped posture. Clin. Biomech. 8, 295–301.

Snijders, C.J., Slagter, A.H.E., Strik van, R., et al., 1995. Why leg-crossing? The influence of common postures on abdominal muscle activity. Spine 20 (18), 1989–1993.

Stewart, T.D., 1984. Pathologic changes in aging sacroiliac joints. Clin. Orthop. Relat. Res. 183, 188.

Sturesson, B., Selvik, G., Udén, A., 1989. Movements of the sacroiliac joints. A roentgen stereophotogrammetric analysis. Spine 14, 162–165.

Sturesson, B., Udén, A., Vleeming, A., 2000a. A radiostereometric analysis of movements of the sacroiliac joints during the standing hip flexion test. Spine 25 (3), 364–368.

Sturesson, B., Udén, A., Vleeming, A., 2000b. A radiostereometric analysis of the movements of the sacroiliac joints in the reciprocal straddle position. Spine 25 (2), 214–217.

Svensson, H.O., Andersson, G.B.J., Hagstad, A., Jansson, P.O., 1990. The relationship of low-back pain to pregnancy and gynaecologic factors. Spine 15, 371–375.

van Wingerden, J.P., Vleeming, A., Snijders, C.J., Stoeckart, R., 1993. A functional–anatomical approach to the spine–pelvis mechanism: interaction between the biceps femoris muscle and the sacrotuberous ligament. Eur. Spine J. 2, 140–144.

Vleeming, A., Stoeckart, R., 2007. The role of the pelvic girdle in coupling the spine and the legs: a clinical-anatomical perspective on pelvic stability. In: Vleeming, A., Mooney, V., Stoeckart, R. (Eds.), Movement, Stability and Lumbopelvic Pain. Elsevier, pp. 113–137.

Vleeming, A., Stoeckart, R., Snijders, C.J., 1989a. The sacrotuberous ligament: a conceptual approach to its dynamic role in stabilizing the sacroiliac joint. Clin. Biomech. 4, 201–203.

Vleeming, A., Wingerden van, J.P., Snijders, C.J., et al., 1989b. Load application to the sacrotuberous ligament: influences on sacroiliac joint mechanics. Clin. Biomech. 4, 204–209.

Vleeming, A., Stoeckart, R., Volkers, A.C.W., Snijders, C.J., 1990a. Relation between form and function in the sacroiliac joint. 1: Clinical anatomical aspects. Spine 15, 130–132.

Vleeming, A., Volkers, A.C.W., Snijders, C.J., Stoeckart, R., 1990b. Relation between form and function in the sacroiliac joint. 2: Biomechanical aspects. Spine 15 (2), 133–136.

Vleeming, A., Wingerden van, J.P., Dijkstra, P.F., et al., 1992a. Mobility in the SI-joints in old people: a kinematic and radiologic study. Clin. Biomech. 7, 170–176.

Vleeming, A., Buyruk, H.M., Stoeckart, R., et al., 1992b. An integrated therapy for peripartum pelvic instability. Am. J. Obstet. Gynecol. 166 (4), 1243–1247.

Vleeming, A., Pool-Goudzwaard, A.L., Stoeckart, R., et al., 1995. The posterior layer of the thoracolumbar fascia: its function in load transfer from spine to legs. Spine 20, 753–758.

Vleeming, A., Pool-Goudzwaard, A., Hammudoghlu, D., et al., 1996. The function of the long dorsal sacroiliac ligament: its implication for understanding LBP. Spine 21 (5), 556–562.

Vleeming, A., de Vries, H.J., Mens, J.M.A., van Wingerden, J.P., 2002. Possible role of the long dorsal sacroiliac ligament in women with peripartum pelvic pain. Acta Obstet. Gynecol. Scand. 81, 430–436.

Vleeming, A., Albert, H.B., Ostgaard, H.C., Sturesson, B., Stuge, B., 2008. European guidelines for the diagnosis and treatment of pelvic girdle pain. [Review] [155 refs]. Eur. Spine J. 17 (6), 794–819.

Walheim, G.G., Selvik, G., 1984. Mobility of the pubic symphysis. In vivo measurements with an electromechanic method and a roentgen stereophotogrammetric method, Clin. Orthop. Relat. Res. 191, 129–135.

Weisl, H., 1955. The movements of the sacroiliac joints. Acta Anat. (Basel) 23, 80.

Willard, F.H., 2007. The muscular, ligamentous and neural structure of the lumbosacrum and its relationship to low back pain. In: Vleeming, A., Mooney, V., Stoeckart, R. (Eds.), Movement, Stability and Lumbopelvic Pain. Elsevier, pp. 5–45.

2.3

Anatomy of the pelvic floor

Ruth Lovegrove Jones

CHAPTER CONTENTS

There is increasing evidence that the pelvic floor muscles (PFM) perform multiple functions such as: continence and pelvic organ support (DeLancey 1990, Howard et al. 2000); sexual function (Baytur et al. 2005); respiration (Hodges et al. 2007); spinal stability; and containment of intra-abdominal pressure (IAP) (Hemborg et al. 1985, Pool-Goudzwaard et al. 2004, Smith et al. 2008). The physiological mechanisms by which they perform these roles are not clearly understood, predominately due to a lack of suitable instrumentation. The pelvic floor (PF) remains, particularly from a biomechanical perspective, an understudied region of the body (Ashton-Miller & DeLancey 2007). PF dysfunction for certain encompasses both urinary and faecal incontinence, pelvic organ prolapse (POP) and pelvic pain (Martins et al. 2007). It is a significant problem for both women and men and has been termed the hidden epidemic (DeLancey 2005), with estimates in the USA indicating that between 21% and 26% of American women have at least one PF disorder, with the greatest percentage experiencing urinary incontinence (Nygaard et al. 2008). PF dysfunction affects between 300 000 and 400 000 American women so severely that they require surgery, and 30% of those will require re-operations (Olsen et al. 1997, Boyles et al. 2003). Similar prevalence data of PF dysfunction are currently unavailable in the UK.

Given the multipurpose role of the PFM, the motor control challenge of the PFM will be immense and the efficiency of the PFMs would not only rely upon the anatomical integrity of the PF, but would depend on the central nervous system (CNS) response to satisfy hierarchical demands of function. The CNS must interpret the afferent input and generate a coordinated response so that the muscle activity occurs at the right time, with the appropriate level of force.

A combination of neuropathic changes, muscle, fascial or connective tissue damage is most likely responsible for the development of PF disorders yet the precise mechanisms remain controversial (Shafik et al. 2005, Ashton-Miller & DeLancey 2007, Petros 2007, Smith et al. 2007). The PF is an intricate, complicated structure, and by virtue of its anatomical position makes it a challenging area to study. The support mechanisms of the PF are responsible for the maintenance of continence and prevention of POP during rises of IAP (Ashton-Miller & DeLancey 2007), so functionally it not only has to allow the passage of urine and faeces at the appropriate time, it must also prevent incontinence. The PF is essential for sexual activity, conception, fertility and vaginal delivery (Herschorn 2004, Delancey 2005). More recently the PF has been implicated in contributing to spinal stability and respiration

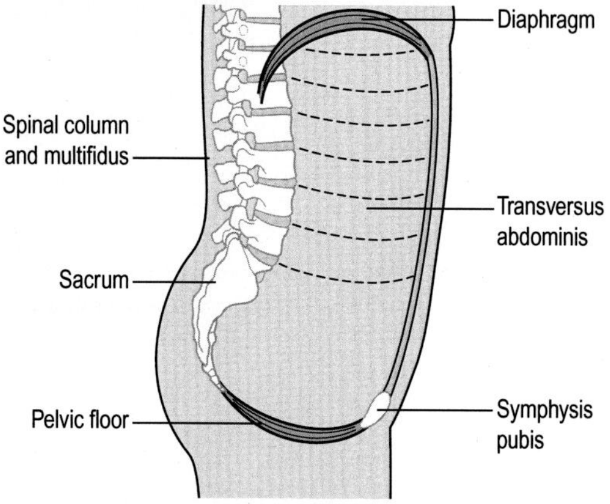

Figure 2.3.1 • Schematic of the lumbopelvic cylinder in which the respiratory diaphragm forms its top, transversus abdominis the sides and pelvic floor the bottom

(Hodges et al. 2007). The lumbopelvic cylinder is closed inferiorly by the PF, the respiratory diaphragm forms the top, the transversus abdominis the sides and the spinal column runs through the middle, supported posteriorly by segmental attachments of lumbar multifidus, anteriorly by segmental attachments of psoas and the abdominal muscles (Figure 2.3.1).

The following sections describe the gross anatomy of the PF and organs. Further details and a practical PF anatomy guide for the palpating physician can be found in Chapter 13.

Pelvic floor muscles

The PFM is the collective name for the muscles of the PF; unfortunately throughout the literature, there still remains lack of consensus regarding their description and terminology. A recent review of the literature revealed over 16 different overlapping terms for different parts of the muscle, yet the anatomy was found to be very consistent amongst different studies (Kearney et al. 2004). Kearney et al. concluded that confusion could be limited by standardizing terminology based upon origin and insertion points of the muscle. Therefore, for the purposes of this book, wherever possible, nomenclature is based upon origin-insertion (attachment) points.

The deep PFM: Levator ani muscle

The levator ani is covered by connective tissue on its superior and inferior surfaces, and with the corresponding muscle from the opposite side it is often referred to as the pelvic diaphragm. It provides the main muscular support for the pelvic viscera and is divided into two parts: the *puboviscerai* muscle and the *iliococcygeal* muscle. Two hiatuses are found in the midline: an anterior urogenital hiatus allows passage of the urethra and in females the vagina, and a posterior hiatus for passage of the anal canal.

The *pubovisceral muscle* is a thick U-shaped muscle which arises from the pubic bones on either side of the midline, and a band of fascia, the arcus tendineus levator ani (ATLA), laterally (Figure 2.3.2).

It passes behind the rectum forming a sling-like arrangement, attaching to the walls of the vagina, or fascial sheath of the prostate and urethra in the male, the perineal body and anal sphincter. The pubovisceral muscle can then be divided into three main components based upon the anatomical attachments: puborectalis, pubovaginalis or levator prostate in the male and pubococcygeus (Figure 2.3.3). In the female, the puborectalis portion passes beside the vagina with some attachment to the lateral vaginal walls. Some other fibres insert into the rectum, and others pass behind the anorectal junction. The fibres of the pubovaginalis pass between the vagina and pubis, connecting to the fascia that supports the urethra. Pubococcygeus only comprises a small proportion of the levator complex, although clinicians have often referred to the entire pubovisceral

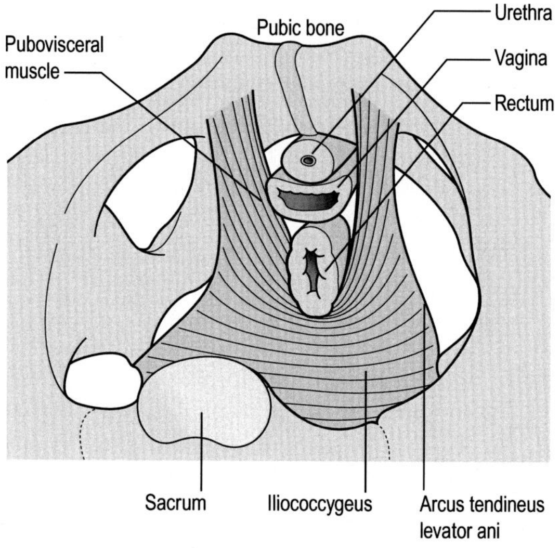

Figure 2.3.2 • Levator ani muscle seen from above. Adapted, with permission from Elsevier North-Holland, from Kearney et al. (2004). © DeLancey 2003).

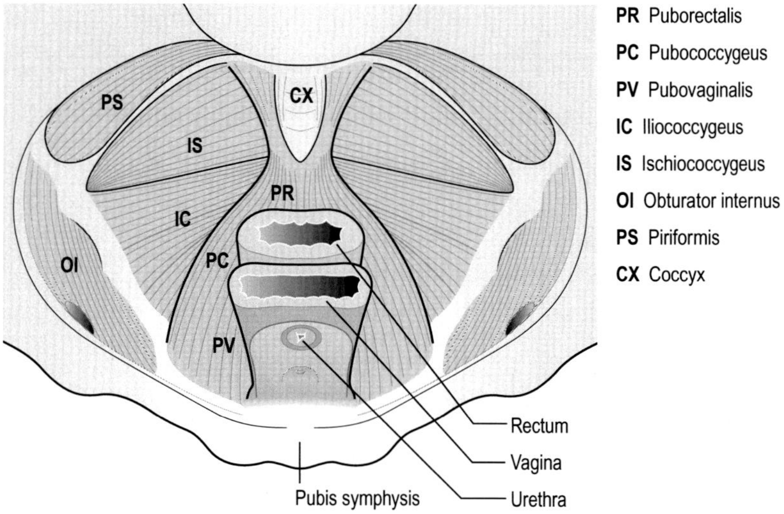

Figure 2.3.3 • Schematic of the pelvic floor illustrating the orientation of the horizontal clock: coccyx at 12 o'clock, and perineal body at 6 o'clock. Reproduced courtesy of Maeve Whelan, Specialist Womens Health Physiotherapist, Dublin, Ireland

muscle as pubococcygeus. Its fibres pass from the pubic bones to the coccyx, with some extending behind the rectum and to the anal canal.

The *iliococcygeal muscle* is attached from one side wall of the pelvis to the other via fascia described below, and forms a horizontal shelf on which the pelvic organs rest.

The ischiococcygeus is not technically part of the PFM, but forms the remainder of the pelvic diaphragm posteriorly, attaching to the ischial spine, the coccyx and lower part of the sacrum (Figure 2.3.3).

The superficial PFM and perineal body

Along with the connective tissue membrane surrounding them, the superficial PFM is often called the perineal membrane or urogenital diaphragm (Figures 2.3.4, 2.3.5). In the female, the perineal membrane lies level with the hymenal ring and attaches the urethra, vagina and perineal body to the ischiopubic rami.

The perineal body is a fibromuscular structure containing smooth muscle, elastic fibres and nerve endings in the middle of the perineum, between the urogenital and anal hiatuses (Figures 2.3.4, 2.3.5). Fibres of the rectum and anal sphincter, superficial PFM and levator ani also extend into the perineal body (Herschorn 2004). There is no consensus over the anatomical configuration of these muscles and fascia (Oelrich 1983, DeLancey 1999) yet the striated muscle fibres are generally thought of as the transverse perinei superficialis, urogenital sphincters (compressor urethrae, urethrovaginal) and external anal sphincters (Figures 2.3.4, 2.3.5, 2.3.6). The bulbocavernous and ischiocavernosus are the most superficial layer of the PF and have a mainly sexual function (Peschers & DeLancey 2008).

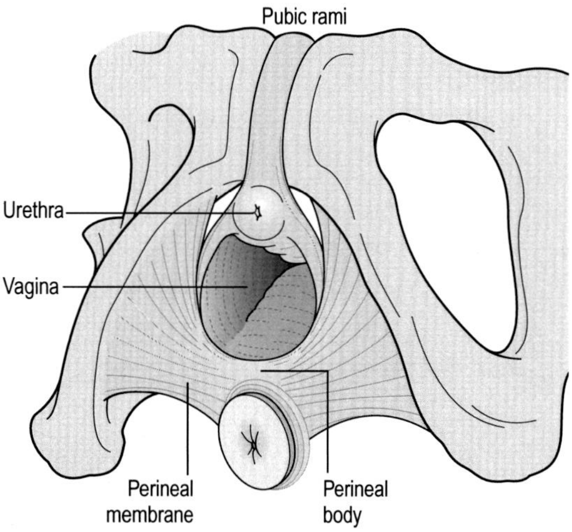

Figure 2.3.4 • Perineal membrane spans the arch between the ischiopubic rami with each side attached to the other through their connection in the perineal body. Reproduced from DeLancey (1999) Am. J. Obstet. Gynecol. 180(4):815–823, with permission.

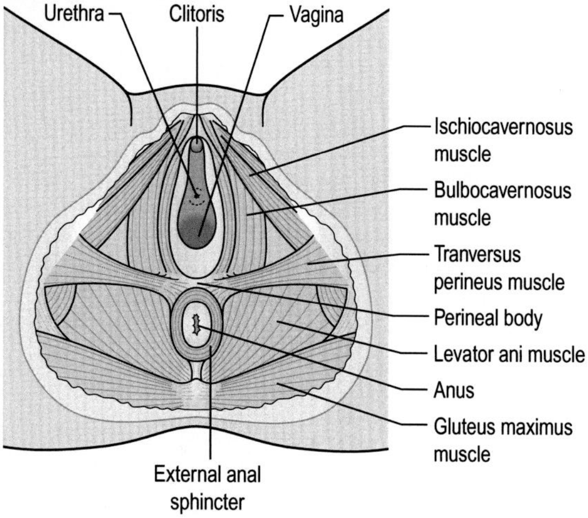

Figure 2.3.5 • Superficial muscles of the pelvic floor. Reproduced from Drake (2009) Gray's Anatomy Student Edition, Churchill Livingston.

Endopelvic fascia

The endopelvic fascia is the collective name given to the connective tissue that attaches the bladder, urethra, vagina and uterus to the pelvic walls (Figure 2.3.6). The pelvic sidewall attachment of the endopelvic fascia is called the arcus tendineus fascia pelvis (ATFP) which is attached to the pubic bone ventrally and to the ischial spine dorsally (Ashton-Miller et al. 2001).

The ATFP is well-defined anteriorly, and lies approximately 3 cm below the levator ani muscle. Posteriorly it is more like a broad sheet of fascia, blending with the endopelvic fascia, and merges with the levator ani. Near the spine, the ATFP fuses with the ATLA which is the band of fascia that the levator ani arises from (Figure 2.3.6).

Pelvic viscera

Bladder and urethra

The lower urinary tract can be divided into the bladder (or detrusor) and urethra, with the junction of these two continuous structures termed the bladder (vesical) neck or urethrovesical junction (Figure 2.3.7). The bladder is attached by ligaments and fascia to the side walls of the pelvis and pubic bones. Anteriorly in males the bladder neck is attached to the posterior surface of the pubic symphysis by the puboprostatic ligament, and in females the pubovesical ligament.

The urethra is a highly vascular multilayered tube approximately 0.6 cm in diameter and 3–4 cm in length in females (Strohbehn et al. 1996) and longer in the male (18–22 cm). In the female, the outer layer of the urethra is formed by the muscle of the striated urogenital sphincter whose fibres lie predominately in a circular orientation in the upper

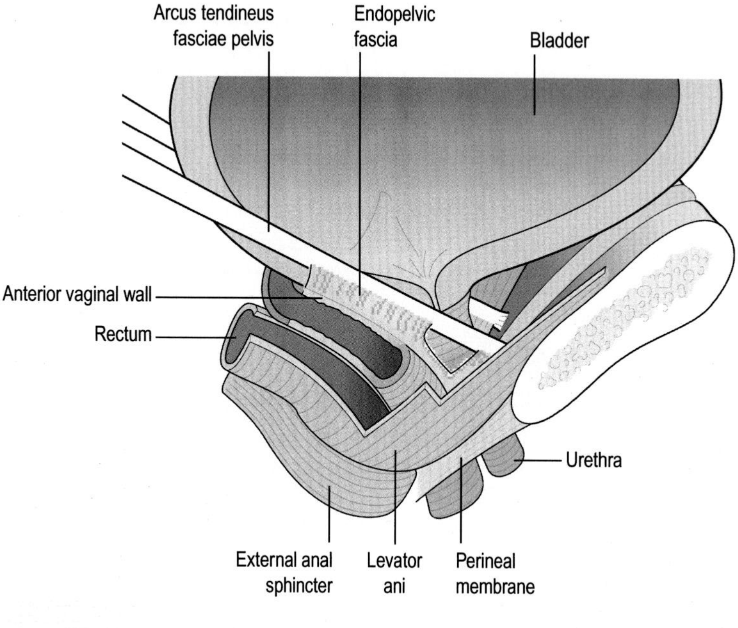

Figure 2.3.6 • Lateral view of the pelvic floor structures seen from the side in the standing position, cut lateral to the midline

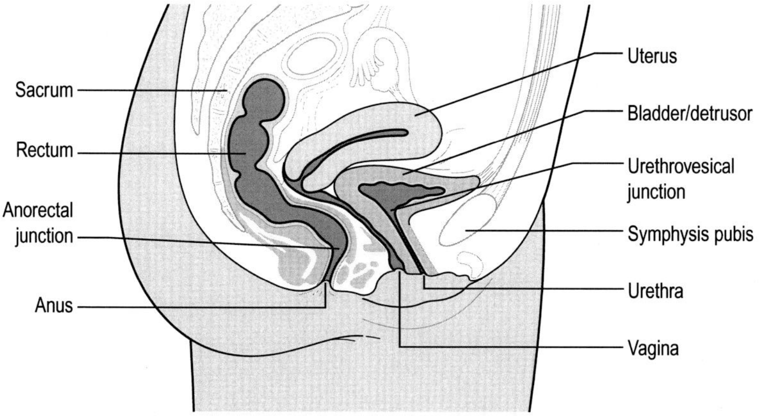

Figure 2.3.7 • Sagittal cross-section of female pelvis indicating main pelvic viscera and bony landmarks. Copyright and courtesy of Maeve Whelan, Specialist Womens Health Physiotherapist, Dublin, Ireland

two-thirds of the urethra. The striated urogenital sphincter muscle region of the ventral urethral wall has three component parts: the sphincter urethrae, the compressor urethrae and the urethrovaginal sphincter (Figure 2.3.8).

The smooth muscle of the urethra is present in the upper four-fifths of the urethra, lies inside the striated urogenital sphincter and is contiguous with the bladder. The orientations of the inner fibres are longitudinal whilst the outer layers are circular (Strohbehn et al. 1996) (Figure 2.3.9).

In the female urethra, closure pressure is known to be developed principally by contraction of the smooth and striated muscle (Perucchini et al. 2002). All elements of the striated urogenital sphincter muscle are found in the ventral urethral wall, whereas the dorsal wall contains only the sphincter urethrae because the urethrovaginal sphincter and the compressor urethrae diverge from the urethral wall to pass laterally toward the ischiopubic ramus and the vaginal wall (Oelrich 1983).

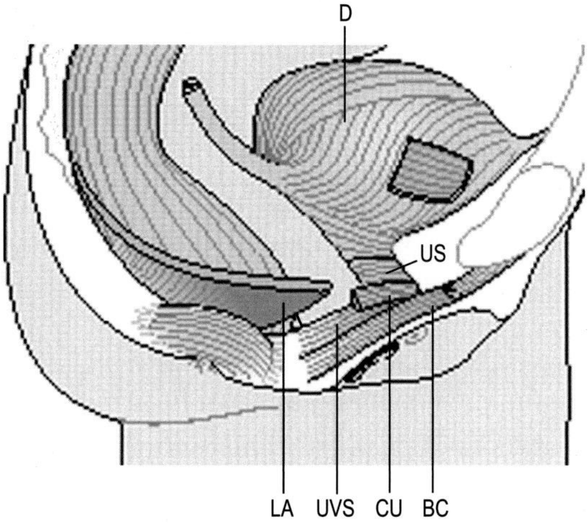

Figure 2.3.8 • Lateral view of urethral and pelvic floor muscular anatomy. BC, bulbocavernosus; CU, compressor urethrae; D, detrusor; LA, levator ani; US, urethral sphincter; UVS, urethrovaginal sphincter. Reproduced, with permission, from DeLancey (2004)

In the male, the urethra can be described in four parts: preprostatic, prostatic, membranous and the penile urethra. The preprostatic urethra extends from the internal urethral orifice to the superior part of the prostate gland and contains an internal urethra sphincter. The prostatic urethra runs through the prostate gland and is where the urinary and reproductive tracts merge. The short membranous part passes through the urogenital diaphragm and is surrounded by circular fibres of the sphincter urethrae. The penile urethra is the longest part of the urethra, which extends the length of the corpus spongiosum of the penis, opening onto the external urethral orifice at the tip of the penis.

Prostate

The prostate is a firm, partly glandular and partly muscular body, the base of which lies at the bladder neck, and the apex at the urogenital diaphragm. A thin filmy layer of connective tissue separates the prostate and seminal vesicles from the rectum posteriorly. Skeletal muscle fibres from the urogenital diaphragm extend into the prostate at the apex and up to the midprostate anteriorly (Hammerich et al. 2009). Further details of the prostate can be found in Chapter 12.

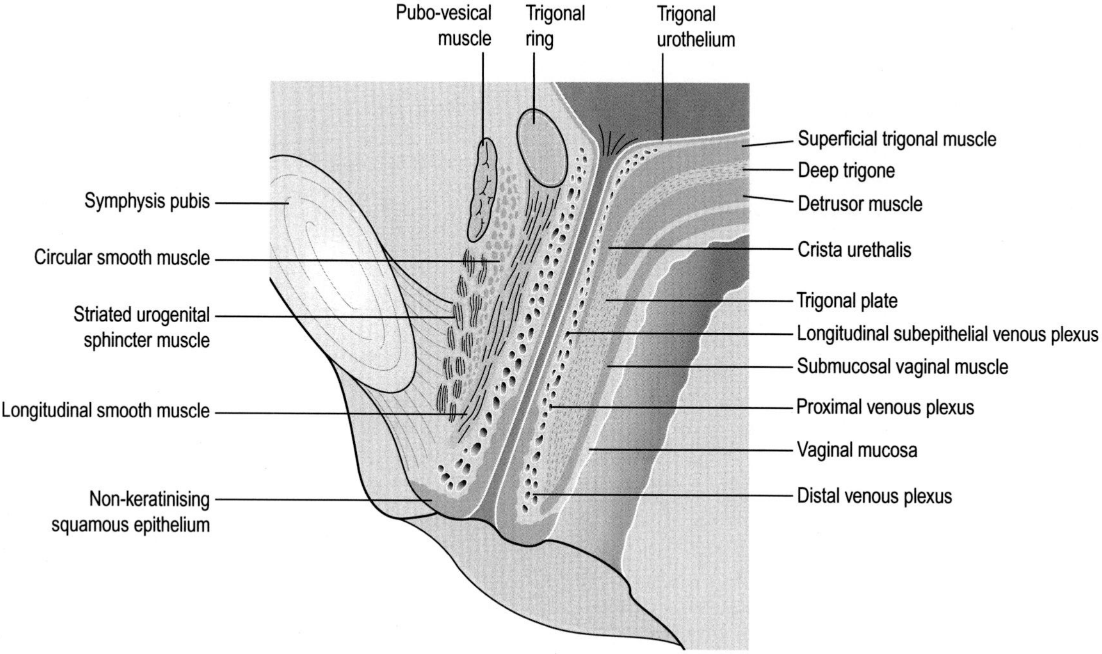

Figure 2.3.9 • Anatomy of the urethra shown in longitudinal section. Reproduced, with permission, from Strohbehn et al. (1996). Magnetic resonance imaging anatomy of the female urethra: a direct histologic comparison. Obstet. Gynecol. 88(5), 750–756.

Vagina and uterus

The vagina is a fibromuscular structure, resting on the rectum, lying posterior to the urethrovesical system (see Figure 2.3.7). It is attached laterally to the vaginal walls by combination of fascia and connective tissue containing smooth muscle, elastic fibres nerves and vessels. The distal third of the vagina is fused with the urethra anteriorly, the perineal body posteriorly, and the perineal membrane and PFM laterally (Peschers & DeLancey 2008). The uterus lies behind and above the bladder, in front of the rectum. The neck of the uterus is the cervix, which is directly attached to the vaginal wall.

Penis, scrotum and testes

The penis is anatomically divided into two continuous areas: the external body and the root (Figure 2.3.10). The root comprises a right and a left crus, which lies medial to the corresponding ischiopubic ramus; between the crura lies the bulb of the penis attached to the perineal membrane. Forming the body of the penis are three cylindrical masses of erectile tissue: the right and left corpus cavernosa, continuing from the crura, and the corpus spongiosum, continuing from the bulb of the penis. Each mass is covered by a layer of fascia, the tunica albuginea, and external to this is the deep fascia of the penis, Buck's fascia, which binds the erectile masses together. The scrotum and scrotal tissue overlie the base of the penis. Deep to the skin is the superficial (dartos) fascia of the scrotum. The septum of the scrotum formed by the dartos fascia extends up to the deep Buck's fascia of the penis creating the sac separating right from left. Deep to the dartos fascia each side is the cremaster muscle and fascia and deeper again is the testis. Extending upwards from the testis are the spermatic tissue, arteries and veins (see Figure 2.3.10).

Rectum and anal canal

The anterior wall of the rectum lies directly behind the posterior vaginal wall of the vagina in the female (Figure 2.3.2) and the base of the bladder in men. The rectum begins at the level of the third sacral vertebrae, is the lowest part of the gastrointestinal tract and is continuous above with the sigmoid colon and below with the anal canal and anorectal junction, which is at the level of the pelvic diaphragm.

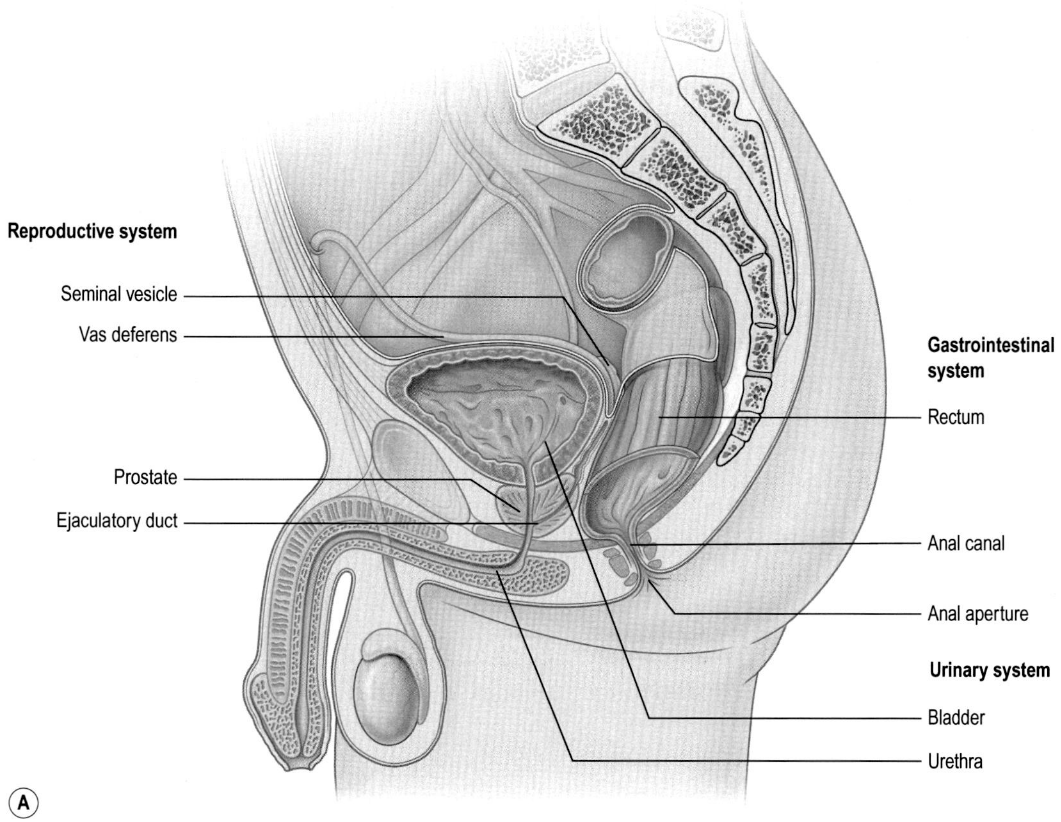
Reproductive system
Seminal vesicle
Vas deferens
Prostate
Ejaculatory duct
Gastrointestinal system
Rectum
Anal canal
Anal aperture
Urinary system
Bladder
Urethra
A

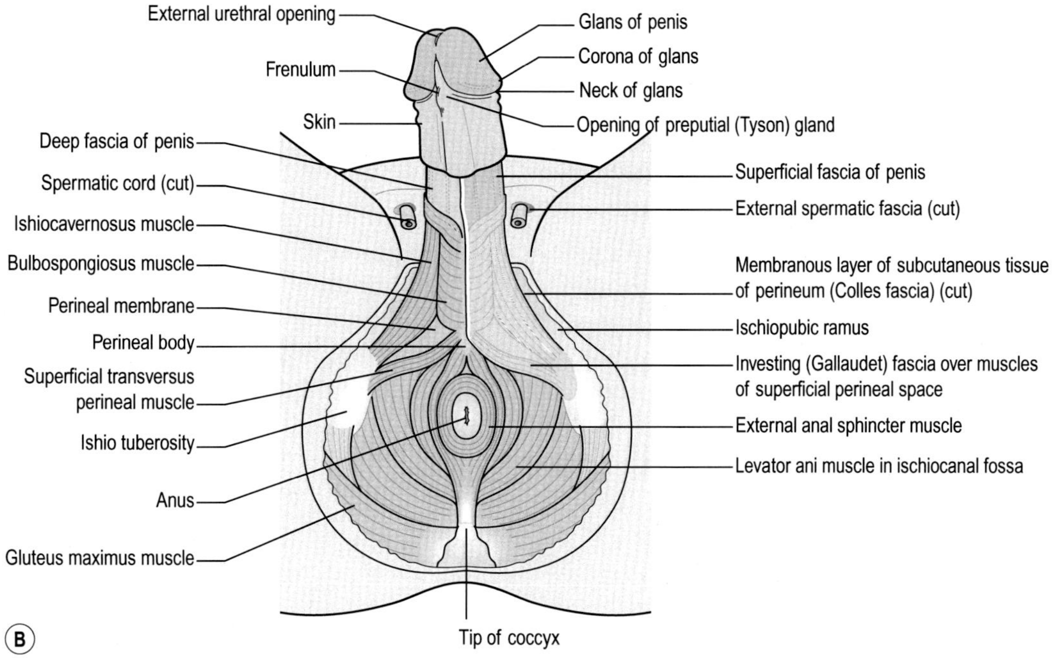
External urethral opening
Frenulum
Skin
Deep fascia of penis
Spermatic cord (cut)
Ishiocavernosus muscle
Bulbospongiosus muscle
Perineal membrane
Perineal body
Superficial transversus perineal muscle
Ishio tuberosity
Anus
Gluteus maximus muscle
Glans of penis
Corona of glans
Neck of glans
Opening of preputial (Tyson) gland
Superficial fascia of penis
External spermatic fascia (cut)
Membranous layer of subcutaneous tissue of perineum (Colles fascia) (cut)
Ischiopubic ramus
Investing (Gallaudet) fascia over muscles of superficial perineal space
External anal sphincter muscle
Levator ani muscle in ischiocanal fossa
Tip of coccyx
B

Figure 2.3.10 • Schematic anatomy of the male pelvic floor (A) and penis (B)

The rectum and its contents are supported by the pelvic floor muscles. The rectum is composed of a circular and longitudinal layer of smooth muscle. At its distal end, the circular layer thickens to form the internal anal sphincter. The *external anal sphincter* is placed outside the internal sphincter, between which are fused longitudinal fibres of the intestinal wall and PFM (Figures 2.3.5, 2.3.6, 2.3.7) (Peschers et al. 1997).

Innervation of the pelvic organs and PFM

Neural control of pelvic organs is affected by a unique coordination of somatic and autonomic motor nervous systems; sensory information and feedback is supplied by both visceral and somatic sensory fibre systems (Enck & Vodusek 2006).

The somatic innervation is largely from the lumbar, sacral and coccygeal plexus. The anterior divisions of the lumbar, sacral and coccygeal nerve roots form the lumbosacral plexus with L1–L4 in the lumbar plexus and L4–S4 in the sacral plexus. The skin of the lower trunk, perineum and proximal thigh is innervated by the iliohypogastric (L1), ilioinguinal (L1), and genitofemoral (L1–L2) nerves and the lateral femoral cutaneous (L2–L3) nerve innervates the lateral thigh.

The obturator (L2–L4) nerve contributes mainly to pelvic wall innervations and it traverses with the vessels along the lateral pelvic wall emerging to the medial compartment of the thigh via the obturator canal. It also innervates the muscles and skin of the medial thigh and skin of the medial lower leg. The sacral plexus ends in multiple peripheral nerves that innervate the additional muscles and skin of the buttocks and lower limbs.

The sciatic (L4–S3) and pudendal nerves (S2–S4) (described in detail in Chapter 13) are the two main nerves arising from the sacral plexus, although the posterior femoral cutaneous nerve (S1–S3/4) gives rise to the inferior cluneal and perineal branches and has been implicated in chronic pelvic pain (CPP) (Darnis et al. 2008, Tubbs et al. 2009) (Figure 2.3.11).The pudendal nerve carries motor, sensory and autonomic fibres; consequently both afferent and efferent pathways can be affected by its injury (Gray et al. 1995). The coccygeal plexus overlies the coccygeus muscle and comprises small nerves from S4 and S5 and the coccygeal nerves. It is thought to supply the coccygeus

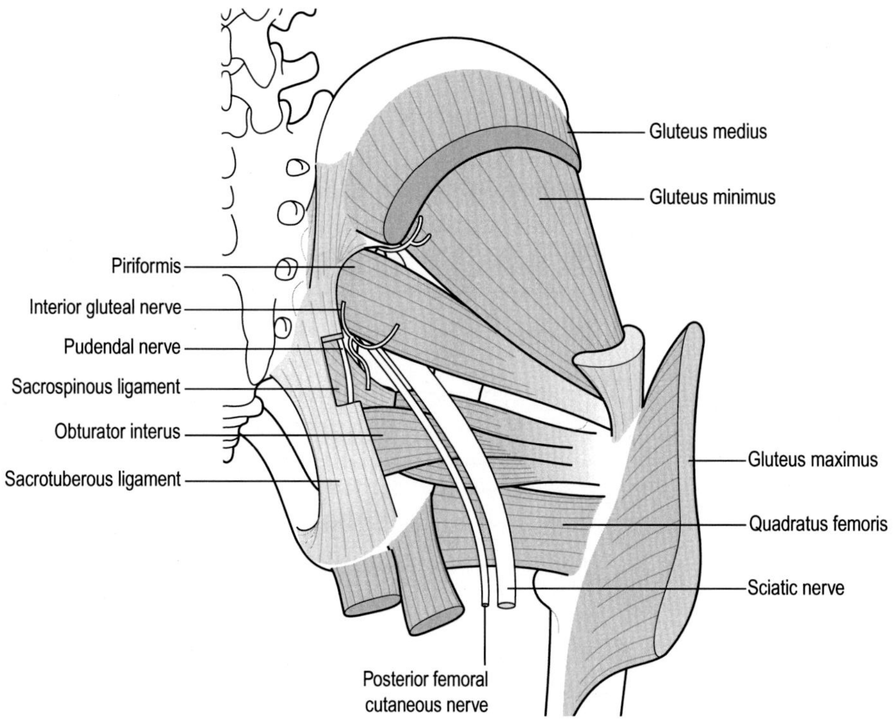

Figure 2.3.11 • Schematic diagram showing the relationship between the muscles and ligaments of the pelvis and the sciatic and pudendal nerves.

muscle, part of the levator ani muscle, the sacrococcygeal joint and a small region of skin between the coccyx and anus (Pattern & Hughes 2008).

The levator ani muscles have constant myoelectric activity and are composed of smooth and striated muscle fibres (Shafik et al. 2002), approximately two-thirds of which are type I (Gosling et al. 1981) reflecting their predominately support function (Shafik et al. 2003). Although there are differences of opinion regarding the exact innervation of the PFM, there is consensus that the nerve supply is from the pudendal nerve with direct branches from the sacral nerves S3–S4 (Shafik 2000, Guaderrama et al. 2005, Grigorescu et al. 2008). It is thought that the PFM predominantly contract or relax en masse (Shafik 1998). Yet due to the separate, though identical innervation of each individual muscle, there may also exist the capacity for voluntary selective activity by which an individual muscle might behave independently from the others (Shafik 1998, Kenton & Brubaker 2002).

The autonomic nerves help control micturition, defecation and sexual intercourse. The sympathetic nerves arise from the lumbar splanchnic nerves and parasympathetic nerves from the pelvic splanchnic nerves. The superior and inferior hypogastric plexuses form the major sympathetic supply to the pelvic viscera. The superior hypogastric plexus receives contributions from the lumbar splanchnic nerves (L3–L4) and divides into the left and right hypogastric nerve on the anterior surface of the sacrum (Drake 2005). They are then joined by the pelvic splanchnic nerves and are therefore a mixed plexus of sympathetic, parasympathetic fibres and visceral afferents (Pattern & Hughes 2008). In general it is thought that the pelvic splanchnic nerves are a combination of efferent fibres from S2–S4 and visceral afferent fibres, supplying the pelvic viscera, descending and sigmoid colon. The pelvic sympathetic innervation produces vasomotor effects, inhibits peristaltic contraction of the rectum and stimulates contraction of the internal genitals during orgasm, producing ejaculation in the male (Pattern & Hughes 2008). Parasympathetic innervation causes contraction of the bladder and rectum for micturition and defecation and clitoral or penile erection (Pattern & Hughes 2008). The pelvic visceral afferents travel with the parasympathetic fibres to the spinal ganglia (S2–S4). Nociceptive visceral afferents (NVAF) from the prostate, seminal vesicles, vagina, cervix, distal sigmoid colon and rectum follow the parasympathetic fibres to the spinal ganglia. NVAF from the bladder, ovaries and uterus travel with the sympathetic fibres to the inferior thoracic and superior lumbar spinal ganglia (Pattern & Hughes 2008). However, in clinical practice with paraplegic patients, sometimes the picture appears more complex.

In summary, when evaluating the patient with pelvic floor pain, it is important to include lumbar and sacral roots, the lumbosacral plexus, individual peripheral nerves, and the sympathetic chain.

These three chapters discussed the anatomical structures that have the potential to be involved with CPP. However, as discussed at the beginning, it is important for the reader not to focus solely on the end organ that they may perceive to be at fault. The next chapter therefore describes the biological basis of chronic pain mechanisms.

References

Ashton-Miller, J.A., DeLancey, J.O.L., 2007. Functional anatomy of the female pelvic floor. Reproductive Biomechanics Annals of the New York Academy of Sciences 1101, 266–296.

Ashton-Miller, J.A., Howard, D., DeLancey, J.O.L., 2001. The functional anatomy of the female pelvic floor and stress continence control system. Scand. J. Urol. Nephrol. Suppl. 35 (207), 1–7.

Baytur, Y.B., Deveci, A., Uyar, Y., Ozcakir, H.T., Kizilkaya, S., Caglar, H., 2005. Mode of delivery and pelvic floor muscle strength and sexual function after childbirth. Int. J. Gynaecol. Obstet. 88 (3), 276–280.

Boyles, S.H., Weber, A.M., Meyn, L., 2003. Procedures for urinary incontinence in the United States, 1979–1997. Am. J. Obstet. Gynecol. 189 (1), 70–75.

Darnis, B., Robert, R., Labat, J.J., Riant, T., Gaudin, C., Hamel, A., et al., 2008. Perineal pain and inferior cluneal nerves: Anatomy and surgery. Surg. Radiol. Anat. 30 (3), 177–183.

DeLancey, J.O.L., 1990. Anatomy and physiology of urinary continence. Clin. Obstet. Gynecol. 33 (2), 298–307.

DeLancey, J.O.L., 1999. Structural anatomy of the posterior pelvic compartment as it relates to rectocele. Am. J. Obstet. Gynecol. 180 (4), 815–823.

DeLancey, J.O., 2005. The hidden epidemic of pelvic floor dysfunction: achievable goals for improved prevention and treatment. [Review] [9 refs]. Am. J. Obstet. Gynecol. 192 (5), 1488–1495.

Drake, R., 2005. Gray's Anatomy. Churchill Livingstone, London.

Enck, P., Vodusek, D.B., 2006. Electromyography of pelvic floor muscles. J. Electromyogr. Kines. 16 (6), 568–577.

Gray, H., Williams, P.L., Bannister, L.H., 1995. Gray's anatomy: the anatomical basis of medicine and surgery, thirty-eighth ed. Churchill Livingstone, NewYork.

Gosling, J.A., Dixon, J.S., Critchley, H.O., Thompson, S.A., 1981. A comparative study of the human external sphincter and periurethral levator ani muscles. Br. J. Urol. 53 (1), 35–41.

Grigorescu, B.A., Lazarou, G., Olson, T.R., Downie, S.A., Powers, K., Greston, W.M., et al., 2008. Innervation of the levator ani muscles: description of the nerve branches to the pubococcygeus, iliococcygeus, and puborectalis muscles. Int. Urogynecol. J. 19 (1), 107–116.

Guaderrama, N.M., Liu, J., Nager, C.W., Pretorius, D.H., Sheean, G., Kassab, G., et al., 2005. Evidence for the innervation of pelvic floor muscles by the pudendal nerve. Obstet. Gynecol. 106 (4), 774–781.

Hammerich, K., Ayala, G., Wheeler, 2009. Anatomy of the prostate gland and surgical pathology of prostate cancer. In: Hedvig, H., Scardino, P. (Eds.), Prostate Cancer. Cambridge University Press.

Hemborg, B., Moritz, U., Lowing, H., 1985. Intra-abdominal pressure and trunk muscle activity during lifting. IV. The causal factors of the intra-abdominal pressure rise. Scand. J. Rehabil. Med. 17 (1), 25–38.

Herschorn, S., 2004. Female pelvic floor anatomy: the pelvic floor, supporting structures, and pelvic organs. Reviews in Urology 6 (Suppl.), S10.

Hodges, P.W., Sapsford, R., Pengel, L.H., 2007. Postural and respiratory functions of the pelvic floor muscles. Neurourol. Urodyn. 26 (3), 362–371.

Howard, D., Miller, J.M., DeLancey, J.O., Ashton-Miller, J.A., 2000. Differential effects of cough, valsalva, and continence status on vesical neck movement. Obstet. Gynecol. 95 (4), 535–540.

Kearney, R., Sawhney, R., DeLancey, J.O.L., 2004. Levator ani muscle anatomy evaluated by origin-insertion pairs. Obstet. Gynecol. 104 (1), 168–173.

Kenton, K., Brubaker, L., 2002. Relationship between levator ani contraction and motor unit activation in the urethral sphincter. Am. J. Obstet. Gynecol. 187 (2), 403–406.

Martins, J.A.C., Pato, M.P.M., Pires, E.B., Natal Jorge, R.M., Parente, M., Mascarenhas, T., 2007. Finite element studies of the deformation of the pelvic floor. Reproductive Biomechanics Annals of the New York Academy of Sciences 1101, 316–334.

Nygaard, I., Barber, M.D., Burgio, K.L., Kenton, K., Meikle, S., Schaffer, J., et al., 2008. Prevalence of symptomatic pelvic floor disorders in US women. JAMA 300 (11), 1311–1316.

Oelrich, T.M., 1983. The striated urogenital sphincter muscle in the female. Anat. Rec. 205 (2), 223–232.

Olsen, A.L., Smith, V.J., Bergstrom, J.O., Colling, J.C., Clark, A.L., 1997. Epidemiology of surgically managed pelvic organ prolapse and urinary incontinence. Obstet. Gynecol. 89 (4), 501–506.

Pattern, D., Hughes, J., 2008. Anatomy of the Urogenital Pain Systems. In: Urogenital Pain in Clinical Practice. Informa Healthcare, pp. 23–43.

Perucchini, D., DeLancey, J.O.L., Ashton-Miller, J.A., Peschers, U., Kataria, T., 2002. Age effects on urethral striated muscle: I. Changes in number and diameter of striated muscle fibers in the ventral urethra. Am. J. Obstet. Gynecol. 186 (3), 351–355.

Peschers, U.M., DeLancey, J.O.L., 2008. Anatomy. In: Haslam, J., Laycock, J. (Eds.), Therapeutic Management of Incontinence and Pelvic Pain. second ed. Springer, pp. 9–20.

Peschers, U.M., DeLancey, J.O., Fritsch, H., Quint, L.E., Prince, M.R., 1997. Cross-sectional imaging anatomy of the anal sphincters. Obstet. Gynecol. 90 (5), 839–844.

Petros, P.E., 2007. The anatomy and dynamics of pelvic floor function and dysfunction. In: The Female Pelvic Floor Function dysfunction and management according to the integral theory. second ed Springer, Heidelberg.

Pool-Goudzwaard, A., van Dijke, G.H., van, G.M., Mulder, P., Snijders, C., Stoeckart, R., 2004. Contribution of pelvic floor muscles to stiffness of the pelvic ring. Clin. Biomech. 19 (6), 564–571.

Shafik, A., 1998. A new concept of the anatomy of the anal sphincter mechanism and the physiology of defecation: Mass contraction of the pelvic floor muscles. Int. Urogynecol. J. Pelvic Floor Dysfunct. 9 (1), 28–32.

Shafik, A., 2000. Neuronal innervation of urethral and anal sphincters: surgical anatomy and clinical implications. [Review] [88 refs]. Curr. Opin. Obstet. Gynecol. 12 (5), 387–398.

Shafik, A., Asaad, S., Doss, S., 2002. The histomorphologic structure of the levator ani muscle and its functional significance. Int. Urogynecol. J. 13 (2), 116–124.

Shafik, A., Doss, S., Asaad, S., 2003. Etiology of the resting myoelectric activity of the levator ani muscle: Physioanatomic study with a new theory. World J. Surg. 27 (3), 309–314.

Shafik, A., Ahmed, I., Shafik, A.A., El-Ghamrawy, T.A., El-Sibai, O., 2005. Surgical anatomy of the perineal muscles and their role in perineal disorders. Anat. Sci. Int. 80 (3), 167–171.

Smith, M.D., Coppieters, M.W., Hodges, P.W., 2007. Postural response of the pelvic floor and abdominal muscles in women with and without incontinence. Neurourol. Urodyn. 26 (3), 377–385.

Smith, M.D., Russell, A., Hodges, P.W., 2008. Is there a relationship between parity, pregnancy, back pain and incontinence? Int. Urogynecol. J. 19 (2), 205–211.

Strohbehn, K., Quint, L.E., Prince, M.R., Wojno, K.J., DeLancey, J.O., 1996. Magnetic resonance imaging anatomy of the female urethra: a direct histologic comparison. Obstet. Gynecol. 88 (5), 750–756.

Tubbs, R., Miller, J., Loukas, M., Shoja, M., Shokouhi, G., Cohen-Gadol, A., 2009. Surgical and anatomical landmarks for the perineal branch of the posterior femoral cutaneous nerve: implications in perineal pain syndromes. J. Neurosurg. 111, 332–335.

Chronic pain mechanisms

3

Andrew Paul Baranowski

CHAPTER CONTENTS

This chapter looks at some of the definitions and talks about the triggers that may result in chronic pelvic pain (CPP) and some of the predisposition and maintenance factors that may place an individual at risk for developing CPP. Whereas these triggers, predisposing and maintenance factors will have a biological basis, we also have to consider the biological basis of the pain mechanisms, acute and chronic, in their own right.

Defining chronic pelvic pain

Several groups have tried to tackle the issue of defining CPP and discussions are ongoing. The Urogenital Pain Special Interest Group of The International Association for the Study of Pain (IASP) are currently proposing the following:

Chronic Pelvic Pain is chronic/persistent pain perceived* in structures related to the pelvis of either men or women. It is often associated with negative cognitive, behavioural, sexual and emotional consequences as well as with symptoms suggestive of lower urinary tract, sexual, bowel or gynaecological dysfunction.

*Perceived indicates that the patient and clinician, to the best of their ability from the history, examination and investigations (where appropriate), have localized the pain as being perceived in the anatomical pelvic area.

They go on to say:

In the case of documented nociceptive pain that becomes chronic/persistent through time, pain must have been continuous or recurrent for at least 6 months. *That is it can be cyclical over a six month period, such as the cyclical pain of dysmenorrhoea. Six months is arbitrary; however, six months was chosen because three months was not considered long enough if we include cyclical pain conditions.* If non-acute and central sensitization pain mechanisms are well documented,

Continued

then the pain may be regarded as chronic, irrespective of the time period.

Chronic Pelvic Pain may be subdivided into those conditions with well defined classical pathology (such as infection and cancer) and those where no obvious pathology are found.

For the purpose of this classification the terms **Specific Disease Associated Pelvic Pain** is proposed for the former and **Chronic Pelvic Pain Syndrome** is used for the latter.

Chronic Pelvic Pain Syndrome definition

Chronic Pelvic Pain Syndrome (CPPS) is the occurrence of chronic pelvic pain where there is no proven infection or other obvious local pathology that may account for the pain. It is often associated with negative cognitive, behavioural, sexual and emotional consequences as well as with symptoms suggestive of lower urinary tract, sexual, bowel or gynaecological dysfunction.

CPPS is a subdivision of Chronic Pelvic Pain (see above).

The implications of the above for clinical management are huge. Essentially pain perceived to be both chronic and sited within the pelvis is associated with a wide range of causes and associated symptoms that must be investigated and managed in their own right. For this to occur, patients with CPP must have access to the appropriate resources through multispeciality (e.g. urology, urogynaecology, gynaecology, neurology and pain medicine) and multidisciplinary (e.g. medical doctor, nurse, psychology and physiotherapy) teams (Baranowski et al. 2008b) (see Chapter 8.1).

Chronic pelvic pain syndrome: The cause

It is important to realize the difference between *trigger*, *predisposition* and *maintenance factors* and how these may relate to the mechanism for the perceived pain and associated other symptoms.

Over the years there has been a great emphasis on the triggers for the chronic pain and much work has focused on local pathology, such as infection and local irritation with inflammation. This has resulted in a number of inappropriate outcomes (Abrams et al. 2006, Baranowski 2008a):

1. Over-investigation of the end-organ as the source of pain;
2. Inappropriate treatment of the end-organ (e.g. the overuse of antibiotics and even the removal of organs);
3. A spurious classification system that encourages the above.

A small group of patients may be able to identify the exact trigger. However, in many ways triggers are not important, as they are probably numerous, transient and can not be avoided. Ongoing and repeated investigations for the 'cause' are associated with a worse prognosis.

Triggers do not result in CPPS in all persons, though the proportion is unknown. It is now accepted that as well as triggers we need to consider predisposing factors and maintenance factors.

Genetics may play a role in predisposing patients to chronic pain, though the exact nature is not fully worked out. Other predisposing factors may include childhood experiences, negative sexual encounters and sexual violence, stress and other social factors, personality traits, as well as physical disability and medical illness. Some of these factors as well as precipitating inappropriate pain responses may also maintain the pain once started.

Maintenance is thus a complex issue. All chronic pain is associated with emotional and behavioural consequences (Sullivan et al. 2006, Nickel et al. 2008). The perceived severity of the pain understandably will be a major decisive factor as to how distressed and disabled the patient is. However, there is a cycle of events, where depression and catastrophizing are poor prognostic factors in their own right and clinical experience suggests that if these issues are not managed no progress in managing the pain will be made. Issues with work, relationships, sex and loss of meaning of life also appear to be as important. All of these factors can produce inappropriate maladaptive coping mechanisms such as inappropriate pain-contingent resting cycling with overactivity and as a result widespread total body pain, increased disability and increased distress.

Chronic pelvic pain syndrome: The mechanisms

There are many texts describing the mechanisms of chronic pain at a cellular level and neurobiological level (Vecchiet et al. 1992, Pezet & McMahon 2006, Nickel et al. 2008). The mechanisms for somatic, visceral and neurological tissue may overlap, but there are some important differences. As well as this science being applied to the patient the biopsychosocial model alluded to above needs to be integrated into the model.

All the structures within the pelvis and some outside of the pelvis (e.g. thoracolumbar junction) may, when stimulated, result in pain perceived in the pelvis. Recurrent activation of the nervous system may be associated with both peripheral and central sensitization.

The main consequences of the above science for the clinician are:

1. Lower threshold activation of peripheral nociceptors with increased pain perception;
2. Increased receptive field;
3. Patients become aware of stimuli not normally perceived – hyperaesthesia;
4. Stimuli that are normally not painful become perceived as painful – allodynia;
5. Cross-over hypersensitivity occurs (viscero-visceral hyperalgesia, visceromuscular hyperalgesia);
6. Central-mediated functional abnormalities of the viscera (e.g. abnormal function of the bowel with alternating diarrhoea and constipation);
7. Central-mediated changes in peripheral structure (e.g. Hunner's ulcers, peripheral oedema and change in vasculature);
8. Neurobiological psychological consequences.

(Vecchiet et al. 1992; Giamberardino 2005; Pezet & McMahon 2006; Baranowski et al. 2008b).

A case history may best illustrate these points:

A patient develops an acute cystitis, infection may never be proven and stress, increased pelvic floor muscle tension is a possible cause for the initial symptoms. Perhaps there is a background of a negative sexual encounter (often there is not) and predisposing genetics, The ongoing pain results in central sensitization involving excitatory amino acid receptors such as N-methyl-D-aspartate (NMDA) and α-amino-3-hydroxy-5-methyl-4-isoxazole epropionic acid (AMPA). The patient feels that their bladder is never empty (aware of stimuli not normally perceived), and holding on to their urine produces pain (stimuli that are normally not painful become perceived as painful). Investigations of the bladder do not reveal infection, but the bladder is inflamed and swollen (central-mediated changes in peripheral structure). The pain appears to spread and the vulvar region becomes very sensitive with evidence of allodynia (increased receptive field). The patient describes erratic bowel habit, this may be due to the treatment; however, irritable-bowel-type symptoms due to central-mediated functional abnormalities of the viscera are also a possibility. The patient develops muscular pain (partly due to visceromuscular hyperalgesia but also due to inappropriate resting and cycles of over- and underactivity). As you might expect, depression, anxiety and anger set in; much of this may be secondary to the low quality of life and the pain but physical neurobiological changes may also be involved.

The initial trigger may involve any structure: somatic (cutaneous/muscular), visceral or neurological. The symptoms may remain well focused in that area, such as in the organ-based pain syndromes (e.g. bladder pain syndrome, vulvar pain syndrome, testicular pain syndrome) or in a specific muscle or local group of muscles. A patient may present at any stage in the above story and with a focus of pain within either a single or multiple system(s)/organ(s). The balance between afferent and efferent (functional) abnormalities is not linear and as a consequence some patients may present with primarily sensory and others with primarily functional phenomena. Patients may present with primarily pain perceived in one area and functional abnormalities in another. As well as these changes occurring or perceived within the pelvis, symptoms may be found elsewhere. For instance, bladder pain syndrome is associated with Sjögren's and many pelvic pain conditions are associated with endocrine and immune deficiency as well as fibromyalgia and chronic fatigue syndrome (Abrams et al. 2006).

Mechanisms for chronic pelvic pain

Chronic pelvic pain mechanisms may involve:

1. Ongoing acute pain mechanisms (Linley et al. 2010) (such as those associated with inflammation or infection) – which may involve somatic or visceral tissue. This chapter will concentrate primarily on the visceral pain mechanisms;
2. Chronic pain mechanisms, which especially involve the central nervous system (McMahon et al. 1995);
3. Emotional, cognitive, behavioural and sexual responses and mechanisms (Binik & Bergeron 2001, Tripp et al. 2006). These will be covered in Chapter 4.

Table 3.1 illustrates some of the differences between the somatic and visceral pain mechanisms. They

Table 3.1 Comparison between visceral and somatic pain

	Visceral pain	Somatic pain
Effective painful stimuli	Stretching and distension, producing poorly localized pain	Mechanical, thermal, chemical and electrical stimuli, producing well-localized pain
Summation	Widespread stimulation produces a significantly magnified pain	Widespread stimulation produces a modest increase in pain
Autonomic involvement	Autonomic features (e.g. nausea and sweating) frequently present	Autonomic features less frequent
Referred pain	Pain perceived at a site distant to the cause of the pain is common	Pain is well-localized
Referred hyperalgesia	Referred cutaneous and muscle hyperalgesia common, as is involvement of other viscera. *This is very important* (see below)	Hyperalgesia tends to be localized
Innervation	Low-density, unmyelinated C fibres and thinly myelinated A fibres	Dense innervation with a wide range of nerve fibres
Primary afferent physiology	Intensity coding. As stimulation increases afferent firing increases with an increase in sensation and ultimately pain	Two-fibre coding. Separate fibres for pain and normal sensation
Silent afferents	50–90% of visceral afferents are silent until the time they are switched on. These fibres are very important in the central sensitization process	Silent afferents present in lower proportions
Central mechanisms	Play an important part in the hyperalgesias, viscerovisceral, visceromuscular and musculovisceral hyperalgesias. Sensations not normally perceived become perceived and non-noxious sensations become painful	Responsible for the allodynia and hyperalgesia of chronic somatic pain
Abnormalities of function	Central mechanisms associated with visceral pain may be responsible for organ dysfunction (see below)	Somatic pain associated with somatic dysfunction
Central pathways and representation	As well as classical pathways, there is evidence for a separate dorsal horn pathway and central representation	Classical pain pathways

underlie some of the mechanisms that may produce the classical features of visceral pain; in particular, the referred pain and the referred hyperalgesias.

Ongoing peripheral visceral pain mechanisms as a cause of chronic pelvic pain

In most cases of chronic pelvic pain *ongoing* tissue trauma, inflammation or infection are not present (Hanno et al. 2005, Abrams et al. 2006, Baranowski et al. 2008a). However, conditions that produce recurrent trauma, infection or ongoing inflammation may result in CPP in a small proportion of cases. It is for this reason that the early stages of assessment will include looking for these pathologies (Van de Merwe & Nordling 2006, Fall et al. 2010). Once excluded, ongoing investigations for these causes are rarely helpful and indeed may be detrimental.

When acute pain mechanisms are activated by a nociceptive event, as well as direct activation of the peripheral nociceptor transducers, sensitization of those transducers may also occur, magnifying the afferent signalling. Afferents that are not normally active may also become activated by the change, that is there may be activation of the so-called silent afferents. Whereas these are mechanisms of acute pain the increased afferent barrage of impulses underlie the mechanisms for chronic pain where the increased afferent signalling is often a trigger for the chronic pain mechanisms that maintain the perception of pain in the absence of ongoing peripheral pathology (see below) (Vecchiet et al. 1992).

There are a number of mechanisms by which the peripheral transducers may exhibit an increase in sensibility.

1. Modification of the peripheral tissue, which may result in the transducers being more exposed to peripheral stimulation.
2. There may be an increase in the chemicals that stimulate the receptors of the transducers (Pezet & McMahon 2006).
3. There are many modifications in the receptors that result in them being more sensitive.
   In general the effect of 1 and 2 is to lower threshold and of 3 to increase responsiveness.

Some of the chemicals responsible for the above changes may be released from those cells associated with inflammation, but the peripheral nervous system may also release chemicals in the form of positive and inhibitory loops (Cevero & Laird 2004).

Nerve growth factor (NGF) is an important trophic factor necessary during development for the growth and survival of sympathetic neurons, sensory neurons and neurons in the central nervous system. Associated with local tissue trauma, mast cells, macrophages, keratinocytes and T cells all release NGF, which can then interact with its receptors, TrkA, on nerve endings. It may both directly activate primary afferents but also indirectly such as through the use of bradykinin (Petersen et al. 1998). The result is an increase in response of the primary afferent with multiple action potentials being generated in response to a stimulus as opposed to one or two. The TrkA–NGF complex formed on the afferent neuron may also be transmitted centrally where it may alter gene expression. Such long-term gene modification may underlie some of the mechanisms of chronic NGF-induced hypersensitivity.

Adenosine triphosphate (ATP) is thought to be released in increased amounts from certain viscera when stimulated by noxious stimuli. As well as this increased ATP producing an increased stimulation of ATP receptors, when inflammation is present the ATP receptors have their properties changed so that there is an increased response per unit of ATP contributing to the nociceptor activation. ATP is thought to act on P2X3 purine receptors which are found on visceral afferents and small-diameter dorsal root ganglion neurons.

Substance P and other neurokinins (McMahon & Jones 2004) act on afferent tachykinin receptors, such as TRPV1 a transducer for noxious heat and protons, and are thought to play a primary role in inflammatory hyperalgesia. In particular, possibly due to proto-oncogene activation, inflammation is associated with an increase in TRPV1 channel density. As well as this, inflammation may also change the sensitivity of the channel so that it is activated at thresholds that would normally be subliminal. For instance, it has been suggested that this receptor for heat pain may be activated at normal body temperature. Substance P may be released from small fibre afferent neurons as a part of an antidromic response, but there may also be direct mechanisms involving direct depolarization of the nerve terminals.

Voltage-gated ion channels (such as tetrodotoxin-resistant sodium channel, NaV1.8) are also implicated in peripheral sensitization. These channels open or close in response to changes in membrane potential. The voltage-gated sodium channel is a complex channel with multiple subunits. The alpha subunit contains the voltage sensor and the ion channel. The alpha subunit is composed of a number of alpha subunit variants that affect its sensitivity to changes in the membrane potential and will also alter ion flow. Changes in these alpha subunits may thus sensitize the neuron associated with the channel. The beta subunit is also considered important by an effect on the action potential as well as by other possible mechanisms. Changes in potassium and calcium voltage-gated channels may also underlie a part of the mechanism responsible for peripheral sensitization.

Second messenger pathways within the primary afferents enable amplification of peripheral singles. In general these pathways are balanced out by others that are responsible for reducing any activation. During chronic pain these mechanisms may become imbalanced. Classical second messengers signalling pathways involve protein kinase which via an elaborate series of chemical activations cause a release of calcium within the neuron. There are probably a number of other mechanisms that may also release calcium, and nitric oxide has been implicated in some of these. As well as producing rapid-onset short-lived changes, activation of this messenger system may produce longer-term changes via alterations of transcription and translation at a genetic level.

Spinal mechanisms of visceral pain and sensitization: Central sensitization (Roza et al. 1998, Giamberardino 2005)

The above mechanisms illustrate some of the mechanisms behind peripheral sensitization. These mechanisms and the recruitment of previously silent nociceptive neurons may be maintained even after injury has healed. As a consequence, ongoing nociceptive information may continue arriving at the spinal cord despite no peripheral 'pathology'. The large ongoing stimulus provided by these mechanisms may then result in a long-term increase in the excitability of the dorsal horn neurons. The mechanisms responsible for this increased excitability produce what is known as central sensitization. Once established central sensitization may be self-perpetuating even if the ongoing peripheral signalling stops or may be maintained by low-threshold fibre activation, e.g. light touch (allodynia).

There are essentially three processes at the spinal cord level that are probably involved in central sensitization. Changes in existing protein activity (post-translational processing) will be the earliest changes (minutes); however, changes in genetic transcription of proteins and even structural changes in neuron connectivity may also have roles to play. These latter changes may occur within days (Nazif et al. 2007).

The chemicals involved in the early phase include a number of neurotransmitters including glutamate, substance P, calcitonin gene-related peptide, prostaglandin E2 (PGE2) and brain-derived neurotrophic factor (BDNF) as well as many others (Cevero & Laird 2004).

Glutamate is an important agent in this process. Increased levels of glutamate, due to recurrent afferent nociceptive fibre activity, remove the magnesium ion block of NMDA. This allows calcium ions to enter the primary afferent with enhanced depolarization. Glutamate also binds to AMPA, which may be another pathway by which it increases intracellular calcium. Other transmitters/modulators released centrally include substance P acting on neural kinin receptors, PGE2 combining to endogenous prostanoid receptors and BDNF acting on tyrosine kinase B receptors which may also increase intracellular calcium. In this situation the calcium ions act to lower the threshold for second-order neuron firing with increased signalling being transmitted to the higher centres.

The second importance of this increase in calcium ions is in *post-translational processing*; this usually involves the addition of phosphate groups to some of the protein's amino acids, by enzymes known as kinases. It is the increase in *calcium* through the above mechanisms that activates these kinases. Phosphorylation can dramatically alter the properties of a protein, typically lowering the threshold at which channels open but also the channel remains open for longer. The result is that a stimulus produces a magnified evoked response.

Visceral hyperalgesia

Central sensitization (Nazif et al. 2007) is responsible for a decrease in threshold and increase in response duration and magnitude of dorsal horn neurons. It is associated with an expansion of the receptive field. As a result it increases signalling to the central nervous system and effects what we perceive from a peripheral stimulus. As an example, for cutaneous stimuli light touch would not normally produce pain. When central sensitization is present light touch may be perceived as painful (allodynia). In visceral hyperalgesia (so called because the afferents are primarily small-fibre), visceral stimuli that are normally subthreshold and not usually perceived may be perceived; for instance, with central sensitization, stimuli that are normally subthreshold may result in a sensation of fullness and a need to void the bladder or to defecate. Stimuli normally perceived may be interpreted as painful and stimuli that are normally noxious may be magnified (true hyperalgesia) with an increased perception of pain. As a consequence, one can see that many of the symptoms of the bladder pain syndrome (formally known as interstitial cystitis) and irritable bowel syndrome may be explained by central sensitization. A similar explanation exists for the muscle pain of fibromyalgia.

Supraspinal modulation of pain perception

It is important to appreciate that nociception is the process of transmitting to those centres involved in perception information about a stimulus that has the potential to cause tissue damage. Pain is far more complex and involves the perception of a nociceptive event but also the emotional response (Rabin et al. 2000). Pain is defined by IASP as 'an unpleasant sensory and emotional experience associated with actual or potential tissue damage, or described in terms of such damage' (Merskey & Bogduk 1994). Modulation of nociceptive pathways may occur throughout the whole of the neuroaxis (spinal cord through to higher centre) and in the periphery and spinal cord involves the mechanisms described above. The brain may also effect the modulation at spinal cord level.

Higher-centre modulation of spinal nociceptive pathways

It is now well-accepted that there are both *descending pain-inhibitory* and *descending pain-facilitatory pathways* that originate from the brain (Melzack et al. 2001). The midbrain periaqueductal grey (PAG), just below the thalamus, plays an important part in spinal modulation. It receives inputs from those centres associated with thought and emotion. Projections from the PAG (via several relay systems) to the dorsal horn can inhibit nociceptive messages from reaching conscious perception by spinal mechanisms. The PAG and its associated centres may also be involved in 'diffuse noxious inhibitory controls' (DNIC). DNIC is when a nociceptive stimulus in an area well away from the receptive fields of a second nociceptive stimulus can prevent or reduce pain from that second area. This is thought to be the mechanism for the paradigm of counterirritation.

Several neurotransmitters and neuromodulators are involved in descending pain-inhibitory pathways. The main contenders are the opioids, 5-hydroxytryptamine and noradrenaline (norepinephrine).

The pathways and chemicals for the facilitatory modulation are even less well understood, but the mechanisms are well accepted.

Neuromodulation and psychology

The psychological areas are those areas involved in emotions, thought and behaviour. They may not be distinct centres but more of a network. Some of these processes may be highly sophisticated and others fundamental in evolutionary terms. The interaction between these areas and nociception is complex. As indicated above, many of the areas involved in the psychological side interact with the PAG and this is thus one mechanism by which they may influence nociceptive transmission at the spinal level. At the spinal level, visceral nociception is dependent upon a system of intensity coding. That is, when it comes to the viscera the primary afferents for normal sensations and nociception are the same small fibres arriving at the spinal cord, and the difference between a normal message and a noxious one depends upon the number of afferent signals transmitted to the dorsal horn (as opposed to the dual fibre, Aδ/C fibre for nociception and Aβ for light touch, seen in somatic tissue). Because of this intensity coding system it is thought that visceral pain is more prone to psychological modulation at the spinal level than is seen in somatic tissue.

There is also a complex network of supratentorial interactions involving psychology that may play a significant role in nociception/pain neuromodulation at the higher level. These higher interactions may both reduce or facilitate the nociceptive signal reaching the consciousness and the pain perception; they will also modulate the response to the nociceptive message and hence the pain experience.

Functional MRI imaging has indicated that the psychological modulation of visceral pain probably involves multiple pathways. For instance, mood and distraction probably act through different areas of the brain when involved in reducing pain (Fulbright et al. 2001).

This psychological modulation may act to reduce nociception within a rapid time frame but may also result in a long-term vulnerability to chronic visceral pain through long-term potentiation (learning). This involvement of higher-centre learning may be both at a conscious or subconscious level and is clearly established as being significant in the supratentorial neuroprocessing of nociception and pain. Long-term potentiation (Rygh et al. 2002) may also occur at any level within the nervous system so that pathways for specific stimuli or combinations of stimuli may become established, resulting in an individual being vulnerable to perceiving sensations that would not normally bother other individuals.

Stress is an intrinsic or extrinsic disturbing force that threatens to disturb the homeostasis of an organism and can be real (physical) or perceived (psychological). Stress induces an adaptive response involving the endocrine, autonomic nervous and immune systems and these systems in turn appear to have feedback loops. Long-term potentiation is one proposed mechanism by which the nervous system learns, and stress can modify the nervous system by this process so that there are long-term abnormalities or potential abnormalities within these systems. It is this process that may be responsible for the effect of early life and significant life events as potential associated factors with chronic pain syndromes. It is through all of these factors that stress can play a significant role in nociceptive and pain neuromodulation with the increased perception of pain as well as the more general effect that stress may have on coping skills (Savidge & Slade 1997). Significant life events will include, rape, sexual abuse, sexual trauma and sexual threat such as during internment or torture. These events may produce long-term physical changes in the central nervous system (biological response) as well as having an effect on a patient's emotional, cognitive, behavioural and sexual responses (Raphael et al. 2001, McCloskey & Raphael 2005, Anda et al. 2006).

Autonomic nervous system

The role of the autonomic nervous system in chronic pain is poorly understood; however, there is good evidence that afferent fibres may develop a sensitivity to sympathetic stimulation both at the site of injury and more centrally, particularly the dorsal horns. In visceral pain the efferent output of the central nervous system may be influenced by central changes (once more those changes may be throughout the neural axis), such modification of the efferent massage may produce significant functional problems of the end-organ and as a result stimulate peripheral nociceptors.

Endocrine system

The endocrine system is involved in visceral function. Pain and the subsequent stress response will thus affect endorgan visceral function. The hypothalamic–pituitary axis (HPA) and corticotropin-releasing hormone (CRH) from the hypothalamus which stimulates the release of adrenocorticotropic hormone (ACTH) from the pituitary are key steps. An up-regulation of CRH has been implicated in several pain states such as rectal hypersensitivity to rectal distension. In this model an action of CRH on mast cells has been suggested.

Significant life events and in particular early life events may alter the development of the HPA and the chemicals released. Increased vulnerability to stress may occur following such events and is thought to be partly due to increased CRH gene expression. A range of stress-related illnesses have been suggested, irritable bowel syndrome and bladder pain syndrome being examples. There is also evidence accumulating to suggest that the sex hormones may also modulate both nociception and pain perception.

Genetics and chronic pain

An individual who has had one chronic pain syndrome is more likely to develop another. Family clusters of pain conditions are also observed and animals can be bred that are more prone to what appears to be a chronic pain state. A whole range of genetic variations have been described that may explain the pain in certain cases, many of these to do with subtle changes in transmitters and their receptors. However, the picture is more complicated in that development, environment and social factors will also influence the situation.

Clinical paradigms and chronic pelvic pain (Baranowski 2008b, Giamberardino & Costantini 2009)

1. *Referred pain* is frequently observed and its identification is important both for diagnosis and treatment. Referral is usually considered as being to the somatic tissues, either somatic to somatic, or visceral to somatic. However, there is no reason as to why the 'pain' cannot also be perceived within the vague distribution of an organ with the nociceptive signal having arisen from a somatic area. That is, it is quite plausible that a patient may consider a 'pain' to be arising from an organ, when in fact the nociceptive source is in a somatic tissue. Referred pain may occur as a result of several mechanisms but the main theory is one of convergence-projection. In the convergence-projection theory afferent fibres from the viscus and the somatic site of referred pain converge onto the same second-order projection neurons.

The higher centres receiving messages from these projection neurons are unable to separate out the two possible sites for the origin of the nociceptive signal.

2. *Referred pain to somatic tissues with hyperalgesia in the somatic tissues*; this is of particular importance to this book. Hyperalgesia refers to an increased sensitivity to normally painful stimuli. Kidney stones passed via the ureter have been a very good model. Research with this model in both man and animals has demonstrated that this extremely painful visceral pathology can produce changes in referred muscle areas, and even in subcuticular tissue and skin. Therefore in patients that have passed a renal stone, somatic muscle hyperalgesia is frequently present, even a year following the expulsion of the stone. Pain to non-painful stimuli (allodynia) may also be present in certain individuals. Somatic tissue hyperaesthesia has been described to be associated with urinary and bilary colic, irritable bowel syndrome, endometriosis, dysmenorrhoea and recurrent bladder infection. This hyperaesthesia may manifest itself as skin allodynia, subcuticular tenderness to pinching and muscle tenderness to deep pressure. Vulvar pain syndromes (previous terms have included vulvar vestibulitis, essential vulvadynia) are examples of cutaneous allodynia that in certain cases may be associated with visceral pain syndromes such as the bladder pain syndrome. Referred pain with hyperalgesia is thought to be due to central sensitization of the converging viscerosomatic neurons. Following a nociceptive insult, an acute high-frequency afferent barrage of signalling from a viscus produces the central sensitization with an increased transmission of signals to the central nervous system from the viscus. Somatic afferent fibres converging on this same sensitized central area would also be increased in their central transmission and this combined with the convergence-projection theory results in perceived somatic pain and also the hyperalgesia response. The central sensitization would also stimulate efferent activity that would explain the trophic changes so often found in the somatic tissues.
3. *Visceral hyperalgesia*. The increased perception of stimuli applied to a viscus is known as visceral hyperalgesia. The term hyperalgesia should really only be applied to an increased perception of a noxious stimulus. However, as visceral primary afferents, both for normal sensation and nociception, are small fibres, the term visceral hyperalgesia is often used for both non-noxious and noxious stimuli. The mechanisms behind visceral hyperalgesia are thought to be responsible for irritable bowel syndrome, bladder pain syndrome and dysmenorrhoea. The mechanisms involved will often be an acute afferent input (such as due to an infection) followed by long-term central sensitization. The autonomic nervous system, endocrine system, immune system and genetics may all influence the situation.
4. *Viscerovisceral hyperalgesia* is thought to be due to two or more organs with overlapping sensory projections. From the pelvic pain perspective it is interesting how the bladder afferents overlap with the uterine afferents and the uterine afferents with the colon afferents.

The above clinical paradigms and mechanisms illustrate the complex nature of CPP. By understanding those mechanisms we can see how triggers in a vulnerable patient combined with predisposing factors and maintenance factors can set up the situation where a patient can activate some very complex mechanisms that result in the individual experiencing chronic, persistent pain. These mechanisms that facilitate noxious afferent transmission can also affect cognition, emotion, behaviour, sexual and efferent function of the nervous system. The more central effects will interact with the noxious signalling to either facilitate or inhibit it and the whole processing will affect the patient's experience and hence quality of life. Due to the widespread sensitization process afferents from further afield can be magnified so that, as well as local hyperalgesia, viscerovisceral and viscerosomatic hyperalgesia may occur and dysfunctional efferent activity may result in peripheral somatic and visceral end-organ trophic changes.

The above gives a good explanation for the patient with dysmenorrhoea and a past history of social and sexual stress who following an acute urinary tract infection develops urinary frequency associated with urge and pain perceived in the bladder. Muscle hyperalgesia develops in the abdominal muscles and clinical examination shows similar changes in the pelvis and spinal muscles. Frank allodynia results in dyspareunia and the patient has symptoms consistent with irritable bowel syndrome. Over time the patient develops autoimmune and endocrine problems...

References

Abrams, P., Baranowski, A.P., Berger, R.E., et al., 2006. A new classification is needed for pelvic pain syndromes – are existing terminologies of spurious diagnostic authority bad for patients? J. Urol. 175 (6), 1989–1990.

Anda, R.F., Felitti, V.J., Bremner, J.D., et al., 2006. The enduring effects of abuse and related adverse experiences in childhood - A convergence of evidence from neurobiology and epidemiology. Eur. Arch. Psychiatry Clin. Neurosci. 256 (3), 174–186.

Baranowski, A.P., Abrams, P., Berger, R.E., et al., 2008a. Urogenital pain - time to accept a new approach to phenotyping and, as a consequence, management. Eur. Urol. 53, 33–36.

Baranowski, A.P., Abrams, P., Fall, M., 2008b. Urogenital Pain in Clinical Practice. Informa Healthcare, New York.

Binik, I., Bergeron, S., 2001. Chronic vulvar pain and sexual functioning. National Vulvodynia Association News (Spring), 5–7.

Cervero, F., Laird, J.M., 2004. Understanding the signalling and transmission of visceral nociceptive events. J. Neurobiol. 61 (1), 45–54.

Fall, M., Baranowski, A.P., Elneil, S., et al., members of the European Association of Urology (EAU) Guidelines Office, 2010. EAU Guidelines on Chronic Pelvic Pain. Eur. Urol. 57, 35–48.

Fulbright, R.K., Troche, C.J., Skudlarski, P., Gore, J.C., Wexler, B.E., 2001. Functional MR imaging of regional brain activation associated with the affective experience of pain. AJR Am. J. Roentgenol. 177 (5), 1205–1210.

Giamberardino, M.A., 2005. Visceral pain. Pain 2005: Clinical Updates XIII (6), 1–6.

Giamberardino, M.A., Costantini, R., 2009. Visceral pain phenomena in the clinical setting and their interpretation. In: Giamberardino, M.A. (Ed.), Visceral pain, clinical, pathophysiological and therapeutic aspects. Oxford University Press.

Hanno, P., Baranowski, A.P., Rosamilia, A., et al., 2005. International Continence Society guidelines on chronic pelvic pain. International Consultation on Incontinence (ICI).

Linley, J.E., Rose, K., Ooi, L., Gamper, N., 2010. Understanding inflammatory pain: ion channels contributing to acute and chronic nociception. Pflugers Arch. 2010 Feb 17 [Epub ahead of print].

McCloskey, K.A., Raphael, D.N., 2005. Adult perpetrator gender asymmetries in child sexual assault victim selection: results from the 2000 National Incident-Based Report System. J. Child Sex Abuse 14 (4), 1–24.

McMahon, S.B., Jones, N.G., 2004. Plasticity of pain signaling: role of neurotrophic factors exemplified by acid-induced pain. J. Neurobiol. 61 (1), 72–87.

McMahon, S.B., Dmitrieva, N., Koltzenburg, M., 1995. Visceral pain. Br. J. Anaesth. 75 (2), 132–144.

Melzack, R., Coderre, T.J., Katz, J., et al., 2001. Central neuroplasticity and pathological pain. Ann. N. Y. Acad. Sci. 933, 157–174.

Merskey, H., Bogduk, 1994. Classification of Chronic Pain, second ed. IASP Press, Seattle.

Nazif, O., Teichman, J.M., Gebhart, G.F., 2007. Neural upregulation in interstitial cystitis. Urology 69 (4 Suppl.), 24–33.

Nickel, J.C., Tripp, D.A., Chuai, S., et al., the NIH-CPCRN Study Group, 2008. Psychosocial parameters impact quality of life in men diagnosed with chronic prostatitis/chronic pelvic pain syndrome (CP/CPPS). Br. J. Urol. 101 (1), 59–64.

Petersen, M., Segond von, B.G., Heppelmann, B., Koltzenburg, M., 1998. Nerve growth factor regulates the expression of bradykinin binding sites on adult sensory neurons via the neurotrophin receptor p75. Neuroscience 83 (1), 161–168.

Pezet, S., McMahon, S.B., 2006. Neurotrophins: mediators and modulators of pain. Annu. Rev. Neurosci. 29, 507–538.

Rabin, C., O'Leary, A., Neighbors, C., et al., 2000. Pain and depression experienced by women with interstitial cystitis. Women Health 31, 67–81.

Raphael, K.G., Widom, C.S., Lange, G., 2001. Childhood victimization and pain in adulthood: a prospective investigation. Pain 92 (1–2), 283–293.

Roza, C., Laird, J.M., Cervero, F., 1998. Spinal mechanisms underlying persistent pain and referred hyperalgesia in rats with an experimental ureteric stone. J. Neurophysiol. 79 (4), 1603–1612.

Rygh, L.J., Tjølsen, A., Hole, K., Svendsen, F., 2002. Cellular memory in spinal nociceptive circuitry. Scand. J. Psychol. 43 (2), 153–159.

Savidge, C.J., Slade, P., 1997. Psychological aspects of chronic pelvic pain. J. Psychosom. Res. 42 (5), 433–444.

Sullivan, M.J., Adams, H., Rhodenizer, T., Stanish, W.D., 2006. A psychosocial risk factor for the prevention of chronic pain and disability following whiplash injury. Phys. Ther. 86, 8–18.

Tripp, D.A., Nickel, C., Wang, Y., et al., the National Institutes of Health – Chronic Prostatitis Collaborative Research Network (NIH-CPCRN) Study Group, 2006. Catastrophizing and pain-contingent rest as predictors of patient adjustment in men with chronic prostatitis/chronic pelvic pain syndrome. J. Pain 7 (10), 697–708.

Van de Merwe, J.P., Nordling, J., 2006. Interstitial cystitis: definitions and confusable diseases. ESSIC meeting 2005 Baden. Eur. Urol. Today March, 6–7, 16–17.

Vecchiet, L., Giamberardino, M.A., de Bigontina, P., 1992. Referred pain from viscera: when the symptom persists despite the extinction of the visceral focus. Adv. Pain Res. Ther. 20, 101–110.

Psychophysiology and pelvic pain

4

Christopher Gilbert Howard Glazer

CHAPTER CONTENTS

Introduction

A tenet of the psychophysiological approach is that certain disorders affect and are affected by both physiology and emotion, or the mind. Many disorders considered to be strictly physical can be either exacerbated or soothed by cognitive and emotional factors. In these cases, correcting a physical imbalance, such as with medication, is not enough; psychophysiological disorders call for psychophysiological interventions.

It is incomplete to try to alter the physiology without addressing the reason for the condition. Like the acoustic howl when a speaker is moved too close to its microphone, psychophysiological disorders often include a 'reaction to the reaction', which in effect traps one in the vicious circle. Thus, anxiety about heartbeat feeds back into the heartbeat, making it faster. Anxiety about breathing further disrupts the breathing. In pelvic pain, anxiety about painful intercourse can alter genital physiology and create the pain that is feared.

In studying the complicated relationship between psychological and physiological factors with regard to chronic pain, researchers have explored certain themes often over the past several decades. Psychological factors, intangible except by their correlates and consequences, may be as objective as blood factors and other physical measures, but they are considered more subjective because of how they must be measured: by self-report, interviews and observation of behaviour, which are all subject to bias. Reliability (consistency of responses over time) and validity of any structured interview or questionnaire can be assessed in the way that blood tests or structural/functional tests can be. For instance, affirmative answers to questions about childhood sexual abuse are far from objective historical data, since they depend first on accurate recall, then willingness to acknowledge and name it as such, and then to acknowledge it in the particular assessment situation. What defines 'abuse' differs from person to person; the term is a label for personal experience, and is subject to interpretation.

Psychophysiology in historical perspective

Any study of 'psychophysiology', the word itself representing an amalgam of mental and physical, must start with the historical roots of mind–body dualism.

Dualism studies the nature of consciousness and its relationship to the physical body, particularly the brain, as the central issue. Dualism argues that the mind is an independently existing substance (physical dualism) or group of independent properties that emerge from (emergent dualism), but cannot be reduced to, the brain. Monism is the position that mind and body are not, by substance, properties, or by development, distinct entities. Reductive physical monism asserts that all mental states and properties will eventually be explained by scientific accounts of physiological processes and states. Most modern philosophers and scientists take a reductive physicalist monism position, asserting that the mind is not separate from the body, and that the physical brain is the fundamental reality. This position has been most influential in the sciences, particularly neurosciences and allied fields such as sociobiology, evolutionary psychology and computer science approaches to artificial intelligence.

Although scientific advances have helped to clarify some mind–body issues, they are far from being resolved. How can the subjective qualities and the essence of a state of consciousness be explained in naturalistic terms? The most recognized modern form of dualism comes from the writings of René Descartes (1641) (see Marenbon 2007), and holds that the mind is a separate mental substance. Descartes clearly identified the mind with consciousness and self-awareness, and distinguished it from the brain, which he identified with intelligence. He was the first to formulate the mind–body problem in the form that it exists today.

Paradoxically, the mind–body issue within the field of psychology became dominated by behaviourism, a form of physical monism, for much of the 20th century. Behaviourism emerged in reaction to the rising popularity of introspection. Introspective reports on one's own mental life cannot be scrutinized by someone else for accuracy, and cannot form the basis of probabilistic predictions. Behaviourists argued that without the possibility of independent confirmation or generalization, psychological data cannot be scientific. The way out was to eliminate the idea of an internal mental life and focus instead on the objective description of observable behaviour. For the behaviourist, mental events manifest only as objective behaviours or behavioural predispositions, allowing an outside observer to predict and explain behaviour.

This type of behaviourism was ultimately dismissed as mechanistic and counterintuitive, ignoring the richness of internal experience. Cognitive-behavioural psychology arose as a direct reaction to the failure of behaviourism. This new version of behaviourism incorporated thoughts, which often triggered behaviour, and reaffirmed the value of internal experience of consciousness and self. In contrast to pure introspection, however, advances in neurosciences began to define cognitive events as both experiential and neurophysiological phenomena. Considering cognitive events as brain states meant that states of consciousness could be studied both by physical scientific methodology and by subjective, experiential methodology. This included investigation of emotional, cognitive, perceptual and motivational events. The line between physical matter and experiential matter became ever thinner with every scientific advance. The increasing success of biology in explaining mental phenomena led to the gradual acceptance of the fundamental claim that every change in mental state involves a change in brain state.

Psychophysiology studies the interaction of mental faculties with specific anatomical regions of the brain, while evolutionary biology studies the origins and development of the human nervous system. Since the 1980s, sophisticated neuroimaging procedures such as functional MRI have furnished increasing knowledge about the workings of the human brain correlated with mental experience. With the expansion of such technology, it seems inevitable that understanding of mental states will be more and more correlated with observable brain events. In clinical practice, this creates the potential to access and alter states that were not previously available. For example, altering blood flow to rhinencephalic structures (brain state) can alter the perception of pain (state of consciousness). Conversely, creating the expectation of loss of control of a situation (state of consciousness) can lead to synaptic neurochemical changes related to anxiety (brain state).

Modern psychophysiological research

Much of the current emphasis is on studying either persistent or transient emotional states together with observations of physiological changes: for instance, the effect of experimental stressors on cortisol secretion. Many studies are simply correlational, with no determination of mechanism or direction of causation. In the study of chronic pelvic pain, childhood sexual abuse emerges often as a critical factor, suggesting that having such a history confers a long-term susceptibility to chronic pelvic pain disorders. The thought style of catastrophic thinking is present more often than chance in cases of chronic pain in general. An increased tendency to avoid movement and sexual activity because of fear of pain is another factor contributing to further disability. Chronic depression and anxiety also correlate with chronic pain.

A central question addressed in psychophysiological research is how emotional, behavioural and cognitive characteristics are related to pelvic floor and lower-abdomen susceptibility to pain. Are there observable malfunctions in visceral tonus, in pelvic circulation, or in muscle function and baseline levels? Or do pain thresholds simply fluctuate according to mental and emotional conditions, without objective physiological differences? This simple question has stimulated much investigation.

Psychophysiological research occupies an area on a continuum which can be described with reference to an analogy: hypothetical aliens observing people driving cars but having no knowledge of how such a process could work. From a distance they might – like the Incas first mistaking Spaniards on horseback for Centaur-like beings – perceive the car–driver combination as a single organism. After further observation, one group of aliens might focus on the workings of the automobile, and they would study the steering linkage and the engine's coupling to the drive train. Another group might study the details of the driver's arms and hands, and the brain that animated them. Another school of thought might take interest in how the driver decides where to drive, and how fast, and even why. A fourth group might study the 'behaviour' of the automobile, how fast, how far, and where it goes, with little concern about how it gets there.

More relevant to clinical concerns, suppose a particular automobile keeps veering out of its lane and hitting the curb. Where should one look for the malfunction? The driver's intent, the driver's sensory system, the driver's muscles and limbs, the steering system, or an uneven road? To the aliens, it might seem that all possibilities should be considered. In this analogy there are several possible levels of analysis, all legitimate, for addressing the fact that people drive cars. Without the existence of both cars and drivers, however, the phenomenon would disappear, so declaring one level of analysis as more objective or closer to the truth seems fanciful.

Psychophysiology's domain is the entire region between the driver's mind and the car's behaviour. An example of a 'psychophysiological' disorder in terms of this analogy might be rapid wear of the brake linings, requiring frequent replacement. A mechanic could examine all the component parts for malfunction, but the ultimate reason might be that the driver, fearful of collision, simply rides the brake excessively. Where, in this case, is the fault?

The psychophysiological approach is complex, requires more complete knowledge of a given disorder and organ system, and may not appeal to extremists at either end of the spectrum, but it can provide a comprehensive understanding of any disorder that has both somatic and emotional aspects. This understanding will increase the options for clinical treatment.

The origin and maintenance of medically unexplained chronic pelvic pain appears to be multidetermined and intertwined with psychological factors. Two reviews of the subject reached similar conclusions:

> The symptoms of CP/CPPS appear to result from an interplay between psychological factors and dysfunction in the immune, neurological and endocrine systems.
>
> (Pontari & Ruggieri 2004)

> The aetiology of medically unexplained chronic pelvic pain is disputed but likely to be multifactorial. A history of interpersonal difficulties and a stressful life is common, and comorbid psychiatric disorders occur frequently.
>
> (Kirste et al. 2002)

A wide variety of provocative events can lead to localized acute tissue reactions with resulting nociceptive pain. This acute pain most often resolves on resolution of the provocative factors. In the presence of organic and psychological predisposition this pain may become chronic pain with the addition of neuropathic elements to the nociceptive factors. With urogenital pain, psychological, sexual and functional states are adversely affected adding a psychophysiological element to the chronic pain. Figure 4.1 depicts some potential relationships among biological and psychological factors in chronic pelvic pain.

What follows is a summary of representative research findings in support of the generalizations above, along with some speculations and assumptions guiding both research and treatment.

Prostate and pelvic pain

One recent study (Ullrich et al. 2007) of benign prostate hyperplasia (BPH) implicated the hypothalamic-pituitary-adrenal (HPA) axis and sympathetic nervous system reactivity in prostate enlargement. Eighty-three men with BPH underwent an experimental stress task (public speaking, videotaped). The degree of stress was defined physiologically as rises

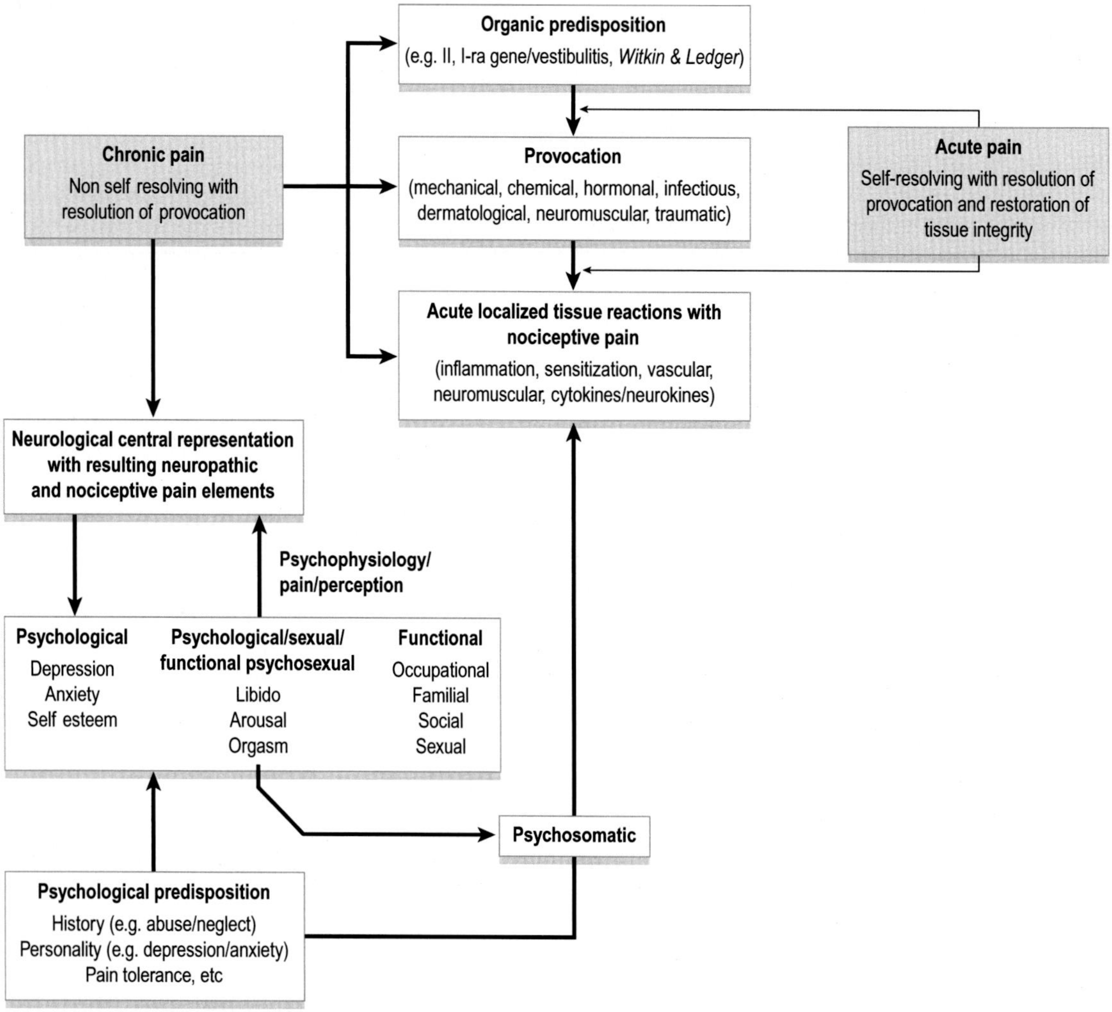

Figure 4.1 • Idiopathic lower urogenital tract disorders model

in cortisol and blood pressure. Personal appraisal of the situation was not assessed. Subjects showing stronger stress responses were found to have larger prostate volume and more objective and subjective indications of urinary tract dysfunction. Among the hypotheses for this relationship were decreased apoptosis (slowed prostatic cell death) as a result of chronically greater sympathetic input; increased pelvic floor muscle tension; greater prostate contractility (stimulated by exogenous epinephrine and norepinephrine); and stress-induced hyperinsulinaemia promoting prostate growth. Not all BPH cases involve pain, but when pain is present it can stimulate the sympathetic system, create a feedback loop, and add to the problem.

Anderson et al. (2005, 2008, 2009) compared men with chronic pelvic pain syndrome (CPPS) with asymptomatic controls for evidence of differences in stress levels. Various psychological tests revealed more perceived stress and anxiety in the CPPS patients, plus more somatization, hostility, interpersonal sensitivity and paranoid ideation. Salivary cortisol on awakening was also measured and found to be significantly higher in the pain patients. This rise in cortisol is thought to indicate the hippocampus preparing the HPA axis for anticipated stress. Cortisol has been found to be higher in situations such as waking on the day of a dance competition (Rohleder et al. 2007), in high-school teachers reporting higher job strain (Steptoe et al. 2000), and waking on work days compared with weekends (Schlotz et al. 2004).

Anderson and Wise have advanced an explanation of chronic, otherwise unexplained pelvic pain as frequently stemming from myofascial trigger points (Wise & Anderson 2008) (see Chapter 16). In their view, much long-term pelvic pain develops from the shortening and tensing of pelvic muscles, eventually creating and then aggravating trigger points, and this condition can be treated with manual release techniques. The more complete treatment, however, involves cultivating a skill for dropping into deep relaxation along with changing attention ('paradoxical relaxation') in a way that contradicts the usual tensing and bracing against pain. This is achieved (in their programme) by progressively more muscular and emotional self-calming.

Trigger points were shown to be exacerbated by stressful emotion (Hubbard & Berkoff 1993, McNulty et al. 1994). EMG was recorded from an upper trapezius trigger point along with a signal from an adjacent area of the muscle without a trigger point. As emotional stress increased, the trigger point EMG increased its voltage even though the rest of the muscle did not. Also, described in Chen et al. (1998) was a demonstration of how electrical activity associated with trigger points in rabbits was abolished by phentolamine, a sympathetic antagonist. This supports the role of the autonomic nervous system in maintaining trigger points, and also is congruent with the cited research on the aggravating effect of negative emotion (anxiety) on trigger points (Simons 2004). Wise and Anderson's protocol for pelvic pain treatment includes both thorough relaxation training and manual release of trigger points. One is temporarily curative, the other preventive.

Alexithymia and pelvic pain

The word 'alexithymia' refers to a relative inability to name feelings, or to verbally elaborate on feeling states. Its Greek roots belie its recent creation, less than 40 years ago, by psychiatrist Peter Sifneos (1973). The phenomenon and the concept existed long before its final naming. Physicians and psychotherapists had noted for many years the tendency of some patients to use very few words to describe their feelings; complex emotional states were reduced to simple terms such as 'feeling bad' or 'upset' without elaboration. This difficulty with feelings includes reflecting on them, naming them, discussing them and expressing them.

Alexithymia seems to be a trait rather than a state, an enduring and stable aspect of behaviour seen by many as a disability. It is the opposite of the concepts 'emotional intelligence' and being 'psychologically minded'. Alexithymics tend toward concrete thinking and restricted imagination. Knowing when their physical sensations and symptoms are emotionally based (rapid heart beat, changes in face temperature, agitated breathing) is not easy for the alexithymic person.

Researchers have pursued correlations between high scores on alexithymia scales such as the Toronto Alexithymia Scale (Bagby et al. 2006) and other problems such as dissociation, Asperger's, autism, substance abuse, anorexia nervosa, somatic amplification and somatoform disorders. A functional disconnection between the two cerebral hemispheres or a right hemisphere deficit has been suggested, with incomplete evidence (Tabibnia & Zaidel 2005).

Most research on chronic pain and alexithymia has found a correlation between them. Celikel and Saatcioglu (2006) found that female chronic pain patients scored more than twice as high on alexithymia scales as controls, and there was also a positive correlation between alexithymia scores and duration of pain. Since the study design was not intended to distinguish direction of causation, it is conceivable that prolonged pain damages the right hemisphere, interfering with full experiencing and transfer of emotional material.

Porcelli et al. (1999) found a strong association between alexithymia and functional gastrointestinal disorders (66% had high alexithymia scores, whereas the population average is below 10%), and later (Porcelli et al. 2003) demonstrated that higher alexithymia scores predicted worse treatment outcome. Although anxiety and depression also predicted worse treatment outcome, the alexithymia scores were stable and independent of anxiety and depression, suggesting a unique contribution to failure to improve.

Hosoi et al. (2010) studied 129 patients with chronic pain from muscular dystrophy. Degree of alexithymia was significantly associated with higher pain intensity and more pain interference. Finally, Lumley et al. (1997) compared chronic pain patients to patients seeking treatment for obesity and nicotine dependence, to control for the variable of 'treatment-seeking'. As predicted, the chronic pain patients scored higher on the alexithymia measures than either of the other groups. They also had higher levels of psychopathology, which can by itself confound and weaken treatment programmes for chronic pain.

There are few theories as to how alexithymia specifically contributes to chronic pelvic pain states;

however, the value of patients both naming and differentiating feeling states at the conscious verbal level is emphasized. A person who routinely does this is likely to consider the material objectively, to process, express, and otherwise deal with material that is commonly relegated to the 'unconscious' domain. This effective processing of feelings has vast potential influence on automatic (autonomic) functioning by differentiating true physical threat from the much more common triggers for social anxiety or symbolic threats. Local pelvic circulation, adjustments in pelvic floor muscle tension, and changes in breathing are subject to the flux of emotions until they are released from functional service. Strong negative emotions associated with traumatic memories, apprehension, sexual conflict and accidents of elimination can influence the complex structures and functions of the pelvic region.

Processing of emotional experience often involves revisiting traumatic or otherwise disturbing memories, which can be done alone or with the help of a friend, relative or therapist. Psychologist James Pennebaker has led the way in a body of research that repeatedly confirms the value of simply writing about undisclosed experiences and the deep feelings that have been kept private (Berry & Pennebaker 1993; Pennebaker 1997). This process of transforming inchoate memories and feelings into a linear, word-based account of an experience seems to be a key step in 'adjusting' to something unpleasant. Part of the value of psychotherapy lies in providing a safe forum for verbalizing one's feelings about something for the first time, and this activity has therapeutic value regardless of response from another person.

This self-adjusting activity, however, is precisely what the individuals describable as 'alexithymic' are not good at. Their poverty of verbal labels for body sensations related to emotional states is their defining characteristic, and may block necessary processing of experiences in real time. Emotional adjustment and acceptance benefit from review, reflection, hindsight, considering contextual factors, and if possible, 'normalization' by an accepting and supportive listener. Pennebaker (2004) has concluded that undisclosed disturbing experiences cause persistent conflict, partly over-suppressing them; the topic stimulates ruminative worry, and this eventually has ill-health effects. Graham et al. (2008) showed that in a large group of chronic pain patients, writing about their anger constructively resulted in better control over both pain and depression, compared with another chronic pain group asked to write about their goals. Junghaenel et al. (2008) also studied the effects of written self-disclosure on chronic pain patients, and found that only those with 'interpersonally distressed' characteristics (denoting deficient social support, feeling left alone, etc.) benefited from the expressing of emotional events.

The role of a listener is apparently optional; Pennebaker's research protocol, extended and repeated by many other researchers over the past 20 years, does not include feedback from another person, but studies only the actual expression, whether through writing, speaking into a tape recorder, or even using sign language or dance. Expression may represent a transfer of affective material from the relatively mute minor (usually right) cerebral hemisphere to the major, speech-dominant hemisphere. The full powers of judgement, rational perspective and philosophical acceptance depend primarily on the major hemisphere, which is dominated by words. So the alexithymic person is at a disadvantage for this process. As a result, strong emotional experiences may remain unprocessed and unexamined. The physiological aspects of this condition may continue to reverberate, causing inappropriate responses to emotion provoking stimuli and situations.

The main thrust of research with alexithymia has been in the areas of somatizing, trying to characterize the 'psychosomatic' patient as deficient in this way. One of the largest surveys of this association, studying over 5000 Finnish citizens, found a clear association between somatization and alexithymia (Mattila et al. 2008). Factors such as depression, anxiety and sociodemographic variables were controlled for, and the association remained. The TAS-20 factor scale labeled 'Difficulty Identifying Feelings' was the strongest common denominator between alexithymia and somatization.

So an apparent deficit in cognitive processing of emotional material seems firmly associated with somatization in general, and unexplained chronic pain in particular. Why this should be so is a larger research question. Meanwhile, anything that helps lessen the gap for an individual between the non-verbal and verbal domains is likely to help process affects and experiences that otherwise continue to cause bodily distress.

Pain catastrophizing and fear-avoidance

Pain is neither a simple stimulus nor a simple response; it is bound up with expectations, memories, interpretations and emotional associations, and the final experience of pain will be altered by all those factors. For example, changing one's initial fearful alarm reaction to a new pain by interpreting it differently ('it's only a nuisance, but not harmful') improves the reaction to pain mentally and physically. Consider the shift in mental state when a household smoke alarm goes off. At first the occupants fear a fire and are 'alarmed', but if they then discover a malfunction in the alarm system, or perhaps that smoke from cooking has set the alarm off, the distress dissolves into annoyance. Physically the sound is just as loud, but the emotion is completely changed, and most aspects of the physiological response are reversed.

Many instances of chronic pelvic pain have an obscure or unknown aetiology, and are associated with other symptoms such as comorbid psychiatric conditions (anxiety, depression), and a tendency toward emotion-triggered multiple somatic complaints over time ('somatizing'). Treating such patients as if they have bona fide medical conditions, when such evidence is lacking, is at best incomplete. Such patients may respond to analgesic medications, but they often respond better to a biopsychosocial approach which addresses interpersonal factors, anxiety, apprehension and catastrophic thinking about the meaning of the pain, plus attention to muscle-bracing, movement and breathing patterns, and sensory awareness (Haugstad et al. 2006).

'Pain catastrophizing' is a psychological variable easily measured by questionnaires such as the Pain Catastrophizing Scale (PCS) (Sullivan et al. 1995, 2001) or the Pain Anxiety Symptoms Scale (McCracken et al. 1992, Burns et al. 2000). These scales quantify negative expectations about pain and include subfactors such as helplessness, degree of suffering and disability expected, estimated ability to cope with the pain, and feeling overwhelmed.

Sample comments from questions from the PCS include:

> 'I keep thinking about how badly I want the pain to stop.'
>
> 'There is nothing I can do to reduce the pain.'

The high-catastrophizing pain patient typically feels that the pain justifies their drastic response, and they do not see their reaction as adjustable. Since pain magnitude is entirely subjective and so far not measurable by objective standards, this attitude is hard to dispute. Since there are genetic and other individual differences in pain perception, a one-to-one correspondence between stimulus intensity (degree of damage on X-ray, degree of nerve impingement, etc.) and the subjective response is not likely. Even within the same person, certain factors can augment or diminish pain intensity within seconds. These factors arise from both psychology and physiology.

Pain catastrophizing as a cognitive process may get stronger as pain gets worse, but it also varies independently of pain intensity. For example, in a prospective study, Flink et al. (2009a) studied childbirth and pain. Eighty-eight women were assessed for pain catastrophizing before they gave birth. Those scoring higher in this variable reported subsequent higher pain and poorer physical recovery (measured as activity levels) as compared with those with lower pre-birth pain catastrophizing scores. Since this was not an intervention study, it could be argued that the high-scoring women knew that their pain would be worse. But intervention studies which alter pain catastrophizing have been successful in altering various aspects of the reaction to pain (Voerman et al. 2007, van Wilgen et al. 2009).

Training patients to reduce pain catastrophizing is a standard part of cognitive-behavioural therapy in comprehensive pain management programmes, and the results in many patients are comparable to medication or other medical interventions. Learning to reduce catastrophizing, regardless of the source of the pain, can favourably affect avoidance behaviour, muscle bracing, medication use, general activity and subjective distress.

Smeets et al. (2006) studied chronic low back pain patients going through either physical or cognitive-behavioural treatment, and found that in both intervention groups, pain catastrophizing was a mediating variable for improvement in pain intensity and disability. Thorn et al. (2007) used a RCT design with wait-list control to study the response of chronic headache sufferers to cognitive change techniques, with particular attention to changes in catastrophic thinking. The active treatment group had significant improvements in affect, anxiety and self-efficacy regarding headache management. About half of them also had clinically meaningful reductions in headache indicators that did not occur in the control group.

Tripp et al. (2006) studied certain characteristics in 253 men with chronic prostatitis/chronic pelvic pain syndrome (CP/CPPS). Magnitude of both sensory pain and affective pain could be predicted by degree of what was termed 'helpless catastrophizing'.

The physiological mediators in pain catastrophizing are largely unknown, but Wolff et al. (2008) showed that the combination of higher paraspinal muscle tension and high catastrophizing predicted high reported pain levels. Muscle tension in this study was not a simple mediating factor, but if resting low back tension was already high, then the co-occurrence of catastrophic thinking amplified the perception of back pain.

Lowering pain intensity is not the only desirable treatment outcome. A study of reducing pain in patients in an emergency deparement (Downey & Zun 2009) instructed patients in slow deep breathing, and in this brief intervention found no significant reduction in pain as estimated by the patients, but there were still significant improvements in rapport with treating physicians, greater willingness to follow the recommendation and numerous statements that the intervention was useful. Another study of back pain patients (Flink 2009b) showed that practising breathing exercises had not so much effect on actual pain levels as it did on less catastrophizing and pain-related distress, along with greater acceptance of the pain condition.

Hypervigilance and fear of movement

One related psychological variable relevant to pain perception is called 'hypervigilance'. This can be measured in several ways, including magnitude of startle response. The factor of unpredictability, basically an absence of reliable threat cues, seems to amplify vigilance, and the Pain Vigilance and Awareness Questionnaire is designed to measure the vigilance specifically for pain (Roelofs et al. 2003). Hypervigilance was also assessed in a group of 54 young male patients one day before chest-correction surgery (Lautenbacher et al. 2009). Subjective ratings of pain intensity 1 week later were significantly predicted by degree of hypervigilance; the more watchful the patients were, the more pain they reported.

The Tampa Scale of Kinesiophobia (TSK) measures fear of movement instead of fear of pain directly (French et al. 2007). This shows a conditioning effect in which the organism with repeated noxious experiences becomes sensitive to earlier and earlier cues. So if a certain pelvic movement causes pain, the fear of pain will inhibit that movement. Some people generalize from this association more drastically than others: perhaps from only that one particular pelvic movement to all related pelvic movements, or – 'just to be safe' – nearly any body movement at all.

Sample items from the TSK scale include:

> 'Simply being careful not to make unnecessary movements is the safest thing I can do to prevent back pain.'
>
> 'Back pain always means the body is injured.'

All these questionnaires seem to tap slightly different aspects of a central quality related to fear and avoidance. As Roelofs et al. put it (2003): 'With regard to the convergent validity, the Pain Vigilance and Awareness Questionnaire was highly correlated with related constructs such as the Pain Catastrophizing Scale (PCS), Pain Anxiety Symptoms Scale (PASS), and Tampa Scale of Kinesiophobia (TSK)'. What such questionnaires tap is related to anxiety, broadly conceived, and with components of depression such as helplessness and loss of hope. Pain studies may not differentiate subcategories of these broader conditions and so end up blaming anxiety and depression for exacerbating chronic pain.

Avoidance of sexual activity

The correlation between degree of pelvic pain and normal sexual activity is not as great as one might think. Emotional factors that facilitate or inhibit sexual activity are many, and include capacity for sustained intimacy, gender identity, general sense of self-worth, baseline desire, relationship quality and comfort with sex in general. Prolonged avoidance of sex can result from a short-sighted withdrawal from situations associated with pain, past or present. Deconditioning through disuse can occur just as easily in sex organs as in the legs or back muscles. Desrochers et al. (2010) found that baseline fear of pain and catastrophizing were strong predictors of eventual success in a programme targeting provoked vulvodynia, and success included return to normal sexual activity. Desrochers et al. (2009) also presented evidence that psychological variables such as catastrophizing, hypervigilance and fear of pain predicted sexual impairment in women with provoked vestibulodynia. This means that pain magnitude is not linearly correlated with sexual functioning; actual pain is only part of the picture, sometimes overshadowed by cognitive and affective variables. There is a wide range of variability between loss of sexual desire and intensity of sexual pain.

Reissing et al. (2004) investigated the accuracy of the usual criteria for diagnosis of vaginismus, which is usually considered a simple muscle spasm problem. Using the factors of degree of vaginal spasm and pain, women previously diagnosed with vaginismus were not significantly different from women with vulvar vestibulitis syndrome, but they could be differentiated by higher vaginal muscle tone (with lower muscle strength) and more defensive and avoidant distress behaviours. The authors concluded: 'These data suggest that the spasm-based definition of vaginismus is not adequate as a diagnostic marker for vaginismus. Pain and fear of pain, pelvic floor dysfunction, and behavioral avoidance need to be included in a multidimensional reconceptualization of vaginismus'.

It is relevant that sexual desire and arousal are autonomically regulated functions which are physiologically and psychologically mutually exclusive. Acute fear can cause extreme pelvic floor muscle relaxation and urinary and bowel incontinence because bodily resources are redirected to 'fight or flight' mechanisms, and away from regulation of elimination and reproductive organs. Therefore the psychological factors, including conditioned avoidance and biased expectations of discomfort, are integral to female pelvic pain problems. They should be addressed along with strictly physiological factors, which even if normalized do not automatically heal problems in the psychological realm which impair natural sexual function.

For instance, a large study in China surveyed 291 men with chronic prostatitis and pelvic pain for degree of anxiety and depression as they underwent a 6-week treatment programme. Other factors expected to affect treatment outcome were also assessed: age, a prostatitis symptom index, and leukocyte count. None of these were predictive of treatment success, but the psychological variables of anxiety and depression were. The authors concluded: 'Such psychological obstacles as anxiety and depression play an important role in the pathogenesis, development and prognosis of CP/CPPS'. The psychophysiological link in this case is unknown, but may involve chronic restriction of pelvic or prostate circulation (Li et al. 2008).

Finally, the variable of self-efficacy has been found to be correlated with both chronic pain and alexithymia. Physical self-efficacy – meaning roughly self-confidence in one's physical capacity – is modifiable to a degree, with favourable health consequences. A study by Pecukonis (2009) found two initial differences between a sample of patients with chronic intractable back pain and a matched control group. The pain group was significantly higher in alexithymia and lower in physical self-efficacy (self-estimate of strength, endurance and ability to perform physically). Foster et al. (2010) found that 'pain self-efficacy' was a strong predictor of recovery from chronic pain, independently of depression, pain catastrophizing and fear of movement. Having a self-concept that includes resilience and capacity to recover is important for participating fully in treatment programmes for any kind of chronic pain.

This quality was pinpointed also in Albert Bandura's 1987 study teaching subjects to withstand experimental pain, using cognitive techniques to boost self-efficacy. The study design included the opioid-blocking chemical naloxone to control for the effects of opiate pain medication administered at certain points. The outcome supported the value of cognitive training to boost pain control. In the author's words: '. . .subjects who expressed efficacious judgments regarding their ability to manage pain experienced as much relief from their symptoms as subjects receiving opioid analgesics or placebo' (Bandura et al. 1987).

Experimentally induced pain differs from natural chronic pain in that it is usually introduced into a non-compromised nervous system. Research subjects can be screened out if they have a chronic pain condition. As pain persists over time, phenomena such as central and peripheral sensitization, kindling, windup and allodynia typically develop, amplifying and complicating the pain sensations. All this constitutes malfunction of the pain-detection system.

The advantage of an experimental pain stimulus is that its intensity and location can be adjusted in order to measure pain thresholds, usually via a thermal stimulus or by intramuscular hypertonic saline infusions. In one such study (Chalaye et al. 2009) pain intensity diminished, as measured by subject ratings (subjective thresholds), in response to slow deep breathing at a rate of six per minute. Another result in that study was the increase in heart rate variability, which correlates with increased vagal tone and general lowering of arousal.

In the varied populations targeted above (headache, back pain and childbirth) there was clear evidence of a specific cognitive variable affecting both pain intensity and degree of disability. In most cognitive-behavioural interventions for any kind of pain, catastrophic thinking and its variants are not addressed in isolation, but as part of an array of techniques including relaxation, re-appraisal, controlled breathing, acceptance, cognitive reframing, distraction and general education about mind–body influences in chronic pain. Much of the important pain-related psychophysiological research has been done on chronic back pain, but patients with pelvic pain are probably not substantially different to the other patient populations discussed; they have the same brain and nervous system, and are presumably subject to the same emotional stresses and imbalances. So until more pelvis-specific research is done, it is reasonable to tentatively generalize the conclusions and treatment methods to patients with pelvic pain.

Identifying these psychological factors in chronic pain patients does not imply the presence of mental illness or require psychotherapy. It simply acknowledges the role of emotions in the pain-modulating system. In the absence of an organized, multidisciplinary treatment team, the essential facts may be conveyed one-on-one, along with suggestions for changing the emotional factors. Such an intervention is far better than none, and can bring about lasting improvements in chronic pain – improvements which medication alone may never achieve. For example, it may be helpful for the patient with CPP to consider the following principles of chronic pain treatment programmes:

- Chronic pain is best treated with a combined approach that includes attention to thinking, emotions and behaviour, as well as medicine and physical therapy.
- Stressful emotions can aggravate pain conditions. Denying feelings or pushing them away will not block their effects.
- Think about what else besides pain provokes your worst anxiety and stress. Look for situations and feelings that coincide with your pain getting worse.
- Learn to relax, physically and mentally, instead of tensing up with pain. This will give you more control over the pain and your reactions to it.
- Don't over-react to what hasn't even happened yet. Expecting the worst when it rarely happens activates more physical upset, which can amplify pain reception.
- Activity keeps your body healthier and will stimulate more healing. Don't avoid movement on the chance that it might hurt.
- Practice breathing slowly to compose yourself. Find ways to feel secure and calm, because this will work against pain.
- Regardless of pelvic pain, avoiding sex can make things worse. The system benefits from normal activity.
- Try writing about your deepest feelings, the things you never told anybody. There's no need to show it to anyone; just read it back to yourself.
- Do some reading about chronic pain and figure out how you can participate in your own treatment. Doctors can't do it all.

Defensiveness, emotional denial and repression

This group of inter-related psychological variables refers to how individuals manage negative emotions, whether personally related (shame, guilt, blame), by denying faults and stress, or by denying negative feelings such as anger and hostility. Burns (2000a) thoroughly reviewed the concept of emotional repression in relation to chronic pain, updating it from its roots in psychoanalysis, and incorporated modern research to make it relevant to current understandings of chronic pain. The conceptual gap between such subjective variables as blocking or denying negative feelings and experiencing somatic pain has been narrowed by psychophysiological research. The evidence supports such a connection in cases where denial of negative feelings coincides with high physiological and/or behavioural reactivity to stress. This mismatch apparently gives rise to conflict, with physiological effects, and correlates with increased pain and poor response to multidisciplinary pain management programmes (Burns 2000b).

Anger suppression was found to increase pain sensitivity in normal subjects without chronic pain. Subjects were asked to perform an arithmetic task and suppress both their experience and expression of anger during an experimentally manipulated 'harassment' condition. Compared to subjects not given such instructions, the anger-suppressors reported higher pain levels in response to the cold pressor (ice water) test. Whether this would also apply to chronic pelvic pain is unknown, but the manipulation may be generalizable to naturally occurring situations involving the need to conceal anger and frustration.

Placebo-nocebo chemistry as psychophysiology

The information presented so far about psychological influences on pain may seem to be floating in conceptual space, lacking a link to physiology. But in the case of pain, much is known about the interaction between mind and body, and relaxation, broadly defined, is at the centre of the pain mechanisms. Relaxation seems effective for reducing and coping with pain of any sort. This includes not only releasing muscles, but also creating greater peace of mind: lower anxiety, less stress, and less apprehension about the pain getting worse. Although multidisciplinary pain programmes routinely teach cognitive change techniques and various kinds of relaxation, they usually operate empirically without too much concern about how the techniques work physiologically.

The relaxation effect acts like a mental lever, affecting the entire pain modulation system. Pain intensity can be adjusted not only with opiates, but also by altering the naturally occurring endogenous opiates (endorphins) and their receptors (Hoffman et al. 2005). Emotional changes accompanying relaxation also affect the proportions of other pain-related biochemicals, such as GABA, cholecystokinin (CCK), dopamine and adrenaline (epinephrine).

Work with mu-opioid receptors has revealed that endorphins serve a more complex role than simply muffling pain. Endorphins also affect motivation and behaviour: low endorphin levels stimulate more alertness and vigilance, preparation for defence, sharper memory, faster reflexes for actions such as limb withdrawal, and a general increase in qualities favouring survival and mobilization of energy. High endorphin levels, in contrast, are associated with somnolence, reduced vigilance, and a sense of well-being. Memory and alertness are reduced, as well as pain sensitivity (Fields 2004).

Endorphins and other pain-related chemicals can be manipulated by triggering expectations in experimental subjects, both humans and animals. Conditioned placebos of any sort will diminish pain (for instance, a cue that has been associated with a pain-relieving injection). Using a 'nocebo' (an inert substance or stimulus that creates the expectation of worse pain) will make pain worse (Benedetti 2006, Benedetti et al. 2005, 2007). Even words of warning before an injection – 'This might hurt a little' – will increase pain perception more than will reassurance or distraction. These rapid adjustments to pain intensity are created by alterations in mu-opioid receptor sensitivity as well as changes in endorphin release. There are also changes in the anterior cingulate cortex, periaqueductal grey,and other brain sites known to be involved in pain modulation. Finally, administering morphine also turns off certain pain-gating cells in the rostral ventromedial nucleus and facilitates descending inhibitory circuits which inhibit dorsal horn neurons (Wager 2007). fMRI and PET scans of opioid receptor sites have confirmed the actions of pain-gating neurons (Scott et al. 2007).

Other chemicals involved in pain-modulation include adrenaline (epinephrine), which also stimulates alertness and lowers sensory thresholds, and CCK, which blocks morphine and stimulates not only pain but bodily changes collectively termed 'fight or flight'. CCK is actually used in research to stimulate panic attacks. Dopamine raises the expectation of pleasure or relief, and helps to enhance placebo effect.

Table 4.1 shows the relevant chemistry and interactions.

Expecting relief, some version of 'help is on the way!' reduces the sense of danger and emergency, and tips the balance of pain-related chemicals away from pain and suffering, toward pain suppression. One notable exception is fear-induced analgesia, which occurs when stress is intense and current rather than anticipatory. Sustaining an injury, for example, brings temporary numbness, and presumably allows the animal to cope with the situation without distraction from pain. But anxiety and apprehension will do the opposite: increase pain along with all the other survival-related changes.

Table 4.1 Biochemicals involved in the placebo and nocebo responses

Chemical	Action	Boosts pain	Suppresses pain
Cholecystokinin (CCK)	Blocks endorphins, increases vigilance and anxiety	X	
Endorphins	Activate mu-opioid receptors; good feelings; weakens memory and vigilance		X
Dopamine	Part of reward system; reinforcer		X, indirectly, boosts placebo
Gamma-aminobutyric acid (GABA)	Reduces brain activation; calms emotions		X
Adrenaline	Increases alertness, anxiety; boosts memory	X	

So relaxation, distraction, meditation and cognitive change are all to a degree pain-reducers, while apprehension, bracing, worrying, etc. agitate the organism. This agitation prompts stronger pain as a part of a general boosting of the behavioural and psychological changes to maximize survival. The psychological variables previously discussed – pain catastrophizing, pain vigilance, low self-efficacy, and kinesiophobia – all have similar effects on the pain modulation system: they stimulate the survival system at the expense of rest and recovery. This is the modern psychophysiology of pain, far beyond tight muscles and fast breathing. So teaching chronic pain patients to create positive expectations, confidence and relaxation modifies the pain-alarm system, ultimately calming the biochemistry and brain activity that supports continued pain.

Effects of physical and sexual abuse

Researchers examining this variable sometimes distinguish early from later (adult) physical abuse and sexual abuse, although they can overlap. Lampe et al. (2003) concluded that 'Childhood physical abuse, stressful life events, and depression had a significant impact on the occurrence of chronic pain in general, whereas childhood sexual abuse was correlated with CPP only'.

Vulvodynia may be a distinctly different disorder than CPP. Reed et al. (2000), generalizing from a small sample, described evidence that vulvodynia patients were not significantly different from control subjects in most psychological or historical variables. Those with chronic pelvic pain, however, were more likely to report a history of sexual or physical abuse, depression and more somatic complaints. Bodden-Heidrich et al. (1999) supported this distinction between the two diagnoses, finding in a comparison of vulvodynia with CPP patients that the latter as a group showed more history of sexual abuse and 'severe psychological problems'.

A study (Heim et al. 1998) of CPP using neuroendocrine assessment of HPA axis activity implicated blunted cortisol response. Compared with normals, a large proportion of CPP subjects reported physical and/or sexual abuse history, and post-traumatic stress disorder-like symptoms were commonly reported. There were similarities to other long-term disorders such as fibromyalgia, rheumatoid arthritis and chronic fatigue syndrome. Reduced cortisol response to stressful conditions impairs energy availability, promotes pain and inflammation by allowing prostaglandins to rise, and permits more of the damaging effects of the stress response, including autoimmunity and susceptibility to chronic pain. The authors concluded that abuse history seems to promote, in many cases, a long-term maladjustment in endocrine aspects of the stress response system, making chronic pain disorders, including CPP, more likely.

Collett et al. (1998) found that the lifetime incidence of sexual abuse was significantly higher in women with CPP, but physical abuse history was comparable in CPP patients and women with non-pelvic chronic pain complaints. Walker et al. (1992) studied psychological characteristics of women with CPP and noted a higher likelihood of dissociation as a coping mechanism, compared with a control group. Women with CPP had more evidence of current psychological distress, somatization, lower vocational and social functioning, and amplification of physical symptoms. In this study also, they were significantly more likely to have experienced severe childhood sexual abuse.

Somatization

Two articles from Austria recommended routine evaluation for psychological aspects of CPP. Maier et al. (1999) summarized experience with 220 women with CPP who were examined in collaboration between the Department of Obstetrics & Gynaecology and the Psychosomatic Department in the St. Johann's Hospital of Salzburg. The patients received both laparoscopic examination and psychological evaluation; the researchers found that somatization was a frequent explanation for the symptoms. Standard somatic medicine, according to the authors, could not explain the discrepancies between the intensity of reported pain and the pathophysiology. They recommended continued engagement of the patients in order to facilitate psychotherapy or consideration of psychological input to the problem. The alternative outcome, ignoring psychological features, carries the risk of 'chronification of CPP in patients approached only in somatic terms'.

Greimel & Thiel (1999), at the University Hospital in Graz, Austria, put forth a similar view: that emphasizing medical approaches to CPP increases the patient's belief that medical (pharmaceutical, surgical) remedies will give them relief. In their view, the majority of CPP patients have evidence of somatoform disorder, which calls for psychological interventions rather than medical.

In making decisions about CPP treatment, psychosocial factors could be considered from the beginning, but more usually the medical approach is started first, to 'rule out' physical aetiology before psychological and behavioural intervention is even considered. This issue was addressed by one study by Peters et al. (1991) which compared the outcomes of these two approaches. One group of CPP patients began with laparoscopic examination to look for somatic problems before doing anything else. The second group was examined for many factors simultaneously: psychological, physiotherapeutic, dietary, environmental and somatic. At one-year follow-up, those receiving the second ('integrated') approach had done significantly better with pain management, and laparoscopic assessment seemed to add little to the results. This conclusion may indicate the advantage of not biasing patients toward a medical solution; otherwise, if no clear-cut medical disorder is found, the patients must re-orient to considering psychological, behavioural and experiential history factors. They can easily feel prematurely cast out and stereotyped.

Carrico et al. (2008) approached interstitial cystitis as amenable to guided imagery, and mounted a study in which guided imagery specific to interstitial cystitis (IC) was developed, recorded and given to IC patients. The recordings contained imagery and suggestions for healing the bladder, relaxing pelvic floor muscles and quieting the nerves supplying the pelvic area. Recordings were to be listened to twice a day for 25 minutes, while the control group simply relaxed for the same amount of time. Results clearly favoured the imagery group, who had significantly more reduced pain, urinary urgency and other symptoms of IC compared with the control group. This approach is remarkably simple and inexpensive, yet brought respectable results to many of the participants.

In the above summaries, researchers nearly always make a dichotomous distinction between 'medical' and 'psychological', or 'somatic' and 'psychogenic'. This distinction perpetuates the notion that a given disorder has its source in either one or the other domain. Yet most of these studies at least speculate about a biological mechanism responsible for the clinical improvements, and also acknowledge the physiological ramifications of trauma, anxiety, depression, etc.

An improvement on the 'somatic/psychogenic' dichotomy might be to estimate the relative contributions of somatic and emotional factors. Given that the HPA axis responds to cognitive changes such as expecting danger or anticipating pain, it could be the primary mind-to-body transduction system. Cognitions can trigger a rapid switch to sympathetic dominance, withdraw vagal tone, initiate appropriate emotions and prepare the body for a physical challenge. Muscle bracing, altered breathing and circulation patterns, endocrine changes, and aggravation of trigger points are all biological responses to psychological shifts. Trying to suppress these factors pharmaceutically may be insufficient to affect the more central source of the problem.

Acknowledgement

We acknowledge with gratitude the help from Dr. Hallie Robbins DO, in the initial conceptualization and organization of this chapter.

This chapter has described how CPP is affected by both physiology and emotion, and suggested that cognitive and emotional factors can both exacerbate or sooth nociception. It appears that biological, socio-cultural and psychosocial aspects determine an individual's response to a variety of potential pain triggers. The next chapter describes the relationship between gender and pain, including the role of sex hormones in CPP, and questions whether women are in general more susceptible than men to experience CPP.

References

Anderson, R.U., Wise, D., Sawyer, T., Chan, C., 2005. Integration of myofascial trigger point release and paradoxical relaxation training treatment of chronic pelvic pain in men. J. Urol. 174 (1), 155–160.

Anderson, R.U., Orenberg, E.K., Chan, C.K., Morey, A., Flores, V., 2008. Psychometric profiles and hypothalamic-pituitary-adrenal axis function in men with chronic prostatitis/chronic pelvic pain syndrome. J. Urol. 179, 956–960.

Anderson, R.U., Orenberg, E.K., Morey, A., Chavez, N., Chan, C.A., 2009. Stress induced hypothalamus-pituitary-adrenal axis responses and disturbances in psychological profiles in men with chronic prostatitis/chronic pelvic pain syndrome. J. Urol. 182 (5), 2319–2324.

Bagby, R.M., Taylor, G.J., Parker, J.D.A., Dickens, S., 2006. The development of the Toronto Structured Interview for Alexithymia: Item selection, factor structure, reliability and concurrent validity. Psychother. Psychosom. 75, 25–39.

Bandura, A., O'Leary, A., Taylor, C.B., Gauthier, J., Gossard, D., 1987. Perceived self-efficacy and pain control: opioid and nonopioid mechanisms. J. Pers. Soc. Psychol. 53 (3), 563–571.

Benedetti, F., 2006. The biochemical and neuroendocrine bases of the hyperalgesic nocebo effect. J. Neurosci. 26 (46), 12014–12022.

Benedetti, F., Mayberg, H.S., Wager, T.D., Stohler, C.S., Zubieta, J.K., 2005. Neurobiological mechanisms of the placebo effect. J. Neurosci. 25 (45), 10390–10402.

Benedetti, F., Lanotte, M., Lopiano, L., Colloca, L., 2007. When words are painful: unraveling the mechanisms of the nocebo effect. Neuroscience 147 (2), 260–271.

Berry, D.S., Pennebaker, J.W., 1993. Nonverbal and verbal emotional expression and health. Psychother. Psychosom. 59 (1), 11–19.

Bodden-Heidrich, R., Küppers, V., Beckmann, M.W., Ozörnek, M.H., Rechenberger, I., Bender, H.G., 1999. Psychosomatic aspects of vulvodynia. Comparison with the chronic pelvic pain syndrome. J. Reprod. Med. 44 (5), 411–416.

Burns, J.W., 2000a. Repression in chronic pain: an idea worth reconsidering. Appl, Prevent. Psychology 9, 173–190.

Burns, J.W., 2000b. Repression predicts outcome following multidisciplinary treatment of chronic pain. Health Psychol. 19 (1), 75–84.

Burns, J.W., Mullen, J.T., Higdon, L.J., Wei, J.M., Lansky, D., 2000. Validity of the pain anxiety symptoms scale (PASS): prediction of physical capacity variables. Pain 84 (2–3), 247–252.

Carrico, D.J., Peters, K.M., Diokno, A.C., 2008. Guided imagery for women with interstitial cystitis: results of a prospective, randomized controlled pilot study. J. Altern. Complement. Med. 14 (1), 53–56.

Celikel, F.C., Saatcioglu, O., 2006. Alexithymia and anxiety in female chronic pain patients. Ann. Gen. Psychiatry 5, 13.

Chalaye, P., Goffaux, P., Lafrenaye, S., Marchand, S., 2009. Respiratory effects on experimental heat pain and cardiac activity. Pain Med. 10 (8), 1334–1340.

Chen, J.T., Chen, S.M., Kuan, T.S., Chung, K.C., Hong, C.Z., 1998. Phentolamine effect on the spontaneous electrical activity of active loci in a myofascial trigger spot of rabbit skeletal muscle. Arch. Phys. Med. Rehabil. 79 (7), 790–794.

Collett, B.J., Cordle, C.J., Stewart, C.R., Jagger, C., 1998. A comparative study of women with chronic pelvic pain, chronic nonpelvic pain and those with no history of pain attending general practitioners. Br. J. Obstet. Gynaecol. 105 (1), 87–92.

Desrochers, G., Bergeron, S., Khalifé, S., Dupuis, M.J., Jodoin, M., 2009. Fear avoidance and self-efficacy in relation to pain and sexual impairment in women with provoked vestibulodynia. Clin. J. Pain 25 (6), 520–527.

Desrochers, G., Bergeron, S., Khalifé, S., Dupuis, M.J., Jodoin, M., 2010. Provoked vestibulodynia: psychological predictors of topical and cognitive-behavioral treatment outcome. Behav. Res. Ther. 48 (2), 106–115.

Downey, L.V., Zun, L.S., 2009. The effects of deep breathing training on pain management in the emergency department. South. Med. J. 102 (7), 688–692.

Fields, H., 2004. State-dependent opioid control of pain. Nat. Rev. Neurosci. 5 (7), 565–575 (review).

Flink, I.K., Mroczek, M.Z., Sullivan, M.J., Linton, S.J., 2009a. Pain in childbirth and postpartum recovery: the role of catastrophizing. Eur. J. Pain 13 (3), 312–316.

Flink, I.K., Nicholas, M.K., Boersma, K., Linton, S.J., 2009b. Reducing the threat value of chronic pain: A preliminary replicated single-case study of interoceptive exposure versus distraction in six individuals with chronic back pain. Behav. Res. Ther. 47 (8), 721–728.

Foster, N.E., Thomas, E., Bishop, A., Dunn, K.M., Main, C.J., 2010. Distinctiveness of psychological obstacles to recovery in low back pain patients in primary care. Pain 148 (3), 398–406.

French, D.J., France, C.R., Vigneau, F., French, J.A., Evans, R.T., 2007. Fear of movement/(re)injury in chronic pain: a psychometric assessment of the original English version of the Tampa scale for kinesiophobia (TSK). Pain 127 (1–2), 42–51.

Graham, J.E., Lobel, M., Glass, P., Lokshina, I., 2008. Effects of written anger expression in chronic pain patients: making meaning from pain. J. Behav. Med. 31 (3), 201–212.

Greimel, E.R., Thiel, I., 1999. Psychological treatment aspects of chronic pelvic pain in the woman. Wien. Med. Wochenschr. 149 (13), 383–387 [Article in German].

Haugstad, G.K., Haugstad, T.S., Kirste, U.M., et al., 2006. Posture, movement patterns, and body awareness in women with chronic pelvic pain. J. Psychosom. Res. 61 (5), 637–644.

Heim, C., Ehlert, U., Hanker, J.P., Hellhammer, D.H., 1998. Abuse-related posttraumatic stress disorder and alterations of the hypothalamic-pituitary-adrenal axis in women with chronic pelvic pain. Psychosom. Med. 60 (3), 309–318.

Hoffman, G.A., Harrington, A., Fields, H.L., 2005. Pain and the placebo: what we have learned. Perspect. Biol. Med. 48 (2), 248–265.

Hosoi, M., Molton, I.R., Jensen, M.P., et al., 2010. Relationships among alexithymia and pain intensity, pain interference, and vitality in persons with neuromuscular disease: considering the effect of negative affectivity. Pain 149 (2), 273–277.

Hubbard, D.R., Berkoff, G.M., 1993. Myofascial trigger points show spontaneous needle EMG activity. Spine (Phila Pa 1976) 18 (13), 1803–1807.

Junghaenel, D.U., Schwartz, J.E., Broderick, J.E., 2008. Differential efficacy of written emotional disclosure for subgroups of fibromyalgia patients. Br. J. Health Psychol. 13 (Pt 1), 57–60.

Kirste, U., Haugstad, G.K., Leganger, S., Blomhoff, S., Malt, U.F., 2002. Chronic pelvic pain in women. Tidsskr. Nor. Laegeforen.

122 (12), 1223–1227 (article in Norwegian).

Lampe, A., Doering, S., Rumpold, G., et al., 2003. Chronic pain syndromes and their relation to childhood abuse and stressful life events. J. Psychosom. Res. 54 (4), 361–367.

Lautenbacher, S., Huber, C., Kunz, M., et al., 2009. Hypervigilance as predictor of postoperative acute pain: its predictive potency compared with experimental pain sensitivity, cortisol reactivity, and affective state. Clin. J. Pain 25 (2), 92–100.

Li, H.C., Wang, Z.L., Li, H.L., et al., 2008. Correlation of the prognosis of chronic prostatitis/chronic pelvic pain syndrome with psychological and other factors: a Cox regression analysis [Article in Chinese]. Zhonghua Nan Ke Xue 14 (8), 723–727.

Lumley, M.A., Asselin, L.A., Norman, S., 1997. Alexithymia in chronic pain patients. Compr. Psychiatry 38 (3), 160–165.

Maier, B., Akmanlar-Hirscher, G., Krainz, R., Wenger, A., Staudach, A., 1999. Chronic pelvic pain – a still too little appreciated disease picture. Wien. Med. Wochenschr. 149 (13), 377–382 (article in German).

Marenbon, J., 2007. Medieval Philosophy: an historical and philosophical introduction. Routledge, London.

Mattila, A.K., Kronholm, E., Jula, A., Salminen, J.K., Koivisto, A.M., Mielonen, R.L., et al., 2008. Alexithymia and somatization in general population. Psychosom. Med. 70 (6), 716–722.

McCracken, L.M., Zayfert, C., Gross, R.T., 1992. The Pain Anxiety Symptoms Scale: development and validation of a scale to measure fear of pain. Pain 50 (1), 67–73.

McNulty, W.H., Gevirtz, R.N., Hubbard, D.R., Berkoff, GM., 1994. Needle electromyographic evaluation of trigger point response to a psychological stressor. Psychophysiology 31 (3), 313–316.

Pecukonis, E.V., 2009. Physical self-efficacy and alexithymia in women with chronic intractable back pain. Pain Manag. Nurs. 10 (3), 116–123.

Pennebaker, J.W., 1997. The Healing Power of Expressing Emotions. Guilford Press, NY.

Pennebaker, J.W., 2004. Writing to Heal. New Harbinger Press, Oakland CA.

Peters, A.A., van Dorst, E., Jellis, B., van Zuuren, E., Hermans, J., Trimbos, J.B., 1991. A randomized clinical trial to compare two different approaches in women with chronic pelvic pain. Obstet. Gynecol. 77 (5), 740–744.

Pontari, M.A., Ruggieri, M.R., 2004. Mechanisms in prostatitis/chronic pelvic pain syndrome. J. Urol. 172 (3), 839–845.

Porcelli, P., Taylor, G.J., Bagby, R.M., De Carne, M., 1999. Alexithymia and functional gastrointestinal disorders: A comparison with inflammatory bowel disease. Psychother. Psychosom. 68, 263–269.

Porcelli, P., Bagby, R.M., Taylor, G.J., De Carne, M., Leandro, G., Todarello, O., 2003. Alexithymia as predictor of treatment outcome in patients with functional gastrointestinal disorders. Psychosom. Med. 65, 911–918.

Reed, B.D., Haefner, H.K., Punch, M.R., et al., 2000. Psychosocial and sexual functioning in women with vulvodynia and chronic pelvic pain. A comparative evaluation. J. Reprod. Med. 45 (8), 624–632.

Reissing, E.D., Binik, Y.M., Khalifé, S., Cohen, D., Amsel, R., 2004. Vaginal spasm, pain, and behavior: an empirical investigation of the diagnosis of vaginismus. Arch. Sex. Behav. 33 (1), 5–17.

Roelofs, J., Peters, M.L., McCracken, L., Vlaeyen, J.W., 2003. The pain vigilance and awareness questionnaire (PVAQ): further psychometric evaluation in fibromyalgia and other chronic pain syndromes. Pain 101 (3), 299–306.

Rohleder, N., Beulen, S.E., Chen, E., Wolf, J.M., Kirschbaum, C., 2007. Stress on the dance floor: the cortisol stress response to social-evaluative threat in competitive ballroom dancers. Pers. Soc. Psychol. Bull. 33 (1), 69–84.

Schlotz, W., Hellhammer, J., Schulz, P., Stone, A.A., 2004. Perceived work overload and chronic worrying predict weekend-weekday differences in the cortisol awakening response. Psychosom. Med. 66 (2), 207–214.

Scott, D.J., Stohler, C.S., Egnatuk, C.M., Wang, H., Koeppe, R.A., Zubieta, J.K., 2007. Individual differences in reward responding explain placebo-induced expectations and effects. Neuron 55 (2), 325–336.

Sifneos, P.E., 1973. The prevalence of 'alexithymic' characteristics in psychosomatic patients. Psychother. Psychosom. 22 (2), 255–262.

Simons, D.G., 2004. Review of enigmatic MTrPs as a common cause of enigmatic musculoskeletal pain and dysfunction. J. Electromyogr. Kinesiol. 14 (1), 95–107.

Smeets, R.J., Vlaeyen, J.W., Kester, A.D., Knottnerus, J.A., 2006. Reduction of pain catastrophizing mediates the outcome of both physical and cognitive-behavioral treatment in chronic low back pain. J. Pain 7 (4), 261–271.

Steptoe, A., Cropley, M., Griffith, J., Kirschbaum, C., 2000. Job strain and anger expression predict early morning elevations in salivary cortisol. Psychosom. Med. 62, 286–292.

Sullivan, M.J.L., Bishop, S.R., Pivik, J., et al., 1995. The pain catastrophizing scale: development and validation. Psych. Assessment 7 (4), 524–532.

Sullivan, M.J.L., Thorn, B., Haythornthwaite, J.A., et al., 2001. Theoretical perspectives on the relation between catastrophizing and pain. Clin. J. Pain 17, 52–64.

Tabibnia, G., Zaidel, E., 2005. Alexithymia, interhemispheric transfer, and right hemispheric specialization: a critical review. Psychother. Psychosom. 74 (2), 81–92.

Thorn, B.E., Pence, L.B., Ward, L.C., et al., 2007. A randomized clinical trial of targeted cognitive behavioral treatment to reduce catastrophizing in chronic headache sufferers. J. Pain 8 (12), 938–949.

Tripp, D.A., Nickel, J.C., Wang, Y., et al., National Institutes of Health-Chronic Prostatitis Collaborative Research Network (NIH-CPCRN) Study Group, 2006. Catastrophizing and pain-contingent rest predict patient adjustment in men with chronicprostatitis/chronic pelvic pain syndrome. J. Pain 7 (10), 697–708.

Ullrich, P.M., Lutgendorf, S.K., Kreder, K.J., 2007. Physiologic reactivity to a laboratory stress task among men with benign prostatic hyperplasia. Urology 70 (3), 487–492.

van Wilgen, C.P., Dijkstra, P.U., Versteegen, G.J., Fleuren, M.J., Stewart, R., van Wijhe, M., 2009. Chronic pain and severe disuse syndrome: long-term outcome of an inpatient multidisciplinary cognitive behavioural program. J. Rehabil. Med. 41 (3), 122–128.

Voerman, G.E., Sandsjö, L., Vollenbroek-Hutten, M.M., et al., 2007. Changes in cognitive-behavioral factors and muscle activation patterns after interventions for work-related neck-shoulder complaints: relations with discomfort and disability. J. Occup. Rehabil. 17 (4), 593–609.

Wager, T.D., 2007. Placebo effects on human mu-opioid activity during pain. Proc. Natl. Acad. Sci. 104 (26), 11056–11061.

Walker, E.A., Katon, W.J., Neraas, K., Jemelka, R.P., Massoth, D., 1992. Dissociation in women with chronic pelvic pain. Am. J. Psychiatry 149 (4), 534–537.

Wise, D., Anderson, R.A., 2008. Headache in the Pelvis, fifth ed. National Center for Pelvic Pain, Occidental, CA.

Wolff, B., Burns, J.W., Quartana, P.J., Lofland, K., Bruehl, S., Chung, O.Y., 2008. Pain catastrophizing, physiological indexes, and chronic pain severity: tests of mediation and moderation models. J. Behav. Med. 31 (2), 105–114.

Gender and chronic pelvic pain

5

Maria Adele Giamberardino Giannapia Affaitati
Raffaele Costantini

CHAPTER CONTENTS

Introduction

Pain arising from the pelvic area, especially recurrent or chronic, is very frequent epidemiologically, and an important reason for patients seeking medical care. Benign or malignant in nature, it can be of different origins (i.e. musculoskeletal, neuropathic or visceral), but that deriving from internal organs is undeniably a prominent form, responsible not only for chronic suffering of patients but also for notable disability (Hubscher et al. 2007, Moore & Kennedy 2007). This chapter is intended to focus on the clinical profile, pathophysiology and treatment of paradigmatic forms of non-cancer pain from the pelvic viscera, with particular attention to recurrent/chronic pain from the reproductive area in both females and males. As an indispensable premise to this topic, general considerations will be made on the role of sex hormones on pain perception in the context of gender differences in pain.

The use of the terms 'sex' and 'gender' has generated much debate in the literature (LeResche 1999), some suggesting that 'sex' should strictly refer to biological aspects of the person and gender to his/her psychosocial identity (Snidvongs & Holdcroft 2008).

However, since strong mutual influences between biological and psychosocial aspects are undeniable in determining individuals' responses to a variety of triggers, including those for pain, the terms 'sex' and 'gender' will here be used interchangeably.

Gender and pain: The role of sex hormones

After being neglected for a long period of time, the relationship between gender and pain has in recent decades become the subject of a huge number of studies in both the experimental and clinical context (Fillingim et al. 2009). Epidemiological investigation clearly shows that a number of clinical pain conditions – especially chronic – are more frequent in women than in men (e.g. chronic tension headache, migraine, facial and temporomandibular pain, musculoskeletal pain, pain from osteoarthritis and rheumatoid arthritis, and fibromyalgia) (Kuba &

Quinones-Jenab 2005). Many of these show symptom fluctuations with the phases of the female cycle during the reproductive years, mostly with increased pain in the perimenstrual period (Allais & Benedetto 2004, Pamuk & Cakir 2005, Heitkemper & Chang 2009).

Women also present more intense and long-lasting pain complaints than men even for conditions occurring with similar frequency in the two sexes. In addition, there is also some suggestion that pain intensity expressed postoperatively and after several interventional procedures may be more intense in women compared to men (Filllingim et al. 2009).

Differences between the two sexes have also been found in experimental pain; though the results of the various studies in the literature are not always unequivocal, on the whole the bulk of human research performed in this area indicates greater pain sensitivity in women than in men in relation to the majority of pain modalities applied at both somatic and visceral levels (Arendt-Nielsen et al. 2004). More recent clinical investigation has focused on the women's compared with the men's responses to analgesic medications – especially opioids and NSAIDs – and to their side-effects (Fillingim & Gear 2004). They have shown significant differences in some cases, though more studies (with more homogeneous protocols) are needed in this specific field to completely clarify the issue (Snidvongs & Holdcroft 2008).

These sex differences in clinical (mostly) and experimental pain as well as in response to pain therapy are likely to be complex and multifactorial, involving a number of biological, sociocultural and psychological variables whose thorough and detailed analysis is far beyond the scope of this text (see Fillingim et al. (2009) for review). Attention will, however, be paid to sex hormones, as they are obviously among the major candidates to explain sex differences in pain (Fillingim & Ness 2000).

Sex hormones and pain

The three main sex hormones (i.e. oestrogen, progesterone and testosterone) are functionally active in both sexes, but their absolute levels and temporal fluctuations differ considerably in males and females (Berkley 1997, Berkley & Holdcroft 1999, Cairns & Gazerani 2009). Females undergo vast hormonal changes during puberty, pregnancy and menopause and cyclic hormonal fluctuations during the ovarian cycle in the reproductive phase of life. Males are instead exposed to less marked fluctuations in hormone levels across the lifespan, with the most significant change being the reduction of testosterone with ageing (Fillingim et al. 2009). Among the many body function parameters influenced by sex hormones, pain perception holds an important place, although there is not always universal agreement about how and to what extent this happens throughout the lifespan nor about the pathophysiology of these differences (Giamberardino 2000). In women, many painful conditions vary in their incidence, disappearance and prevalence as a function of puberty, pregnancy, menopause and ageing and, as already mentioned, during the reproductive years different forms of pain also vary with the phase of the menstrual cycle, mostly exacerbating in the perimenstrual period. In men, some pain disorders also show different profiles in the various stages of life (Berkley 2005, Cairns & Gazerani 2009, Fillingim et al. 2009).

Progesterone is mostly associated with analgesia because some pain conditions in humans – such as migraine and temporomandibular pain – disappear or improve during pregnancy or the midluteal phase of the menstrual cycle, and other pains are reduced in animals during lactation (when progesterone levels are high), and some anaesthetics are progesterone-based (e.g. alphaxolone) (Berkley & Holdcroft 1999, Silberstein 2004, LeResche et al. 2005, Brandes 2006, Craft 2007). Oestrogen has also been associated with analgesia, since some pain conditions increase when oestrogen decreases. For instance, as the oestradiol level sharply declines postpartum, the frequency of migraine attacks increases (Sances et al. 2003) and after the menopause, when oestrogen declines, several pain complaints – such as orofacial pain and vaginal pain – increase (LeResche et al. 2003, Fillingim et al. 2009). Similarly, testosterone promotes analgesia, its decline with ageing in men being consistently associated with an increase in a number of pains, such as angina or muscle pain (Berkley & Holdcroft 1999, Vecchiet 2002). For each of these examples, however, either a lack of effects or contrasting examples can be found, such as the decrease in postmenopausal women of musculoskeletal pain, chronic widespread pain and fibromyalgia, and in postmenopausal women and older men of abdominal pain (including irritable bowel syndrome, IBS) migraine and tension headaches, in parallel with a decrease in oestrogen, progesterone and testosterone. Another example is the emergence of cluster headaches in men at puberty, when testosterone increases (Berkley & Holdcroft 1999, LeResche et al. 2003, Kuba & Quinones-Jenab 2005). Exogenous hormone use has also been associated with change in several pain patterns. Women under oral contraceptive treatment have an increased risk for development of temporomandibular (TMD) pain and carpal tunnel syndrome.

Postmenopausal women under hormone replacement are at increased risk of back pain and TMD pain (LeResche et al. 1997, Ferry et al. 2000, Musgrave et al. 2001), but also discontinuation of this therapy is associated with higher levels of reported pain or stiffness (Ockene et al. 2005). Likewise, after sustained oestradiol administration, migraine attacks are precipitated by oestradiol withdrawal (Lichten et al. 1996). An interesting study in transsexuals taking hormones to acquire characteristics of the opposite sex has shown changes in pain responses, with over 30% of those taking oestradiol/antiandrogen developing chronic pain and 50% of those taking testosterone reporting improvement of chronic pain (headache) present before start of treatment (Aloisi et al. 2007). Thus both administration and withdrawal of exogenous oestrogens – but not testosterone – appear associated with an increased risk of chronic pain.

All these apparent contradictions can, at least partially, be accounted for by the fact that the overall hormonal effects on clinical pain expression depend more on the concentration of one hormone relative to the others than on its absolute values (Fillingim et al. 2009; see also Giamberardino 2000). The modulation of pain perception by sex hormones is probably the result of a combination of factors, among which the hormonal influences on metabolism (with implications for drug action), the immune system (with implications for painful autoimmune diseases, up to nine times more common in women), trauma-induced inflammation (modulated by sex hormones), the hypothalamic–pituitary axis (with implications for the interactions between stress and pain), and nervous and cardiovascular systems (Fillingim et al. 2002, al'Absi et al. 2004, Aloisi & Bonifazi 2006, Craft 2007, Straub 2007).

As already discussed, however, sex hormone effects on pain perception cannot be separated from the many other variables that affect pain modulation. Of particular importance are social and cultural factors, which can entail profound diversities in men and women (both patients and physicians) in their attitude towards and approach to painful symptoms, especially regarding particular forms of pain such as those arising from the pelvic area (see below) (Myers et al. 2003).

Visceral pelvic pain

The global incidence of pelvic pain is six times higher in women than in men, the difference being mostly due to pain originating from internal organs (Luzi 2002, Moore & Kennedy 2007). Viscera of the pelvic cavity belong to the genital, digestive and urinary tracts. The genital organs include ovaries, Fallopian tubes, uterus and upper vagina in women, ejaculatory ducts and vas deferens in men; the digestive organs consist of the sigmoid colon, rectum and a few coils of the small intestine; the urinary organs include the terminal parts of the ureters, the urinary bladder and pelvic urethra (Giamberardino 2000). Pain arising from the various organs of the pelvic cavity can be classified into three main categories:

1. Pelvic pain from sex-specific internal organs (female or male reproductive organs);
2. Pelvic pain from non-sex-specific internal organs (pelvic portion of the digestive and urinary tracts); and
3. Mixed pelvic pain (originating from both the reproductive organs and the digestive and/or urinary tracts, as well as from non-visceral structures) (Box 5.1).

Each of the recurrent/chronic visceral pain conditions from the pelvic area has its own specificities; however, common characteristics exist, which are typical of visceral pain in general. A brief summary of these characteristics is provided in the section below.

Box 5.1

Visceral pelvic pain

Sex-specific visceral organs

- Female reproductive organs (dysmenorrhoea, endometriosis, pelvic inflammatory disease)
- Male reproductive organs (prostatodynia, chronic orchialgia)

Non-sex-specific visceral organs

- Pelvic digestive tract (irritable bowel syndrome)
- Pelvic urinary tract (interstitial cystitis)

Multiple organs ('mixed')

- Chronic pelvic pain
- Viscerovisceral hyperalgesia

Visceral pain

The clinical presentation of pain from internal organs typically varies with time. In the first phases of a visceral algogenic process the symptom is very aspecific, always perceived in the same site – along the midline of the thorax or abdomen – whatever the viscus in question. It is vague and poorly discriminated, often described more as a sense of oppression or malaise rather than frank pain, and is accompanied by marked neurovegetative signs and emotional reactions (*true visceral pain*) (Procacci et al. 1986, Giamberardino 2005). In a second phase – after a few minutes or a few hours in the first episode or in a subsequent episode – it becomes *referred* to somatic structures of the body wall, in areas that are neuromerically connected to the viscus in question. Examples are the left chest area and ipsilateral upper limb for the heart, the lumbar region–flank–anterior abdomen spreading to the groin for renal colics, the upper right abdominal quadrant radiating towards the back at the inferior angle of the scapula for biliary colics, or the lowest abdominal quadrants and sacral region for pain from the female reproductive organs. In this phase, the symptom is very similar to that originating directly from the somatic structures; its visceral origin can thus be difficult to identify. In the referred pain area, hyperalgesia (i.e. an increased sensitivity to painful stimuli) typically develops. This is mostly localized in the skeletal muscle layer, but during particularly prolonged and/or intense processes it spreads upward to also involve the overlying superficial somatic tissues – the subcutis first, and finally the skin. Cutaneous hypersensitivity can become frank allodynia (pain perceived for normally non-painful stimuli) in extreme cases, as happens in peritonitis from painful abdominal conditions, such as a perforated appendicitis. Vice versa, in the course of the healing process of the painful visceral condition, the desensitization of the somatic area of referral proceeds from the surface downwards; the skin is the first to normalize and then the subcutis, with the muscle keeping some degree of residual hyperalgesia for a very long period of time (Giamberardino & Cervero 2007). The characteristics and temporal evolution of the referred hyperalgesia have been deducted from a number of studies in patients with visceral pains of various origin, such as urinary/biliary colics (from calculosis or diskinesia), IBS, dysmenorrhea, endometriosis. Most of this research has employed a combination of both clinical and instrumental procedures to assess the hypersensitivity, the latter involving measurement of pain thresholds to various stimuli (thermal, mechanical, chemical and electrical). Hyperalgesia is demonstrated by a significant lowering in pain detection threshold (Vecchiet et al. 1989, 1992, Giamberardino et al. 1994, 2001, 2005, Caldarella et al. 2006).

The global outcome of the studies performed indicates that hyperalgesia only appears in visceral conditions that are painful, irrespective of the nature of the visceral trigger (organic or dysfunctional), but is absent in any organic condition that is not algogenic. As already mentioned, the hyperalgesia is mostly a muscle phenomenon, involving the overlying subcutis and skin tissues only in more severe cases. Muscle hyperalgesia occurs early in the course of the visceral algogenic process (i.e. a few painful episodes are sufficient for it to manifest), and is accentuated by repetition of the episodes as the degree of pain threshold lowering becomes progressively more pronounced. Furthermore, it is of long duration; it normally outlasts the spontaneous pain – being detectable in the pain-free interval – and in most cases even the primary insult in the internal organ, though in a milder form. For instance, the majority of patients with urinary colics from calculosis who have passed the stone still present some degree of referred muscle hyperalgesia in the lumbar region months or even years after elimination (Vecchiet et al. 1992, Giamberardino et al. 1994).

Referred hyperalgesia is usually accompanied by trophic changes of local deep somatic wall tissues, mostly consisting of increased thickness of the subcutis and decreased thickness/section area of muscle, the latter testifying a tendency towards atrophy of muscle layers. These can be documented by clinical means (i.e. pinch palpation) but better quantified by ultrasonography. In symptomatic urinary and biliary calculosis, in fact, a significant increase in subcutis thickness and a significant decrease in muscle thickness have been found in the referred area (lumbar region and cystic point area, respectively) with respect to the contralateral non-affected area (Giamberardino et al. 2005, Giamberardino & Cervero 2007). Like the hyperalgesia, also trophic changes are set off by the algogenic impulses from the affected organ, since they are not detected in non-painful organic visceral conditions such as asymptomatic gallbladder calculosis. Unlike the hyperalgesia, however, they are not modulated by the extent of algogenic impulses from the visceral organ. In fact, they have been shown not to increase with the repetition of the painful episodes or decrease with their cessation; they seem to be a rather on–off phenomenon (Giamberardino 2005).

Referred pain with hyperalgesia has been attributed to phenomena of central sensitization involving viscerosomatic convergent neurons (Woolf & Salter 2000). The afferent barrage from the affected organ would increase the activity and response properties of these neurons, thus enhancing the central effect of the normal input from the somatic area of pain referral and accounting for the hyperalgesia (*convergence-facilitation theory*) (Cervero & Laird 2004, Sengupta 2009). (See discussion of these issues in Chapter 3.)

The visceral input would also activate a number of reflex arcs, whose afferent branch is represented by sensory fibres from the organ and whose efferent branch would be somatic towards the skeletal muscle and sympathetic towards the subcutis and skin of the referred area. Activation of these reflexes would contribute to the secondary hyperalgesia and also account for the local trophic changes (see Giamberardino et al. 2005). Hyperalgesia and trophic changes can be typically detected in referred pain areas from pelvic internal organs, as will be reported in the following sections.

Pelvic pain from sex-specific internal organs

Pain conditions from sex-specific visceral organs appear more frequently in women than in men, due to the more complex make-up of the pelvic region in females and the number of pathophysiological conditions directly or indirectly linked to their reproductive function (see Giamberardino 2000). Paradigmatic examples are primary dysmenorrhoea, chronic pain from endometriosis and pelvic inflammatory disease. There are, of course, also several examples of pain conditions of the reproductive organs in men (e.g. prostatitis, epididymitis, etc.); one of the most typical is chronic testicular pain, which represents an important medical problem from both a diagnostic and a therapeutic point of view (Wesselmann et al. 1999).

Pain from the female reproductive organs

Primary dysmenorrhoea

Primary dysmenorrhoea is defined as cyclic pain associated with menses in the absence of any documentable organic condition in the pelvic cavity. It is extremely common, estimated to occur in over 50% of all menstruating women in the world (Proctor & Farquhar 2006). The pain is believed to be caused by relative uterine ischaemia from hypercontractility of the myometrium, which is in turn the result of excess prostaglandins (prostaglandins would act by increasing uterine contractility and also by sensitizing nerve endings to the pain-producing effects of other compounds, such as bradykinins). By increasing the input towards the central nervous system, peripheral sensitization due to these mechanisms would then also favour the occurrence of central sensitization phenomena (Hubscher et al. 2007).

Symptoms usually start a few hours or days before bleeding, worsen as the menstrual flow begins and can last throughout the entire period of menses. Usually cramp-like in nature, the pain is typically perceived in the midportion of the lower abdomen but may also involve the lower back and upper thighs. Neurovegetative signs and emotional reactions, typical of visceral pain perception (i.e. nausea, vomiting, changes in heart rate, diarrhoea and anxiety) may precede or accompany the pain. Some dysmenorrhoeic patients also have midcycle pain (Giamberardino 2008). Pain of primary dysmenorrhoea can be very intense and, like other forms of pain from internal organs, is usually accompanied by tissue hypersensitivity in the somatic area of referral. This phenomenon was quantified in psychophysical studies in dysmenorrhoeic versus non-dysmenorrhoeic women using the technique of pain threshold measurement to electrical stimulation of skin, subcutis and muscle. Thresholds of all three tissues were lower than normal in dysmenorrhoeic women with respect to non-dysmenorrhoeic women, but the reduction was particularly accentuated in the muscle (rectus abdominis). The reduction was present not only in the painful period but also in the intervals between the cycles, testifying to the long duration of the hyperalgesic phenomenon. The muscle decrease proved more pronounced in women who had suffered from dysmenorrhoea for many years compared with women with dysmenorrhoea of recent onset, which, considering the repetitive nature of the condition, corresponds to a high or low number of painful episodes, respectively (Giamberardino et al. 1997).

Apart from hyperalgesia in the area of pain referral, however, dysmenorrhoeic women also showed a certain degree of muscle hypersensitivity in other body regions (diffuse muscle hyperalgesia), similar to the pattern observed in women affected with fibromyalgia (Russell & Larson 2009). Indeed, dysmenorrhoea is a significantly more frequent occurrence in fibromyalgia patients than in the general population (women with fibromyalgia syndrome have a fivefold higher probability to have dysmenorrhoea) (Shaver et al. 2006), a circumstance that has triggered scientific speculation about a common pathophysiological feature in the two conditions, consisting of a tendency to develop a state of central sensitization (Giamberardino 2008), which a generalized lowering in pain threshold would be proof of. Fibromyalgia is not the only frequent comorbidity for dysmenorrhoea. It is estimated, in fact, that about 50% of dysmenorrhoea patients have comorbidities also with other chronic pain conditions, such as IBS, interstitial cystitis (IC) or headache (Altman et al. 2006, Stanford et al. 2007, Watier 2009).

It is worth noting that also these conditions are characterized by a tendency to a generalized hypersensitivity to painful stimuli, thus suggesting once more that dysmenorrhoea is part of the wide spectrum of the so-called 'functional disorders' whereby central sensitization phenomena play a crucial role (Giamberardino 2008). Primary dysmenorrhoea needs to be differentiated from the pain complaints of premenstrual syndrome (PMS), a recurrent disorder occurring in the luteal phase of the menstrual cycle, estimated to affect up to 75% of women of childbearing age (Zaafrane et al. 2007). This disorder, a complex of somatic and psychological symptoms, is still incompletely explained pathophysiologically, but it has recently been put into relationship with overbreathing, a typical female syndrome (Slatkovska et al. 2006, Sauty & Prosper 2008; see also Chapters 11 and 12); in women with PMS the sensitivity of the respiratory centre to CO_2 would be increased more than normal by secretory products of the corpus luteum, resulting in hyperventilation. In addition, Ott et al. (2006) suggest that: 'some symptoms of PMS may be caused by chronic hyperventilation'. Treatment of primary dysmenorrhoea is mainly performed with NSAIDs, although it is estimated that over 30% of women fail to show any improvement. Other measures are vitamins, magnesium, oral contraceptives and, in extreme cases, surgery (e.g. presacral neurectomy) (Proctor & Farquhar 2006).

Endometriosis

Endometriosis is defined as the presence of endometrial tissue in abnormal locations in the abdominal/pelvic cavity. This condition is estimated to affect 7–10% of all women of reproductive age in the world, with the most common sites of endometrial lesions being ovaries, uterine tubes, cul-de-sac, supporting ligaments of the uterus, pelvic peritoneum, rectovaginal septum, cervix and bowel surface (Berkley et al. 2005). The pathophysiology of endometriosis is still partly unknown. Hypotheses are retrograde menstruation, lymphatic system spread or haematogenous spread (Hubscher et al. 2007).

The clinical presentation of endometriosis is variable as regards pain. Though all women with the condition present infertility or subfertility, vaginal hyperalgesia and dyschezia, not all have spontaneous pain. Some are entirely asymptomatic, a number of them have secondary dysmenorrhoea, others show chronic pelvic pain (CPP). There is usually no correlation between the extent of the lesions and the amount of pain experienced, with minor lesions sometimes being the reason for intense pain and major lesions being asymptomatic. The mechanisms of pain are also not completely known, but probably involve more than one factor, including excess prostaglandin production, increased peritoneal sensitivity, chemical irritation of the peritoneum and bleeding in sites of endometriosis (Berkley 2005).

Like primary dysmenorrhoea sufferers, women with symptomatic endometriosis present abdomino-pelvic hyperalgesia, especially at muscle level, and also a generalized state of deep tissue hypersensitivity (Bajaj et al. 2003). As for primary dysmenorrhoea, it is worth noting that also endometriosis presents a high degree of co-morbidity with other pain conditions characterized by a generalized hypersensitivity to pain. In fact, women with endometriosis have higher rates of fibromyalgia (5.9 versus 3.4%, $P < 0.0001$), headache (endometriosis is significantly more common in migraineurs than in controls: 22% vs 9.6%, $P < 0.01$) but also IBS, IC and vulvodynia (Chung et al. 2005, Tietjen et al. 2007, Nyholt et al. 2009). Treatment of endometriosis remains a challenge for the medical community as no therapeutic option so far available has proven completely satisfactory. The choice is among pituitary inhibitory hormones, danazol, high-dose progesterone for medical treatment; laser during laparoscopy, surgical severance of the uterocervical plexus of the superior hypogastric plexus (presacral neurectomy) for the non-medical treatment. Symptomatic treatment of secondary dysmenorrhoea is similar to that for primary dysmenorrhoea, mainly with NSAIDs. A new possibility currently under evaluation in animal models involves drugs reducing blood supply to the ectopic growths (Ferrero et al. 2006).

Pelvic inflammatory disease

Pain associated with infection and inflammation of the female reproductive organs (pelvic inflammatory disease, PID) is of great clinical significance and a common cause of infertility, chronic pain and ectopic pregnancy (Haggerty & Ness 2008). It is the most common gynaecologic reason for admission to hospital in the USA; each year, in fact, at least 1 million American women are diagnosed with PID and more than 200 000 are hospitalized, with substantial healthcare costs (Wesselmann et al. 1999, Ross 2008, Sweet 2009). An ascending genital infection is generally the primary cause of PID. The aetiology is multimicrobial, including both sexually transmitted organisms – primarily *Neisseria gonorrhoeae* and *Chlamydia trachomatis* – and microorganisms found in the endogenous flora of the vagina and cervix, including anaerobic and facultative bacteria, many of which are associated with bacterial vaginosis (Haggerty & Ness 2008, Sweet 2009). Genital tract mycoplasms, mostly *Mycoplasma genitalium*, may also be implicated. Serious consequences of these upper genital inflammations include chronic pelvic pain in about 30% of patients (Moore & Kennedy 2007); it is estimated that while overall a woman has about a 5% risk of having chronic pelvic pain in her lifetime, patients with a previous diagnosis of PID have a fourfold increased risk of this complication (Ryder 1996). As for other forms of visceral pain, in PID, severe hyperalgesia often develops in muscles of the lower abdominal quadrants and pelvic area. This hyperalgesia normally outlasts the spontaneous pain and persists for a long time, to the point that the affected women may remain chronically hypersensitive in these somatic areas (Giamberardino 2000). Diagnosis of PID is challenging, mostly resulting from a combination of symptoms and signs and documentation of a polymicrobial aetiology. Due to the potential of serious sequelae, a low threshold for diagnosis and thus of treatment of acute PID is recommended (Haggerty & Ness 2008). Therapy should consist of wide-spectrum antibiotic regimens (oral or parenteral) that provide adequate coverage against the implicated microorganisms (Sweet 2009).

Pain from the male reproductive organs (See also Chapters 12 & 15)

Prostatitis/prostatodynia

Among the various forms of prostatitis, as defined by the NIH (Wagenlehner et al. 2009), chronic prostatitis, also called chronic pelvic pain syndrome (CPPS), is one of the most relevant regarding the pain problem. This syndrome is defined as pelvic pain for more than 3 of the previous 6 months, urinary symptoms and painful ejaculation, without documented urinary tract infections from uropathogens. It affects 10–15% of the male population. The aetiology is poorly understood. It is probably the consequence of an infectious or inflammatory initiator that results in neurological injury and eventually pelvic floor dysfunction (increased pelvic muscle tone). It is important to operate a differential diagnosis with chronic bacterial prostatitis through cultural examination. The therapy involves firstly a 4–6-week course of a fluoroquinolone, which provides relief in 50% of cases, and secondly NSAIDs and α-blockers for urinary symptoms. Pelvic floor training/biofeedback is also used. Minimally invasive surgical treatment may be necessary for treatment of refractory patients (Hubscher et al. 2007, Murphy et al. 2009).

Chronic orchialgia

Chronic orchialgia is defined as 'intermittent or constant, unilateral or bilateral testicular pain lasting >3 months that significantly interferes with the daily activities'. It may occur at any age but the majority of patients are 20–30 years old (Granitsiotis & Kirk 2004). It is one of the most vexing problems for men and their treating physician (Wesselmann et al. 1999, Hubscher et al. 2007). The exact incidence and prevalence of this chronic pain syndrome are not known. The majority of patients are in their mid- to late 30s but chronic testicular pain has been described from adolescence to old age. In nearly 25% of the patients with this condition pain starts spontaneously in the absence of a clear precipitating event. Secondary causes of chronic orchialgia include infection, tumour, testicular torsion, varicocele, hydrocele, spermatocele, trauma or previous surgery. Referred pain from the ureter or the hip has also been reported as a cause of testicular pain, although other aetiologies cannot be excluded (Hubscher et al. 2007). Chronic orchialgia can be unilateral or bilateral. Some patients have constant pain; in others the pain is intermittent, either spontaneous or precipitated by certain movements or pressure on the testis. The pain may be confined to the scrotal contents or radiate to the groin, penis, perineum, abdomen, legs and back. The diagnosis is based on the clinical history and physical examination (urological/neurological). Treatment of this kind of patient requires identification of the underlying aetiology. However, when this is not possible (in 25% of cases, as already stated) several medical and non-medical treatments have proven beneficial, for instance a trial of antibiotics and NSAIDs (possible occult inflammatory processes), low-dose antidepressants, anticonvulsants, opiates or lumbar sympathetic blocks. Complete resolution of the symptomatology is, however, difficult (Sinclair et al. 2007, Baranowski 2009).

Pelvic pain from non-sex-specific visceral organs

Numerous pain conditions can affect the pelvic portion of the digestive and urinary tracts. We report here two paradigmatic examples of conditions for which no specific 'organic' cause has, to date, been identified: IBS and IC.

Irritable bowel syndrome

IBS is a chronic episodic medical condition characterized by abdominal/pelvic pain or discomfort and altered bowel habits in the absence of a detectable organic disease. It may present with diarrhoea and/or constipation, and is part of the spectrum of functional gastrointestinal disorders. IBS has a prevalence of 9–23% in the general population and accounts for up to 50% of diagnoses made by gastroenterologists. It affects women four times more than men, with a female predominance also in greater symptom severity. Its age distribution is unclear; some studies report a higher prevalence in the young and a decrease with age. This condition has a large impact on quality of life, with consequent high direct and indirect healthcare costs (Chang et al. 2006; Chang & Harris 2007). The pathophysiology of IBS is still incompletely known but is probably complex and multifactorial. A sensory disturbance has been hypothesized, in terms of an altered processing of the painful signal (visceral hyperalgesia), though it is still debated if this disturbance occurs primarily in the central nervous system or is triggered, at least initially, by a peripheral event, such as an infection (*peripheral sensitization followed by central sensitization*). Among specific molecules possibly involved in pain pathogenesis of IBS, serotonin (5-HT) has received most attention as it is an important player in the normal peristaltic reflex of the gut and can also sensitize visceral nociceptors and facilitate transient receptor potential family V receptor 1 (TRPV1) function. The role of a genetic predisposition is controversial (Mathew & Bhatia 2009, Van Oudenhove & Qasim 2009). IBS diagnosis is at present performed on the basis of Rome III criteria, i.e. recurrent abdominal pain or discomfort of at least 3 days/month in the last 3 months associated with two or more of the following: improvement with defecation, onset associated with a change in frequency of stools, onset associated with a change in form (appearance) of stool. The criteria need to be fulfilled for the last 3 months with symptom onset at least 6 months prior to diagnosis (see Grundmann & Yoon 2010). Alarm symptoms (e.g. weight loss, fever, rectal bleeding, steatorrhoea, lactose/gluten intolerance) suggest the possibility of a structural disease, such as colon cancer, inflammatory bowel disease or malabsorption disorders (e.g. coeliac sprue), but do not necessarily exclude a diagnosis of IBS. The onset of IBS is usually precipitated by disruption of gastrointestinal function secondary to infection, dietary factors, lifestyle changes or psychological stress (IBS patients report a higher prevalence of sexual, physical and emotional abuse compared to healthy individuals). The spontaneous pain is described as a cramping, aching abdominal sensation whose severity ranges from mild and intermittent to severe and continuous. It can be precipitated by meals and improved by defecation. In female patients it is influenced by the menstrual cycle, with an increase immediately before and during menses. The abdominal painful areas typically enlarge with the progression of the disease. Abdominal pain is also evoked by intestinal transit (e.g. postprandial colonic contractions, unnoticed by controls) and endoscopic procedures. A number of clinical conditions occur more frequently in IBS than in the general population (comorbidities), such as psychiatric disorders (prevalence 40–90% in IBS patients), FMS (prevalence 31.6% in women with IBS), recurrent/chronic pelvic pain (prevalence of dysmenorrhoea 50% in women with IBS), chronic fatigue syndrome, interstitial cystitis, back pain, temporomandibular joint pain, headache (see Giamberardino 2008). IBS patients have abnormal reactivity to painful stimuli at both visceral and somatic level, particularly (1) lowered pain thresholds to mechanical and electrical stimuli of the gut in the majority of cases (visceral hyperalgesia) and (2) lowered pain thresholds in skin, subcutis and muscle *in somatic abdominal areas of pain referral.* In *somatic areas outside the sites of pain referral*, pain thresholds are lowered in subcutis and muscle while controversial results have been found in skin, with normal, higher than normal or lower than normal pain thresholds (thermal, mechanical electrical stimuli) (Caldarella et al. 2006). IBS typically lasts for the entire life of the patient, though a mild control of the symptoms can be achieved through treatment. This is typically multimodal, involving: appropriate diet (careful analysis of potential food triggers), traditional pharmacologic therapy (including bulking agents, antispasmodics, tricyclic antidepressants and other psychotropic agents, and laxatives), serotoninergic agents (5-HT3 receptor antagonists, 5-HT4 receptor agonists, combination 5-HT4 agonist and 5-HT3 antagonist), behavioural and psychological therapy (Heizer et al. 2009) .

Interstitial cystitis/painful bladder syndrome

Interstitial cystitis is a clinical syndrome characterized by urinary frequency and urgency, nocturia and suprapubic pain, without an identifiable organic cause, such as a bacterial infection (Theoharides et al. 2008). Reports on its prevalence (0.01–0.5% or higher) and female/male ratio (from 5:1 to 10:1) vary in different studies due to variations in disease definition and diagnostic criteria in the course of the years (Parsons et al. 2007). The typical age of onset is 40 years. It is a vexing condition and it normally takes 5–7 years and four or five specialist consultations for patients to receive a diagnosis. Over 70% of patients with IC present painful comorbidities: dysmenorrhoea, CPP, IBS, fibromyalgia and other rheumatic diseases (Alagiri et al. 1997; see also Giamberardino 2008). The aetiology and pathogenesis of IC are still undetermined. The present theories involve: deficiency in the surface glycosaminoglycan–mucin layer, allowing increased amounts of some unspecified toxic substance to permeate the bladder wall, causing inflammation (and eventually ulcers: Hunner's ulcers) and pain; altered immunologic response/allergic reaction (elevated number of intravesical mast cells); neurogenic disorder (i.e. a chronic neurogenic inflammation of the bladder); and nociceptive disorder (visceral hyperalgesia). According to the latter, IC would not substantially differ from conditions like IBS, where after an initial triggering event determining visceral hyperalgesia, the hypersensitivity then continues to be sustained by central mechanisms of amplification of the pain signal (central sensitization) (Kelada & Jones 2007). The symptoms of IC are of variable intensity, but can reach devastating levels in some cases: intense suprapubic burning pain, urgency, incontinence, vaginal pain on intercourse, increased urinary frequency up to 60 times/day and 30 times/night (CPP). Symptoms are often triggered by some foods, they are progressive and worsen with time. They can greatly compromise the quality of life and be the cause of severe depression. The diagnosis is based on the clinical features and exclusion of other causes, cystoscopy only being confirmatory. The therapy to date is empirical, palliative and often scarcely effective. Changes in dietary habits, such as avoiding coffee, chocolate, alcohol, etc. are recommended, together with psychotherapy, drugs (e.g. tricyclic antidepressants) and intravesical instillations of hyaluronic acid (Nickel 2000).

Mixed pelvic pain

This category includes substantially two groups of conditions: CPP of mixed origin and pain from viscerovisceral hyperalgesia (Giamberardino 2008).

Chronic pelvic pain of mixed origin

This is a typical female condition, defined as pain in the lowest abdominal quadrants that persists for at least 6 months, continuous or intermittent, not exclusively associated with menstruation or sexual intercourse. It affects over 25% of all gynaecological patients and was estimated to be the cause of 5–10% of all laparoscopies and 20% of all hysterectomies up to 10 years ago. Though its aetiology is scarcely known, it is thought to be due to a combination of pelvic algogenic conditions, visceral (mostly dysmenorrhoea/endometriosis, but also IBS or IC), musculoskeletal and neuropathic. The therapy is still highly unsatisfactory, as a consequence of the limited knowledge about pathophysiological mechanisms (Chung et al. 2005, Altman et al. 2006, Butrick 2007, Montenegro et al. 2008).

Chronic pelvic pain from visceroviseral hyperalgesia

Viscerovisceral hyperalgesia is a phenomenon consisting of an enhancement of painful symptoms, both direct and referred, due to the interaction between two affected internal organs that have at least partially overlapping sensory projections, for instance heart and gallbladder (common projections: T5), but more specifically in the case of pelvic pain, uterus and colon (T10–L1), or uterus and urinary tract (T10–L1) (Giamberardino et al. 2010). Women with dysmenorrhoea and IBS have been shown to complain of more menstrual pain and referred pelvic muscle hyperalgesia than women with dysmenorrhoea without IBS. They also report more abdominal pain from intestinal transit and referred abdominal muscle hyperalgesia than women with IBS without dysmenorrhoea. Effective hormonal treatment of dysmenorrhoea results in improvement also of IBS symptoms, while dietary treatment of IBS, if able to improve IBS, is also capable of ameliorating pain from dysmenorrhoea. Similarly, women with dysmenorrhoea and urinary calculosis report more menstrual pain, urinary colics and referred pelvic and lumbar muscle hyperalgesia than women with either dysmenorrhoea or urinary calculosis only, over a comparable period of time. Effective hormonal treatment of dysmenorrhoea improves the urinary pain, while calculosis treatment via extracorporeal shock wave lithotripsy also relieves the dysmenorrhoea (see Giamberardino & Cervero 2007). Thus the concomitance of two painful conditions in different internal organs sharing at least part of their central sensory projection causes an enhancement of pain symptoms from both districts. The notable therapeutic implication is that the typical pain from one district can be modulated by treating not only the specific condition of that district but also that of the other organ. Of importance is that viscerovisceral hyperalgesia also occurs when one of the two visceral disorders is latent with respect to pain. For instance, asymptomatic endometriosis (discovered by chance at laparoscopy performed for infertility reasons) enhances pain perception from the urinary tract in women with urinary calculosis; over a comparable period of time, women with the two conditions complain of more colics and referred lumbar muscle hyperalgesia than women with urinary calculosis only. Laser treatment of endometriosis improves the urinary pain (Giamberardino et al. 2001). Mechanisms behind viscerovisceral hyperalgesia remain to be fully established. However, since viscerovisceral convergences have been documented in the central nervous system between different internal organs (e.g. afferent fibres from uterus, urinary bladder, vagina and colon converge upon the same sensory neurons), it is plausible that sensitization of these neurons occurs, due to the increased input from one internal organ (Berkley 2005, Pezzone et al. 2005, Winnard et al. 2006, Malykhina 2007, Brumovsky & Gebhart 2010). As a result, the central effect of the input from the second organ would be enhanced. Since neurons receiving visceral inputs also constantly receive somatic projections, the referred phenomena are also amplified (Cervero 2000). It is interesting to note that viscerovisceral hyperalgesia at pelvic level seems to occur preferentially in women. This circumstance triggers a number of questions about women being more prone than men to develop chronic pelvic pain conditions (see section below).

Are women more susceptible than men to chronic pain?

As so far discussed, pelvic pain is by no doubt much more frequent in women than in men, mostly in relation to the higher complexity of structure and function of the reproductive area. But are women also more prone than men to develop chronic pain conditions from this and other areas? Berkely (2005) raised the interesting point that one contributing factor to pain sex differences derives from the vagina and cervix providing ready access to internal pelvic structures, and thus ready access also to the entrance of a number of infectious agents (i.e. viruses, bacteria, etc.). This entails a greater propensity to develop a number of pelvic inflammatory conditions that, in turn, can increase the vulnerability in women of the T10–L1 (innervating uterus and cervix) and S2–S4 (innervating vagina and cervix) segments to morbidity (Bonica 1990). Repeated/persistent input from the periphery can then lead to central sensitization phenomena responsible for the evolution of pelvic pain conditions towards chronicity and also, by spreading of sensitization to other segments, to the development of more generalized pain states (such as fibromyalgia) which women present much more frequently than men (Abeles et al. 2007).

Whether or not the initiating factor is represented by infectious agents from the vaginal canal, as in Berkley's hypothesis, the fact remains that the high number of acute/recurrent pain events from sex-specific organs in women – linked to their reproductive physiology – is a potential trigger for central neuroplastic changes in the pelvic segments. This, in turn, also facilitates phenomena of viscerovisceral hyperalgesia in the same domain, with mutual exacerbation of symptoms from the reproductive organs, and digestive and urinary tracts in the area, predisposing women compared with men to developing more complex and persisting painful conditions (Giamberardino 2008).

Further research in the field, also employing animal models of relevant pelvic pain conditions, such as the models of uterine inflammation and of endometriosis plus ureteral calculosis in the female rat (Wesselmann et al. 1998, Giamberardino et al. 2002), is needed to further elucidate mechanisms behind the higher susceptibility of women to chronic visceral pain.

Conclusion

The clinical examples provided show how pain from the pelvic area holds a prominent place in the context of all pains of visceral origin. This is particularly true for women who not only have more frequent forms of pain from this area but also present more intricate and long-lasting clinical pictures with respect to men. It would be too simplistic to attribute the major burden of pelvic pain in women entirely to the pathophysiological role of the reproductive organs and sex hormones, given the complexity of other factors (e.g. genetic, psychological, sociocultural) that play a role in pain differences between the two sexes (Wiesenfeld-Hallin 2005, Bernardes et al. 2008, Buskila 2007, Fillingim et al. 2009, Paras et al. 2009). The powerful impact of the reproductive area on the experience of visceral pain in the life of every woman is, however, undeniable. This is due not only to the various sex-specific organ pains but also to the numerous pains from other districts that are 'facilitated' by central nervous system bombardment from this area. This concept has an important clinical implication: maximal attention and early treatment should be provided for any even minimal algogenic state – of the reproductive organs in women – also to prevent the development of complicated pain pictures from multiple sources (Wesselmann & Czakanski 2001). In this respect, the attitude to adopt is exactly the opposite of the one traditionally held in medical practice in many contexts, that is to underestimate and undertreat pelvic pain in women because this pain is regarded as 'physiological' or 'normal' (Reddish 2006). Pelvic pain should be afforded full dignity for careful investigation and thorough management as 'no pain is ever normal' either in women or in men.

This chapter has explored how, in addition to genetic, psychological, sociocultural factors, gender differences such as the reproductive organs and sex hormones can influence the experience of CPP. The next chapter discusses the musculoskeletal contributions to CPP, including posture, movement and sport.

References

Abeles, A.M., Pillinger, M.H., Solitar, B.M., Abeles, M., 2007. Narrative Review: The Pathophysiology of Fibromyalgia. Ann. Intern. Med. 146, 726–734.

al'Absi, M., Wittmers, K.L., Ellestad, D., et al., 2004. Sex differences in pain and hypothalamic-pituitary-adrenocortical responses to opioid blockade. Psychosom. Med. 66, 198–206.

Alagiri, M., Cottiner, S., Ratner, V., Slade, D., Hanno, P.M., 1997. Interstitial cystitis, unexplained associations with other chronic disease and pain syndromes. Urology 49, 52–57.

Allais, G., Benedetto, C., 2004. Update on menstrual migraine: from clinical aspects to therapeutical strategies. Neurol. Sci. 25 (Suppl. 3), S229–S231.

Aloisi, A.M., Bonifazi, M., 2006. Sex hormones, central nervous system and pain. Hormon. Behav. 50, 1–7.

Aloisi, A.M., Bachiocco, V., Costantino, A., et al., 2007. Cross-sex hormone administration changes pain in transsexual women and men. Pain 132 (1), S60–S67.

Altman, G., Cain, K.C., Motzer, S., Jarrett, M., Burr, R., Heitkemper, M., 2006. Increased symptoms in female

IBS patients with dysmenorrhea and PMS. Gastroenterol. Nurs. 29, 4–11.

Arendt-Nielsen, L., Bajaj, P., Drewes, A.M., 2004. Visceral pain: gender differences in response to experimental and clinical pain. Eur. J. Pain 8, 465–472.

Bajaj, P., Bajaj, P., Madsen, H., Arendt-Nielsen, L., 2003. Endometriosis is associated with central sensitization: a psychophysical controlled study. J. Pain 4, 372–380.

Baranowski, A.P., 2009. Urogenital pain. In: Giamberardino, M.A. (Ed.), Visceral Pain: clinical, pathophysiological and therapeutic aspects. Oxford University Press, Oxford, pp. 83–93.

Berkley, K.J., 1997. Sex differences in pain. Behav. Brain Sci. 20, 371–380.

Berkley, K.J., 2005. A life of pelvic pain. Physiol. Behav. 86, 272–280.

Berkley, K.J., Holdcroft, A., 1999. Sex and gender differences in pain. In: Wall, P.D., Melzack, R. (Eds.), Textbook of Pain, fourth ed. Churchill Livingstone, Edinburgh, London, New York, Philadelphia, St Louis, Sydney, Toronto, pp. 951–965.

Berkley, K.J., Rapkin, A.J., Papka, R.E., 2005. The pains of endometriosis. Science 308, 1587–1589.

Bernardes, S.F., Keogh, E., Lima, M.L., 2008. Bridging the gap between pain and gender research: A selective literature review. Eur. J. Pain 12, 427–440.

Bonica, J.J., 1990. Applied anatomy relevant to pain. In: Bonica, J.J. (Ed.), The Management of Pain, vol. 1. Lea & Febiger, Philadelphia, London, pp. 133–158.

Brandes, J.L., 2006. The influence of oestrogen on migraine: a systematic review. JAMA 295, 1824–1830.

Brumovsky, P.R., Gebhart, G.F., 2010. Visceral organ cross-sensitization – An integrated perspective. Auton. Neurosci. 153, 106–115.

Buskila, D., 2007. Genetics of chronic pain states. Best Pract. Res. Clin. Rheumatol. 21, 535–547.

Butrick, C.W., 2007. Patients withchronic pelvic pain: endometriosis or interstitial cystitis/painful bladder syndrome? JSLS 11, 182–189.

Cairns, B.E., Gazerani, P., 2009. Sex-related differences in pain. Maturitas 63, 292–296.

Caldarella, M.P., Giamberardino, M.A., Sacco, F., et al., 2006. Sensitivity disturbances in patients with irritable bowel syndrome and fibromyalgia. Am. J. Gastroenterol. 101, 2782–2789.

Cervero, F., 2000. Visceral pain – central sensitization. Gut 47 (IV), 56–57.

Cervero, F., Laird, J.M., 2004. Understanding the signaling and transmission of visceral nociceptive events. J. Neurobiol. 61, 45–54.

Chang, L., Harris, L., 2007. Irritable bowel syndrome and functional abdominal pain syndromes: Clinical features and management. In: Pasricha, P.J., Willis, W.D., Gebhart, G.F. (Eds.), Chronic Abdominal and Visceral Pain. Informa Healthcare, New York, London, pp. 357–372.

Chang, L., Toner, B.B., Fukudo, S., Guthrie, E., Locke, G.R., Norton, N.J., et al., 2006. Gender, age, society, culture, and the patient's perspective in the functional gastrointestinal disorders. Gastroenterology 130, 1435–1446.

Chung, M.K., Chung, R.P., Gordon, D., 2005. Interstitial cystitis and endometriosis in patients with chronic pelvic pain: The "Evil Twins" syndrome. JSLS 9, 25–29.

Craft, R.M., 2007. Modulation of pain by oestrogens. Pain 132 (Suppl. 1), S3–S12.

Ferrero, S., Ragni, N., Remorgida, V., 2006. Antiangiogenic therapies in endometriosis. Br. J. Pharmacol. 149, 133–135.

Ferry, S., Hannaford, P., Warskyj, M., Lewis, M., Croft, P., 2000. Carpal tunnel syndrome: a nested case-control study of risk factors in women. Am. J. Epidemiol. 15, 566–574.

Fillingim, R.B., Gear, R.W., 2004. Sex differences in opioid analgesia: clinical and experimental findings. Eur. J. Pain 8, 413–425.

Fillingim, R.B., Ness, T.J., 2000. Sex-related hormonal influences on pain and analgesic responses. Neurosci. Biobehav. Rev. 24, 485–501.

Fillingim, R.B., Browning, A.D., Powell, T., Wright, R.A., 2002. Sex differences in perceptual and cardiovascular responses to pain: the influence of a perceived ability manipulation. J. Pain 4, 439–445.

Fillingim, R.B., King, C.D., Ribeiro-Dasilva, M.C., Rahim-Williams, B., Riley III, J.L., 2009. Sex, gender, and pain: a review of recent clinical and experimental findings. J. Pain 10, 447–485.

Giamberardino, M.A., 2000. Sex-related and hormonal modulation of visceral pain. In: Fillingim, R.B. (Ed.), Sex, Gender, and Pain. Progr Pain Res Man, vol. 17. IASP Press, Seattle, pp. 135–163.

Giamberardino, M.A., 2005. Visceral pain. Pain: Clinical Updates 13, 1–6.

Giamberardino, M.A., 2008. Women and visceral pain: Are the reproductive organs the main protagonists? Mini-review at the occasion of the "European Week Against Pain in Women 2007". Eur. J. Pain 12, 257–260.

Giamberardino, M.A., Cervero, F., 2007. The neural basis of referred visceral pain. In: Parischa, P.J., Willis, W.D., Gebhart, G.F. (Eds.), Chronic abdominal and visceral pain: theory and practice. Informa Healthcare, New York, London, pp. 177–192.

Giamberardino, M.A., de Bigontina, P., Martegiani, C., Vecchiet, L., 1994. Effects of extracorporeal shock-wave lithotripsy on referred hyperalgesia from renal/ureteral calculosis. Pain 56, 77–83.

Giamberardino, M.A., Berkley, K.J., Iezzi, S., de Bigontina, P., Vecchiet, L., 1997. Pain threshold variations in somatic wall tissues as a function of menstrual cycle, segmental site and tissue depth in non-dysmenorrheic women, dysmenorrheic women and men. Pain 71, 187–197.

Giamberardino, M.A., De Laurentis, S., Affaitati, G., Lerza, R., Lapenna, D., Vecchiet, L., 2001. Modulation of pain and hyperalgesia from the urinary tract by algogenic conditions of the reproductive organs in women. Neurosci. Lett. 304, 61–64.

Giamberardino, M.A., Berkley, K.J., Affaitati, G., et al., 2002. Influence of endometriosis on pain behaviors and muscle hyperalgesia induced by a ureteral calculosis in female rats. Pain 95, 247–257.

Giamberardino, M.A., Affaitati, G., Lerza, R., Lapenna, D., Costantini, R., Vecchiet, L., 2005. Relationship between pain symptoms and referred sensory and trophic changes in patients with gallbladder pathology. Pain 114, 239–249.

Giamberardino, M.A., Costantini, R., Affaitati, G., et al., 2010. Viscerovisceral hyperalgesia: characterization in different clinical models. Pain 151, 307–322.

Granitsiotis, P., Kirk, D., 2004. Chronic testicular pain: an overview. Eur. Urol. 45, 430–436.

Grundmann, O., Yoon, S.L., 2010. Irritable bowel syndrome: Epidemiology, diagnosis and treatment: An update for health-care practitioners. J. Gastroenterol. 25, 691–699.

Haggerty, C.L., Ness, R.B., 2008. Diagnosis and treatment of pelvic inflammatory disease. Womens Health (Lond.) 4, 383–397.

Heitkemper, M.M., Chang, L., 2009. Do fluctuations in ovarian hormones affect gastrointestinal symptoms in women with irritable bowel syndrome? Gend. Med. 6 (Suppl. 2), 152–167.

Heizer, W.D., Southern, S., McGovern, S., 2009. The role of diet in symptoms of irritable bowel syndrome in adults: a narrative review. J. Am. Diet. Assoc. 109, 1204–1214.

Hubscher, C.H., Chadha, H.K., Kaddumi, E.G., 2007. Pelvic pain syndromes: pathophysiology. In: Pasricha, P.J., Willis, W.D., Gebhart, G.F. (Eds.), Chronic Abdominal and Visceral Pain, Theory and Practice. Informa Healthcare, New York, London, pp. 463–477.

Kelada, E., Jones, A., 2007. Interstitial cystitis. Arch. Gynecol. Obstet. 275, 223–229.

Kuba, T., Quinones-Jenab, V., 2005. The role of female gonadal hormones in behavioral sex differences in persistent and chronic pain: clinical versus preclinical studies. Brain Res. Bull. 66, 179–188.

LeResche, L., 1999. Gender considerations in the epidemiology of chronic pain. In: Crombie, I.K. (Ed.), Epidemiology of Pain. IASP Press, Seattle, WA, pp. 43–52.

LeResche, L., Saunders, K., Von Korff, M.R., Barlow, W., Dworkin, S.F., 1997. Use of exogenous hormones and risk of temporomandibular disorder pain. Pain 69, 153–160.

LeResche, L., Manel, J.J., Sherman, B., Gandara, S.F., Dworkin, S.F., 2003. Changes in temporomandibular pain and other symptoms across the menstrual cycle. Pain 106, 253–261.

LeResche, L., Sherman, J.J., Huggins, K., Saunders, K., Manci, L.A., Lenz, G., et al., 2005. Musculoskeletal orofacial pain and other signs and symptoms of temporomandibular disorders during pregnancy: a prospective study. J. Orofac. Pain 19, 193–201.

Lichten, E.M., Lichten, J.B., Whitty, A., Pieper, D., 1996. The confirmation of a biochemical marker for women's hormonal migraine: The depo-oestradiol challenge test. Headache 36, 367–371.

Luzi, G.A., 2002. Chronic prostatitis and chronic pelvic pain in men: aetiology, diagnosis and management. J. Eur. Acad. Dermatol. Venereol. 16, 253–256.

Malykhina, A.P., 2007. Neural mechanisms of pelvic organ cross-sensitization. Neuroscience 149, 660–672.

Mathew, P., Bhatia, S.J., 2009. Pathogenesis and management of irritable bowel syndrome. Trop. Gastroenterol. 30, 19–25.

Montenegro, M.L., Vasconcelos, E.C., Candido Dos Reis, F.J., Nogueira, A.A., Poli-Neto, O.B., 2008. Physical therapy in the management of women with chronic pelvic pain. Int. J. Clin. Pract. 62, 263–269.

Moore, J., Kennedy, D., 2007. Pelvic pain syndromes: Clinical features and management. In: Pasricha, P.J., Willis, W.D., Gebhart, G.F. (Eds.), Chronic Abdominal and Visceral Pain, Theory and Practice. Informa Healthcare, New York, London, pp. 479–493.

Murphy, A.B., Macejko, A., Taylor, A., Nadler, R.B., 2009. Chronic prostatitis: management strategies. Drugs 69, 71–84.

Musgrave, D.S., Vogt, M.T., Nevitt, M.C., Cauley, J.A., 2001. Back problems among postmenopausal women taking oestrogen replacement therapy. Spine 26, 1606–1612.

Myers, C.D., Riley III, J.L., Robinson, M.E., 2003. Psychosocial contributions to sexcorrelated differences in pain. Clin. J. Pain 19, 225–232.

Nickel, J.C., 2000. Interstitial cystitis. Etiology, diagnosis, and treatment. Can. Fam. Physician 46, 2430–2434, 2437–2440.

Nyholt, D.R., Gillespie, N.G., Merikangas, K.R., Treloar, S.A., Martin, N.G., Montgomery, G.W., 2009. Common genetic influences underlie comorbidity of migraine and endometriosis. Genet. Epidemiol. 33, 105–113.

Ockene, J.K., Barad, D.H., Cochrane, B.B., et al., 2005. Symptom experience after discontinuing use of oestrogen plus progestin. JAMA 294, 183–193.

Ott, H.W., Mattle, V., Zimmermann, U.S., Licht, P., Moeller, K., Wildt, L., 2006. Symptoms of premenstrual syndrome may be caused by hyperventilation. Fertil. Steril. 86, 1001.e17–1001.e19.

Pamuk, O.N., Cakir, N., 2005. The variation in chronic widespread pain and other symptoms in fibromyalgia patients. The effects of menses and menopause. Clin. Exp. Rheumatol. 23, 778–782.

Paras, M.L., Murad, M.H., Chen, L.P., et al., 2009. Sexual abuse and lifetime diagnosis of somatic disorders: a systematic review and meta-analysis. JAMA 302, 550–561.

Parsons, J.K., Kurth, K., Sant, G.R., 2007. Epidemiologic issues in interstitial cystitis. Urology 69, 5–8.

Pezzone, M.A., Liang, R., Fraser, M.O., 2005. A model of neural cross-talk and irritation in the pelvis: implications for the overlap of chronic pelvic pain disorders. Gastroenterology 128, 1953–1964.

Procacci, P., Zoppi, M., Maresca, M., 1986. Clinical approach to visceral sensation. In: Cervero, F., Morrison, J.F.B. (Eds.), Visceral Sensation. Progress in Brain Research, vol. 67. Elsevier, Amsterdam, pp. 21–28.

Proctor, M., Farquhar, C., 2006. Diagnosis and management of dysmenorrhoea. BMJ 332, 1134–1138.

Reddish, S., 2006. Dysmenorrhea. Aust. Fam. Physician 35, 842–849.

Ross, J.D., 2008. Pelvic inflammatory disease. Clin. Evid. (Online) 2008 Mar 10: pii, 1606.

Russell, I.J., Larson, A.A., 2009. Neurophysiopathogenesis of fibromyalgia syndrome: a unified hypothesis. Rheum. Dis. Clin. North Am. 35, 421–435.

Ryder, R.M., 1996. Chronic pelvic pain. Am. Fam. Physician 54, 2225–2232.

Sances, G., Granella, F., Nappi, R.E., Fignon, A., Ghiotto, N., Polatti, F., et al., 2003. Course of migraine during pregnancy and postpartum: a prospective study. Cephalalgia 23, 197–205.

Sauty, A., Prosper, M., 2008. The hyperventilation syndrome. Rev. Med. Suisse 4, 2500, 2502–2505.

Sengupta, J.N., 2009. Visceral pain: the neurophysiological mechanism. Handb. Exp. Pharmacol. 194, 31–74.

Shaver, J.L., Wilbur, J., Robinson, F.P., Wang, E., Buntin, M.S., 2006. Women's health issues with fibromyalgia syndrome. J. Womens Health (Larchmt) 15, 1035–1045.

Silberstein, S.D., 2004. Headaches in pregnancy. Neurol. Clin. 22, 727–756.

Sinclair, A.M., Miller, B., Lee, L.K., 2007. Chronic orchialgia: consider gabapentin or nortriptyline before considering surgery. Int. J. Urol. 14, 622–625.

Slatkovska, L., Jensen, D., Davies, G.A., Wolfe, L.A., 2006. Phasic menstrual cycle effects on the control of breathing in healthy women. Respir. Physiol. Neurobiol. 154, 379–388.

Snidvongs, S., Holdcroft, A., 2008. Gender differences in responses to medication and side effects of medication. PCU XVI, 1–4.

Stanford, E.J., Dell, J.R., Parsons, C.L., 2007. The emerging presence of interstitial cystitis in gynecologic patients with chronic pelvic pain. Urology 69, 53–59.

Straub, R.H., 2007. The complex role of oestrogens in inflammation. Endocr. Rev. 28, 521–574.

Sweet, R.L., 2009. Treatment strategies for pelvic inflammatory disease. Expert. Opin. Pharmacother. 10, 823–837.

Theoharides, T.C., Whitmore, K., Stanford, E., Moldwin, R., O'Leary, M.P., 2008. Interstitial cystitis: bladder pain and beyond. Expert. Opin. Pharmacother. 9, 2979–2994.

Tietjen, G.E., Bushnell, C.D., Herial, N.A., Utley, C., White, L., Hafeez, F., 2007. Endometriosis is associated with prevalence of comorbid conditions in migraine. Headache 47, 1069–1078.

Van Oudenhove, L., Qasim, A., 2009. Gastrointestinal pain. In: Giamberardino, M.A. (Ed.), Visceral pain: clinical, pathophysiological and therapeutic aspects. Oxford University Press, Oxford, pp. 71–81.

Vecchiet, L., 2002. Muscle pain and aging. J. Musculoskelet. Pain 10, 5–22.

Vecchiet, L., Giamberardino, M.A., Dragani, L., ALbe-Fessard, D., 1989. Pain from renal/ureteral calculosis: evaluation of sensory thresholds in the lumbar area. Pain 36, 289–295.

Vecchiet, L., Giamberardino, M.A., de Bigontina, P., 1992. Referred pain from viscera: when the symptom persists despite the extinction of the visceral focus. Adv. Pain Res. Ther. 20, 101–110.

Wagenlehner, F.M., Naber, K.G., Bschleipfer, T., Brähler, E., Weidner, W., 2009. Prostatitis and male pelvic pain syndrome: diagnosis and treatment. Dtsch. Arztebl. Int. 106, 175–183.

Watier, A., 2009. Irritable bowel syndrome and bladder-sphincter dysfunction. Pelvi-perineologie 4 (2), 136–141.

Wesselmann, U., Czakanski, P.P., 2001. Pelvic pain: a chronic visceral pain syndrome. Curr. Pain Headache Rep. 5, 13–19.

Wesselmann, U., Czakanski, P.P., Affaitati, G., Giamberardino, M.A., 1998. Uterine inflammation as a noxious visceral stimulus: behavioral characterization in the rat. Neurosci. Lett. 246, 73–76.

Wesselmann, U., Burnett, A.L., Heinberg, L.J., 1999. The urogenital and rectal pain syndromes. Pain 73, 269–294.

Wiesenfeld-Hallin, Z., 2005. Sex differences in pain perception. Gend. Med. 2, 137–145.

Winnard, K.P., Dmitrieva, N., Berkley, K.J., 2006. Cross-organ interactions between reproductive, gastrointestinal, and urinary tracts: modulation by estrous stage and involvement of the hypogastric nerve. Am. J. Physiol. Regul. Integr. Comp. Physiol. 291, R1592–R1601.

Woolf, C.J., Salter, M.W., 2000. Neuronal plasticity: increasing the gain in pain. Science 288, 1765–1769.

Zaafrane, F., Faleh, R., Melki, W., Sakouhi, M., Gaha, L., 2007. An overview of premenstrual syndrome. J. Gynecol. Obstet. Biol. Reprod. (Paris) 36, 642–652.

Musculoskeletal causes and the contribution of sport to the evolution of chronic lumbopelvic pain

6

Bill Taylor   Ruth Lovegrove Jones   Leon Chaitow

CHAPTER CONTENTS

Introduction

Although it is generally accepted that movement changes with pain, there is little agreement regarding the processes that underlie movement changes and their relevance to rehabilitation of musculoskeletal pain (Hodges & Moseley 2003, Tsao et al. 2010). Additionally, one of the main difficulties in the diagnosis of pain in the pelvis is the overlap of signs and symptoms in various conditions, including medical conditions not directly related to musculoskeletal injuries (Nam & Brody 2008). As discussed in Chapters 1, 2, 3, 8 and 12, these can include urinary tract infection, prostatitis and other urinary, bowel and sexual dysfunctions. The urological, neurological, muscular, skeletal and fascial systems may all have a role to play to varying degrees, and consideration of each is necessary to provide a more accurate diagnosis, and a more valid paradigm on which to base treatment. Furthermore, as discussed in Chapter 2, pain perceived to be within the pelvis can be referred from the thoracolumbar spine, sacroiliac joint and the hip (Lee 2004), and since the body operates as a complete movement system, each component of the system is capable of influencing distal and proximal regions.

In this chapter, the authors consider the concept of movement as a physiological system, and describe a method of assessment based on analysis of a patient's movement (dys)function, combined with an assessment of their injury history and pain presentation (Sahrmann 2002). Rehabilitation is then focused upon restoring efficient movement patterns, improving function, and less on treating the pain per se. Manual therapists have traditionally used the client's pain patterns and physical findings, such as pain provocation tests, to identify structures contributing to mechanical pain. However, in the presence of central sensitization and neurogenic pain mechanisms, the reliability of such a pathoanatomical assessment to identify the sources of pain can be limited, particularly as the relationship between pain and the state of the tissues becomes weaker as pain persists (Moseley 2007). Classification of movement patterns, used to identify the mechanical causes of pain, may be similarly limited in the presence of central sensitization, where any mechanical stimulus may be sufficient to generate a painful response. At all times then, current pain physiology, and other contributing factors to chronic pelvic pain (CPP), as discussed in Chapters 1, 2 and 3, need to be considered when assessing the movement system. The role of clinical reasoning is further described in Chapter 7.

Assessment of the movement system

As discussed in Chapters 1 and 2, the movement system is modulated by many factors from across somatic, psychological and social domains (Moseley 2007). It is recognized that the nervous system is likely to coordinate muscle activity to meet the demands for stable movement, so it will not only be affected by the task, posture or movement direction, but potentially the real or perceived risk of injury (Hodges & Cholewicki 2007). Motor changes have been documented to occur throughout the movement system, at the motoneuron level and coordination of muscle behaviour, to changes in organization of the motor cortex (for a review see Tsao et al. 2010). Strategies adopted during pain and injury can increase protection of injured or painful parts, but can have mechanical consequences that may prolong pain states, or result in a higher incidence of recurrence (Hodges & Moseley 2003, van Dieen et al. 2003). In controlled clinical trials, rehabilitation of these motor changes has been linked to clinical improvement, resulting in improvements in pain and dysfunction (Cowan et al. 2003, Ferreira et al. 2006). More recently such improvements have also been shown to be associated with recovery of plastic changes at the motor cortex (Tsao et al. 2010).

Various classifications for the analysis of movement and the sub-classification of movement dysfunction have been proposed (McGill 2002, Sahrmann 2002, McKenzie & May 2003, O'Sullivan 2005) and in some instances are gaining good evidence of validity and reliability (Van Dillen et al. 1998, 2003, Dankaerts et al. 2006, Harris Hayes et al. 2009, 2010). It is beyond the scope of this chapter to describe the benefits and limitations of each classification system; however it is reasonable to suggest that the multidimensional problem of chronic low back and pelvic pain should also encompass biopsychosocial principles (Linton 2000, Waddell 2004, Woby et al. 2004, 2007) which are discussed in Chapter 7. The following section describes the evaluation, classification, and subsequent rehabilitation of lumbopelvic movement disorders based upon the work of Sahrmann (2002).

Sahrmann (2002) suggested a classification system for the analysis of lumbopelvic movement and the subsequent prescription of treatment based on clinically assessed movement system dysfunction. A central tenant of the system is that 'faulty movement can induce pathology, not just be a result of it, and musculoskeletal pain syndromes are seldom caused by isolated events but are the consequence of habitual imbalances in the movement system' (Sahrmann 1993). Therefore, specific postures and movements that produce pain need to be identified and corrected, as misalignment and aberrant movement patterns might result in further pain and future recurrences (Van Dillen et al. 2003).

The objective examination has two major components:

1. The patient reports the response of symptoms to the movement pattern tested, i.e. whether there is an increase or decrease in symptoms;
2. Assessment of bony and/or joint alignment, in various positions, as outlined in Table 6.1.

There are several unique components to this examination system:

1. The effect of active limb movements on spinal movements and symptoms;
2. The relative timing of movements of the spine and proximal joints during limb and trunk movements;
3. The effect on symptoms of modifying lumbar alignment or movement during repetition of a previously symptomatic test (Van Dillen et al. 2003).

Table 6.1 Items from original examination (Van Dillen et al. 1998) proposed as important for classification of mechanical low back pain organized by test position, symptom behaviour with variations of the test position or movements within the test position, and clinical judgements of quality of alignment or movement

Test position	Symptom behaviour with	Judgement of alignment or movement
Standing	• Standing • Posterior pelvic tilt against wall • Forward bending • Corrected† forward bending • Return from forward bending • Corrected return from forward bending • Side bending	• Shape of the lumbar curve (with and without flexible ruler) • Asymmetry of the lumbar curve • Regularity of the lumbar curve (with and without flexible ruler) • Swayback posture • Lumbar flexion • Lumbar extension • Relative flexibility* • Hip extension • Lumbar extension • Pelvic and shoulder sway • Asymmetrical lumbar region movement
Sitting	• Sitting with lumbar region flat • Sitting with lumbar region flexed • Sitting with lumbar region extended • Knee extension • Corrected knee extension	• Lumbar region rotation or pelvic rotation‡
Supine	• Hips and knees flexed • Hips and knees extended	
Hook (crook) lying	• Hip abduction with lateral rotation • Corrected hip abduction with lateral rotation	• Relative flexibility
Prone	• Prone • Corrected prone • Knee flexion • Hip rotation • Hip extension	• Relative flexibility • Asymmetrical pelvic rotation • Relative flexibility • Asymmetrical pelvic rotation
Quadruped	• Natural alignment • Corrected alignment • Arm lifting • Rocking backward • Corrected rocking backward • Rocking forward	• Lumbar region alignment • Asymmetry of the lumbar region • Alignment of hip joint • Asymmetrical lumbar region rotation • Relative flexibility • Pelvic rotation or tilt

*A judgement of relative flexibility refers to a judgement made by the examiner about the relative timing of movement of the lumbar region and the proximal joints when the patient performs a trunk or a limb movement. In general, a patient exhibits a relative flexibility impairment if the lumbar region moves in the first 50% of the range of the overall movement or excessively during the overall movement.

†Corrected test items are follow-up items in which the lumbar region is repositioned to achieve a neutral alignment, or movement of the lumbar region is restricted relative to what was observed with the previous symptomatic test item. The effect of the changes in alignment and movement on symptoms is assessed.

‡Because rotation and side-bending are coupled motions in the lumbar region, items that refer to judgements of alignment and movement of lumbar region rotation or pelvic rotation include side-bending alignment or movement.

The information obtained from this assessment allows the patient to be categorized into one of five different categories, named after the type of mechanical factors hypothesized to be factors in the contribution of mechanical low back pain (MLBP) (Van Dillen et al. 2003):

1. Lumbar flexion;
2. Lumbar extension;
3. Lumbar rotation;
4. Lumbar rotation with extension;
5. Lumbar rotation with flexion.

Although the classifications are termed lumbar movement impairments, the analysis is technically of the lumbopelvic region. Additionally as discussed in Chapters 1, 2 and 3, not only do proximal regions of dysfunction affect distal segments of the movement system, the lumbar spine refers pain to the pelvis and hip and CPP definitions involve the pelvis, anterior abdominal wall, lower back and/or buttocks (ACOG 2004, Fall et al. 2010).

The musculoskeletal factors that need to be considered include the passive and active stiffness of the lumbopelvic spine and hips which will be influenced by muscle and fascial systems, all under neuronal control. Assessment of the neural system is therefore also critical, as irritability of, and the ability of the nerve trunk to glide along its neural canal, will affect the perceived length of the muscle (Hall et al. 1998; Walsh et al. 2009). Structural differences such as bony variation of the pelvis and femur, imbalances of strength, length, timing and magnitude of recruitment of the trunk and hip muscles will also need to be assessed during test movements, as well as specific functional activities.

1. *Lumbar flexion syndrome*: the primary dysfunction in this syndrome is that the lumbar spine range of motion into flexion is more flexible than the hip range of motion into flexion. The habitual movement of the individual is towards flexion with spinal movements and movements of the extremities. The spinal alignment tends to be relatively flexed in different postures (Figure 6.1) and symptoms are elicited and/or aggravated when the patient moves towards the flexed position. When movement into flexion is restricted the symptoms are abolished or diminished. The syndrome is more common in individuals between the ages of 18 and 45 and is more common in males. Habitually flexed work postures or repeated forward bending are often reported, and there is increased relative stiffness in the hip extensors (particularly the hamstrings) relative to the erector spinae (Sahrmann 2002).

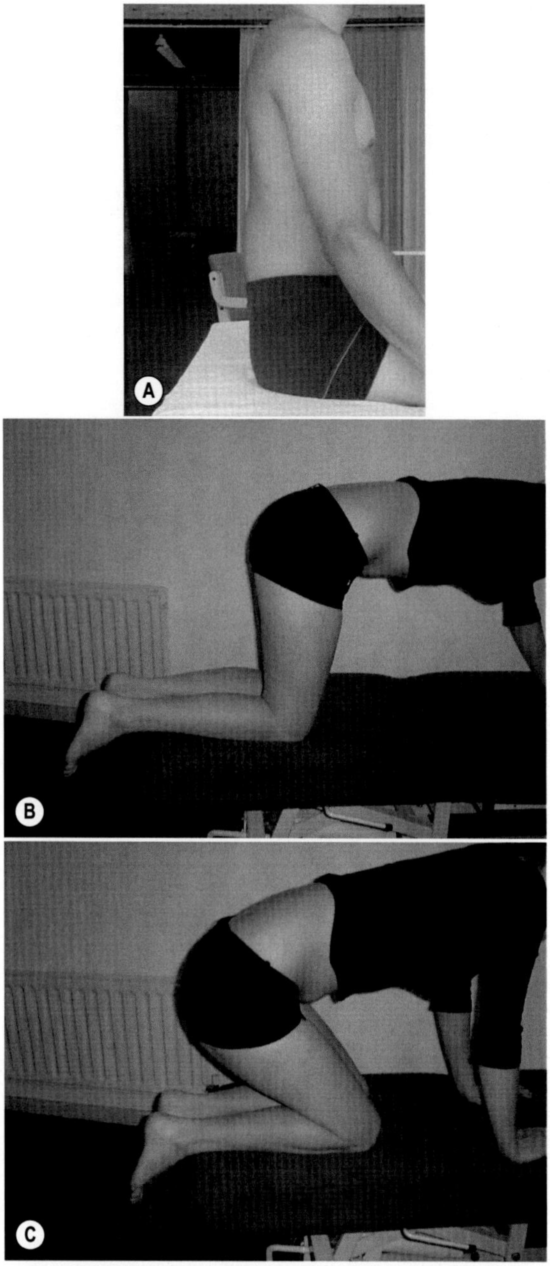

Figure 6.1 • (A) Sitting, (B) quadrupled and (C) backward rocking in relative lumbar spine flexion

2. *Lumbar extension syndrome*: the primary dysfunction in this syndrome is that the lumbar spine range of motion into extension is more flexible than the hip range of motion into extension. Functionally this means that the lumbar spine can extend more readily than the hip extensors can extend the hip (Sahrmann 2002). The hip flexor muscles therefore exert an anterior shear force on

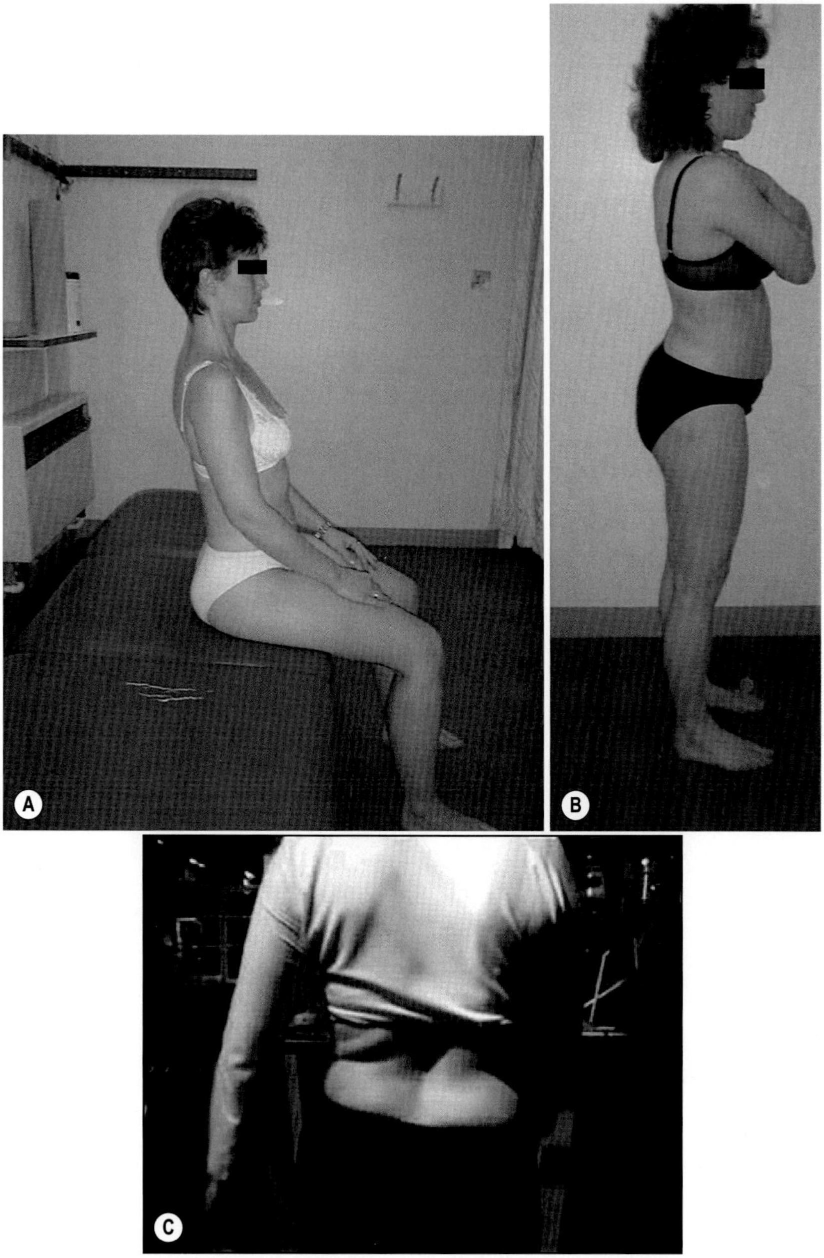

Figure 6.2 • (A) Sitting (B) standing and (C) walking in relative lumbar spine extension

the lumbar spine, as well as a forward rotation moment on the innominates bilaterally. The patient's habitual movement is towards extension with spinal movements and movements of the extremities (Figure 6.2). When movement into extension is restricted the symptoms are abolished or diminished (Sahrmann 2002). The patients are usually over 55 years of age, and there is no reported gender bias. This pattern is often found in patients with acute recurrent low back pain or chronic ongoing low back pain (Sahrmann 2002).

3. *Lumbar rotation syndrome*: this syndrome describes a three-dimensional dysfunction of a spinal segment. The primary dysfunction is increased lumbar segmental rotation, side-flexion and translation, relative to other spinal segments (Sahrmann 2002) (Figure 6.3). These three motions occur together, due to the complex

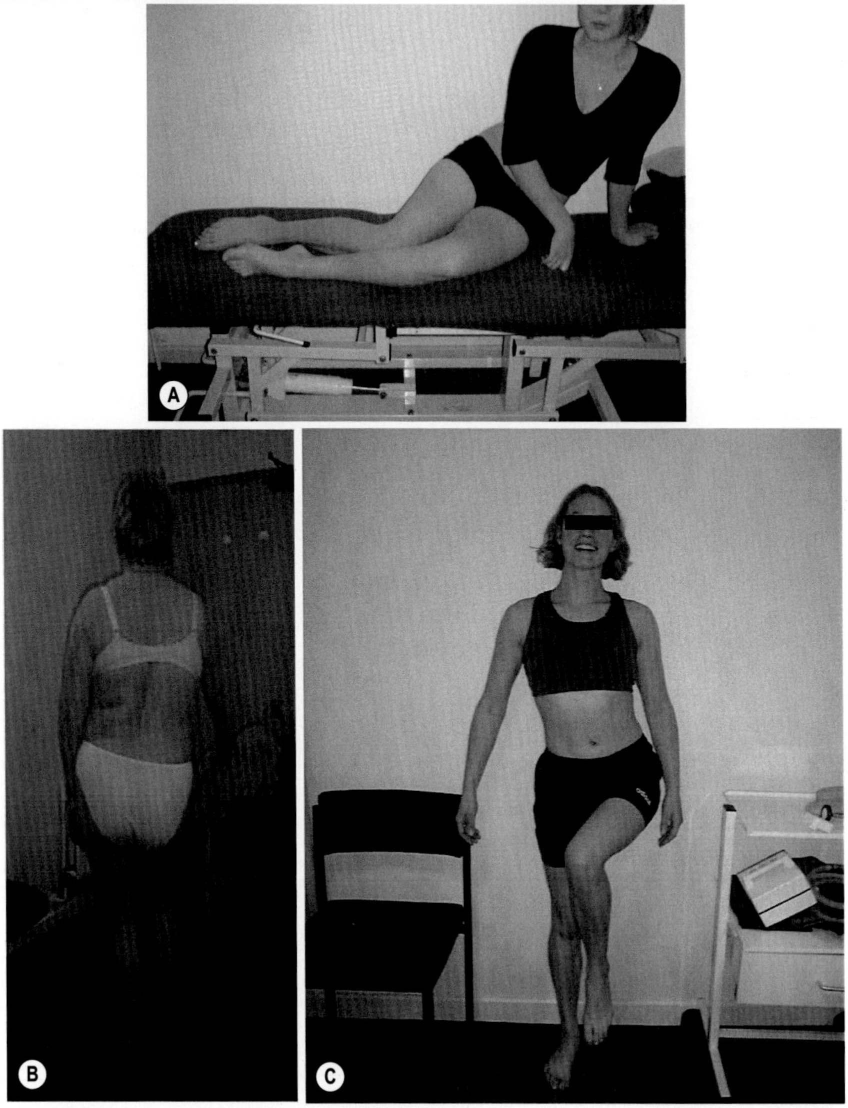

Figure 6.3 • (A) Sitting, (B) standing and (C) hip flexion in relative lumbar spine rotation

interaction of the shape of the Z-joint articular surface, the control of the ligamentous restraint systems, and the flexibility of segmental and global muscle system (White & Punjabi 1990). Clinical spinal instabilities usually involve increased arthrokinematic glides, and fit into this group. The rotational stress on the lumbar spine can be produced directly via lumbar spinal rotation/side-flexion/translation or, indirectly, rotation of the pelvis can produce a relative rotation of the lumbar spine segments (White & Punjabi 1990). In certain patients there is an observable rotation of the lumbar spine whilst in others there is no obvious dysfunction (Sahrmann 2002.) The signs and symptoms are similar to those described for lumbar flexion syndrome; however, they are elicited with spinal rotation, and diminished when lumbar rotation is restricted (Van Dillen et al. 2003).

4. *Lumbar rotation with flexion*: in response to spinal or extremity movement, the patient moves the lumbar spine in the direction of rotation and flexion. The lumbar spine tends to assume a flexed and rotated position in habitual postures. Symptoms are often unilateral, are aggravated by postures involving flexion and rotation and are eased by limitation of flexion and rotation. Symptoms are often aggravated when sitting to standing and functional movements that involve more than one plane (Sahrmann 2002).

5. *Lumbar rotation with extension*: in response to spinal or extremity movement, the patient moves the spine in the direction of rotation with extension. The lumbar spine tends to assume an extended and rotated position with habitual postures. Symptoms are often unilateral and elicited by extension rotation movements of the lumbar spine (Sahrmann 2002). This syndrome is more common in patients over the age of 55 and with a history of chronic low back and pelvic pain. It is also more common in those individuals who participate in sports that involve significant amounts of torsion in the lumbar spine, e.g. golf, squash, tennis and racquetball (Harris-Hayes et al. 2009).

Common postural types (see Kendall et al. 2005, Sahrmann 2002)

Ideal standing posture (Figure 6.4) can be described as a position where:
- A marker on the lateral tip of the acromion, the midpoint of the greater trochanter, the tip of the lateral malleolus, all line up to form an angle of approximately 180°
- The lumbar lordosis, thoracic kyphosis, and pelvic tilt are in neutral
- *Lumbar neutral*: the spinal curve should be 20–30°, there should be less than 1.5 cm (1/2″) difference in prominence of the (L) and (R) region 5 cm (2″) lateral from the spinous process
- *Pelvis neutral*: the line between anterior superior iliac spine (ASIS) and posterior superior iliac spine (PSIS) is within 15° of horizontal line (may vary in women). No lateral tilt or rotation
- *Hip neutral*: no angle between peak of iliac crest, to greater trochanter to line along thigh
- *Knee neutral*

Kyphotic lordotic standing posture (see Figure 6.2B) can be described as a position where:
- A marker on the lateral tip of the acromion, the midpoint of the greater trochanter, the tip of the lateral malleolus, all line up to form an angle greater than 195°, the back is swayed back, the hips swayed forward
- *Lumbar lordosis*: inward curve increased in depth, greater than 30°
- *Thoracic kyphosis*: often increased in depth
- *Pelvis anterior pelvic tilt*: ASIS is 20° lower than PSIS
- *Hips flexed*: Hip angle of flexion, between peak of iliac crest to greater trochanter, to line along thigh is more than 10°

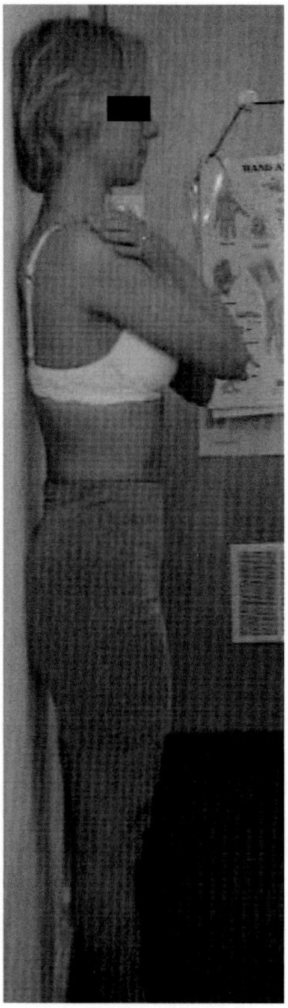

Figure 6.4 • Ideal standing posture

Sway standing posture (Figure 6.5) can be described as a position where:

- A marker on the lateral tip of the acromion, the midpoint of the greater trochanter, the tip of the lateral malleolus, all line up to form an angle less than 165°; the back is swayed back or the hips swayed forward
- *Lumbar lordosis*: often decreased in length.
- *Thoracic kyphosis*: often increased in length, shoulders more than 5 cm posterior to greater trochanter
- *Pelvis neutral to posterior pelvic tilt*: for posterior pelvic tilt, ASIS is 20° higher than PSIS
- *Hips extended*: hip angle of extension, between peak of iliac crest, to greater trochanter to line along thigh is more than 10°
- *Knees hyperextended*: backward bowing of knee joint; tibia may be posterior to femur

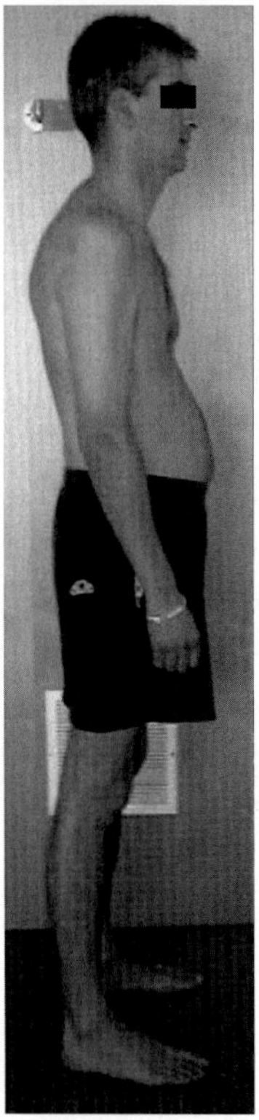

Figure 6.5 • Sway standing posture

Flat back standing posture (Figure 6.6) can be described as a position where:

- A marker on the lateral tip of the acromion, the midpoint of the greater trochanter, the tip of the lateral malleolus, all line up to form an angle of approximately 180°
- *Lumbar lordosis*: flat, absent inward curve (may be normal in men)
- *Thoracic kyphosis*: flat, absent outward curve
- *Pelvis neutral to posterior pelvic tilt*: for posterior pelvic tilt, ASIS is 20° higher than PSIS
- *Hips neutral to extended*: hip angle of extension, between peak of iliac crest, to greater trochanter to line along thigh is more than 10°
- *Knees neutral to hyperextended*: Backward bowing of knee joint, tibia may be posterior to femur

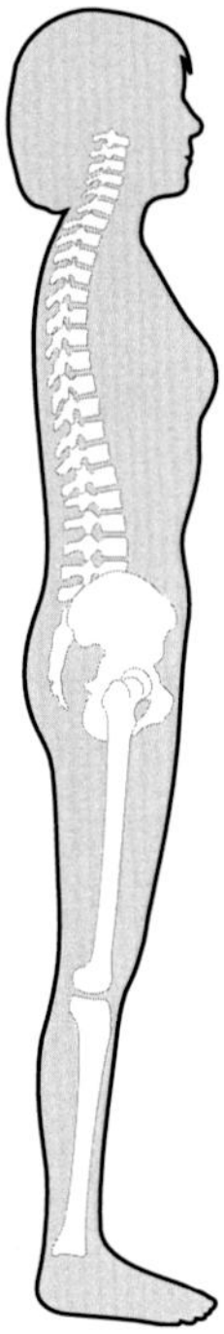

Figure 6.6 • Flat back standing posture

Asymmetry (Figure 6.7): any of the postural shapes above with:

- *Paraspinal asymmetry*: (L) and (R) paraspinal regions from lumbar spinous processes to 5 cm lateral are greater than 1.5 cm difference in prominence
- *Scoliosis/rib hump*: ribs more prominent on one side
- *Lateral tilt*: one iliac crest is more than 1.5 cm higher than other iliac crest (Figure 6.7A,B)
- *Rotation*: ASIS on one side is anterior to ASIS on other side
- *Lateral shift*: the pelvis is shifted away from the midline (Figure 6.7C)

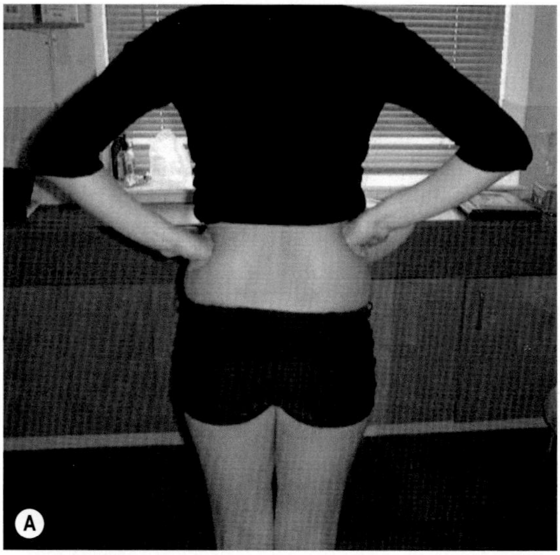

Figure 6.7A • Lateral tilt from behind

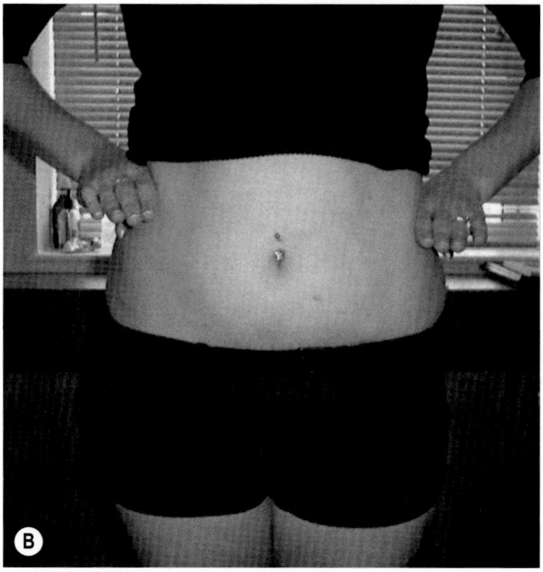

Figure 6.7B • Lateral tilt from front

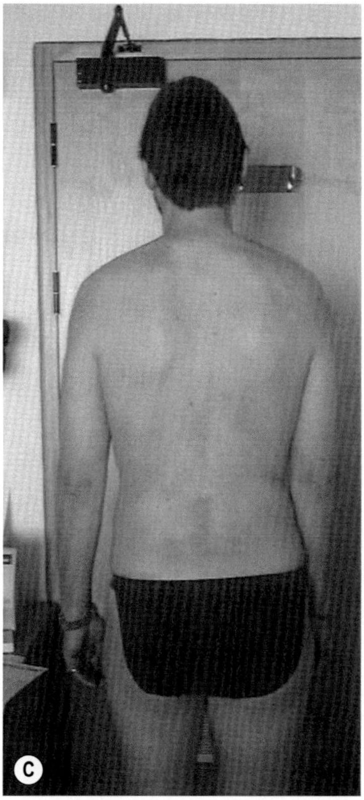

Figure 6.7C • Lateral shift from behind

Table 6.2 shows the proposed MLBP categories with the associated signs, symptoms and general treatment guidelines. Although it should be stressed that this movement assessment system has not yet been fully validated, the construct validity of the movement impairment-based classification system provided support for three out of the five categories (Van Dillen et al. 2003) and recently the inter-tester reliability based on this classification system has been shown to be substantial (Harris-Hayes & Van Dillen 2009).

The aim of the assessment is to identify the postural alignment strategies and the habitual movement patterns which may contribute to the individual's presenting condition. Each syndrome has specific key tests, which help identify the alignment strategies assumed by the individual and confirm the direction of the movement patterns. The patient is then observed during performance of symptom-provoking functional activities, to determine if the same strategies are repeated. Functional instruction is then directed toward modifying the patient's preferred strategies. Exercise prescription is directed toward correcting the patient-preferred movement and alignment strategies identified on examination. Emphasis is on modifying the strategies that (1) are symptom-provoking and (2) can be modified to decrease the patient's symptoms during the examination (Van Dillen et al. 2003). This systematic approach is repeated in order to classify movement impairment syndromes of the hip and is described later in this chapter (Table 6.3). It should also be emphasized that, in the authors' opinion, if the client holds negative beliefs and attitudes associated with pain, such as exhibiting fear-avoidance behaviours without an understanding of current pain biology, the way in which these corrective exercises are explained could contribute to their fear of movement and potentially make their pain problem worse. In this instance, addressing the patients' attitudes, beliefs and understanding needs to be the therapists' main priority (O'Sullivan 2005).

Table 6.2 Proposed mechanical low back pain categories with associated signs and symptoms and general treatment guidelines (taken from Van Dillen et al. 2003)

Category	Associated signs and symptoms	General treatment guidelines
Flexion	Tendency for the patient to move the lumbar spine in the direction of *flexion* with movements of the spine or extremities. Lumbar spine alignment tends to be *flexed* relative to neutral with the assumption of postures. Symptoms occur or increase with positions and movements associated with flexion of the lumbar spine. Symptoms are decreased with restriction of lumbar flexion	*Functional instruction*: 1. Bed positioning/mobility: Don't curl your spine as you sit up in bed. Roll to your side and push yourself up with your arms to come to sitting 2. Sitting: Sit with your back supported, your shoulders over your hips, your hips and knees level, or your knees positioned lower than your hips. You may need a small towel roll in your lower back region for support. Don't sit slumped 3. Sit to stand: Scoot yourself to the edge of the chair keeping your back upright. Get up against the edge of the chair before sitting down. Don't bend in your back getting up and down. Bend the hips and knees 4. Standing: Don't stand with your pelvis swayed forward *Exercise*: 1. Train trunk muscles (paraspinals and abdominals) to work isometrically with performance of limb movements (e.g. standing against a wall, flex shoulders while keeping lumbar region neutral) 2. Training to isolate hip flexion without lumbar spine flexion (e.g. rock backward in quadruped keeping lumbar region neutral) 3. Exercise to increase flexibility of any muscles contributing to lumbar flexion (e.g. stretch gluteus maximus while supine keeping lumbar region supported in neutral) 4. Exercise to shorten muscles that may assist in reducing lumbar spine flexion alignment (e.g. iliopsoas strengthening in sitting while keeping lumbar region neutral) *Support*: 1. Taping of lumbar region to discourage lumbar flexion 2. Use of abdominal support, particularly during activities that encourage lumbar flexion

Table 6.2 Proposed mechanical low back pain categories with associated signs and symptoms and general treatment guidelines (taken from Van Dillen et al. 2003)—cont'd

Category	Associated signs and symptoms	General treatment guidelines
Extension	Signs and symptoms are similar to those described for flexion except that they are associated with *extension* of the lumbar spine. Symptoms are decreased with restriction of lumbar extension	*Functional instruction*: 1. Bed positioning/mobility: Position a pillow(s) under your knees when back lying or under your abdomen when face lying. Slide your legs up so your hips and knees are bent. Avoid allowing your back to arch when you move your legs. Roll to your side moving your trunk and legs together. Drop your legs over the side of the bed as you push yourself up to sitting or lower yourself to side lying 2. Sitting: Sit with your back and feet supported and your hips and knees level. Relax your back against the chair. Don't sit on the edge of the chair 3. Sit to stand: Come forward in chair by pushing with your hands while keeping your back slightly rounded. Lean forward. Push with your legs. As you straighten up don't arch your back; pull in your abdominals. Lean forward when you lower yourself into the chair to sit 4. Standing: Occasionally lean up against a wall with your knees and hips bent slightly. Pull in your abdominals and relax your back against the wall *Exercise*: 1. Training of trunk muscles to work isometrically with performance of limb movements (particularly abdominals) 2. Training to perform hip extension without increased lumbar region extension (e.g. perform return-from-forward bending emphasizing hip extension over lumbar extension) 3. Exercise to increase flexibility of any muscles contributing to lumbar region extension (e.g. bend knee in prone while keeping lumbar region stationary to stretch hip flexors) 4. Exercise to shorten muscles that may assist in reducing lumbar spine extension alignment (e.g. pull in lower abdominals while standing with back against wall and knees and hips flexed slightly)
Rotation	Signs and symptoms are similar to those described for flexion except that they are associated with rotation of the lumbar spine. Symptoms are decreased with restriction of lumbar rotation	*Functional instruction*: 1. Bed positioning/mobility: When side lying, place a pillow(s) between your knees and a towel roll in the area between your ribs and pelvis on the side you are sleeping. Slide your legs up so your hips and knees are bent. Roll to your side moving your trunk and legs together. Drop your legs over the side of the bed as you push yourself up to sitting or lower yourself to side lying. Don't side bend or rotate your trunk as you get up or down from bed 2. Sitting: Sit with your back supported. Don't rotate or side bend your trunk to one side. Don't lean on an elbow for support. Don't cross your legs or sit on one leg. Don't shift from side to side as you sit for prolonged periods 3. Sit to stand: Don't move forward by rotating one hip forward at a time 4. Standing: Don't stand on one leg. Stand with your weight evenly distributed over both legs *Exercise*: 1. Training of trunk muscles (particularly lateral abdominals) to work isometrically with performance of limb movements (e.g. lift one arm in quadruped while holding trunk stationary) 2. Training to isolate hip rotation and hip abduction and adduction without lumbar region rotation or side bending (e.g. laterally rotate and abduct hip in side lying while holding trunk stationary)

Continued

Table 6.2 Proposed mechanical low back pain categories with associated signs and symptoms and general treatment guidelines (taken from Van Dillen et al. 2003)—cont'd

Category	Associated signs and symptoms	General treatment guidelines
		3. Exercise to increase flexibility of any muscles contributing to lumbar region rotation or side bending (e.g. laterally rotate one hip in prone while holding pelvis stationary) 4. Exercise to shorten muscles contributing to lumbar region rotation or sidebending on one side (e.g. laterally rotate and abduct a hip in side lying with pillows between the knees while holding pelvis stationary) *Support*: 1. Taping of lumbar spine region to discourage lumbar region rotation 2. Use of abdominal support, particularly during activities that encourage lumbar region rotation
Rotation with flexion	Tendency for the patient to move the lumbar spine in the direction of *rotation and flexion* with movements of the spine or extremities. Lumbar spine alignment tends to be flexed and rotated relative to neutral with the assumption of postures. Symptoms (often unilateral) occur or increase with positions and movements associated with rotation and flexion of the lumbar spine. Symptoms are decreased with restriction of lumbar rotation and flexion	The same as for the rotation and flexion categories with an emphasis on (1) symmetry of performance of functional activities, (2) attaining symmetry of muscle activity and flexibility with exercises, and (3) support to discourage flexion and asymmetry of alignment and movement of the lumbar region
Rotation with extension	Signs and symptoms are similar to those described for rotation with flexion except that they are associated with **rotation and extension** of the lumbar spine. Symptoms (often unilateral) are decreased with restriction of lumbar rotation and extension	The same as for the extension and the rotation categories with an emphasis on (1) symmetry of performance of functional activities, (2) attaining symmetry of muscle activity and flexibility with exercises, and (3) support to discourage extension and asymmetry of alignment and movement of the lumbar region

Lumbopelvic cylinder and chronic pelvic pain

In the presence of postural changes, respiratory demands, lumbopelvic pain (LPP) and stress incontinence, muscles of the lumbopelvic cylinder (LPC) are altered (Hemborg et al. 1985, Hodges & Richardson 1996, 1998, Hides et al. 1996, Moseley et al. 2002, Hodges & Gandevia 2000, O'Sullivan et al. 2002, Jones et al. 2006, Hodges et al. 2007, Dickx et al. 2008). However, it appears that skilled voluntary activation of muscles with altered motor recruitment can reduce pain, disability and recurrence rate for musculoskeletal conditions (Hides et al. 2001, Cowan et al. 2003, Ferreira et al. 2006), restore motor co-ordination including automatic postural adjustments (Cowan et al. 2003, Tsao & Hodges 2007, 2008), reversing cortical reorganization in people with recurrent pain (Tsao et al. 2010). These findings suggest then, that in addition to the five categories of movement dysfunction described above, muscles of the LPC should be evaluated and rehabilitated, when appropriate, in patients with CPP, although to date there is no scientific trial that has evaluated this clinical approach in this sub-group of chronic pain patients.

The pelvic floor muscles (PFM) form the bottom of the LPC, with the respiratory diaphragm its top, and transversus abdominis (TrA) the sides. The spinal column is part of this cylinder and runs through the middle, supported posteriorly by segmental attachments of lumbar multifidus and anteriorly by segmental attachments of psoas (posterior fasciculii) to the abdominal muscles (Jones 2001). Intra-abdominal pressure (IAP) is generated by co-activation of the PFM, the diaphragm and the abdominal muscles (Hemborg et al. 1985, Hodges & Gandevia 2000), implying that co-ordinated co-activation of the muscles of the LPC is necessary in order to balance the functional demands of continence, respiration and lumbopelvic stability (Hemborg et al. 1985, Hodges & Gandevia 2000, Pool-Goudzwaard et al. 2004, Hodges et al. 2007). Muscles of the LPC work at low levels at all times and increase their activity when the central nervous system can predict timing of increased load, such as occurs in coughing, lifting or limb movements (Constantinou & Govan 1982, Moseley et al. 2002, Barbic et al. 2003). Further details regarding the diaphragm (Chapter 9) and the PFM (Chapter 13) will be found in the appropriate chapters, while the next section describes the assessment and rehabilitation of muscles of the LPC.

Assessment and rehabilitation of muscles of the lumbopelvic cylinder

Voluntary activation of TrA independently from other trunk muscles (Richardson et al. 1999)

Activation of TrA

- Palpate approximately two fingers' breadth down from the anterior superior iliac spine (ASIS) along the inguinal ligament, and one finger's breadth medially
- Ask the patient to breathe in, then on the out-breath to relax and let go of the stomach. Ask the patient to then draw in the low lateral abdominal wall (below the umbilicus) as if to pull the stomach away from the pant (knicker) elastic and breathe normally (Figure 6.8)

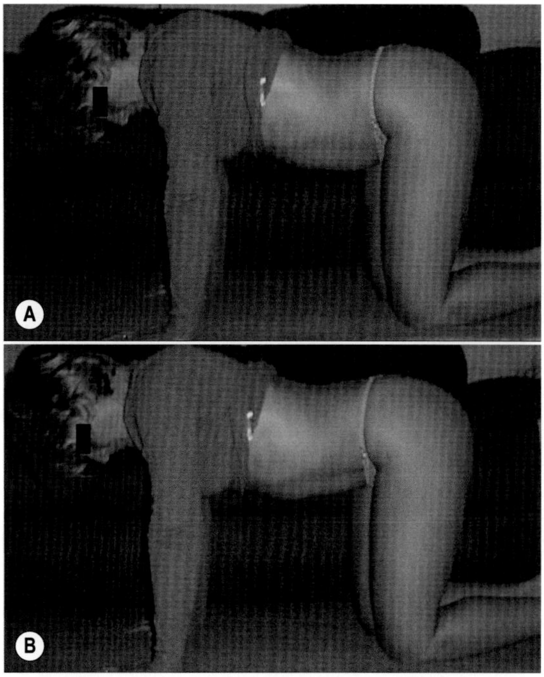

Figure 6.8 • (A) Relaxed abdomen in 4 point kneeling; (B) activation of TrA

Continued

- Palpate for a symmetrical tensioning, without excessive bulging, underneath the palpating fingertips, or verify with real-time ultrasound imaging to observe thickening and shortening of the abdominal muscle (Hodges et al. 2003)
- Once the patient can activate TrA with minimal activity of the abdominal muscles, they should hold the contraction, whilst breathing normally, for up to 10 seconds
- Three sets of ten repetitions, twice a day, has been shown to be effective (Tsao & Hodges 2008)

Common substitution patterns or faults

- Movement of the trunk or pelvis out of a neutral position
- Asymmetry
- Breath holding, apical breathing
- Drawing in of the upper abdominal wall
- Rib cage depression with a decrease of the infrasternal angle
- Lateral flaring or bulging of the waist
- Excessive superior, inferior or lateral movement of the umbilicus
- Bearing down of the pelvic floor (Valsalva)

Facilitation techniques for TrA

- Alternative starting positions such as crook lying, 4-point kneeling, side lying, standing, sitting forward lean, prone
- Visualize the lower abdomen as an old-fashioned corset, and as the stays are drawn in, the waist narrows and flattens, into an hourglass shape
- Ensure that the abdomen is relaxed to start with, often easier in sitting or standing forward lean, 4-point kneeling, prone
- Tactile feedback: ask the patient to put one hand above the umbilicus and one hand below, as soon as movement is felt above the umbilicus, drawing in should cease. Tactile feedback: ask patient to palpate you, noting the difference between bulging and tensioning, then to self-palpate
- Facilitation using the PFM which can be particularly useful for asymmetry of contraction (Chapter 13) as can psoas activation (described later)

Assessment and rehabilitation of muscles of the lumbopelvic cylinder

Voluntary activation of pelvic floor muscles (Laycock & Jerwood 2001, Messelink et al. 2005)

Activation and facilitation of PFM

- In a supine, crook lying position with a pillow under the head and legs supported, the International Continence Society (ICS) guidelines to facilitate a PFM contraction are 'squeeze the muscles of the pelvic floor as if attempting to stop the flow of urine or prevent wind or flatus escaping' (Messelink et al. 2005)
- Recent research and clinical experience have suggested that the addition of 'squeeze around the back passage, as if you were trying to prevent breaking wind (flatus), bring that feeling forward towards the urethra/pubic bone and then lift, as if you were elevating the PFM, whilst breathing normally' elicits a consistent PFM contraction, resulting in a cranioventral lift of the PFM and pelvic organs (Lovegrove Jones 2010)
- With consent, confirm the ability of the volunteer to perform an elevating, sustained PFM contraction by vaginal or rectal palpation, real-time perineal (Figure 6.9) or transabdominal ultrasound (Figure 6.10).

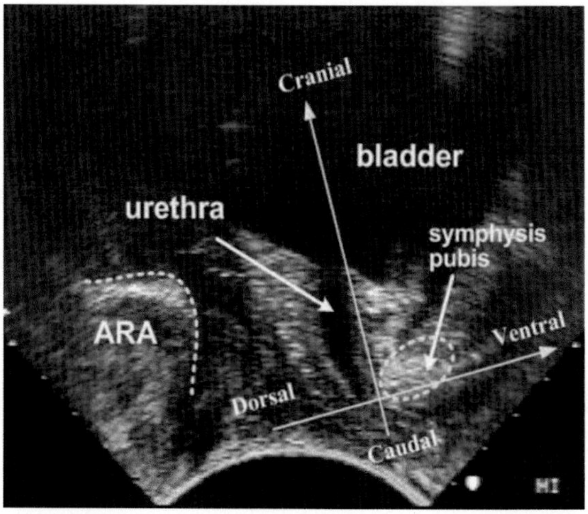

Figure 6.9 • Typical perineal ultrasound image. Voluntary activation of PFM produces a cranioventral lift of the pelvic floor and organs. ARA, anorectal angle

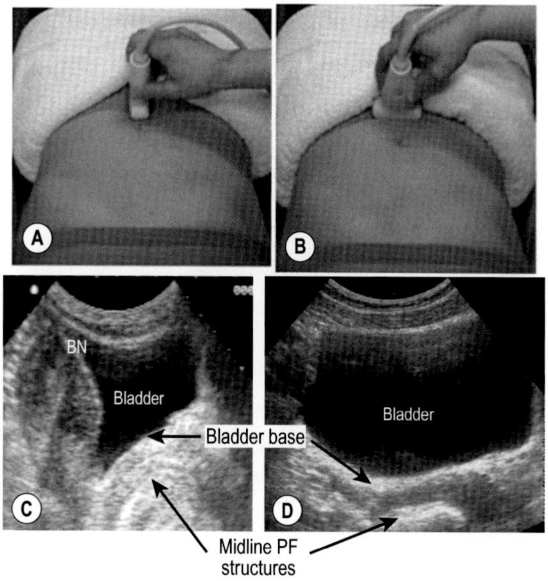

Figure 6.10 • Transabdominal ultrasound transducer placement for (A) sagittal and (B) transverse ultrasound imaging of the bladder. Reproduced from Whittaker (2007) Ultrasound Imaging for Rehabilitation of the Lumbopelvic Region: A Clinical Approach. Typical sagittal (C) and transverse (D) plane transabdominal view of the bladder, bladder base and midline pelvic floor (PF) structures. BN, bladder neck

The patient should have a sensation of a 'lifting' rather than 'bearing down' contraction, which can also be verified by observation of the perineum 'lifting'. If verification is not possible in any of the ways described, palpating abdominally, approximately two fingers' breadth down from the ASIS along the inguinal ligament and one finger's breadth medially, as in the evaluation of a TrA contraction above, will give an indication of whether co-activation of TrA and the PFM has occurred. Recent evidence has indicated the presence of co-activation in healthy continent and incontinent women (Sapsford et al. 2001, Urquhart et al. 2005, Jones et al. 2006)

- Once the patient can activate the PFM they should hold the contraction whilst breathing normally for up to 10 seconds. The co-ordination of a pelvic floor contraction and normal relaxed breathing seems to be very difficult for some subjects. If this is the case then repeated practice is advised, using low effort. The ability to voluntarily relax the PFM after contraction (Messelink et al. 2005), particularly with PFM overactivity, is essential and the presence of pain on voluntary contraction should be noted (see Chapter 13)

Voluntary activation of deep segmental lumbar multifidus

(Richardson et al. 1999)

Activation of multifidus

- In prone lying (often over a pillow is helpful), palpate the medial paraspinal muscles at each segmental level in turn, just to the side of the lumbar vertebrae and let them sink firmly into the muscle
- Instruct the patient to take a breath in, then on the breath out to relax and let go of the stomach. Slowly and gently hollow and pull up the lower stomach towards the spine, and gently swell the muscles into the palpating fingertips
- Palpate for a symmetrical tensioning, underneath the palpating fingertips or verify with real-time ultrasound imaging to observe thickening of the muscle (Hides et al. 1992)
- Once the patient can activate multifidus they should hold the contraction whilst breathing normally for up to 10 seconds

Common substitution patterns or faults

- Asymmetry of contraction
- Breath holding
- Bracing and increasing IAP with overactivation of abdominals resulting in movement of the trunk or pelvis out of a neutral position into spinal flexion or posterior tilt

Facilitation techniques for multifidus

- Visualization of the muscle as deep triangles that extend down and out from each of the spinous processes
- Instruct the patient to feel the contraction on you first, to understand the concept of an isometric swelling contraction
- Other starting positions such as side lying, standing or sitting
- In standing, move from a position of upright standing to sway, palpating the differences in tension of the medial paraspinals

Continued

- In standing, palpate the dysfunctional multifidus with one hand and lift the opposite arm forward and away from the body from 0° to 90°, palpating the superficial fibres changes in tension. Sustain the contraction when multifidus activity decreases. Maintain active muscle tension during slow, repetitive arm flexion. Maintain this multifidus contraction and keep tension in the muscle during slow arm movements with relaxed breathing (Figure 6.11A)
- In walk stance, with full weight on the rear foot, palpate the tension in the dysfunctional multifidus muscle on the rear foot side, and move the body weight forward onto the front foot. Multifidus should activate just after heel lift. Try to sustain the contraction during slow weight transfer with relaxed breathing (Figure 6.11B)

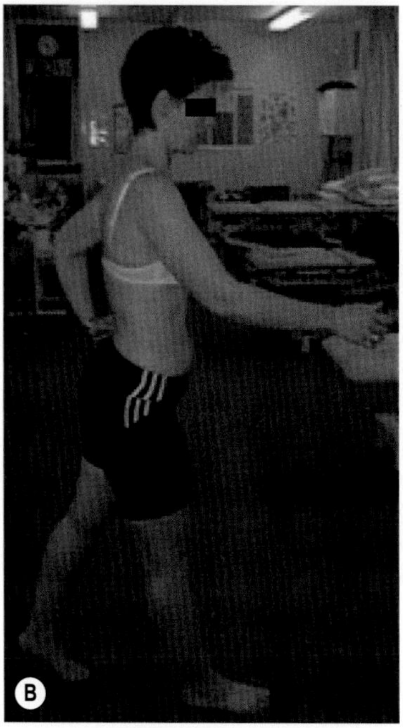

Figure 6.11B • Walk stance

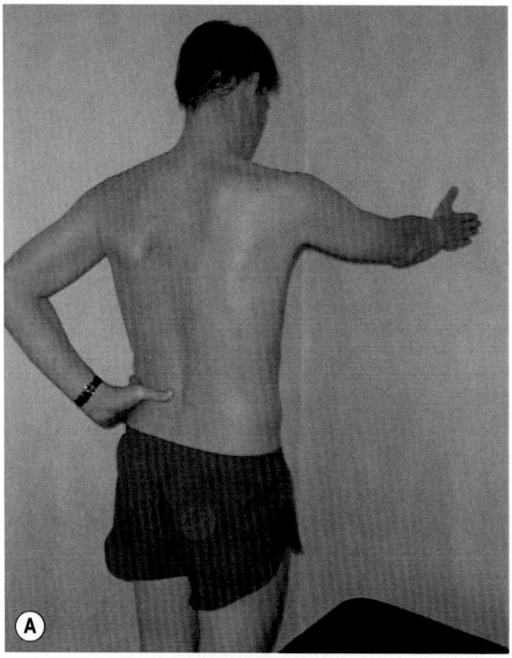

Figure 6.11A • Contralateral arm lift

Voluntary activation of the posterior fasciculii of psoas
(Gibbons et al. 2002)

Activation and facilitation of the posterior fasciculii of psoas

- With both the lumbar spine and hip in neutral, gently distract the femur in supine or side lying (Figure 6.12). Maintain the distraction and instruct the patient to take a breath in, then on the out-breath to relax and let go of the stomach, whilst slowly and gently drawing in or shortening the hip into the acetabulum without moving the pelvis or lumbar spine. It may be helpful to push the femur into the acetabulum several times to give the sensation of the action required
- Then palpate both the anterior superior iliac spine (ASIS) and the soft tissue below in the anterolateral groin (5 cm below the ASIS). The upper finger assesses for control of movement of the pelvis and maintenance of the lumbopelvic neutral position while the lower finger checks for excessive activity in rectus femoris and sartorius
- Once the therapist is confident that the patient is able to activate the muscle, the patient lies in prone on the plinth with one leg firmly extended to help maintain balance, and the other leg hanging freely over the edge with the foot on the floor. The side with the leg hanging freely is the side to be assessed. In pelvis and lumbar neutral with the trunk muscles relaxed, each lumbar vertebral level is manually palpated to assess the relaxed joint play displacement in the transverse and anterior directions. When the patient then facilitates the psoas contraction, each vertebral level is repalpated to assess the contracted joint play in the transverse and anterior directions. Ideally, there should be a significant palpable increase in resistance to manual displacement (stiffness) at each level

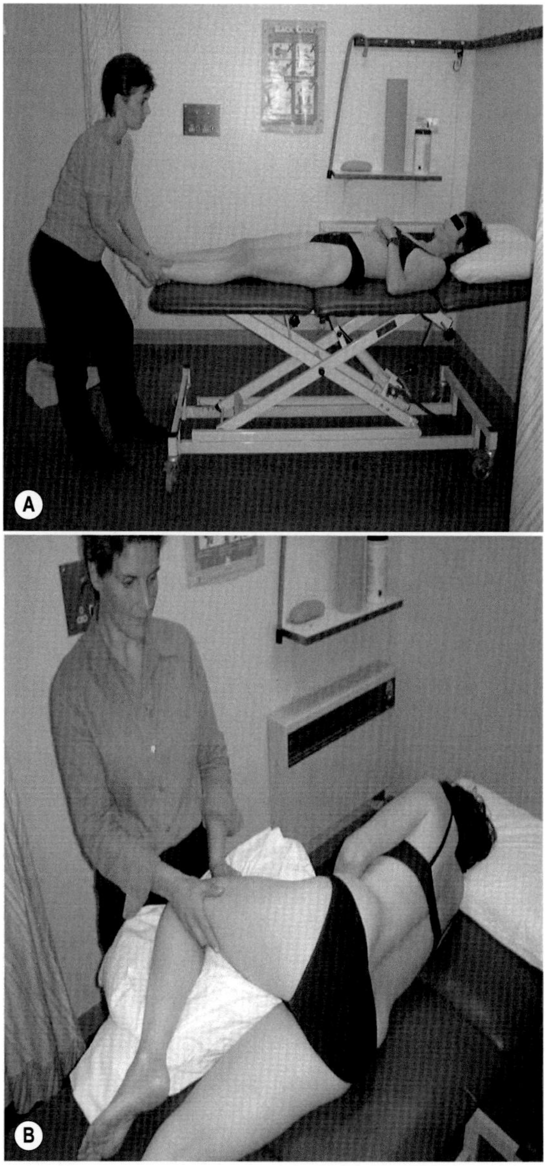

Figure 6.12 • Facilitation of the longitudinal action of posterior fasciculii of psoas muscle in (A) supine and (B) side lying

Common substitution patterns or faults

- Movement of the trunk or pelvis out of a neutral position
- Pushing down with the contralateral leg to provide stability for the trunk
- Dominant or excessive activation of rectus femoris, tensor fascia lata or trunk muscles indicated by a resistance to passive rotation of the hip or pelvis. Suggest that the patient uses less effort

Integration of voluntary activation of the lumbopelvic cylinder into function

When muscles of the LPC are working efficiently, voluntary and involuntary activation of any one muscle, should elicit a co-contraction with the others. Although this has been shown with TrA, multifidus and the PFM (Sapsford et al. 2001, Richardson et al. 2002, Urquhart et al. 2005, Jones et al. 2006), to date this has not been scientifically verified with posterior fasciculii of psoas muscle. However, in the authors' clinical opinion, particularly when asymmetry of contraction is observed in the PFM or TrA contraction, using the methods to elicit a psoas contraction has been effective to facilitate activation (of TrA or PFM) on the deficient side. Once the patient is able to elicit a satisfactory co-contraction of the muscles of the LPC, the activation of these muscles should be incorporated into previously aggravating static postures and functional tasks (O'Sullivan et al. 1997). The ability to immediately perform a task without pain with the addition of a voluntary activation of any of the muscles of the LPC can be a powerful rehabilitation tool, significantly reduce fear of movement, and change attitudes and beliefs about what the pain means to the patient. However, skilled training of sustained voluntary activation of TrA in supine, without integrating into function, was sufficient to reduce pain, disability and create reorganization of the motor cortex in individuals with recurrent low back pain (Tsao & Hodges 2008, Tsao et al. 2010).

The neural system and chronic pelvic pain

As discussed in Chapters 2, 3 and elsewhere, the nervous system is likely to coordinate muscle activity to meet the demands for stable movement, so it will not only be affected by the task, posture, movement direction, but potentially by high real, or perceived, risk of injury (Hodges & Cholewicki 2007). The assessment of the relative stiffness of the global pelvic and hip musculature and muscles of the LPC will therefore allow the *current* relative stiffness between the proximal and distal movement systems to be evaluated, so that treatment can then be targeted at the specific dysfunction. Another potential confounding variable in the assessment of muscle length and relative stiffness is the range of motion of joints associated with the muscle (Kendall et al. 2005). Hence in order to accurately assess the length of a muscle, knowledge of the underlying joint range of motion is essential. Muscle tissue consists of both contractile and non-contractile components, and a shortened muscle may be due to decreased length in the non-contractile component, increased tone in the contractile component, or neurogenic/neuropathic components. As mentioned earlier, assessment of the neural system is crucial to the full understanding of pelvic dysfunction as the ability of the nerve trunk to glide along its neural canal, will influence the perceived length of the muscle (Hall et al. 1998, Walsh et al. 2009). As described in Chapter 2, there are a number of significant nerves around the pelvis which are associated with CPP, and some of them are amenable to direct assessment, such as the sciatic, femoral and pudendal nerves. For example in lumbar-pelvic flexion dysfunction, the hips will be relatively stiff in flexion compared to the lumbopelvic spine. Whether this is due to, for example, short, stiff hamstrings, long erector spinae, or an irritable sciatic nerve will need to be assessed by the examiner. Similarly, in lumbopelvic extension dysfunction, one or more of the hip flexors could be stiff relative to the abdominal muscles, or the client may have restricted hip motion due to joint degeneration, or the femoral nerve may also restrict hip extension, and will need to be evaluated. To differentiate muscle stiffness from increased neural mechanosensitivity limiting the apparent length of a muscle, the use of differentiation via slump testing, cervical spine movement or ankle dorsiflexion will be essential (Hall et al. 1998, Walsh & Hall 2009, Walsh et al. 2009).

Additionally, as discussed in Chapter 14, patients with CPP experience changes in the fascial system which may result in restrictions of neural or soft tissue movement. Assessment of this system will rely upon skilled observation of the tissues surrounding the pelvic region: especially the areas of the anterior thigh, inguinal region, anterior abdominal and trunk region, posterior trunk region, peri-perineal area and transperineal area. Clinical reasoning is explored further in Chapter 7.

Sporting activities and chronic pelvic pain

As discussed above, musculoskeletal causes of CPP are many and varied, but sport and leisure activities can result in an increased risk of sustaining an injury, particularly when the activities in question are excessively pursued early in life (Antolak et al. 2002). Failure to recognize and diagnose musculoskeletal injuries in difficult-to-access regions of the pelvis and pelvic floor myofascial system can potentially result in an acute impairment becoming a chronic disability. People with LPP who regularly participate in sports requiring repeated rotation of the trunk and hips have less overall passive hip rotation motion and more asymmetry of rotation between sides, than people without LPP (Van Dillen et al. 2008). These findings suggest that the specific directional demands imposed on the hip and trunk during regularly performed activities may be an important consideration in prevention and intervention of sporting injuries involving the lumbopelvic area.

In general though, studies suggest a therapeutic effect from aerobic exercise in CPP (Giubilei et al. 2007) with inactivity associated with negative long-term effects (Orsini et al. 2006). However there remains some controversy regarding the role of cycling and urogenic disorders (Taylor III et al. 2004, Sommer et al. 2010). Some researchers suggest a significant relationship between cycling-induced perineal compression leading to vascular, endothelial and neurogenic dysfunction with the development of erectile dysfunction (ED) (Sommer et al. 2010), and others imply that the overall prevalence of ED in the cycling community does not appear to be greater than that of historical controls (Taylor III et al. 2004). It should be emphasized that exercise in general and non-impact aerobic-cardiovascular exercise in particular have extensive support in the medical literature over a period of greater than five decades (Brock 2005) and should be encouraged.

The following section discusses the general effect of aerobic activity on CPP followed by specific groin injuries, with a classification of movement impairment syndromes of the hip to aid assessment and rehabilitation. This is followed by a discussion on cycling and other sporting activities associated with CPP.

The effect of aerobic exercise on chronic pelvic pain

A sedentary lifestyle has been shown to be a risk factor for CPP (Orsini et al. 2006). Orsini et al. (2006) analysed surveys from 30 000 Swedish men aged between 45 and 70 years of age and concluded that those men who were physically active at work and pursued an active lifestyle in their leisure time showed a 50% reduction in their risk of severe lower urinary tract symptoms, compared to inactive men. Inactivity of greater than 5 hours a day (at age 30 plus) was associated with a twofold increased risk in developing symptoms. The authors concluded that physical activity in young and late adulthood appears to be associated with a lower risk of moderate and severe urinary tract symptoms. In a double-blind, randomized controlled trial, Giubilei et al. (2007) compared the effects of an aerobic exercise programme (n = 52) versus placebo/stretching and motion exercises (n = 51) on a group of previously sedentary men. The cohort was recruited from a volunteer sample of 231 men who had at least a 12-month diagnosis of chronic prostatitis/CPP syndrome, who had not responded to conventional treatment for CPP and had no contraindications to moderately intense physical exercise. The aerobic exercise protocol included:

- A warm-up and cool-down regimen of slow-paced walking;
- Postural muscle isometric strengthening;
- 40 minutes of fast-paced outdoor walking – at 70–80% maximum heart rate.

The control group performed flexibility and motion exercises for the same length of time and frequency, but exercised at a level of a steady heart rate of 100 beats per minute. The results showed improvement in both groups at the end of the 18-week exercise period; however the improvements in the aerobic exercise group were significantly better compared to those in the placebo/stretching group. Despite the small numbers in the study and the short length of the follow-up, the authors recommended aerobic exercise as a valid treatment option in the treatment of CPP, until further studies could confirm or repudiate their findings.

Specific groin injuries

Sports which include kicking, side-to-side cutting, interval sprinting, rapid or sudden changes of direction, quick accelerations and decelerations, repetitive hip and pelvic girdle rotation with axial loading such as running, golfing, ice hockey, figure skating, football, baseball, ballet, martial arts and gymnastics have a high incidence of groin injuries (Cowan et al. 2003, Verral et al. 2002, Pizzari et al. 2008, Shindle et al. 2007). According to Lovell (1995) in Nam et al. (2008), determining a differential diagnosis is essential, as 27–90% of patients who present with groin pain present with more than one injury. These co-existing injuries are thought to arise due to an initial injury altering the complicated biomechanics of the hip and groin, leading to secondary overuse injuries and/or the close proximity of anatomical elements in the region, predisposing one insult to involve adjacent structures (Morelli & Weaver 2005). Furthermore, in the sporting arena, the primary source of specialist consultation is the orthopaedic surgeon who may perform a wide-ranging assessment of the musculoskeletal system with no real evaluation of pelvic girdle mobility or pelvic floor musculature. The patient is unlikely to be asked about urinary, bowel or sexual dysfunction, and often the patient does not volunteer this information unless prompted. Likewise the urological specialist will provide a thorough assessment and examination of the pelvic floor, bladder and bowel, with no musculoskeletal component to the assessment. As described in previous chapters, many patients with CPP have a complex presentation and may well fit in to more than one diagnostic category, resulting in a 'best fit' diagnosis. If the signs and symptoms do not fit neatly into a diagnostic category then a more creative approach to the assessment of the patient's condition is warranted.

The common types of groin injuries are listed below (see also Table 6.4):

- Ligament and muscle strains/tendonitis/tendonoses/bursitis
  - Iliopsoas
  - Piriformis/obturator internus/obturater externus/gemelli
  - Sartorius/gracilis
  - Adductor magnus/brevis/longus/pectineus/gracilis
  - Hamstring insertional injuries
- Acetabular tears
- Osteitis pubis
- Athletic pubalgia or sports hernias
- Avulsion and stress fractures
  - Anterior inferior iliac spine – rectus femoris and gracilis
  - Adductors at the pubic rami
  - Hamstrings at the ischial tuberosity
  - Femoral neck
  - Pubic rami

- Nerve compression injuries
  - Obturator nerve
  - Femoral nerve
  - Iliohypogastric nerve
  - Genitofemoral nerve
  - Ilioinguinal nerve
  - Lateral femoral cutaneous nerve of the thigh
  - Pudendal nerve

Ligament and muscle strain

The most common site of strain is the musculotendinous junction of the adductor longus or gracilis muscle and is the most common cause of groin pain in the athlete (Reid 1992). The incidence among soccer players is between 10% and 18% (Nielsen & Yde 1989). Muscular and tendinous assessment can be performed using Cyriax's Soft Tissue Tension Differentiation Tests, which involve palpation of the muscle over the area of strain and the elicitation of pain on resisted adduction and passive stretch into abduction (Ombregt et al. 2002). The history of the injury usually provides information about the biomechanical forces involved and the likely tissues involved, and the use of real time ultrasound imaging can help confirm or exclude the diagnosis of tendonosis/tendonitis or muscle tear (Heyde et al. 2005). Care must be taken to differentiate muscle strains and tendonoses/itis from osteitis pubis, sports hernias and nerve entrapment (described below), which can present with similar symptoms (Morelli & Weaver 2005). In cases where athletes recall a traumatic event, which results in the acute onset of symptoms, the diagnosis is more straightforward (Reid 1992). When the onset of symptoms is insidious a definitive diagnosis is difficult to make and often patients in this category are difficult to treat with orthodox protocol for adductor strains. It is these patients who present with ambiguous signs and symptoms that appear to fit into the CPP category as soft tissue differentiation tests can often be equivocal. For example, during active contraction of the adductors, which insert directly into the ramus of the pubis, stress on the symphyseal tissue can reproduce the patient's symptoms and produce a false-positive test. This is usually confirmed by a lack of insertional tenderness and absence of pain on passive stretch (Ombregt et al. 2002). If an adductor strain is suspected, the tear has to be accurately located and this requires accurate and precise knowledge of functional anatomy (Figure 6.13). There is a need to know whether the strain has occurred in the belly of the muscle or the musculotendinous junction rather than the insertion into the pubic bone. This will in part determine how aggressive the treatment programme can be (Fricker 1997), as insertional strains will require an initial period of rest before active rehabilitation can begin (Reid 1992). Decreased abductor range of motion and decreased adductor strength are associated with an increased incidence of adductor strains (Ekstrand & Gillquist 1983, Tyler et al. 2001). Biomechanical abnormalities of the lower limb, imbalance of the surrounding hip musculature, and muscular fatigue have also been hypothesized to increase the risk of adductor strain (Holmich et al. 1999). Prevention programmes focused on eliminating some of these abnormalities have been shown to be effective in professional hockey players, although there have been no controlled clinical studies proving these latter elements to be causative (Tyler et al. 2002).

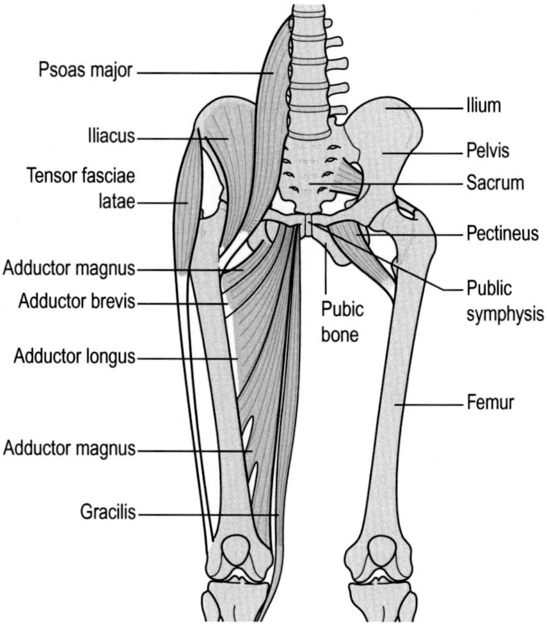

Figure 6.13 • Bony pelvis showing insertion of the adductor group of muscles

Iliopsoas originates from the transverse processes and anterior vertebral bodies of the lumbar vertebrae passing inferiorly to insert on the lesser trochanter of the femur. It traverses the pelvic rim, and crosses the hip joint and it is at this point that the iliopsoas bursa is interposed between the muscle and the underlying bone. The iliopsoas bursa (Figure 6.14) is the largest bursa in the body and has

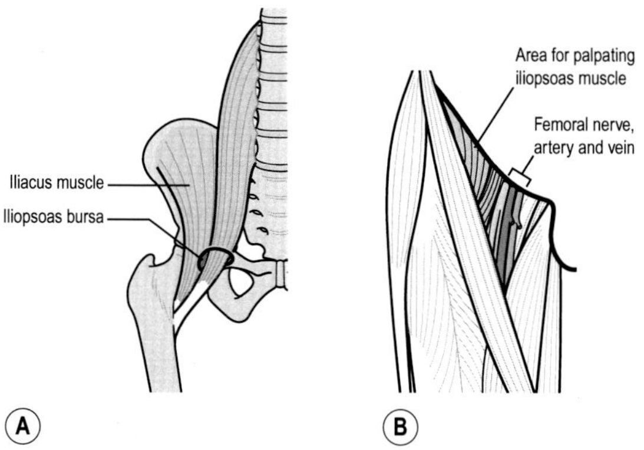

Figure 6.14 • Location of iliopsoas and the bursa (A), and area of palpation (B)

a direct communication with the hip joint in 15% of patients (Standring 2008) and is best visualized on MRI scan (Reid 1992). The bursa and tendon can become irritated as they rub over the iliopectineal eminence of the pubis, particularly in sports requiring a significant use of the hip flexors, so is common amongst football players, ballet dancers, hurdlers and martial arts experts (Hackney 1993). Bursitis can be characterized by a deep groin pain, difficult for patients to localize and to reproduce, which occasionally radiates to the anterior hip. Due to poor localization and reproducibility of the pain, the average time from onset of symptoms to diagnosis is 32–41 months (Johnston et al. 1998). There is tenderness below the lateral inguinal ligament over the femoral triangle, adjacent to the femoral artery, where the musculotendinous junction of the iliopsoas muscle can be palpated (Figure 6.15). The pain can be reproduced by stretching the iliopsoas; however, care must be taken to differentiate the pain in psoas bursitis from femoral nerve irritation and conditions of the hip such as anterior hip impingement syndrome. Pain may also be reproduced when the flexed, abducted, externally rotated hip is extended and brought back into a neutral position (extension test) or have the supine athlete raise his or her heels off the table to about 15° (Morelli & Weaver 2005).

Trigger points associated with the muscles around the pelvis and hip are discussed in Chapter 14.

Acetabular tears and impingements of the hip

Acetabular labral tears are a recently recognized source of hip pain, particularly in the anterior hip or groin region (Lewis & Sahrmann 2006). Femoro-acetabular impingement of the hip is a soft tissue impingement of the acetabular-labrum complex, which may or may not include the capsule, psoas tendon or bursa. Upon further evaluation, studies have indicated that 22% of athletes with groin pain (Narvani et al. 2003) and 55% of patients with mechanical hip pain of unknown aetiology (McCarthy et al. 2001) have a labral tear. Except in cases of specific trauma, the aetiology of labral tears is often difficult to determine and can evade detection by non-invasive means. The pain and disability can be severe, with a sudden onset of symptoms, but an acetabular labral tear should also be suspected when a patient with normal radiographs complains of a long duration of anterior hip pain and clicking, with minimal to no restriction in range of movement (ROM). A wide range of provocative tests have been reported, but typically it is confirmed with pain on passive hip flexion combined with adduction and medial (internal) rotation, and pain with a resisted active straight leg raise (Farjo et al. 1999, Hase & Ueo 1999, McCarthy et al. 2001, Mason 2001, Binningsley 2003). Other reported tests are:

- Flexion with medial rotation alone or combined with adduction or axial compression;
- Flexion with lateral (external) rotation;
- Hip extension alone or combined with medial rotation.

Whether these other tests were performed actively or passively was not specified and the sensitivity and specificity of these tests have yet to be published. In six professional soccer players with anterior labral tears, Saw & Villar (2004) found that all of the players had significant pain with combined hip flexion, medial rotation and adduction. Mitchell et al. (2003) reported that the flexion–abduction–external rotation (FABER) test elicited pain in 88% of patients (15 of 17) with intra-articular pathology, but they did not find any correlation between a positive FABER test result and different types of hip joint pathology.

The wide range of provocative tests may be attributable to differences in the location of the tear. In 56 hips of 55 patients, Fitzgerald (1995) used two different clinical tests that provoked symptoms in 54 patients, depending on tear location. To identify an anterior labral tear, the patient's leg was brought into full flexion, lateral rotation and full abduction and then extended with medial rotation and adduction. To identify a posterior labral tear, the patient's leg

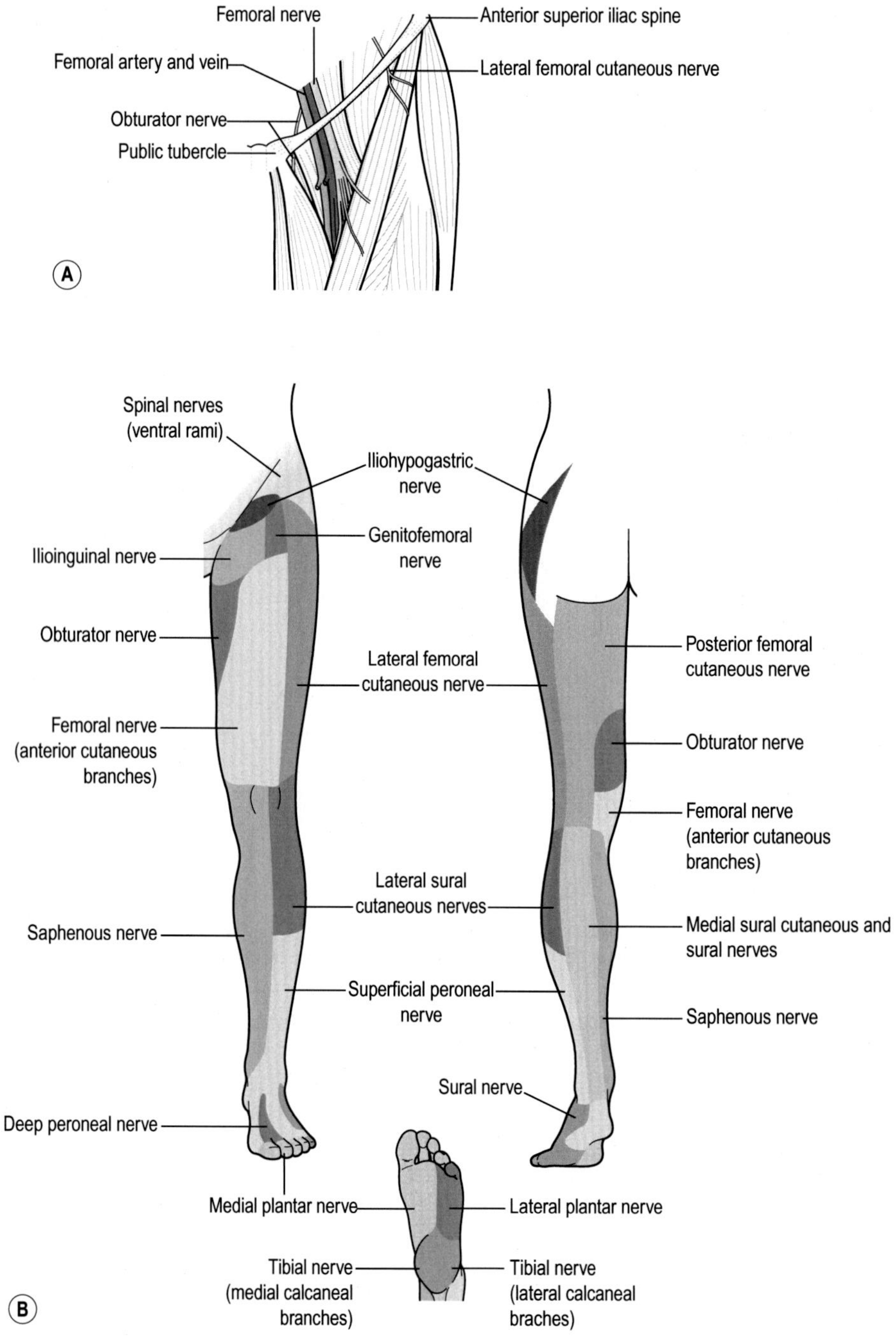

Figure 6.15 • Nerves of the thigh and distribution

was brought into extension, abduction and lateral rotation and then flexed with medial rotation and adduction. If a labral tear is present, these manoeuvres will result in sharp pain with or without a click (Fitzgerald 1995).

Once a labral tear is diagnosed, to date conservative medical treatment has not proven to be effective, and the appropriate physical therapy intervention has yet to be established. Surgical treatment results in short-term improvement, but the long-term outcomes are still unknown (Tyler & Slattery 2010). As labral tears have been associated with a higher risk for joint degeneration, this area warrants further investigation, especially with regard to prevention, early detection, appropriate physical therapy and medical treatment (Lewis & Sahrmann 2006).

Osteitis pubis

The name osteitis pubis (OP) suggests inflammation, however it appears to involve a degenerative rather than an inflammatory process, characterized by symphysis pubis (SP) pain, with occasional referral along the adductor muscles to the hip, superiorly to the lower abdominal region and posteriorly towards the perineum and scrotum in men (Hackney 1993). OP can produce symptoms of exercise-induced pain in the inner thigh and abdominal area which come on gradually and worsen as the activity progresses. Examination reveals tenderness over the SP and this usually needs to be present to confirm a diagnosis (Reid 1992). Confusingly resisted hip adduction or trunk flexion may also reproduce the symptoms, which is usually indicative of muscular lesions. Plain film radiographs commonly reveal sclerosis of the pubic bones; with occasional widening of the symphysis, with laxity on stork views >2 mm (Harris & Murray 1974). However, X-rays have poor construct validity as often changes on X-ray do not correlate with symptoms and there are positive radiographic findings found in asymptomatic individuals (Hackney 1993). Bone and MRI scans correlate better with symptoms than radiographic appearance, with the ability of MRI scans to show bone marrow oedema into the pubic bones and detachment of anterior fascial layer, which is continuous with fascia overlying adductor muscles and the inguinal ligament (Karlsson & Jerre 1997). OP is generally thought of as the end result of an overuse continuum, resulting in excessive and repetitive strain of the SP and pelvis (Cunningham et al. 2007, Pizzari et al. 2008). There is limited evidence of proven risk factors for OP in the literature although greater hip abductor to adductor muscle strength ratios and decreased total rotation range of hip motion have been implicated (Maffey & Emery 2007, Verrall et al. 2001).

Lower-quadrant biomechanical abnormalities such as hypermobility, intrapelvic asymmetry and technique deficits are also said to play a role in the onset of OP, but to date there are no published trials to support this clinical observation (Reid 1992, Pizzari et al. 2008). Some authors also cite mechanical traction of the pelvic muscles (Ashby 1994). Although there is no convincing evidence that steroid injections are of any benefit (Hackney 1993) treatment typically includes general modified activity, physiotherapy in the form of correction of biomechanical abnormalities and muscle stretching, NSAIDs and corticosteroid injections (Holt et al. 1995). It occurs commonly in runners, footballers and in grass hockey goalkeepers and can be difficult to distinguish from adductor strains, with the two conditions frequently occurring simultaneously.

Athletic pubalgia or sports hernias

The diagnosis of a sports hernia or athletic pubalgia (AP) is controversial as there is frequently no clinically detectable inguinal hernia on physical examination and there is currently no consensus as to what specifically constitutes this diagnosis (Swan Jr & Wolcott 2007, Caudill et al. 2008). It has been defined as a set of pelvic injuries involving the abdominal and pelvic musculature outside the ball-and-socket hip joint and on both sides of the pubic symphysis (Meyers et al. 2008, Omar et al. 2008). AP occurs more often in men, although female proportion, age, numbers of sports and soft tissue structures involved have all increased recently (Meyers et al. 2008). Provocative sports usually include activities that involve quick turns whilst the foot is planted, cutting, pivoting, kicking and sharp turns, such as those that occur during soccer, ice hockey, rugby or football or high knee lift action such as in the martial arts, sprinters and hurdlers. Although with focused questioning a specific inciting incident may be identified (Caudill et al. 2008), it usually has no specific traumatic cause and comes on insidiously, with some correlation with OP, weakness of the posterior inguinal wall, a stretched external ring and generalized distension of the anterior abdominal wall (Nam & Brody 2008). Posterior inguinal wall weakening is said to occur from excessive or high repetition shear forces applied through the pelvic attachments of poorly balanced hip adductor and abdominal muscle activation (Caudill et al. 2008). The pain is felt deep in the groin and gradually worsens over time, which may spread along the inguinal ligament into the perineum, rectus abdominis muscles and to the testicles in about 30% of symptomatic individuals (Zimmerman 1988). Further investigations such as MRI, diagnostic ultrasonography and isotope scans are said not to provide any useful data in the assessment of sports hernias except to exclude other conditions (Caudill et al. 2008, Nam & Brody 2008). However, a recent review concluded that large-field-of-view MRI survey of the pelvis, combined with high-resolution MRI of the pubic symphysis provides excellent information about the location, causes and severity of the condition (Omar et al. 2008). MRI depicts patterns of findings in patients with AP including rectus abdominis insertional injury, thigh adductor injury and OP (Zoga et al. 2008). The range of possible pathologies or injuries is very wide and an in-depth knowledge of the pelvic regional anatomy is essential in the diagnosis of this condition. Conservative management consisting of soft tissue and joint mobilization and manipulation, neuromuscular re-education, manual stretching and therapeutic exercise is a viable option (Kachingwe & Grech 2008). A final course of action is surgical exploration of the posterior abdominal wall for defects, which are subsequently repaired. Surgery seems to be more effective than conservative treatment, and laparoscopic techniques generally enable a quicker recovery time than open repair (Brown et al. 2008).

Stress fractures

Although stress fractures are not common, if they do occur the two most frequent sites for these to occur are the femoral neck and the pubic ramus (Morelli & Smith 2001). Stress fractures can be caused by overtraining, which can cause repetitive strain on the underlying bone structure. They are often seen in long distance runners and military recruits, who may be required in their training to cover long distances with less than adequate footwear (Morelli & Smith 2001). Dancers are also subject to stress fractures especially classical ballet dancers, who concurrently may also present with nutritional imbalances (Howse & Hancock 1992). In addition, there are risk factors which predispose individuals to stress fractures: osteoporosis, muscle fatigue, excessive increase in training intensity or duration as well as running on cambered or uneven surfaces (Reid 1992). The pain with stress fractures is exacerbated by activity and diminished by rest; however, pain at rest is indicative of advanced disease. Confirmation of a stress fracture is usually made by MRI scan which has been show to be accurate and reliable in the imaging of these injuries (Ahovuo et al. 2002).

Nerve compression

Several nerves around the groin and pelvis are vulnerable to compression: ilioinguinal; iliohypogastric; lateral femoral cutaneous nerve of the thigh; genitofemoral; obturator (Figure 6.16) and pudendal.

The hip joint itself is supplied by the femoral nerve (which also innervates the iliofemoral ligament and the superior capsule), the obturator nerve (also supplying the pubofemoral ligament), the superior gluteal nerve (which supplies the superior and lateral part of the joint capsule and also the gluteus medius and minimus), and by the nerve to the quadratus lumborum, which supplies the posterior capsule and the ischiofemoral ligament (O'Brian & Delaney 1997). The spinal nerves L2, L3 and L4 can also refer pain to the groin or anterior thigh (Morelli & Weaver 2005).

The ilioinguinal, iliohypogastric and genitofemoral nerves originate from the first lumbar nerve (L1) but the genitofemoral receives additional input from L2

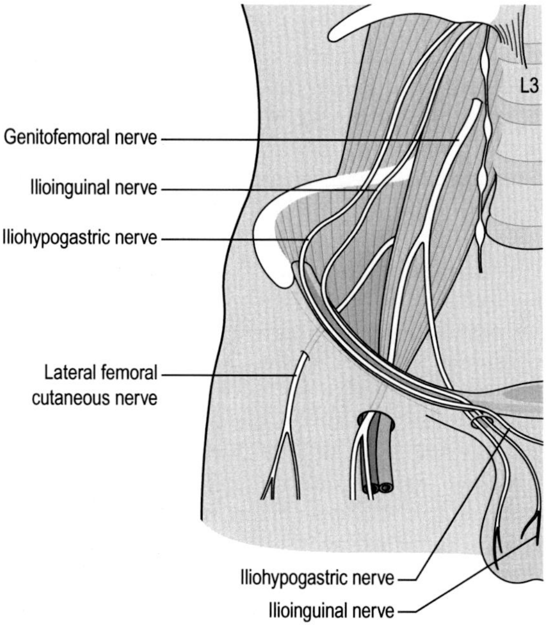

Figure 6.16 • Schematic drawing of the iliohypogastric, ilioinguinal, genitofemoral and lateral femoral cutaneous nerve of the thigh

or L3. There is considerable anatomic variation in the origin and course of these nerves as well as anoverlap of their cutaneous distributions (Aszmann et al. 1997, Akita et al. 1999, Rab et al. 2001). The ilioinguinal branch passes through the inguinal canal, becoming fairly superficial near the superficia inguinal ring, and continues to supply the root of the penis (or labia majora), anterior scrotum, and medial thigh, as does the genitofemoral nerve.The iliohypogastric further divides into two branches: the anterior cutaneous, which carries cutaneous sensation from the lower abdominal and groin region medial to the ASIS; and the lateral cutaneous branch, which receives sensation from the lateral thigh and gluteal region (Morelli & Weaver 2005). In addition to these sensory distributions, the ilioinguinal and iliohypogastric nerves provide motor innervations to the lower abdominal musculature.

Entrapment of the ilioinguinal, iliohypogastric and genitofemoral nerves may result in groin pain or lower abdominal pain that can radiate to the genitals. These nerves can be injured by direct trauma including abdominal surgery such as caesarean section, transvaginal tape for stress incontinence surgery and hernia repairs for overzealous training of the abdominals (Starling & Harms 1989, al-Dabbagh 2002, Murovic et al. 2005, Whiteside & Barber 2005, Vervest et al. 2006, van Ramshorst et al. 2009). Tenderness is often noted 2–3 cm inferior-medial to the ASIS, and hip extension usually produces increased pain or hypoaesthesia in the nerve's distribution (Morelli & Weaver 2005).

Compression of the lateral femoral cutaneous nerve of the thigh or meralgia paraesthetica can occur as it passes under or through the inguinal ligament resulting in a persistent burning sensation, tingling or aching pain, and hypersensitivity or hyposensitivity in the anterolateral aspect of the thigh (Moucharafieh et al. 2008). In addition to sportsmen such as squatting rifle team members and athletes who sustain acute trauma to the area, it has been noted in women who sit for prolonged periods with the involved leg underneath the body (Morelli & Weaver 2005) and more recently in wearers of tight low-cut trousers (Moucharafieh et al. 2008).

The obturator nerve supplies the adductor muscles and the skin over the inner thigh and is increasingly being reported as a source of chronic groin pain in athletes, and usually becomes entrapped in the obturator foramen or by thickened fascia surrounding the adductor muscles – usually adductor brevis (Morelli & Weaver 2005). Symptoms can include deep aching over the adductors or at the pubic bone, but its anatomy makes it difficult to distinguish between adductor strain and obturator nerve entrapment (Morelli & Weaver 2005). Classically the deep ache near the adductor origin of the pubic bone is exacerbated by exercise, subsides with rest, but often resumes with activity, and may radiate down the medial thigh toward the knee. Spasm, weakness and paraesthesia in the area may also occur (Brukner et al. 1999).

Conservative management of nerve compressions, including changes in training regimens, ice, NSAIDs, pharmacological management, local corticosteroid injections and nerve blocks, have been suggested with surgical referral in resistant cases (Brown et al. 2008, Suresh et al. 2008).

The pudendal nerve is commonly seen as a source of CPP due to its course through the levator ani muscle. The treatment and evaluation of pudendal nerve entrapment will be dealt with in Chapter 11.

Similar to the classification of mechanical LPP described earlier, classification of movement-impairment syndromes of the hip provides a systematic process with which to examine and select exercises to provide appropriate prescription and pathology-specific modification of exercise for hip pain (Lewis et al. 2006). A summation of hip classifications organized by test position, symptom behaviour with variations of the test position or movements within the test position, and clinical judgements of quality of alignment or movement are summarized in Table 6.3.

As discussed previously, differentiation of any neural components associated with the limitation of length testing of muscles needs to be evaluated to ensure that the perceived length changes are not due to neural irritation. The next section of the chapter discusses specific sports and CPP including genitourinary symptoms in cycling.

Cycling and genitourinary symptoms in men and women

The reported incidence of bicycling-related urogenital symptoms varies considerably (Leibovitch & Mor 2005) and some question the existence of a relationship between bicycle riding and urogenital symptoms, suggesting that larger case-control studies are required before conclusions can be drawn (Taylor III et al. 2004, Brock 2005). Yet in a recent comprehensive review of the literature, Sommer et al. (2010) conclude that there is a significant risk in relationship to

Table 6.3 Items for classification of hip organized by test position, symptom behaviour with variations of the test position or movements within the test position, and clinical judgements of quality of alignment or movement (taken from Sahrmann 2002)

Test position	Symptom behaviour with	Judgement of femoral alignment or movement
Standing	Standing	*Normal femoral alignment* (long axis of femur orientated 10° lateral to the sagittal plane) with patellae orientated in the frontal plane (facing forward) *Hip flexed*: Hip angle flexion >10°. Suggests short hip flexors *Hip extended*: Hip angle extension >10°. Suggests long iliopsoas, short hamstrings
	Bilateral hip/knee flexion (partial squat)	*Normal*: Knee flexion 45° with heel staying in contact with floor. Knee in line with second toe. Foot pronates (Figure 6.17A) *Hip medial rotation*: Knee moves in line medial to big toe. Suggests poor stability of posterior gluteus medius or overactivity of tensor fascia latae (TFL) (Figure 6.17B) *Hip lateral rotation*: Knee moves in line lateral to fourth toe
	Single leg stance, other leg flexed to 70° (degrees)	*Normal*: No change in hip joint rotation *Hip adduction*: Downward tilting of opposite side of pelvis. Suggests stance side hip abductors weak/long (Figure 6.18) *Pelvic rotation*: towards stance leg. Suggests short hip medial rotators *Hip rotation*: Femur rotates medially. Suggests short long/weak hip lateral rotators
	Forward bending	*Hip flexion*: Men <75°, women <85°. Suggests short stiff hip extensors (Figure 6.19B) *Hip flexion*: >100° or >70° during a standing bow (forward bend with straight back). Suggests long hamstrings and potential for anterior hip impingement (Figure 6.19C)

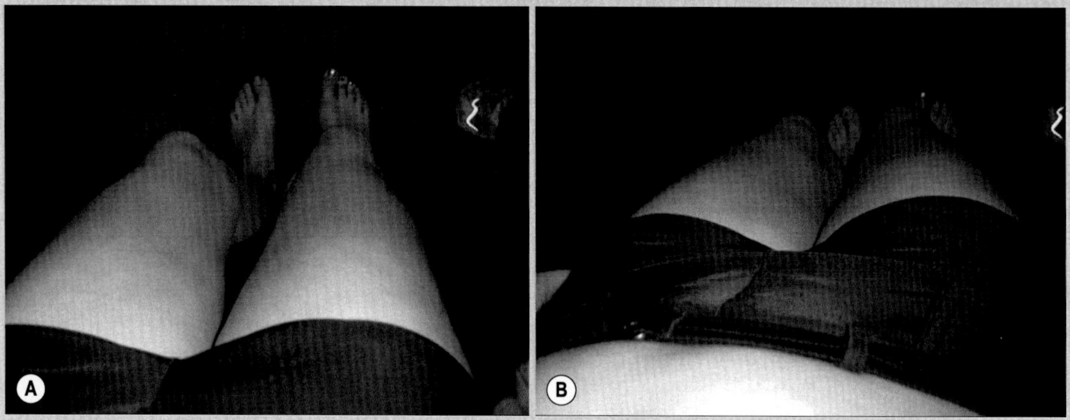

Figure 6.17 • Small knee bend from above. (A) Ideal alignment: knee in line with second toe. (B) Hip medial rotation: knee moves in line medial to big toe. This suggests poor stability of the posterior gluteus medius or overactivity of tensor fascia latae

Table 6.3 Items for classification of hip organized by test position, symptom behaviour with variations of the test position or movements within the test position, and clinical judgements of quality of alignment or movement (taken from Sahrmann 2002)—cont'd

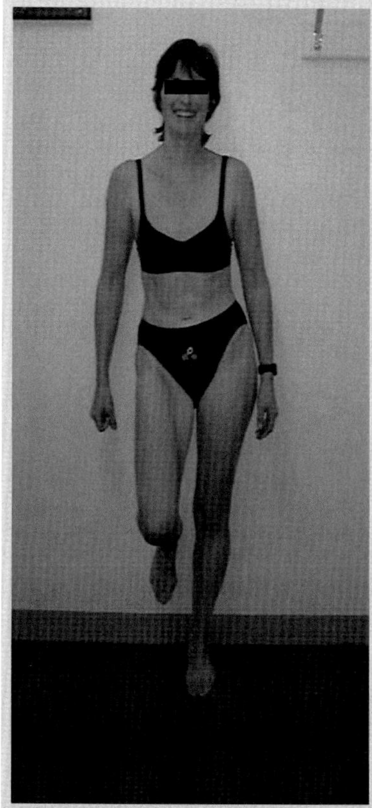

Figure 6.18 • Single leg stance, other leg flexed, downward tilting of opposite side of pelvis. Suggests stance side hip abductors weak/long

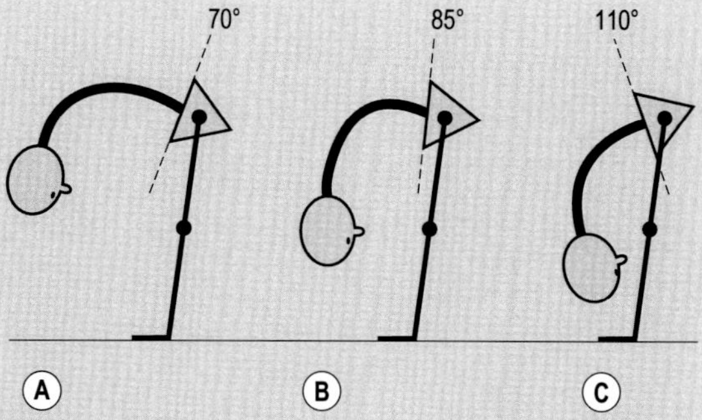

Figure 6.19 • Forward bending. (A) Normal: even flexion throughout the lumbar and thoracic regions with the hips flexing to approximately to 70°. (B) Hip flexion <75° (men) and <85° (women) suggests short stiff hip extensors. (C) Hip flexion >100° suggests long hamstrings and potential for anterior hip impingement

Test position	Symptom behaviour with	Judgement of femoral alignment or movement
Sitting	Sitting knee extension with ankle dorsiflexion	*Knee extends* <75° with hip flexed to 90°. Suggests short hamstrings (differentiate neural component with trunk and cervical flexion) *Hip medially rotates*: Suggests short medial hamstrings, and/or over-activity TFL (Figure 6.20)
	Sitting hip flexion	*Normal*: Hip flexed to 120°, maximum resistance to iliopsoas is tolerated. Muscle long if can resist between 105° and 110° but not 120°. Weak if unable to tolerate resistance at any point in range
	Hip rotation	*Normal*: Hip medial and lateral rotation symmetrical and approximately 30° *Medial rotation* ROM > lateral rotation. Suggests structural variation hip antetorsion when also observed in hip extension. *Lateral rotation* ROM > medial rotation. Suggests structural variation hip retrotorsion when also observed in hip extension

Continued

Table 6.3 Items for classification of hip organized by test position, symptom behaviour with variations of the test position or movements within the test position, and clinical judgements of quality of alignment or movement (taken from Sahrmann 2002)—cont'd

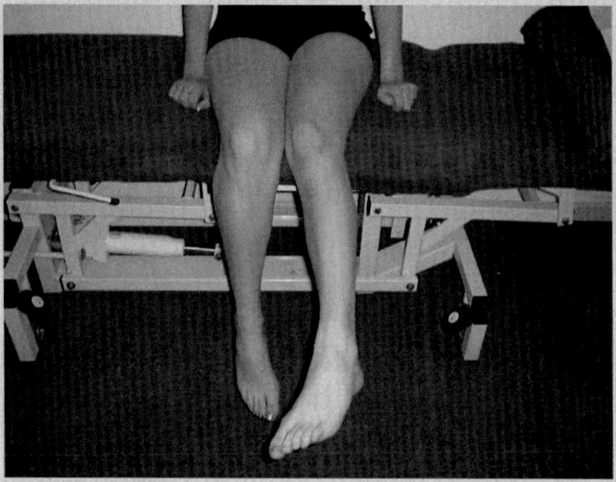

Figure 6.20 • Sitting knee extension with hip flexed to 90°, hip medially rotates; suggests short medial hamstrings and/or overactivity of TFL

Test position	Symptom behaviour with	Judgement of femoral alignment or movement
Supine	Hip flexor length test (modified Thomas)	*Normal*: Extended thigh lies on table with lumbar spine flat. Femur in midline without hip rotation or abduction. Knee flexed to 80° without abduction of tibia or lateral tibial rotation. Hip extended 10° *Short hip flexors*: Thigh does not reach table (Figure 6.21). Abduct hip and extension range increases suggests TFL-ITB (ITB, iliotibial band) short. Passive extension knee range increases, suggest rectus femoris short. Iliopsoas short if hip abducted, knee extended and thigh does not lie on table *Femoral head glides anteriorly*: Suggests iliopsoas long and/or anterior capsule stretched
	Straight-leg raise (SLR)	*Normal*: Greater trochanter (GT) maintains constant axis of rotation (AoR) during passive and active SLR, hip flexes to 80° *Femoral anterior glide*: GT moves anterior and superior (medial rotation and insufficient posterior glide) during active SLR. Suggests stiff posterior structures and/or hamstrings short (Figure 6.22). During passive SLR, GT maintains relatively constant position but examiner needs to control AoR with thumb placed in inguinal crease. Active SLR may produce anterior hip pain, whilst passive SLR pain-free *Femoral medial rotation*: Iliopsoas long, and/or long stiff hip lateral rotators
	Hip abduction/lateral rotation with hip flexed	Limited hip ROM with groin pain
	Unilateral hip flexion, passive and active	*Femoral anterior glide*: Pain in groin, and GT moves anteriorly/superiorly. Restriction GT movement with pressure at inguinal crease, increases resistance to hip flexion Limited hip ROM, flexion $<115°$. Suggests short gluteus maximus/ piriformis/posterior hip joint structures

Table 6.3 Items for classification of hip organized by test position, symptom behaviour with variations of the test position or movements within the test position, and clinical judgements of quality of alignment or movement (taken from Sahrmann 2002)—cont'd

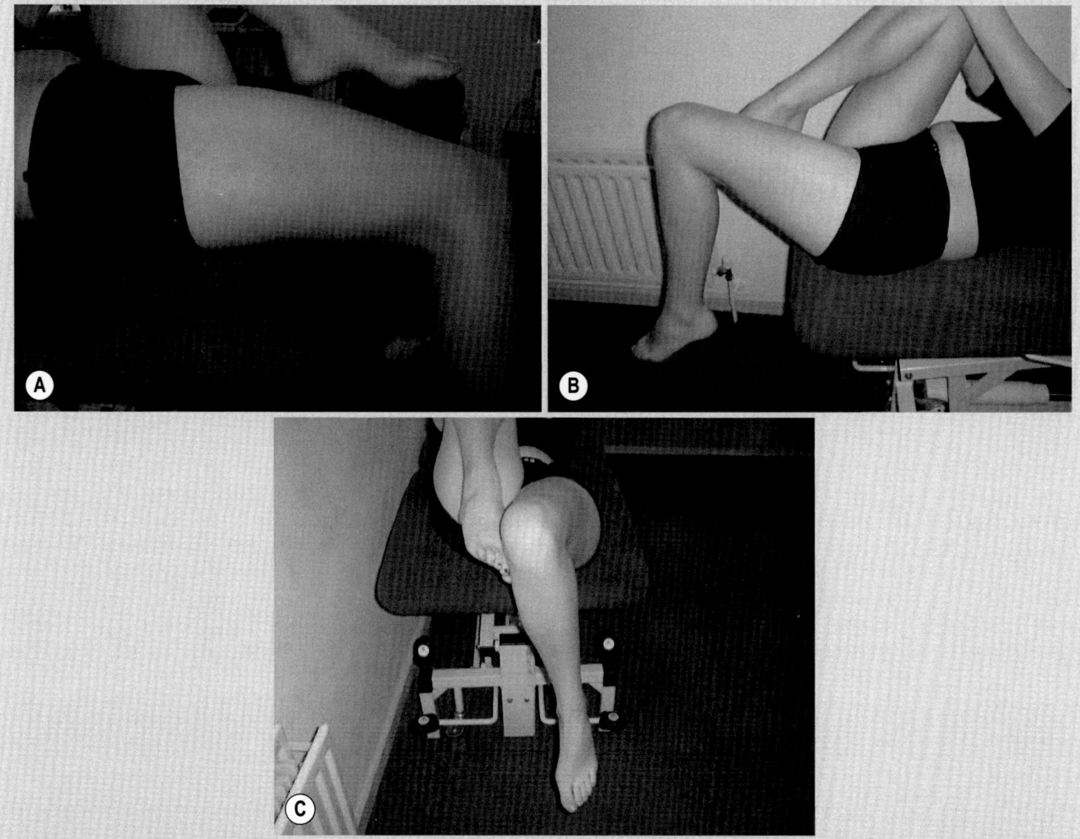

Figure 6.21 • (A) Normal: extended thigh lies on table with lumbar spine flat. Femur in midline without hip rotation or abduction. Knee flexed to 80° without abduction of tibia or lateral rotation. Hip extended 100°. (B,C) Short hip flexors: thigh does not reach table, showing femoral medial rotation and lateral tibial rotation

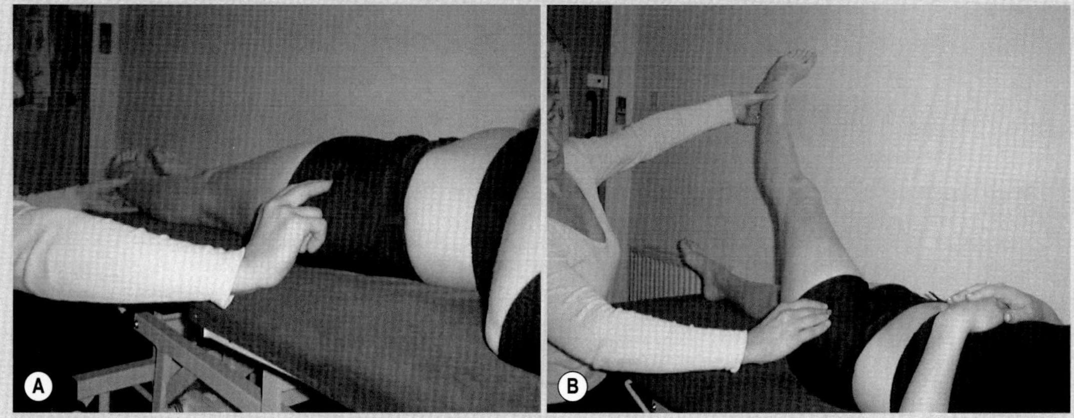

Figure 6.22 • (A) Monitoring greater trochanter (GT), (B) GT moves anterior and superior during active straight leg raise (medial rotation and insufficient posterior glide). Suggests stiff posterior structures and/or short hamstrings

Continued

Table 6.3 Items for classification of hip organized by test position, symptom behaviour with variations of the test position or movements within the test position, and clinical judgements of quality of alignment or movement (taken from Sahrmann 2002)—cont'd

Test position	Symptom behaviour with	Judgement of femoral alignment or movement
Side lying	Hip abduction, other hip positions neutral	*Normal* strength hip abductors (gluteus medius/minimus, TFL): Resisted hip abduction with pressure above ankle, able to tolerate maximum end of range. Long if able to resist after 10–15° adduction. Weak if unable to tolerate any resistance
	Hip abduction with lateral rotation and extension	*Normal* strength posterior gluteus medius: Able to tolerate maximum end of range resistance. Long if able to resist after 10–15° adduction. Weak if unable to tolerate any resistance *Hip flexes* when maximum resistance applied. Suggests TFL overactivity
	Hip adduction (uppermost leg). Starting position: hip abduction, lateral rotation, slight extension with knee extended	*Normal*: Hip adducts 10° Hip adducts <5°, suggests short hip abductors (Figure 6.23) Hip flexes and/or medially rotates. Suggests TFL and/or anterior gluteus medius/minimus short *Femoral lateral glide*: Excessive hip adduction with anterior distal portion of GT. Suggests long hip abductors
	Hip adduction (lowermost leg). Starting position: hip adduction, neutral rotation, flexion/extension with knee extended	*Normal*: Able to tolerate maximum resistance applied to lower thigh. Weak adductors if unable

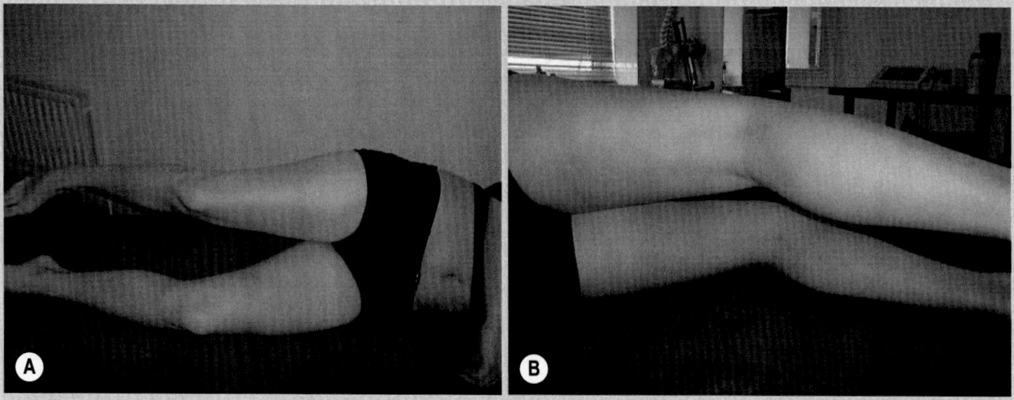

Figure 6.23 • Side lying hip adduction (uppermost leg) from in front (A) and behind (B). Starting position: hip abduction, lateral rotation, slight extension with knee extended; hip adducts <5° suggests short hip abductors

Test position	Symptom behaviour with	Judgement of femoral alignment or movement
Prone	Hip medial rotation	*Normal*: 35° medial rotation without pelvic rotation. Hip ROM is very variable and does not necessarily imply muscle shortness. However <30° check obturators, quadratus femoris, gracilis, piriformis, gemelli, posterior gluteus medius *Structural variation*: <10° medial rotation suggests retroversion of femur. >50° medial rotation suggests antetorsion of femur (Figure 6.24A). Check range in supine to confirm
	Hip lateral rotation	*Normal*: 35° lateral rotation without pelvic rotation. Hip ROM is very variable and does not necessarily imply muscle shortness. However <30° check medial rotators; TFL/ITB, anterior gluteus medius, gluteus minimus

Table 6.3 Items for classification of hip organized by test position, symptom behaviour with variations of the test position or movements within the test position, and clinical judgements of quality of alignment or movement (taken from Sahrmann 2002)—cont'd

Test position	Symptom behaviour with	Judgement of femoral alignment or movement
		Structural variation: <10° lateral rotation suggests antetorsion of femur. >50° lateral rotation suggests retroversion of femur (Figure 6.24B). Check range in supine to confirm *Femoral anterior glide*: GT moves anteriolateral, making wide arc of movement. Suggests TFL/ITB short
	Hip extension with knee extended	*Normal*: 10° hip extension with slight lumbar extension and simultaneous contraction of gluteus maximus and hamstrings *Femoral anterior glide*: GT moves anteriorly. Suggests overactivity of hamstrings, and/or short and stiff TFL and stretched anterior capsule (Figure 6.25)
	Hip extension with knee flexed	*Normal*: 10° hip extension with slight lumbar extension. Short rectus femoris/TFL if hip extension <5°. If unable to maintain hip extension when maximum resistance applied, implies weak/long gluteus

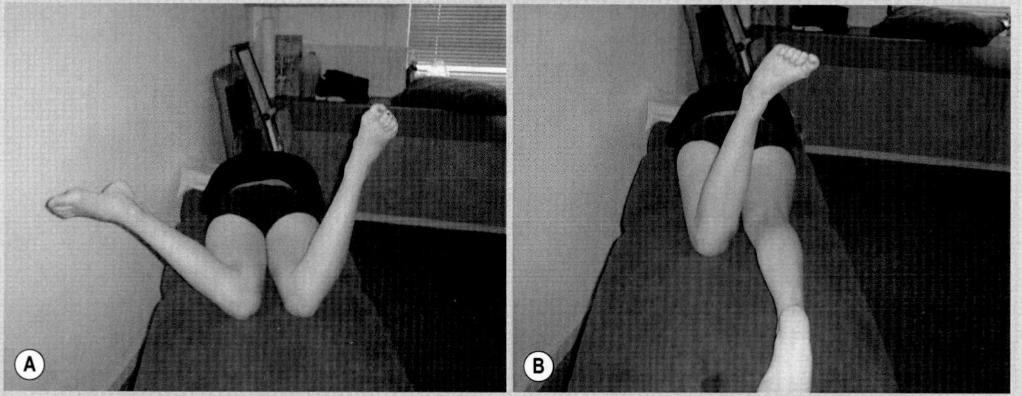

Figure 6.24 • (A) Prone hip medial rotation. (L) Hip >50° medial rotation suggestive of antetorsion/anteversion of femur. (R) Hip just within normal range. (B) Prone hip lateral rotation. Hip ROM is very variable and does not necessarily imply muscle shortness. However, <30° check medial rotators; TFL/ITB, anterior gluteus medius, gluteus minimus; <10° lateral rotation suggests antetorsion of femur. Confirm similar ranges in supine

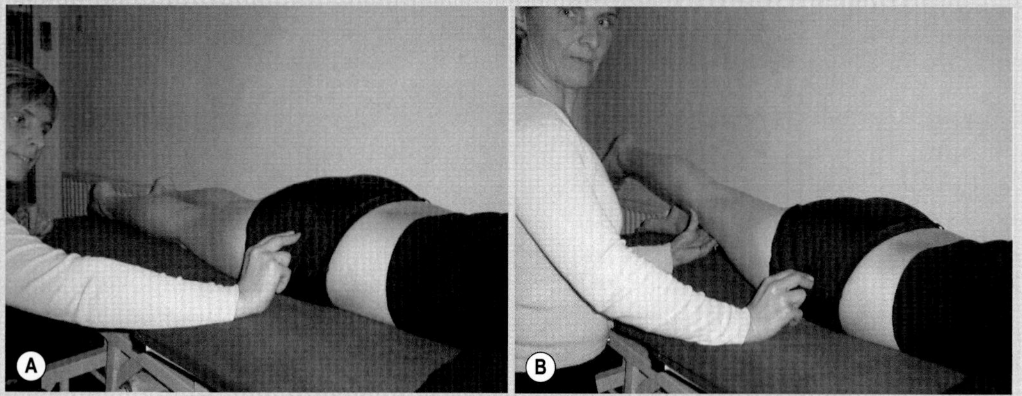

Figure 6.25 • Prone hip extension with knee extended. (A) Therapist monitoring greater trochanter (GT); (B) femoral anterior glide: GT moves anteriorly which suggests overactivity of hamstrings and/or stretched anterior capsule

Continued

Table 6.3 Items for classification of hip organized by test position, symptom behaviour with variations of the test position or movements within the test position, and clinical judgements of quality of alignment or movement (taken from Sahrmann 2002)—cont'd

Test position	Symptom behaviour with	Judgement of femoral alignment or movement
		Femoral anterior glide: GT moves anteriorly. Suggests overactivity hamstrings, and/or stretched anterior capsule
Quadruped	Quadruped	*Normal*: 90° angle between femur and pelvis. Neutral rotation, abduction/adduction <90° or hip lateral rotation suggests short/stiff posterior hip joint capsule, gluteus maximus/piriformis (Figure 6.26A)
	Backward rocking towards heels	*Normal*: Hips flex to heels, no pain. Decreased hip flexion or pelvic rotation implies short/stiff gluteus maximus/piriformis (rotation implies asymmetric stiffness) (Figure 6.26B). Confirm by abducting and/or lateral rotating hips which increases hip flexion

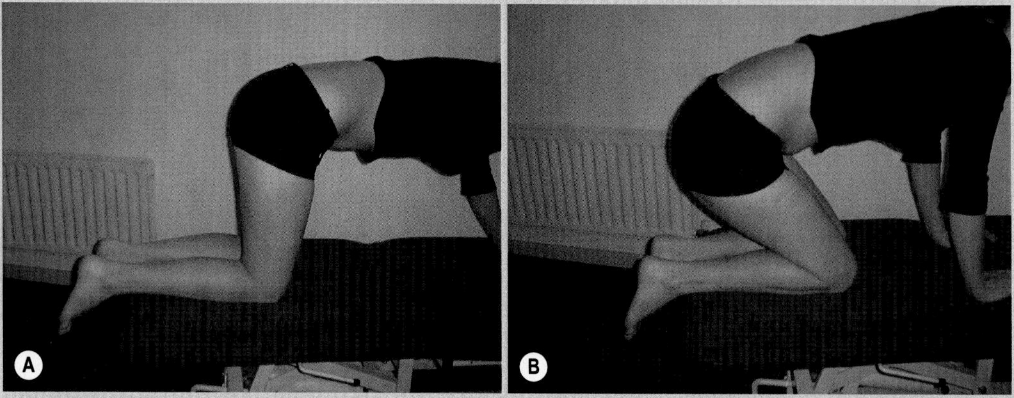

Figure 6.26 • (A) Quadruped <90° angle between femur and pelvis suggests short/stiff posterior hip joint capsule, gluteus maximus/piriformis. (B) Backward rocking heels, hips do not flex to heels, suggestive of decreased hip flexion or pelvic rotation implies short/stiff gluteus maximus/piriformis (rotation implies asymmetric stiffness)

cycling-related urogenital symptoms in both men and women, emphasizing the requirement for further research on bicycle and bicycle seat design. Rather than discourage cycling as an activity this section aims to describe the urogenital symptoms most commonly attributed to cycling, including the hypothesized mechanisms and inform the reader of the potential adjustable bicycle factors to assist the rider who complains of cycling-related urogenital dysfunction.

Symptoms

The most common bicycling-associated urogenital problems are genitalia numbness, followed by ED (Ricchiuti et al. 1999, Leibovitch & Mor 2005, Sommer et al. 2010). Other less common symptoms include CPP, priapism, penile thrombosis, infertility, haematuria, dysuria, difficulty in achieving orgasm, lymphoedema of the labia majora or 'bicyclist's vulva', torsion of spermatic cord, prostatitis, hardened perineal nodules and elevated serum prostate-specific antigen (PSA) (Doursounian et al. 1998, LaSalle et al. 1999, Baeyens et al. 2002, Leibovitch & Mor 2005, Sommer et al. 2010). A summary of important epidemiological studies assessing the impact of bicycle riding on sexual function is shown in Table 6.4.

Potential mechanisms

Compression of the pudendal nerve between the symphysis pubis and the bicycle seat (Goodson 1981) or at its course through Alcock's canal (Amarenco et al. 1987) have been proposed, although several authors have attributed numbness

Table 6.4 Important epidemiological studies assessing the impact of bicycle riding on erectile function/sexual function (Sommer et al. 2010)

Reference	Study population, type of study	Number of subjects	Outcome measurement	Results	Limitations of the study
Andersen et al. 1997	Cross-sectional, bicyclists in a 540-km race	160	Questionnaire	22% had symptoms of pudendal or cavernosal nerves; 20.6% had penile numbness >1 hour, and 6% for >1 week; 13% had impotence (7% for >1 week, 2% for >1 month)	No validated outcome measurement, just observational and descriptive study, self report, small sample size, lack of longitudinal follow-up
Marceau et al. 2001	Cross-sectional survey (MMAS)	1709	Questionnaire interview	OR for erectile dysfunction 1.72; if bike riding, >3 hours/week	Self report, small sample size of bicyclists/sport bicyclists, lack of longitudinal follow-up
Schrader et al. 2002	Bicycle police officers (mean cycling time 5.4 hours/day)	22	Rigiscan, pressure measurement	In cyclists, significantly lower erectile events in sleep, correlated with duration of biking and pressure of the nose of the saddle; 91% had groin numbness	Small sample size, lack of longitudinal follow-up
Schrader et al. 2008	Bicycle police officers using a no-nose saddle for 6 months	90	Questionnaire, Rigiscan, pressure, and biothesiometry	66% reduction in saddle contact pressure, significant improvement in tactile sensation and erectile function	No improvement in Rigiscan after 6 months, no control group, small sample size
Guess et al. 2006	Female premenopausal bicyclists, runners as controls	70	Biothesiometry, questionnaire	Significantly higher vibratory thresholds in bike riders at perineum, posterior vagina, and labia; no negative effect on sexual function	Questionnaire's validity is questionable, small sample size, no longitudinal follow-up, no statistical associations possible, no unathletic control group
Battaglia et al. 2009	Female horseback and mountain bike riders	6	Ultrasonography, questionnaire	Disseminated microlithiasis of the clitoral body in five women	Small sample size, no longitudinal follow-up, no statistical associations possible, unclear clinical significance
Dettori et al. 2004	Prospective cohort study, bicyclists riding 320 km	463	Questionnaire	Cumulative incidence of ED after the ride was 4.2% and 1.8% 1 month after the event; mountain biking and relative height of handlebars were associated with a higher risk of ED; 31% experienced perineal numbness	Sample size too small for valid statistical conclusions (large CI)

A summary of the most important studies showing the impact of bicycle riding on erectile function, nocturnal penile tumescence, clitoral structure, and female sexual function. ED, erectile dysfunction; MMAS, Massachusetts Male Aging Study.

transient ischaemia caused by pressure on the vascular supply of the perineum (Oberpenning et al. 1994, Ricchiuti et al. 1999, Ramsden et al. 2003, Gemery et al 2007) As discussed in Chapters 2 and 11, Alcock's canal is bordered laterally by the ischial spine and medially by the fascial layer of obturator internus muscle. The pudendal nerve leaves the canal ventrally below the ischiopubic ramus and it is thought that pressure on the ramus compresses neural and vascular tissue in Alcock's canal, resulting in penile and perineal paraesthesia often called Alcock's syndrome (Amarenco et al. 1987, Oberpenning et al 1994). Oberpenning et al. (1994) hypothesized that the onset of temporary perineal numbness, which can last 10–20 minutes or more, is due to compression on the perineum, which in turn causes compression on the pudendal nerve and artery. Ricchiuti et al. (1999) reported electromyographic (EMG) evidence of bilateral pudendal nerve injury associated with excessive cycling. They reported that the transient ischaemic episodes to the pudendal nerve and subsequent measurable delays in conduction were rapidly reversible if the ischaemia was of relatively short duration. However, ischaemia of longer than 8 hours duration resulted in significant deterioration of nerve function and would take several weeks for recovery to occur. Although acknowledging that the cause of perineal numbness and ED resulting from bicycle riding is not fully understood, it is suggested to be a result of continuous compression and strain on the pudendal nerve and arteries leading to nerve entrapment and vascular occlusion (Gemery et al. 2007, Sommer et al. 2010).

Leibovitch et al. (2005) postulated that the movements of the pedalling legs in the forward sitting position could result in stretching of the pudendal nerves over the sacrospinal and the sacrotuberous ligaments. This may cause increased tensile and compressive stress on the nerve trunk and a loss of the normal gliding movement of the nerve relative to the adjacent soft tissue and bony structures of the pelvic floor. The gliding movement of nerves in general has been described by Shacklock (2005) as being an essential aspect of the mechanical function of neural tissue, which serves to disperse the tension applied at one point of a nerve to the whole length of a nerve, reducing the forces on the nerve tissue. Neural mechanosensitivity is discussed further in Chapter 14.

Nanka et al. (2007) proposed an alternative mechanism of urogenital dysfunction in cyclists. They suggested that, as the pudendal nerve is protected by a thick layer of fatty tissue extending below the extent of the pubic body in the floor of Alcock's canal, compression of the posterior dorsal nerve of the penis (PDNP) in the sulcus nervi dorsalis penis (SNDP) is the main cause of Alcock's syndrome. They hypothesize that the position of the PDNP close to the pubic ramus and its proximity to the fibres of the suspensory ligament of the penis and the ischiocavernosus body make it more vulnerable to mechanical insult (Nanka et al. 2007). Since a compression neuropathy depends upon mechanical and ischaemic insult they suggest that the PDNP is the mostly likely nerve to be affected, particularly as the PDNP is the only nerve supplying the glans penis, hence able to be the cause of diminished glandular and penile sensitivity (Nanka et al. 2007).

Irrespective of the causative mechanisms, Labat et al. (2008) stated that despite these examples of pudendal nerve compression, very few cyclists go on to develop pudendal neuralgia.

Therapeutic options regarding adjustable bicycle factors

As discussed earlier there remains controversy as to whether alterations in riding habits actually change the prevalence of urogenital symptoms among cyclists (Taylor III et al. 2004). However, in addition to modifying training schedules and rising from the saddle for a brief time periodically to relieve pressure and help re-establish blood flow (Huang et al. 2005), the factors that have been evaluated are adjustments of the saddle, bicycle and body position. There are areas of agreement and inconsistencies in the literature; these factors are addressed in turn.

Saddle design

The design of the bicycle saddle is thought by a number of authors to be a major factor in the aetiology of perineal compression (Rodano et al. 2002, Seong et al. 2002, Sommer et al. 2010). Some saddles have a deep groove or hole connecting the anterior to the posterior part of the saddle and there is disagreement as to whether they are more or less likely to cause neurovascular compression (Rodano et al. 2002, Gemery et al. 2007, Sommer et al. 2010) (Figure 6.27). Saddles without a narrow protruding nose or with a large hole and a shape that allows for proper seating of the ischial tuberosities significantly reduce pressure distributed in the perineal region of cyclists (Schrader et al. 2008, Sommer et al. 2010). However,

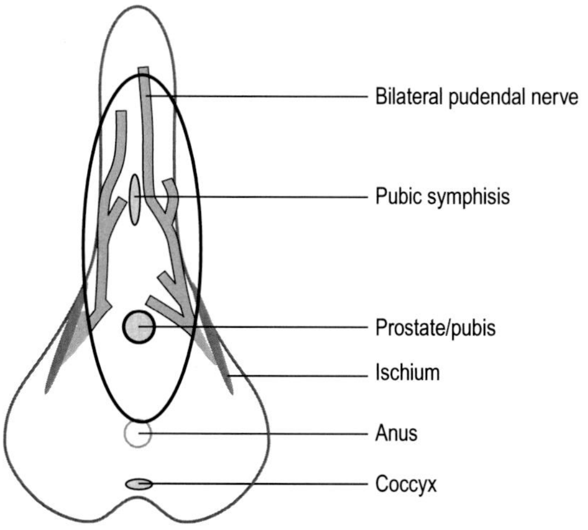

Figure 6.27 • Estimation of the alignment of the human body in the cycle saddle. The helix shows the anatomical area most subjected to injury during cycling. After Rodano et al. 2002

Rodano et al. (2002) argued that there is a *greater* likelihood of perineal numbness with holed or deep-grooved saddles as the load is transferred from the ischiopubic ramus to the perineum, particularly as the edge of the groove frequently corresponds anatomically to the location of the pudendal nerve and artery. Holed saddles present edges in the region where the hole is projected and these edges in saddle design can affect saddle pressure due to the contact of small areas under an elevated compressive load (Carpes et al. 2009). Gemery et al. (2007) stated that a grooved seat allows better preservation of the seat/symphysis space and reduces the compression on the pudendal artery more than a standard saddle. They constructed 3D models from computed tomography scans of one adult male pelvis (a healthy volunteer) and three bicycle seats to assess the influence of the rider's saddle position on vascular compression (Figure 6.29). These models were correlated with lateral radiographs of a seated rider in order to determine potential vascular compression between the bony pelvis and cycle seats at different angles of rider positioning as well as saddle type. They concluded that the rider's position is more important for reducing compression than is seat design alone (see section below on postural adjustment).

Posture and type of bike

Rodano et al. (2002) suggest that, in competitive road and mountain biking, 30–40% of a cyclist's body weight will be loaded through the saddle, but because the body weight is distributed through the pedals, handlebar and saddle the combination of the position of the cyclist on the bicycle, the pedalling action and the body weight distribution will determine the effect on the muscles, ligaments and other structures around the pelvis, including the prostate and neurovascular bundle. Disagreement remains about whether the upright or forward lean posture is most suitable to minimize urogenital distress whilst cycling (Rodano et al. 2002, Gemery et al. 2007, Carpes et al. 2009, Potter et al. 2008, Sommer et al. 2010). Sommer et al. (2010) stated that in the upright-seated position, a reduction in penile blood flow of up to 70% occurs due to compression of the dorsal penile arteries in the perineum. Whereas Gemery et al. (2007) suggested that with the rider leaning forward, greater compression of the internal pudendal artery occurs, immediately below the pubic symphysis (Figures 6.27, 6.28). Rodano et al. (2002) indicated that when the cyclist is in the bent forward race position (Figure 6.29) the pudendal nerve is more likely to be compromised as the greatest pressure is transferred to the anteroposterior section of the saddle.

A study to verify the effect of trunk position and saddle design on saddle pressure in both men and women concluded that it is the masculine anatomy that mainly influences saddle pressure during riding (Carpes et al. 2009). For men the trunk forwards position lowers the values of saddle pressure only for men using the 'holed' saddle, whereas there were no statistical differences comparing saddle pressure between the two trunk positions for women. Differences in centre of gravity, perineal anatomy and pelvic bone shape of men and women may therefore result in gender differences in pressure values from bicycle seats (Potter et al. 2008).

Use of a recumbent cycle has also been shown to produce a smaller decrease in genital oxygen tension; however, in some situations it can be a more difficult and less practical bike to ride (Schrader et al. 2002, Dettori & Norvell 2006). Mountain bicycles have been associated with a greater risk of ED as compared with road bicycles (Dettori et al. 2004); however, the study is weakened by a small cohort size of impotent bicyclists and a high non-responder rate (>20%).

Saddle width

It has been suggested that endothelial injury of the penile artery can occur due to the compressive

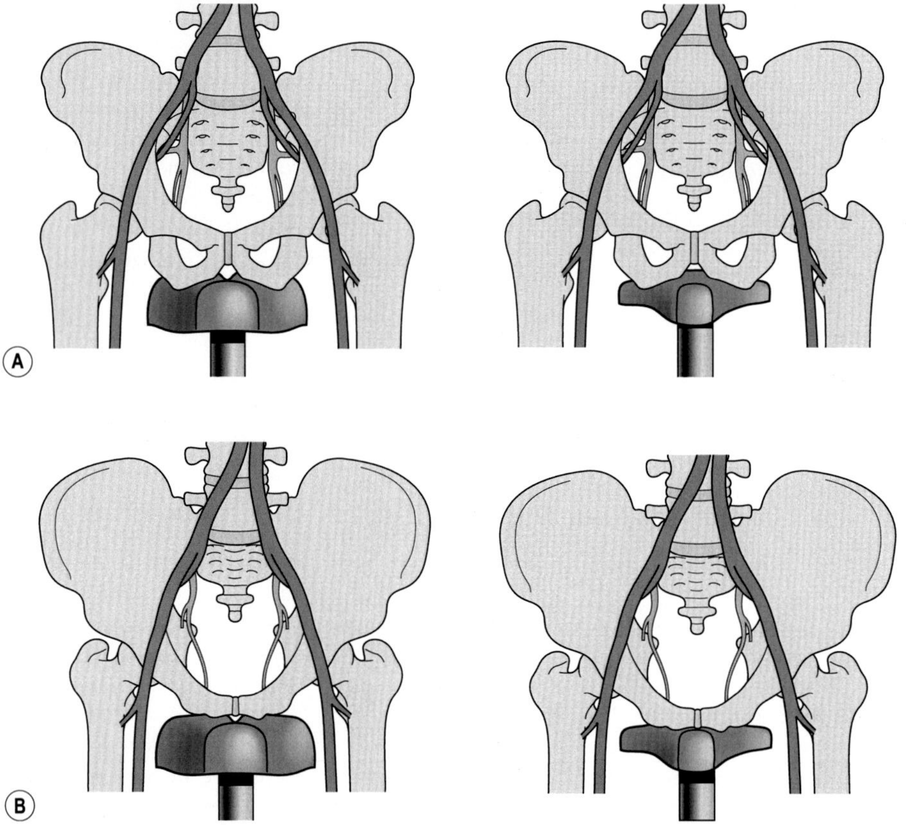

Figure 6.28 • Frontal views with pelvis positions corresponding to (A) a rider in a partial forward lean with arms extended, and (B) a rider in a full forward lean as when using aerodynamic bars. The seats on the left have a central groove (preserving the seat-symphysis space), while the seats on the right are of a flat racing style. There appears to be greater compression during the forward lean, as well as involving use of the racing saddle

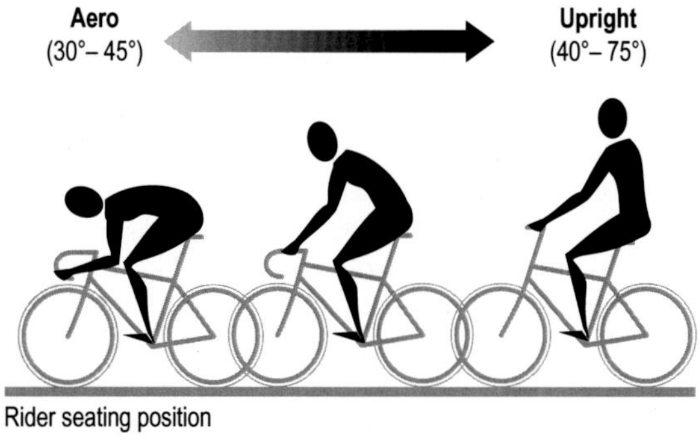

Figure 6.29 • Rider seating position. This figure shows the different seating positions on a bicycle

trauma caused by the pressure of sitting on a bicycle saddle, either by chronic compression of the neurovascular structures in the perineum or when a cyclist slips on to the top bar of a bicycle and land directly on the perineum or the ischiopubic ramus (Sommer et al. 2010). Most cyclists sit on a saddle which is narrower than the space between the ischial tuberosities, causing the load to be borne on the ischiopubic ramus, close to the Alcock's canal which may lead to a compromised blood supply to the penis (Richciutti et al. 1999, Seong et al. 2002, Rodano et al. 2002, Sommer et al. 2010). Seong et al. (2002) also conclude that a narrower saddle significantly reduces penile blood flow and could be the cause of blunt trauma to the perineum, although the small number of subjects (n = 20) and the indirect method used to measure penile blood flow reduces the validity of the study. Weiss (1985) and Bond (1975) both have proposed that transient ischaemia can be caused by compression of structures between the saddle and the symphysis pubis.

Sommer et al. (2010) conclude that the width of the saddle must span at least the distance between the ischial tuberosities, and the saddle must be wide enough for the ischial tuberosities to be situated on the flat back region of the saddle so that they are positioned higher than the soft tissue.

Saddle padding

Cycling on a gel saddle resulted in 37% more loss of penile oxygenation than cycling on an unpadded saddle (Sommer et al. 2010). They hypothesized that this was due to the gel being pressed into the perineal region until the ischial tuberosities encountered resistance as the rider sinks into the saddle. Furthermore, the wider saddle showed 57% better penile oxygenation than the narrow saddle when comparing the same seat position and padding material.

Conclusions

Particularly given the cardiovascular benefits from this low-impact activity, practitioners are urged to balance the risk–benefit ratio of cycling, as they would any intervention in medicine (Brock 2005). Rather than discourage cycling, the authors suggest the reader should emphasize to their patients with urogenital dysfunction strategies that may minimize the potential adverse effects of cycling, such as:

- Rising from the saddle for a brief time periodically, which can relieve pressure and help re-establish blood flow;
- Modifying training schedules;
- Adjusting the posture on the bike or using a different type of bike;
- Modification of the saddle, such as an unpadded, wide, no-nosed saddle; but consideration must be taken regarding the location of the groove or hole.

Running

Whilst running has many beneficial effects such as improving cardiovascular health and improving bone density, there is a risk of injury to the musculoskeletal system due to poor training technique and overtraining (Harrast & Colonno 2010).

Geraci & Brown (2005) report that the most common causes of hip pain in runners are muscle strains and tendinitis, which can be attributable to changes in running speed, sudden change of direction and a sudden increase in weekly or monthly mileage. The athlete presents with acute localized pain, which is found over the muscle–tendon unit on examination. Assessment reveals weakness on resisted testing and pain on passive stretching. There are underlying risk factors for the development of a stress fracture, including increase in frequency, duration or intensity (Harrast et al. 2010). Periodization of training is a coaching technique which builds in rest days to a training programme, after higher-intensity training sessions, and reduces risk of injury. Training in running shoes older than 6 months is a risk factor for stress fracture (Gardner et al. 1988). Stress fractures of the pelvis account for approximately 1–7% of all stress fractures and the most common site for a fracture is the pubic ramus (Frederickson et al. 2006). Patients may present with pubic ramus stress fractures, which may be initially thought of as soft tissue injury to the adductors. The history of onset and analysis of the athlete's training programme should help to avoid this. Hreljac (1999) reported that up to 70% of runners sustain overuse injuries during any one year.

Football

Ekstrand & Gillquist (1983) reported that the incidence of groin pain in soccer players, over a period of one year, was 8%. Other authors have reported the incidence of groin injury in professional footballers is as high as 22% (Werner et al. 2009). They investigated the incidence, pattern and severity of hip and groin injuries in professional footballers over seven consecutive seasons. A total of 628 hip/groin injuries were recorded, accounting for 12–16% of all injuries per season. More than half of the injuries (53%) were classified as moderate or severe (absence of more than a week), the mean absence per injury being 15 days. Re-injuries accounted for 15% of all registered injuries. In the 2005/6 to 2007/8 seasons, 41% of all diagnoses relied solely on clinical examination (Werner et al. 2009). They concluded that hip/groin injuries are common in professional football, and the incidence over consecutive seasons is consistent. They further noted that hip/groin injuries are associated with long absences and many hip/groin diagnoses are based only on clinical examination. A qualitative study by Pizzari et al. (2008) looking at the prevention and management of osteitis pubis in the Australian football league, reported all clubs involved in the study showed a high awareness of the condition and had identified a number of management strategies to combat it, such as rest-modified training, correction of predisposing factors, as well as early detection of onset. As discussed previously in this chapter, there is much debate about the aetiology of adductor-related groin pain.

Ice hockey

Ice hockey is an aggressive contact sport, where the players have to move at great speed on the ice, whilst displaying a very high level of skating ability. The combination of speed, rapid acceleration and deceleration and contact makes for significant potential for injury. Kai et al. (2010) state that groin injuries in hockey make up for 5–7% of all hockey injuries, whilst National Hockey League data revealed that 13–20% of players would suffer a groin injury (Caudill et al. 2008). As in other sports, groin pain in hockey players has multiple aetiologies, which often do not present with unequivocal signs and symptoms. OP is common due to the repetitive changes in direction in combination with bursts of acceleration and deceleration (Kai et al. 2010). Whilst skating the adductor muscles function in adduction and external rotation and adductor pain is often reported as being worse on skating and shooting the puck (Kai et al. 2010). Repetitive motions during hockey, for example during a slapstick manoeuvre, involve ipsilateral hip extension with contralateral trunk rotation and will also predispose the adductor muscles to injury. A slap shot manoeuvre requires rapid twisting motions of the body and abdominal muscle tears occur during these rapid torque-producing movements.

Sports involving repetitive flexion of the hip

Antolak et al. (2002) concluded that CPP may in part be explained by compression of the pudendal nerve, especially when the activities included continued flexion of the hip as occurs during many sports such as American football, weightlifting and wrestling (Antolak et al. 2002). Antolak et al. (2002) hypothesize that as many athletes begin participation in their sport as teenagers, hypertrophy of the muscles of the pelvic floor during these developmental years can cause elongation and remodelling of the ischial spine. This results in rotation of the sacrospinous ligament, causing the sacrotuberous and sacrospinous to be superimposed over each other. Furthermore, during squatting activities or during sitting and rising activities, the pudendal nerve may be stretched over the sacrospinous ligament or the ischial spine, which may produce shearing force on the nerve (Antolak et al. 2002). This can be made worse by the actions of gluteus maximus and the abduction and extension of the hip, for example rising from the squatting position of the baseball catcher or in the rugby scrum or during a ruck.

The following two case studies look at examples of athletes who presented with chronic anterior pelvic girdle pain and chronic posterior thigh pain.

Case study 6.1

A 21-year-old female middle-distance runner complained of a 3-year history of anterior hip and groin pain diagnosed with chronic left-sided osteitis pubis (OP). The athlete first noticed a gradual onset of anterior abdominal wall pain with running which increased in intensity over a number of weeks. It progressively restricted her running ability and finally completely prohibited participation in training. As time progressed, the irritability and severity of the symptoms increased with decreasing levels of activity, including the length of time for symptoms to dissipate. Aggravating factors included pain whilst walking, sitting at a desk studying or in moving vehicles, resulting in a gradual decrease in physical activity with concurrent reduction in conditioning.

Various physical assessments were performed and specialist consultations carried out with no treatment resulting in an improvement in her signs and symptoms. Eventually she become so disabled by her groin pain that she was finding it difficult to attend university lectures, travel on public transport or even private motor vehicles. A MRI scan indicated some bone marrow oedema around the margins of the symphysis pubis, concurrent with findings in OP, but evaluation by a consultant with a special interest in groin problems concluded that despite the changes on MRI scan, there was a large cortical input to the athlete's symptoms. In view of the longevity of her symptoms he suggested that she could not aggravate the situation any further and should return to being as active as possible and disregard the pain.

Assessment revealed a significant shift of the pelvis to the left, with associated apparent leg length discrepancy. There was a visible rotoscoliosis to the right in the lumbar spine, with an apex at L3. Forward flexion was limited by pain and stiffness in the lumbar spine. Left rotation was also limited by pain and stiffness in the lumbar spine. Right rotation reproduced the anterior pubic pain. Arthrokinematic assessment of the mobility segments in the lumbar spine revealed reduced neutral zone motion at the L5–S1 segment, with a blocked articular end feel. There were bony alignment changes in the pelvis with the left innominate positioned in anterior rotation. Arthrokinematic assessment of the sacroiliac joints (SIJ) revealed a significantly diminished neutral zone motion especially in the left-sided SIJ (Lee 2004). There was associated diminished multifidus bulk and active voluntary recruitment. There was also delayed recruitment time in the left gluteus maximus and increased tone in the left hamstrings. Osteokinematic assessment of the hip revealed a fixed flexion deformity of the left hip flexors, and palpable hypertonicity in the hip flexor group and adductor group of muscles. Treatment consisted of a high-velocity manipulation to L5–S1, myofascial release and deep tissue mobilization. Additionally, following treatment to reduce the hip flexor and adductor group hypertonicity, it was assessed that there was underlying diminished length of the flexor and adductor group. These muscle groups were stretched passively and the athlete was prescribed a stretching programme to follow independently. Trigger points were discovered in the proximal third of adductor magnus and the distal third of iliopsoas. These were treated using a modified treatment protocol as described by Travell & Simons (1993).

A unique aspect of the assessment of this athlete was the per rectal assessment of the pelvic floor. This involves a sophisticated digital analysis of the tone, length and function of the pelvic floor muscles and the mobility of the pudendal nerve. This is outlined in detail in Chapters 11 and 13. In this case pubococcygeus (PC) and iliococcygeus (IC) were both found to be hypertonic and short. Trigger points were found in the anterior third of both PC and IC, which reproduced the anterior groin pain reported by the athlete. Assessment of the mobility of the three branches of the pudendal nerve was carried out, and diminished mobility was found in the anterior and perineal branches of the nerve (Chapter 11). Prolonged sustained pressure techniques including Thiele massage and trigger point techniques were applied to the hypertonic PC and IC (Chapter 13). Finally mobilization of the pudendal nerve was carried out, with an emphasis on the perineal and anterior branches (Chapter 11).

On assessment of breathing patterns, the athlete had poor lateral expansion of her lower ribs and a hypertonic diaphragm. The importance of the assessment of an athlete's breathing is discussed fully in Chapter 9. Breathing re-education included awareness and relaxation of upper thorax, lateral costal breathing, teaching inhalation via nasopharyngeal breathing and exhalation via oropharyngeal breathing.

The assessment of the LPC using manual and visual assessment with real-time diagnostic ultrasound, has been discussed earlier in this chapter and the same principles were applied with this athlete. The athlete was found to have hypertonic and weak external and internal oblique muscles, poor contraction of transversus abdominis and weakness of the PFM group. Re-education of the trunk overactivity was performed using the techniques described previously in this chapter.

The athlete was instructed in self-treatment of the internal trigger points and hypertonic PFM, as well as stretches to address shortened muscles as described above. Treatment was initially fortnightly decreasing to monthly and then every 2 months. The treatment was continued for a period of 8 months.

Good outcomes were achieved with regards to improved function, reduced pain levels, reduced hypertonicity in the global muscles and the pelvic floor. Improved pelvic floor function was observed using real-time diagnostic ultrasound imaging and correlated with digital manual examination. The athlete was able to return to a more normal life in activities of daily living, returned to recreational running, and was able to recommence progressive weight training and conditioning in the gym. She remains active and symptom free to date.

Case study 6.2

A 30-year-old male rugby player (loose-head prop) complained of an acute onset of pain in the right hamstring insertion. A sudden tear was felt during a ruck and was attended to pitch side but he returned to play the remainder of the match. The hamstring tightened after the match and the player consulted the team physiotherapist the next day. A torn posterior medial right hamstring was diagnosed and PRICE (protect, relative rest, ice, elevation and elevation) protocol instituted. Over the next few weeks he attended for treatment by the team physiotherapists and treatment was focused primarily on the soft tissue lesion in his hamstring insertion. After initial improvement in his pain and walking ability round week 6 his improvement seemed to plateau. He still experienced a significant restriction in his ability to run even a slow pace. Further treatment over the following 3 months included steroid injections, deep tissue massage to the hamstrings, progressive strengthening programme and acupuncture, but did not result in any further reduction in his pain or improvement in his running ability. MRI revealed an intact hamstring with no evidence of recent or previous tears.

Eight months post-injury he was not making any progress and was still experiencing pain localized to the medial aspect of the right ischial tuberosity, aggravated by clenching his pelvic floor or gluteus maximus. He reported pain on rising from sitting, taking a wider than normal step, climbing stairs, getting out of a car, running, trying to kick a ball. Differential tissue tension testing revealed no indication of contractile or non-contractile lesions in the hamstrings or the adductors. Osteokinematic assessment of the pelvis revealed an up-slip dysfunction of the innominate, with an associated anterior rotation. Arthrokinematic assessment of the sacroiliac joints revealed decreased neutral zone motion, with a fixed articular end-feel. There was a corresponding rotation of the L5 mobility segment to the left. Arthrokinematically the L5 mobility segment revealed a compressed neutral zone, with a fixed articular end feel. There was increased tone in the adductors and hamstrings with associated tenderness on palpation in the proximal to middle third of the adductors and the proximal third of the medial hamstrings. Additionally there was increased tone in the quadratus lumborum (QL), piriformis (P) and obturator internus (OI). There were a significant number of trigger points in these muscles, which when released revealed underlying muscle length changes. Per rectal assessment revealed increased tone in the posterior pelvic floor, specifically IC and the posterior third of PC, with trigger points in the belly of these muscles. Pressure on these trigger points produced pain locally and referred the pain to the site of the medial hamstring pain.

Treatment consisted of high-velocity traction manipulation to the right sacroiliac joint and high-velocity thrust manipulation to the L5–S1 mobility segment. Soft tissue release, via myofascial techniques and trigger point techniques as described in Chapter 11, were performed on the hamstrings, adductors, QL, P and OI and pelvic floor. The athlete was instructed in self-treatment of the external hypertonic muscles and the external trigger points. He was also instructed in techniques to lengthen the adductors, hamstrings and piriformis muscles and QL.

After three treatments he reported no pain in the hamstring and was able to return to a graduated weight training and conditioning programme. He was rugby-fit by the end of 1 month and was able to return to his first team place.

This chapter has described the musculoskeletal contribution to CPP and the potential for increased risk of developing CPP due to sporting activity. However it has also emphasized the benefits of exercise which suggest that aerobic exercise represents a valid treatment option in CPP and it should be further investigated in a larger study with longer follow-up. It has highlighted the difficulty in assessing the various potential contributing factors to CPP, and the overlapping signs and symptoms of pain around the pelvis. The next chapter provides an evidence-based approach, which considers the patient's values and integrates the practitioner's clinical reasoning, skills and the available research evidence into decision-making for appropriate therapeutic interventions in CPP.

References

ACOG Practice Bulletin No. 51, 2004. Chronic pelvic pain. Obstet. Gynecol. 103 (3), 589–605.

Ahovuo, J.A., Kiuru, M.J., Kinnunen, J.J., Haapamäki, V., Pihlajamäki, H.K., 2002. MR imaging of fatigue stress injuries to bones: Intra- and interobserver agreement. Magn. Reson. Imaging 20, 401–406.

Akita, K., Niga, S., Yamato, Y., et al., 1999. Anatomic basis of chronic groin pain with special reference to sports hernia. Surg. Radiol. Anat. 21 (1), 1–5.

al-Dabbagh, A.K., 2002. Anatomical variations of the inguinal nerves and risks of injury in 110 hernia repairs. Surg. Radiol. Anat. 24, 102–107.

Amarenco, G., Lanoe, Y., Perrigot, M., Goudal, H., 1987. Un nouveau syndrome canalaire: la compression du nerf honteux interne dans le canal d'Alcock ou paralysie perineale du cycliste. Presse Med. 160.

Andersen, K.V., Bovim, G., 1997. Impotence and nerve entrapment in long distance amateur cyclists. Acta Neurol. Scand. 95, 233–240.

Antolak Jr., S.J., Hough, D., Pawlina, W., Spinner, R.J., 2002. Anatomical basis of chronic pelvic pain syndrome: compresssion; the ischial spine and pudendal nerve entrapment. Med. Hypotheses 59 (3), 349–353.

Ashby, E.C., 1994. Chronic obscure groin pain is commonly caused by enthesopathy: 'tennis elbow' of the groin. Br. J. Surg. 81, 1631–1634.

Aszmann, O.C., Dellon, E.S., Dellon, A.L., 1997. Anatomical course of the lateral femoral cutaneous nerve and its susceptibility to compression and injury. Plast. Reconstr. Surg. 100, 600–604.

Baeyens, L., Vermeersch, E., Bourgeois, P., 2002. Bicyclist's vulva: Observational study. Br. Med. J. 325, 138.

Barbic, M., Kralj, B., Cor, A., 2003. Compliance of the bladder neck supporting structures: importance of activity pattern of levator ani muscle and content of elastic fibers of endopelvic fascia. Neurourol. Urodyn. 22, 269–276.

Battaglia, C., Nappi, R.E., Mancini, F., et al., 2009. Ultrasonographic and Doppler findings of subclinical clitoral microtraumatisms in mountain bikers and horseback riders. J. Sex. Med. 6, 464–468.

Binningsley, D., 2003. Tear of the acetabular labrum in an elite athlete. Br. J. Sports Med. 37, 84–88.

Bond, R.E., 1975. Distance bicycling may cause ischaemic neuropathy of the penis. Physician Sportsmed. 3, 54.

Brock, G.B., 2005. Editorial comment. Eur. Urol. 47, 286–287.

Brown, R.A., Mascia, A., Kinnear, D.G., et al., 2008. An 18-year review of sports groin injuries in the elite hockey player: clinical presentation, new diagnostic imaging, treatment, and results. Clin. J. Sport Med. 18, 221–226.

Brukner, P., Bradshaw, C., McCrory, P., 1999. Obturator neuropathy. Phys. Sportsmed. 27 (5), 1–5.

Carpes, F.P., Dagnese, F., Kleinpaul, J.F., Martins, E.A., Mota, C.B., 2009. Bicycle saddle pressure: effects of trunk position and saddle design on healthy subjects. Urol. Int. 82, 8–11.

Caudill, P., Nyland, J., Smith, C., Yerasimides, J., Lach, J., 2008. Sports hernias: a systematic literature review. [Review] [104 refs]. Br. J. Sports Med. 42, 954–964.

Constantinou, C.E., Govan, D.E., 1982. Spatial distribution and timing of transmitted and reflexly generated urethral pressures in healthy women. J. Urol. 127 (5), 964–969.

Cowan, S.M., Bennell, K.L., Hodges, P.W., Crossley, K.M., McConnell, J., 2003. Simultaneous feedforward recruitment of the vasti in untrained postural tasks can be restored by physical therapy. J. Orthop. Res. 21, 553–558.

Cunningham, P.M., Brennan, D., O'Connell, M., et al., 2007. Patterns of bone and soft tissue injury at the symphysis pubis in soccer players: observations at MRI. Am. J. Roentgenol. 188, 291–296.

Dankaerts, W., O'Sullivan, P.B., Straker, L.M., Burnett, A.F., Skouen, J.S., 2006. The inter-examiner reliability of a classification method for non-specific chronic low back pain patients with motor control impairment. Man. Ther. 11 (1), 28–39.

Dettori, J.R., Koepsell, T.D., Cummings, P., Corman, J.M., 2004. Erectile dysfunction after a long-distance cycling event: Associations with bicycle characteristics. J. Urol. 172, 637–641.

Dettori, N.J., Norvell, D.C., 2006. Non-traumatic bicycle injuries : a review of the literature. [Review] [51 refs]. Sports Med. 36, 7–18.

Dickx, N., Cagnie, B., Achten, E., et al., 2008. Changes in lumbar muscle activity because of induced muscle pain evaluated by muscle functional magnetic resonance imaging. Spine 33, E983–E989.

Doursounian, M., Catney-Kiser, J., Salimpour, P., et al., 1998. Sexual and urinary tract dysfunction in bicyclists. J. Urol. 159 (Suppl.), 30.

Ekstrand, J., Gillquist, J., 1983. The avoidability of soccer injuries. Int. J. Sports Med. 4 (2), 124–128.

Fall, M., Baranowski, A., Elneil, S., et al., 2010. EAU guidelines on chronic pelvic pain. Eur. Urol. 57, 35–48.

Farjo, L.A., Glick, J.M., Sampson, T.G., 1999. Hip arthroscopy for acetabular labral tears. Arthroscopy 15, 132–137.

Ferreira, P.H., Ferreira, M.L., Maher, C.G., Herbert, R.D., Refshauge, K., 2006. Specific stabilisation exercise for spinal and pelvic pain: a systematic review. [Review] [42 refs]. Aust. J. Physiother. 52, 79–88.

Fitzgerald Jr., R.H., 1995. Acetabular labrum tears: diagnosis and treatment. Clin. Orthop. 311, 60–68.

Frederickson, M., Jennings, F., Beaulieu, C., et al., 2006. Stress fractures in athletes. Top. Magn. Reson. Imaging 17 (5), 309–325.

Fricker, P.A., 1997. Management of groin pain in athletes. Br. J. Sports Med. 31, 97–101.

Gardner, L.I., Dziados, J.E., Jones, B.H., et al., 1988. Prevention of lower extremity stress fractures: a controlled trial of shock absorbent insole. Am. J. Public Health 78, 1563–1567.

Gemery, J.M., Nangia, A.K., Mamourian, A.C., Reid, S.K., 2007. Digital three-dimensional modelling of the male pelvis and bicycle seats: impact of rider position and seat design on potential penile hypoxia and erectile dysfunction. BJU Int. 99, 135–140.

Geraci, M., Brown, W., 2005. Evidence-based treatment of hip and pelvic injuries in runners. Phys. Med. Rehabil. Clin. N. Am. 16, 711–747.

Gibbons, S.G.T., Comerford, M.J., Emerson, P., 2002. Rehabilitation of the stability function of psoas major. Orthopaedic Division Review (Jan/Feb), 7–16.

Giubilei, G., Mondaini, N., Minervini, A., et al., 2007. Physical activity of men with chronic prostatitis/chronic pelvic pain syndrome not satisfied with conventional treatments. Could it represent a valid option? The Physical Activity and Male Pelvic Pain Trial: A double-blind, randomized study. J. Urol. 177, 159–165.

Goodson, J.D., 1981. Pudenadal neuritis from biking. N. Engl. J. Med. 304, 365.

Guess, M.K., Connell, K., Schrader, S., et al., 2006. Genital sensation and sexual function in women bicyclists and runners: Are your feet safer than your seat? J. Sex. Med. 3, 1018–1027.

Hackney, R.G., 1993. The sports hernia: a cause of chronic groin pain. Br. J. Sports Med. 27, 58–62.

Hall, T., Zusman, M., Elvey, R., 1998. Adverse mechanical tension in the nervous system? Analysis of straight leg raise. Man. Ther. 3, 140–146.

Harrast, M.A., Colonno, D., 2010. Stress fractures in runners. Clin. Sports Med. 399–416.

Harris-Hayes, M., Van Dillen, L.R., 2009. The inter-tester reliability of physical therapists classifying low back pain problems based on the movement system impairment classification system. Pm & R 1, 117–126.

Harris-Hayes, M., Holtzman, G.W., Earley, J.A., Van Dillen, L.R., 2010. Development and preliminary reliability testing of an assessment of patient independence in performing a treatment program: standardized scenarios. J. Rehabil. Med. 42, 221–227.

Harris, N.H., Murray, R.O., 1974. Lesions of the symphysis in athletes. BMJ 4, 211.

Hase, T., Ueo, T., 1999. Acetabular labral tear: arthroscopic diagnosis and treatment. Arthroscopy 15, 138–141.

Hemborg, B., Moritz, U., Lowing, H., 1985. Intra-abdominal pressure and trunk muscle activity during lifting. IV. The causal factors of the intra-abdominal pressure rise. Scand. J. Rehabil. Med. 17, 25–38.

Heyde, C.E., Mahheld, K., Stakel, P.F., Kayser, R., 2005. Ultrasonography as a reliable diagnostic tool in old quadriceps tendon ruptures: a prospective multi-centre study. Knee Surg. Sports Traumatol. Arthrosc. 13, 564–568.

Hides, J.A., Cooper, D.H., Stokes, M.J., 1992. Diagnostic ultrasound imaging for measurement of the lumbar multifidus muscle in normal young adults. Physiother. Theory Pract. 8, 19–26.

Hides, J.A., Richardson, C.A., Jull, G.A., 1996. Multifidus muscle recovery is not automatic after resolution of acute, first-episode low back pain. Spine 21, 2763–2769.

Hides, J.A., Jull, G.A., Richardson, C.A., 2001. Long-term effects of specific stabilizing exercises for first-episode low back pain. Spine 26, E243–E248.

Hodges, P.W., Cholewicki, J., 2007. Functional control of the spine. In: Vleeming, A., Mooney, V., Stoeckart, R. (Eds.), Movement, Stability and Lumbopelvic Pain. Elsevier, pp. 489–512.

Hodges, P.W., Gandevia, S.C., 2000. Changes in intra-abdominal pressure during postural and respiratory activation of the human diaphragm. J. Appl. Physiol. 89, 967–976.

Hodges, P.W., Moseley, G.L., 2003. Pain and motor control of the lumbopelvic region: effect and possible mechanisms. J. Electromyogr. Kinesiol. 13, 361–370.

Hodges, P.W., Richardson, C.A., 1996. Inefficient muscular stabilization of the lumbar spine associated with low back pain. A motor control evaluation of transversus abdominis. Spine 21, 2640–2650.

Hodges, P.W., Richardson, C.A., 1998. Delayed postural contraction of transversus abdominis in low back pain associated with movement of the lower limb. J. Spinal Disord. 11, 46–56.

Hodges, P.W., Pengel, L.H., Herbert, R.D., Gandevia, S.C., 2003. Measurement of muscle contraction with ultrasound imaging. Muscle Nerve 27, 682–692.

Hodges, P.W., Sapsford, R., Pengel, L.H., 2007. Postural and respiratory functions of the pelvic floor muscles. Neurourol. Urodyn. 26, 362–371.

Holmich, P., Uhrskou, P., Ulnits, L., et al., 1999. Effectiveness of active physical training as treatment for long-standing adductor-related groin pain in athletes: randomised trial. Lancet 353 (9151), 439–443.

Holt, M., Keene, J., Graf, B., et al., 1995. Treatment of osteitis pubis in athletes: Results of corticosteroid injections. Am. J. Sports Med. 23, 601–606.

Howse, J., Hancock, S., 1992. Dance Technique and Injury Prevention. A&C Black.

Hreljac, A., 1999. Evaluation of lower extremity overuse injury potential in runners. Med. Sci. Sport Exerc. 32, 1653–11641.

Huang, V., Munarriz, R., Goldstein, I., 2005. Bicycle riding and erectile dysfunction: an increase in interest (and concern). [Review] [43 refs]. J. Sex. Med. 2, 596–604.

Johnston, C.A., Wiley, J.P., Lindsay, D.M., et al., 1998. Iliopsoas bursitis and tendinitis: A review. Sports Med. 25 (4), 271–283.

Jones, R.C., 2001. Pelvic floor muscle rehabilitation. Urol. News 5, 1–4.

Jones, R.C., Peng, Q., Shishido, K., Constantinou, C.E., 2006. 2D ultrasound imaging and motion tracking of pelvic floor muscle activity during abdominal manoeuvres in stress urinary incontinent women. Neurourol. Urodyn. Abstract.

Kachingwe, A.F., Grech, S., 2008. Proposed algorithm for the management of athletes with athletic pubalgia, (sports hernia): A case series. J. Orthop. Sports Phys. Ther. 38, 768–781.

Kai, B., Lee, K.D., Andrews, G., Wilkinson, M., Forster, B.B., 2010. Puck to pubalgia: imaging of groin pain in professional hockey players. Can. Assoc. Radiol. J. 6, 74–79.

Karlsson, J., Jerre, R., 1997. The use of radiography, MRI and ultrasound in the diagnosis of hip, pelvis and groin injuries. Sports Med. Arthrosc Rev. 5, 268–273.

Kendall, F., McCreary, E., Provance, P., Rodgers, M., Romani, R., 2005. Muscles: Testing and Function with Posture and Pain, fifth ed. Williams & Wilkins.

Labat, J.J., Riant, T., Robert, R., et al., 2008. Diagnostic criteria for pudendal neuralgia by pudendal nerve entrapment (Nantes criteria). Neurourol. Urodyn. 27 (4), 306–310.

LaSalle, M., Salimpour, P., Adelstein, M., Mourtzinos, A., Wen, C., Renzulli, J., et al., 1999. Sexual and urinary tract dysfunction in female bicyclists. J. Urol. 161, 269.

Laycock, J., Jerwood, D., 2001. Pelvic floor muscle assessment: The PERFECT scheme. Physiotherapy 87 (12), 631–642.

Lee, D., 2004. The Pelvic Girdle. Churchill Livingston, Edinburgh.

Leibovitch, I., Mor, Y., 2005. The vicious cycling: bicycling related urogenital disorders. [Review] [62 refs]. Eur. Urol. 47, 277–286.

Lewis, C.L., Sahrmann, S.A., 2006. Acetabular labral tears. Phys. Ther. 86, 110–121.

Linton, S.J., 2000. A review of psychological risk factors in back and neck pain. Spine 25 (9), 1148–1156.

Lovegrove Jones, R.C., 2010. Dynamic Evaluation of Female Pelvic Floor Muscle Function Using 2D Ultrasound and Image Processing Methods. University of Southampton, Faculty of Medicine, Health and Life Sciences. Thesis/Dissertation.

Lovell, G., 1995. The diagnosis of chronic groin pain in athletes: a review of 189 cases. Aust. J. Sci. Med. Sport 27, 76–79.

Maffey, L., Emery, C., 2007. What are the risk factors for groin strain injury in sport? A systematic review of the literature. Sports Med. 37, 881–894.

Marceau, L., Kleinman, K., Goldstein, I., McKinlay, J., 2001. Does bicycling contribute to the risk of erectile dysfunction? Results from the Massachusetts Male Aging Study (MMAS). Int. J. Impot. Res. 13, 298–302.

Mason, J.B., 2001. Acetabular labral tears in the athlete. Clin. Sports Med. 20, 779–790.

McCarthy, J.C., Noble, P.C., Schuck, M.R., et al., 2001. The Otto E. Aufranc Award: the role of labral lesions to development of early degenerative hip disease. Clin. Orthop. 393, 25–37.

McGill, S., 2002. Low Back Disorders. Evidence-Based Prevention and Rehabilitation. Human Kinetics, Champaign, IL.

McKenzie, R., May, S., 2003. The Lumbar Spine: Mechanical Diagnosis & Therapy. second ed. Orthopedic Physical Therapy Products.

Messelink, B., Benson, T., Berghmans, B., Bo, K., Corcos, J., Fowler, C., et al., 2005. Standardization of terminology of pelvic floor muscle function and dysfunction: report from the pelvic floor clinical assessment group of the International Continence Society. Neurourol. Urodyn. 24, 374–380.

Meyers, W.C., McKechnie, A., Philippon, M.J., Horner, M.A., Zoga, A.C., Devon, O.N., 2008. Experience with "sports hernia" spanning two decades. Ann. Surg. 248, 656–665.

Mitchell, B., McCrory, P., Brukner, P., et al., 2003. Hip joint pathology: clinical presentation and correlation between magnetic resonance arthrography, ultrasound, and arthroscopic findings in 25 consecutive cases. Clin. J. Sport Med. 13, 152–156.

Morelli, V., Smith, V., 2001. Groin injuries in athletes. Am. Fam. Physician 64, 1405–1414.

Morelli, V., Weaver, V., 2005. Groin injuries and groin pain in athletes: Part 1. Prim. Care Clin. Office Pract. 32, 163–183.

Moseley, G.L., 2007. Reconceptualising pain according to modern pain science. Phys. Ther. Rev. 12, 169–178.

Moseley, G.L., Hodges, P.W., Gandevia, S.C., 2002. Deep and superficial fibers of the lumbar multifidus muscle are differentially active during voluntary arm movements. Spine 27, E29–E36.

Moucharafieh, R., Wehbe, J., Maalouf, G., 2008. Meralgia paresthetica: a result of tight new trendy low cut trousers ('taille basse'). Int. J. Surg. 6, 164–168.

Murovic, J.A., Kim, D.H., Tiel, R.L., Kline, D.G., 2005. Surgical management of 10 genitofemoral neuralgias at the Louisiana State University Health Sciences Center. Neurosurgery 56, 298–303.

Nam, A., Brody, F., 2008. Management and therapy for sports hernia. [Review] [63 refs]. J. Am. Coll. Surg. 206, 154–164.

Nanka, O., Sedy, J., Jarolim, L., 2007. Sulcus nervi dorsalis penis: Site of origin of Alcock's syndrome in bicycle riders. Med. Hypothesis 69, 1040–1045.

Narvani, A., Tsiridis, E., Tai, C., Thomas, P., 2003. Acetabular labrum and its tears. Br. J. Sports Med. 37, 207–211.

Nielsen, A.B., Yde, J., 1989. Epidemiology and traumatology of injuries in soccer. Am. J. Sports Med. 17 (6), 803–807.

O'Brian, M., Delaney, M., 1997. The anatomy of the hip and groin. Sports Med. Arthrosc. (5), 252–267.

Ombregt, L., Bisschop, P., ter Veer, H.J., 2002. A System of Orthopaedic Medicine, second ed. Churchill Livingstone.

O'Sullivan, 2005. Diagnosis and classification of chronic low back pain disorders: Maladaptive movement and motor control impairments as underlying mechanism. Man. Ther. 10, 242–255.

O'Sullivan, P.B., Phyty, G.D., Twomey, L.T., Allison, G.T., 1997. Evaluation of specific stabilizing exercise in the treatment of chronic low back pain with radiologic diagnosis of spondylolysis or spondylolisthesis. Spine 22, 2959–2967.

O'Sullivan, P.B., Beales, D.J., Beetham, J.A., Cripps, J., Graf, F., Lin, I.B., et al., 2002. Altered motor control strategies in subjects with sacroiliac joint pain during the active straight-leg-raise test. Spine 27, E1–E8.

Oberpenning, F., Roth, S., Leusmann, D.B., van Ahlen, H., Hertie, L., 1994. The Alcock Syndrome. Temporary penile insensitivity due to compression of the pudendal nerve within the Alcock canal. J. Urol. 151, 423–425.

Omar, I.M., Zoga, A.C., Kavanagh, E.C., Koulouris, G., Bergin, D., Gopez, A.G., et al., 2008. Athletic pubalgia and "sports hernia": optimal MR imaging technique and findings. [Review] [75 refs]. Radiographics 28, 1415–1438.

Orsini, N., RashidKhani, B., Andersson, S.O., Karlberg, L., Johansson, J.E., Wolk, A., 2006. Long-term physical activity and lower urinary tract symptoms in men. J. Urol. 176, 2546–2550.

Pizzari, T., Coburn, P.T., Crow, J.F., 2008. Prevention and management of osteitis pubis in the Australian Football League: A qualitative analysis. Phys. Ther. Sport 9, 117–125.

Pool-Goudzwaard, A., van Dijke, G.H., van Gurp, M., Mulder, P., Snijders, C., Stoeckart, R., 2004. Contribution of pelvic floor muscles to stiffness of the pelvic ring. Clin. Biomech. 564–571.

Potter, J.J., Sauer, J.L., Weisshaar, C.L., Thelen, D.G., Ploeg, H.L., 2008. Gender differences in bicycle saddle pressure distribution during seated cycling. Med. Sci. Sports Exerc. 40, 1126–1134.

Rab, M., Ebmer, A.J., Dellon, A.L., 2001. Anatomic variability of the ilioinguinal and genitofemoral nerve: implications for the treatment of groin pain. Plast. Reconstr. Surg. 108, 1618–1623.

Ramsden, C.E., McDaniel, M.C., Harmon, R.L., Renney, K.M., Faure, A., 2003. Pudendal nerve entrapment as a source of intractable perineal pain. Am. J. Phys. Med. Rehabil. 82, 479–484.

Reid, D.C., 1992. Sports Injury Assessment and Rehabilitation. Churchill Livingstone, Edinburgh.

Ricchiuti, V.S., Haas, C.A., Seftel, A.D., Chelimsky, T., Goldstein, I., 1999. Pudendal nerve injury associated with avid bicycling. J. Urol. 162, 2099–2100.

Richardson, C., Jull, G., Hodges, P., et al., 1999. Therapeutic Exercise for Spinal Segmental Stabilization in Low Back Pain. Churchill Livingstone, London.

Richardson, C.A., Snijders, C.J., Hides, J.A., Damen, L., Pas, M.S., Storm, J., 2002. The relation between the transversus abdominis muscles, sacroiliac joint mechanics, and low back pain. Spine 27, 399–405.

Rodano, R., Squadrone, R., Sacchi, M., Marzegan, 2002. Pressure distribution on bicycle saddles (a comparrison between saddles with a "hole" in the perineal area). In: Proceedings of the Symposium of the International Society of Biomechanics in Sports. Milan.

Sahrmann, S.A., 1993. Movement science and physical therapy. J. Phy. Ther. Educ. 7, 4–7.

Sahrmann, S.A., 2002. Diagnosis and Treatment of Movement Impairment Syndromes. Harcourt Health Sciences.

Sapsford, R.R., Hodges, P.W., Richardson, C.A., Cooper, D.H., Markwell, S.J., Jull, G.A., 2001. Co-activation of the abdominal and pelvic floor muscles during voluntary exercises. Neurourol. Urodyn. 20, 31–42.

Saw, T., Villar, R., 2004. Footballer's hip: a report of six cases. J. Bone Joint Surg. Br. 86, 655–658.

Schrader, S.M., Breitenstein, M.J., Clark, J.C., Lowe, B.D., Turner, T.W., 2002. Nocturnal penile tumescence and rigidity testing in bicycling patrol officers. J. Androl. 23, 927–934.

Schrader, S.M., Breitenstein, M.J., Lowe, B.D., 2008. Cutting off the nose to save the penis. J. Sex. Med. 5, 1932–1940.

Seong, S., Park, K., Moon, J., Ry, S., 2002. Bicycle saddle shape affects penile blood flow. Int. J. Impotence Res. 14, 513–551.

Shacklock, M., 2005. Clinical neurodynamics: A new system of musculoskeletal treatment. Elsevier-Butterworth-Heinemann.

Shindle, M.K., Domb, B.G., Kelly, B.T., 2007. Hip and pelvic problems. Oper. Tech. Sports Med. 15, 195–203.

Sommer, F., Goldstein, I., Korda, J.B., 2010. Bicycle riding and erectile dysfunction: a review. J. Sex. Med. 7, 2346–2358.

Standring, S., 2008. Gray's Anatomy: The Anatomical Basis of Clinical Practice. Expert Consult - Online and Print [Hardcover]. Churchill Livingstone, Edinburgh.

Starling, J.R., Harms, B.A., 1989. Diagnosis and treatment of genitofemoral and ilioinguinal neuralgia. World J. Surg. 13 (5), 586–591.

Suresh, S., Patel, A., Porfyris, S., Ryee, M.Y., 2008. Ultrasound-guided serial ilioinguinal nerve blocks for management of chronic groin pain secondary to ilioinguinal neuralgia in adolescents. Paediatr. Anaesth. 18, 775–778.

Swan Jr., K.G., Wolcott, M., 2007. The athletic hernia: a systematic review. [Review] [44 refs]. Clin. Orthop. Relat. Res. 455, 78–87.

Taylor III, J.A., Kao, T.C., Albertsen, P.C., Shabsigh, R., 2004. Bicycle riding and its relationship to the development of erectile dysfunction. J. Urol. 172, 1028–1031.

Travell, J.G., Simons, D.G., 1993. Myofascial pain and dysfunction. Am. Pain Soc. 2, 116–121.

Tsao, H., Hodges, P.W., 2007. Immediate changes in feedforward postural adjustments following voluntary motor training. Exp. Brain Res. 181, 537–546.

Tsao, H., Hodges, P.W., 2008. Persistence of improvements in postural strategies following motor control training in people with recurrent low back pain. J. Electromyogr. Kinesiol. 18, 559–567.

Tsao, H., Galea, M.P., Hodges, P.W., 2010. Driving plasticity in the motor cortex in recurrent low back pain. Eur. J. Pain 14 (8), 832–839.

Tyler, T.F., Nicholas, S.J., Campbell, R.J., et al., 2001. The association of hip strength and flexibility with the incidence of adductor muscle strains in professional ice hockey players. Am. J. Sports Med. 29 (2), 124–128.

Tyler, T.F., Nicholas, S.J., Campbell, R.J., et al., 2002. The effectiveness of a preseason exercise program to prevent adductor muscle strains in professional ice hockey players. Am. J. Sports Med. 30 (5), 680–683.

Tyler, T., Slattery, A., 2010. Rehabilitation of the hip following sports surgery. Clinics Sports Med. 29 (1), 107–126.

Urquhart, D.M., Hodges, P.W., Allen, T.J., Story, I.H., 2005. Abdominal muscle recruitment during a range of voluntary exercises. Man. Ther. 10, 144–153.

van Dieen, J.H., Selen, L.P., Cholewicki, J., 2003. Trunk muscle activation in low-back pain patients, an analysis of the literature. [Review] [141 refs]. J. Electromyogr. Kinesiol. 13, 333–351.

Van Dillen, L.R., Sahrmann, S.A., Norton, B.J., Caldwell, C.A., Fleming, D.A., McDonnell, M.K., et al., 1998. Reliability of physical examination items used for classification of patients with low back pain. Phys. Ther. 78, 979–988.

Van Dillen, L.R., Sahrmann, S.A., Norton, B.J., Caldwell, C.A., McDonnell, M.K., Bloom, N.J., 2003. Movement system impairment-based categories for low back pain: stage 1 validation. J. Orthop. Sports Phys. Ther. 33, 126–142.

Van Dillen, L.R., Bloom, N.J., Gombatto, S.P., Susco, T.M., 2008. Hip rotation range of motion in people with and without low back pain who participate in rotation-related sports. Physical Therapy in Sport 9, 72–81.

van Ramshorst, G.H., Kleinrensink, G.J., Hermans, J.J., Terkivatan, T., Lange, J.F., 2009. Abdominal wall paresis as a complication of laparoscopic surgery. Hernia 13, 539–543.

Verrall, G.M., Slavotinek, J.P., Fon, G.T., 2001. Incidence of pubic bone marrow oedema in Australian rules football players: relation to groin pain. Br. J. Sports Med. 35 (1), 28–33.

Vervest, H.A., Bongers, M.Y., van der Wurff, A.A., 2006. Nerve injury: an exceptional cause of pain after TVT. Int. Urogynecol. J. 17, 665–667.

Waddell, G., 2004. The Back Pain Revolution, second ed. Churchill Livingstone, Edinburgh.

Walsh, J., Hall, T., 2009. Reliability, validity and diagnostic accuracy of palpation of the sciatic, tibial and common peroneal nerves in the examination of low back related leg pain. Man. Ther. 14, 623–629.

Walsh, J., Ther, M., Hall, T., 2009. Agreement and correlation between the straight leg raise and slump tests in subjects with leg pain. J. Manipulative Physiol. Ther. 32, 184–192.

Weiss, B.D., 1985. Non-traumatic injuries among amateur long distance bicyclists. Am. J. Sports Med. 13, 187–192.

Werner, J., Haggland, M., Walden, M., Ekstrand, J., 2009. UEFA injury study: a prospective study of hip and groin injuries in professional football over seven consecutive seasons. Br. J. Sports Med. 43, 1036–1040.

White, A.A., Punjabi, M.M., 1990. Clinical Biomechanics of the SpIne. Lippincott & Co.

Whiteside, J.L., Barber, M.D., 2005. Ilioinguinal/iliohypogastric neurectomy for management of intractable right lower quadrant pain after cesarean section: a case report. J. Reprod. Med. 50, 857–859.

Whittaker, J.L., 2007. Ultrasound Imaging for Rehabilitation of the Lumbopelvic Region: A Clinical Approach. Churchill Livingstone, London.

Woby, S.R., Watson, P.J., Roach, N.K., Urmston, M., 2004. Adjustment to chronic low back pain – the relative influence of fear-avoidance beliefs, catastrophizing, and appraisals of control. Behav. Res. Ther. 42, 761–774.

Woby, S.R., Roach, N.K., Urmston, M., Watson, P.J., 2007. The relation between cognitive factors and levels of pain and disability in chronic low back pain patients presenting for physiotherapy. Eur. J. Pain 11, 869–887.

Zimmerman, G., 1988. Groin pain in athletes. Am. Fam. Physician 17 (12), 1046–1052.

Zoga, A.C., Kavanagh, E.C., Omar, I.M., Morrison, W.B., Koulouris, G., Lopez, H., et al., 2008. Athletic pubalgia and the "sports hernia": MR imaging findings. Radiology 247, 797–807.

The role of clinical reasoning in the differential diagnosis and management of chronic pelvic pain

7

Diane Lee Linda-Joy Lee

Authors' note: The first part of this chapter is adapted from Lee L.J. & Lee D.G. [originally titled Clinical Practice: The reality for clinicians]. Chapter 7 of Lee, L.J. & Lee, D.G., 2011. The Pelvic Girdle, fourth ed. Churchill Livingstone. The Case Study is original to this current chapter.

CHAPTER CONTENTS

Introduction

All health practitioners spend considerable time gaining the knowledge necessary for their chosen career. What types of knowledge are there and what do practitioners need on a daily basis? Knowledge can be categorized as:

1. Propositional, theoretical or scientific knowledge (Higgs & Titchen 1995), also known as declarative knowledge (Jensen et al. 2007);
2. Non-propositional or professional craft knowledge (knowing how to do something) (Higgs & Titchen 1995) or procedural (Jensen et al. 2007). Non-propositional knowledge also includes personal knowledge or knowing oneself as a person and in relationship with others.

Propositional, or declarative, knowledge refers to the content knowledge that one's profession is based on and includes factual information derived from formal research trials. In addition, this category includes theoretical knowledge developed from existing empirical protocols and principles, derived from dialogue with professionals in the same discipline, and logic (Higgs 2004).

Non-propositional, or procedural, knowledge pertains to knowing how to do things pertaining to one's profession (craft and personal knowledge), such as how to mobilize a joint, release a hypertonic muscle, rewire a neural network, train a movement pattern and/or motivate an individual to change. This knowledge is gained through reflection on both professional and personal experiences (what worked, what did not work and how could it have been 'done' or handled differently to achieve a different outcome). Historically, non-propositional knowledge formed the basis for both medicine and allied health professionals including physiotherapy. All treatment is influenced by a practitioner's perspective, their personal knowledge, values and beliefs. This factor contributes to the outcome of an intervention and is often not considered in clinical trials studying the efficacy of a particular treatment (i.e. a trial that aims to identify whether manipulation or exercise is more effective for the treatment of low back pain).

Most practitioners continue to take post-graduate courses or attend professional conferences to improve their knowledge pertaining to clinical theory and research (propositional) as well as their technical skills (non-propositional or craft); however, Rivett & Jones (2004) note that there is a tendency in both courses and conferences to neglect an essential component of daily clinical practice – *clinical reasoning*. How should the practitioner integrate into clinical practice the newly learned scientific and theoretical knowledge? Who is it appropriate for and when is the new skill appropriate to use? Clinical practice is, and always will be, a blend of science and 'art' with a healthy dose of logic and reasoning. Clinical expertise comes from reasoning, reflection, skill acquisition and the continual life-long pursuit of knowledge (propositional (declarative) and non-propositional (procedural and personal)) (Figure 7.1) (Jensen et al. 2007). This takes time, discipline and often mentorship and professional affiliation with both individuals and groups.

Recently, for best practice, there is increasing pressure for practitioners to become evidence-based when making all clinical decisions. However, it appears that this term, evidence-based practice, means different things to different people. What is evidence-based practice and what is its history?

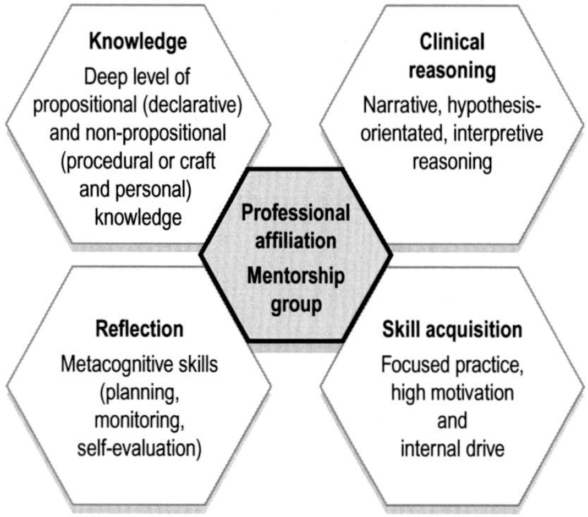

Figure 7.1 • Five components for the development of clinical expertise. Adapted from Jensen et al. (2007). Expertise in Physical Therapy Practice, second ed. Saunders.

Evidence-based practice: Where did it come from? Where is it going?

The term 'evidence-based' was first used in 1990 by David Eddy and 'evidence-based medicine' by Guyatt et al. in 1992. The methodologies used to determine 'best evidence' were largely established by the Canadian McMaster University research group led by David Sackett and Gordon Guyatt. Professor Archie Cochrane, a Scottish epidemiologist, has been credited with increasing the acceptance of the principles behind evidence-based practice (Cochrane 1972). Cochrane's work was honoured through the naming of centres of evidence-based medical research, Cochrane Centers, and an international organization, the Cochrane Collaboration. Since the early 1990s there has been an explosion of research evidence, and accessibility to this evidence has been facilitated for those involved in research or formal study through easy internet access to full-text articles in indexed journals. Unfortunately, access to full-text articles is still limited, or expensive, for clinicians not affiliated with research centres or universities.

Evidence-based medicine categorizes and ranks the different types of clinical evidence. The terms 'levels of evidence' or 'strength of evidence' refer to the protocols for ranking the evidence based on the strength of the study to be free from various biases. The highest level of evidence for therapeutic interventions is a systematic review, or meta-analysis, including only randomized, double-blind, placebo-controlled trials that involve a homogeneous patient population and condition. Expert opinion has little value as evidence and is ranked the lowest due to the placebo effect, the biases inherent in both the observation, and reporting of the cases and difficulties in discerning who is really an expert.

Evidence-based practice (EBP) embraces all disciplines of health care (not just medicine) and has become synonymous with best practice, but what does the term really mean? To some, it appears that EBP means that a clinician can only use assessment tests and treatment techniques/protocols that have been validated through the scientific process with high-ranking studies as valued by the 'levels of evidence'. This is difficult to adhere to for many reasons, one

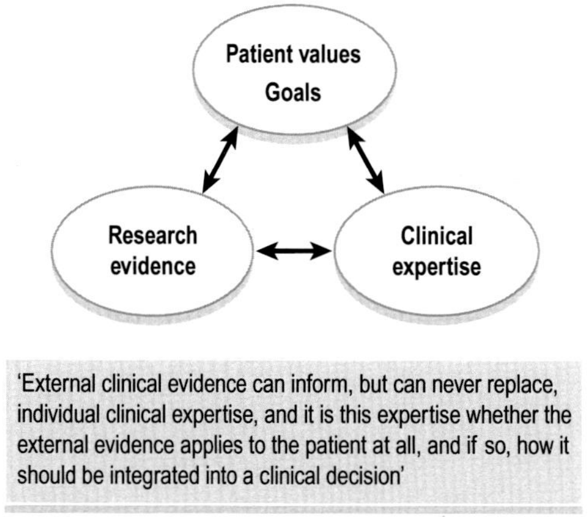
Patient values
Goals
Research evidence
Clinical expertise
'External clinical evidence can inform, but can never replace, individual clinical expertise, and it is this expertise whether the external evidence applies to the patient at all, and if so, how it should be integrated into a clinical decision'

Figure 7.2 • The three components of evidence-based practice as defined by Sackett et al. (2000)

being that there is not enough evidence at this time. Indeed, could there ever be enough scientific evidence for every situation met in clinical practice? Sackett and colleagues define EBP as 'the integration of best research evidence, with clinical expertise and patient values' (Sackett et al. 2000) (Figure 7.2). They note that:

> External clinical evidence can inform, but can never replace individual clinical expertise, and it is this expertise that decides whether the external evidence applies to the patient at all, and if so, how it should be integrated into a clinical decision.

Clinical expertise, as noted above, comprises both propositional (declarative) and non-propositional (procedural, craft and personal) knowledge; in other words, knowing what, and how, to do the right thing at the right time (clinical reasoning and skill). The type of knowledge gained from scientific studies contributes to building only one kind of knowledge. In EBP according to Sackett et al.'s definition, clinical expertise plays an equal role alongside the research evidence. A third component of EBP is the patient's values and goals, which come from the person for whom all of the research and expertise is intended to help.

Recently, the term 'evidence-informed' has surfaced, the intent being to suggest that since there is not enough research evidence for every situation met in clinical practice, the clinician should be informed of what is known and make their clinical decisions accordingly. However, if we adopt Sackett et al.'s definition of EBP, there is no need to modify the term since clinical expertise (reasoning and skill) is considered part of the definition of best practice.

Understanding pain: What do we need to know?

Understanding the neurophysiology of pain mechanisms is essential knowledge for treating patients with pelvic pain. Since the proposal of the gate control theory of pain by Melzack and Wall in 1965, significant advances in pain research and therapy have occurred. It is not our intent to provide an in-depth coverage of this topic here, but instead to highlight key features and establish a common language to be used throughout this chapter. See Chapter 3 for a full discussion of pain mechanisms in general, and as these relate to chronic pelvic pain.

What causes pain? Searching for the pain driver

The search for 'the pain driver' in peripheral tissues began when Descartes, in the 17th century, proposed that specific pathways existed from the peripheral tissues to the passive brain to transmit information notifying the brain of tissue injury. The premise that injury of the tissues (ligaments, connective tissue, bones, nerves, organs, etc.) is the cause of pain is the basis of the *pathoanatomical* or *biomedical* model of pain, and has prevailed in the assessment and treatment of pain until quite recently. This model has led to research and increased understanding about nociception, including the stimuli that can cause it (mechanical, thermal and chemical), which peripheral tissues can be painful and the pain patterns they generate. Clinicians believed that if the tissues could heal or be fixed (by whatever means, including by anaesthetic injection, anti-inflammatory medication, or removal of the offending tissue), then nociception would stop, the pain would go away, and the patient would recover function.

It is now well recognized that the pathoanatomical model is limited in several ways. Pelvic pain commonly exists in the absence of any findings on diagnostic tests (X-ray, CT scan, blood tests, nerve conduction tests, etc.), and damaged tissues can be identified in people who experience no pain (Nachemson 1999, Waddell 2004). Tissues heal and yet the pain experience persists. Furthermore, a focus on only treating 'the painful tissue' neglects to consider that other systems or structures, which may be dysfunctional but *painfree*, could be the underlying cause of excessive mechanical stresses on the painful structures, or the cause of decreased blood flow or nutritional supply. In order to resolve the pain, the *painfree* but *impaired* structures or systems need to be treated for long-term resolution. Identification of what tissue hurts does not provide insight as to *why* it hurts. Finally, significant developments in neuroscience have changed our understanding of what pain is, and have required us to reframe and change our thinking.

We now understand that at any time in one patient there are *many* 'pain drivers' that do not exist solely in the peripheral tissues. Rather than looking for one source of pain, we need to consider that multiple mechanisms are at play in the experience of pain in all our patients. These mechanisms can be broadly separated into *peripherally mediated* (nociception and peripheral neurogenic pain) or *centrally mediated* (related to processing in the central nervous system (CNS)) (Butler 2000), and will be discussed in more detail later in this section.

Classifying pain

Timelines and mechanism of injury

Patients are commonly classified according to the timeline or duration of their pain experience, and the cause or mechanism of their injury. In general, problems are considered to be *acute* if they are within the first 6 weeks to 3 months (depending on the type of tissue injured) after an initiating incident (Brukner & Khan 2002, Magee et al. 2007). Tissue injury results in a known sequence of events aimed at protecting and repairing the damaged structures. These stages of tissue healing occur in three overlapping stages that have been given multiple names but refer to the same processes:

1. Acute inflammatory stage;
2. Subacute or proliferation stage;
3. Chronic or maturation and remodelling stage.

The term *chronic* is often used to indicate the persistence of pain beyond the normal timeline for tissue healing (Bonica 1953, Merskey & Bogduk 1994), as opposed to a stage of the tissue-healing process. In the *Classification of Chronic Pain* (Merskey & Bogduk 1994) published by the International Association for the Study of Pain, it is noted that the normal time of healing 'may be less than one month, or more often, more than six months. With nonmalignant pain, three months is the most convenient point of division between acute and chronic pain, but for research purposes six months will often be preferred.' Chronic pain is also further outlined as 'a persistent pain that is not amenable, as a rule to treatments based upon specific remedies, or to the routine methods of pain control such as non-narcotic analgesics' (Merskey & Bogduk 1994).

More recently, the term *persistent* low back pain has emerged in the literature, to indicate pain that continues past the expected timeframe for tissue healing. Others are suggesting that *acute episodes* of low back pain would be better termed *recurrent episodes* in a *chronic* problem as the underlying mechanisms contributing to recurrent low back pain are likely to be different from a first-time traumatic episode of low back pain, and recurrence of pain after an acute episode is a common problem (Pengel et al. 2003).

Acute pain, especially when related to a specific initiating incident, is commonly perceived as being relatively straightforward in terms of what pain mechanisms are at play. These are generally accepted to be types of peripherally mediated pain (nociceptive or peripheral neurogenic) related to tissue damage and the resultant inflammatory processes are aimed at restoring homeostasis in the body. However, is any pain experience truly simple? Consider the following report:

> A builder aged 29 came to the accident and emergency department having jumped down on to a 15 cm nail. As the smallest movement of the nail was painful he was sedated with fentanyl and midazolam. The nail was then pulled out from below. When his boot was removed a miraculous cure appeared to have taken place. Despite entering proximal to the steel toecap the nail had penetrated between the toes; the foot was entirely uninjured.
>
> (Fisher et al. 1995)

The initial logical hypothesis in this case was that acute trauma to the foot was causing severe nociceptive input from the damaged tissues. However, as physical examination revealed completely intact tissues, this cannot explain the patient's pain experience. Clearly other pain mechanisms were at play, despite the timeline (acute onset) and mode of onset (traumatic) of the pain.

Empirical evidence now exists to explain these kinds of stories. A consistent factor that has emerged from the pain sciences is that the *meaning* of the pain experience, and especially the *threat value* of the experience, is significant. In other words, does the pain signify something harmful or not? While some may continue to function and keep going in spite of pain, others are completely debilitated by the mere thought of the sensation. There is increasing evidence to support that an individual's experience of pain is significantly influenced by the way they think and feel about the situation as a whole, regardless of the severity of tissue injury. The story above illustrates these influences; his pain experience is an example of 100% centrally mediated pain, driven by his beliefs (cognitive dimension) and emotional state (affective dimension) related to the event (having a nail driven through his boot). It is clear that we cannot separate the tissues from the person to which they belong; we are integrated beings and our experience of our body (whether positive or negative) is the result of complex interactions and processes occurring in the brain.

Thus, although the mechanism of onset and timeframes related to the pain experience are important to know, we must take care that this information does not lead us to assume that certain timelines *necessitate* certain pain mechanisms. Acute pain can be largely driven by central mechanisms. Persistent pain can also be largely driven by peripheral mechanisms. That is, persistent or chronic pain states may have central components, but these are not necessarily the dominant mechanism for every patient simply because the pain experience has persisted for a long period of time. While evidence supports that 'the relationship between pain and the state of the tissues becomes less predictable as pain persists (Moseley 2007), we need to remember that the pain experience is uniquely individual. Regardless of whether the pain is a newly occurring event or a persistent experience, it is a multidimensional experience, and thus any person presenting with pain should be evaluated with a framework in mind that allows for the consideration of all these factors. As Butler (2000, p. 53) notes:

> Overlap of mechanisms is the key feature because the boundaries are often fuzzy. There will be differing contributions of mechanisms to the injury state over time, person and injury.

Classification by pain mechanisms

So what are the different biological mechanisms that drive the pain experience? Pain mechanisms can be further categorized (Gifford 1998, Butler 2000) as they relate to:

1. Input into the nervous system;
2. Processing in the nervous system;
3. Output from the nervous and other systems.

The brain receives continuous information from the body and the environment (input mechanisms or all sensory pathways) that is assessed and interpreted (processing at both conscious and unconscious levels) prior to producing a response (output mechanisms). Some of this incoming information is nociceptive. There are many factors that determine an individual's behaviour and pain experience (physical, cognitive, emotional) in response to nociceptive input, including:

- Contextual factors of the immediate circumstance (i.e. how dangerous is this sensation in the light of environmental and internal factors?); as well as
- Past experiences and personal knowledge that collectively contribute to the individual's beliefs, attitudes, emotions and physical responses.

Input mechanisms as they pertain to pain include all the sensory information reaching the CNS from the body internally and externally. This includes nociceptive pain from tissues including bones, ligaments, tendons, muscles, connective tissue, viscera, etc. (Gifford 1998, Butler 2000, Wright 2002) and peripheral neurogenic pain from neural tissue outside of the CNS. Processing occurs in the dorsal root ganglion and in the CNS. In the brain, an individual's thoughts and feelings (cognitions + emotions = perception) are integrated and can influence the output mechanisms, which include:

1. Somatic or motor (altered posture, altered motor control);
2. Autonomic (increased sympathetic response for 'fight or flight');
3. Neuroendocrine (increased stress, heightened emotions, hormonal changes);
4. Neuroimmune.

Thinking within the context of stress biology creates a broader framework for understanding pain. Gifford (1998), in proposing the Mature Organism Model (Figure 7.3), notes that

> ... the sensation of pain is seen as a perceptual component of the stress response whose prime adaptive purpose is to alter our behaviour in order to enhance the processes of recovery and chances of survival. Stress biology and the stress response broadly considers the systems and responses concerned with maintaining homeostasis.
>
> (Gifford 1998)

It has been proposed that continued activation of the stress-regulation systems and excessive or prolonged cortisol output has a destructive effect on peripheral tissues such as muscle, bone and nerve tissue, thereby perpetuating a vicious cycle of stress, pain and tissue injury (Melzack 2005).

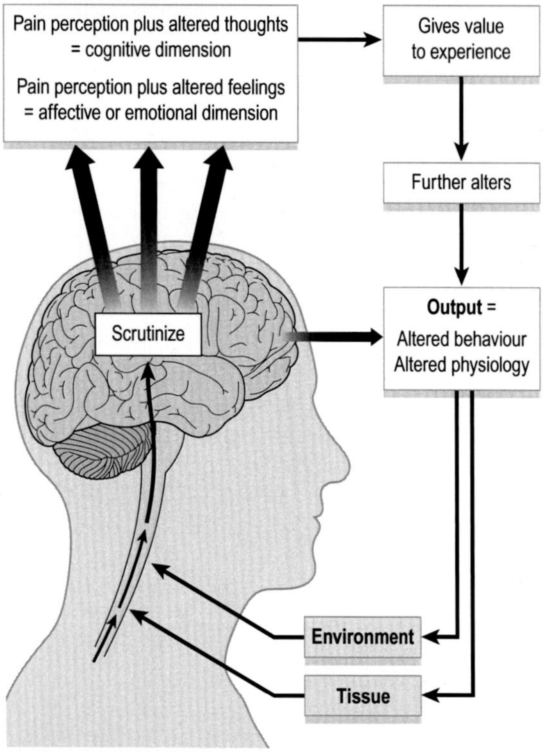

Figure 7.3 • The Mature Organism Model of Gifford (1998). Adapted from Rivett & Jones (2004). Improving clinical reasoning in manual therapy. In: Jones, M.A., Rivett, D. (Eds.), Clinical reasoning for manual therapists, Churchill Livingstone; and Gifford (1998) Physiotherapy 84:27.

In his *Neuromatrix Theory of Pain*, Ronald Melzack (2001, 2005) highlights the need to assess and treat the whole person, not just the painful parts.

> The body is felt as a unity, with different qualities at different times. ... [Together all outputs] produce a continuous message that represents the whole body [which he also describes] as a flow of awareness.
>
> (Melzack 2001, 2005)

Melzack's model has four components (2001, 2005):

1. The body-self neuromatrix – an anatomical substrate in the brain of the body-self;
2. Cyclical processing and synthesis of nerve impulses which produces a neurosignature;
3. The flow of neurosignatures is projected back to areas of the brain, the sentient neural hub, which converts them into the flow of awareness;
4. Activation of an action neuromatrix occurs to provide the pattern of movements to bring about the desired goal.

> The neuromatrix, distributed throughout many areas of the brain, comprises a widespread network of neurons which generates patterns, processes information that flows through it, and ultimately produces the pattern that is felt as a whole body. The stream of neurosignature output with constantly varying patterns riding on the main signature pattern produces the feelings of the whole body with constantly changing qualities. ... The final, integrated neurosignature pattern for the body-self ultimately produces awareness and action.
>
> (Melzack 2005)

Figure 7.4 is a modification of Melzack's representation of the body-self neuromatrix to illustrate the sensorial, cognitive and emotional dimensions of pain. Perhaps the best summary for this section

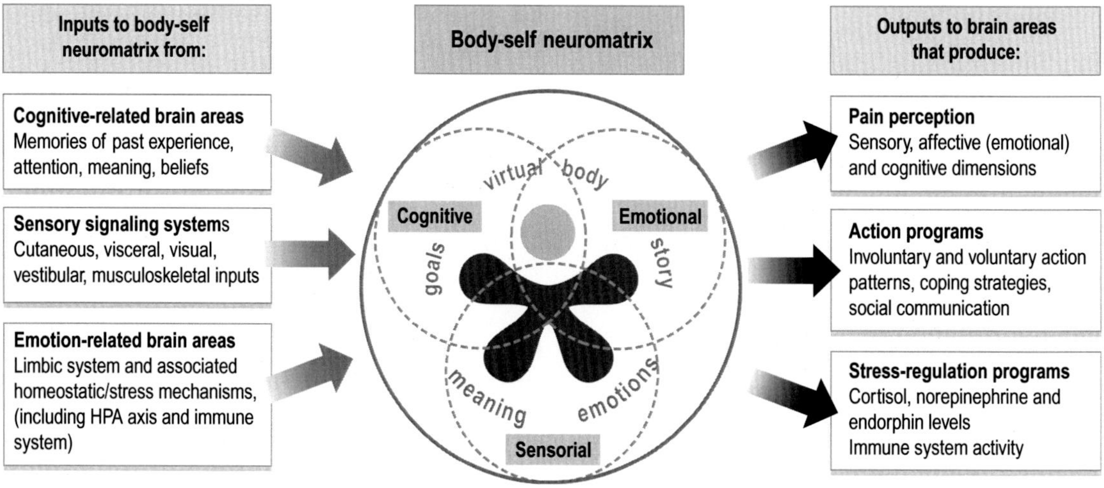

Figure 7.4 • An adaptation of Melzack's Body-Self Neuromatrix (Melzack 2001, 2005). HPA, hypothalamic–pituitary–adrenal

highlighting the broad view we need to take when considering pain comes from this leader in the study of pain himself, Ronald Melzack (2001):

> We have traveled a long way from the psychosocial concept that seeks a simple one-to-one relationship between injury and pain. We now have a theoretical framework in which a genetically determined template for the body-self is modulated by the powerful stress system and the cognitive functions of the brain, in addition to the traditional sensory inputs. The neuromatrix theory of pain – which places genetic contributions and the neural-hormonal mechanisms of stress on a level of equal importance with the neural mechanisms of sensory transmission – has important implications for research and therapy. The expansion of the field of pain to include endocrinology and immunology may lead to insights and new research strategies that will reveal the underlying mechanisms of chronic pain and give rise to new therapies to relieve the tragedy of unrelenting suffering.

It is very clear that as clinicians we need to be aware of all the possible mechanisms that can create pain and to challenge ourselves to have an open mind as we seek to understand each individual's unique pain experience in order to determine which mechanisms are primary and specifically related to their problem in all stages of their rehabilitation process.

Classification and clinical prediction rules: Are we searching for the holy grail?

Given the multidimensional nature of pain, it is not surprising that using pain presentation (location, duration, onset) as the sole means to classify patients and determine best treatment has been ineffective. Fritz and colleagues report that despite over 1000 randomized clinical trials investigating the effectiveness of interventions for the management of low back pain, 'the evidence remains contradictory and inconclusive' (Fritz et al. 2007). One key reason believed to contribute to this state of the evidence is the lack of classification of low back pain patients into subgroups, not only for studying treatment efficacy, but also for determining aetiological and prognostic factors (Leboeuf-Yde et al. 1997, Riddle 1998, Gombatto et al. 2007).

Sahrmann in the late 1980s noted:

> As we all know, general diagnoses such as low back pain or hip pain do not often relate to the cause or to the underlying nature of the condition.
>
> (Sahrmann 1988)

As clinicians have long recognized, it is now widely accepted that patients with pain do not form homogeneous populations, but consist of multiple subgroups with different combinations of underlying impairments (physical and psychosocial), and these subgroups require different treatment approaches for best outcomes. Furthermore, given that multiple factors contribute to pain, it is also unrealistic to expect that one single type of treatment modality will resolve a patient's presenting pain and functional limitations. Thus, the pursuit of valid ways to identify subgroups of patients with pain has become an increasingly prominent theme in the literature over the last three decades.

The classification for lumbopelvic pain has evolved since the pathoanatomically based classification of MacNab (1977) with a variety of patient characteristics proposed for use in creating homogeneous subgroups (McKenzie 1981, Kirkaldy-Willis 1983, Bernard & Kirkaldy-Willis 1987, Coste et al. 1992, Delitto et al. 1995, Sahrmann 2001, O'Sullivan 2005, Reeves et al. 2005, Fritz et al. 2007, O'Sullivan & Beales 2007) (Table 7.1).

O'Sullivan (2005) noted that a limitation of many classification systems is that often only a single dimension (pathoanatomical, psychosocial, neurophysiological, motor control, signs and symptoms, etc.) is used to create subgroups. Classification systems will be most useful in clinical practice if variables across multiple domains are used to create subgroups.

Features that have been incorporated into different systems include (note this is not intended to be an exhaustive list):

- Presence or absence of identifiable underlying pathology (pathoanatomical, peripheral pain generator models);
- Pain presentation (central, unilateral, with or without radiation of symptoms to the lower extremity) (signs and symptoms models);
- Underlying pain mechanisms/neurophysiology;
- Response of pain to movement (centralization or peripheralization) (signs and symptoms models) (movement impairment models);
- Physical impairments such as loss or increase of mobility, altered motor control, altered posture/spinal alignment, and the relationship of symptom provocation to these impairments (motor control models, signs and symptoms models, movement impairment models);

Table 7.1 Multiple proposals for the classification of patients

Model/system	Description	Diagnostic/classification determinants
Pathoanatomical (McNab 1977, Kirkaldy-Willis & Hill 1979, Kirkaldy-Willis 1983, Nachemson 1999)	Focuses on structural changes which occur as a consequence of inflammation, infection, metabolic disorders, trauma and/or disease (pathology-based)	Radiological diagnosis, blood work
Mechanical diagnosis and therapy (The McKenzie Method) (McKenzie 1981)	Directional preference and centralization or peripheralization of pain with repeated movements. Four subgroups: • derangement syndrome • dysfunction syndrome • posture syndrome • other	Rapidly reversible symptoms with repeated movements in a specific direction
Peripheral pain generator model (Laslett & Williams 1994, Laslett et al. 2005)	Attempts to identify the painful peripheral pain-generating structure with the main therapeutic intervention being to block or denervate the nociceptive source	Diagnostic blocks of various peripheral structures seeking to relieve pain
Neurophysiological pain model (Butler 2000)	Generation and maintenance of pain both peripherally and/or centrally mediated (central and/or peripheral sensitization of neural networks)	Subjective examination (confirmed/negated by features of the objective examination)
Psychosocial model (Waddell 2004)	Cognitive and emotional factors such as negative thinking, fear-avoidance behaviours and hypervigilance	Subjective examination
Treatment-based Classification System (Delitto et al. 1995) updated criteria (Fritz et al. 2007)	Intended for patients with acute/acute exacerbation of low back pain (LBP). Patients placed into treatment categories based on patterns of signs and symptoms: • manipulation • specific exercise (flexion, extension, lateral-shift patterns) • stabilization • traction	Subjective examination, objective examination features based on clinical experience and propositional knowledge. Specific exercise grouping based primarily on centralization/peripheralization principles (McKenzie 1981). Updated criteria include disability questionnaire data and is based on CPRs and scientific research. Traction group removed in updated classification
Movement System Impairment System (Sahrmann 2001)	Based on the kinesiopathic model of movement; musculoskeletal pain develops as a result of repeated movements and postural alignments in the same direction across daily activities, causing repeated loading and microtrauma. LBP subgroups: • lumbar flexion • lumbar extension • lumbar rotation • lumbar rotation with flexion • lumbar rotation with extension	Subjective and objective examination aimed to identify the direction of movement and alignment that is related to LBP. Symptoms are monitored in response to standardized movement and alignment tests, along with observation of timing of relative motion of body segments, and the response to modification of alignment/movement

- Response to specific treatments (manipulation, stabilization exercises, specific exercises, traction); and
- Psychosocial and cognitive features such as fear avoidance, coping strategies and beliefs (biopsychosocial models).

In recent years, the development of clinical prediction rules (CPRs) has emerged as another way to classify patients. CPRs are derived statistically with the aim of identifying the combinations of clinical examination findings that can predict a condition or outcome. Thus, they are proposed to be a useful tool to assist in clinical decision-making by improving the accuracy of diagnosis, prognosis or prediction of response to specific treatment protocols (Beattie & Nelson 2006, Cook 2008, Fritz 2009). Development of CPRs in physiotherapy has mainly focused on the response to treatment protocols (Fritz 2009) in order to identify subgroups of patients most likely to respond to a specific treatment approach. It is important to note that, at this time, CPRs are still in their infancy of development and validation, and are not yet at the appropriate stage to be widely applied in clinical practice (Cook 2008).

It has been suggested that CPRs will best impact physiotherapy practice where there is complexity in the clinical decision-making process, and that 'an appeal of CPRs is their potential to make [the] subgrouping process more evidence based and less reliant on unfounded theories and tradition' (Fritz 2009). However, the use of CPRs should be balanced with the knowledge that:

> Clinical prediction rules provide probabilities of a given diagnosis or prognosis but do not necessarily recommend decisions. Clinical prediction rules can be of great value to assist clinical decision-making but should not be used indiscriminately. They are not a replacement for clinical judgment and should complement rather than supplant clinical opinion and intuition.
>
> (Beattie & Nelson 2006)

Research on specific subgroups and development of classification systems will definitely provide a much better understanding of the specific impairments, mechanisms and psychosocial features that characterize subgroups and their response to treatment. As Melzack wrote about the evolution of the gate control theory of pain:

> As historians of science have pointed out, good theories are instrumental in producing facts that eventually require a new theory to incorporate them.
>
> (Melzack 2001)

However, it is important to recognize that there are limitations on how information gained from classification systems, CPRs, clinical trials, and indeed the findings of any scientific study, can be translated and applied to the reality of clinical practice. Firstly, statistical averages tell us about the average response of the group defined by the characteristics used in design of the study. Individual responses may be to a greater or lesser degree than the average, or even in the opposite direction of the reported response. Indeed, practising clinicians are well aware of the many patients they have seen who do not fit the data from clinical trials or other studies. These clinical cases provide valuable insight and can generate questions for further research. Secondly, while the data provide relatively unbiased information, the interpretation and conclusions made from the data, and published alongside the data, are subject to bias just as much as clinical opinion is subject to bias. It is also important to recognize that a *lack* of data or science does not invalidate a technique or approach, nor does it mean that approaches that have been studied are necessarily superior. In clinical practice, application of any classification system/CPR requires care to ensure that it does not create a rigid, narrow mindset. Placing the patient 'in a box' could prevent the clinician from considering other options for treatment that may be greatly beneficial. Neglecting to provide these other options could then result in sub-optimal outcomes.

Consider the one domain of underlying pain mechanism as a way to create subgroups.

Butler (2000) notes that:

> The word "division" can be instant trouble because these mechanisms all occur in a continuum. All pain states probably involve all mechanisms, however in some, a dominance of one mechanism may become obvious. Pain mechanisms are not diseases or specific injuries. They simply represent a process or biological state.

In their classification of pelvic pain disorders, O'Sullivan & Beales (2007) categorize non-specific pelvic pain disorders into two groups: one that has centrally mediated pain, and one that has peripherally mediated pain. Although the group of centrally mediated pain is further classified into those with non-dominant psychosocial factors and those with dominant psychosocial factors, the treatment protocol for the subgroup of centrally mediated pelvic girdle pain is medical management (central nervous system modulation), psychological (cognitive-behavioural therapy), and functional capacity rehabilitation. Specific interventions directed at identified physical impairments in the periphery are not recommended, and yet it is highly unlikely that many patients will have 100% centrally mediated pain. In the authors' experience, even in patients with a strong contributor of central sensitization to their pain experience, careful assessment often reveals specific meaningful tasks that relate to a consistent reproduction of symptoms. It is reasonable to suggest that even if peripheral mechanisms only contribute 20% to the complete picture, addressing that 20% in addition to the other approaches will provide the greatest chance for the best outcome. Furthermore, it is likely that by addressing the physical impairments, psychosocial variables will also be impacted, further advancing the goals of treating drivers of central sensitization. It is also crucial to recognize that our patients change as a result of their changing life circumstances and our interactions with them (both physical and personal). Thus, during the course of treatment continual re-evaluation is necessary to adapt the treatment programme accordingly. Sticking to a rigid plan based on an initial placement into a subgroup may result in the provision of sub-optimal care.

Finally, in our quest for better classification schemes and science to support and test our clinical approaches, it is important to remember that at the end of the day no matter how detailed and well defined our classification schemes, the person presenting to the clinician is a unique *individual* with unique life experiences. There will never be one recipe for treatment that is the best fit for all patients. Furthermore, patient values and beliefs are central to the treatment process, and if they do not want to receive what is considered 'best practice' from the current evidence, we cannot force it on them. Given the same impairment in the tissues, no two individuals will have exactly the same perception and presentation (experience and behaviour) because 'how they manifest their pain or illness is shaped in part by who they are' (Jones & Rivett 2004). A reminder, the highest level of evidence for therapeutic interventions is a systematic review, or meta-analysis, of only randomized, double-blind, placebo-controlled trials which involve a homogeneous patient population and condition. Is this possible in the light of what is known about pain? Do homogeneous populations really exist in clinical practice?

Science can provide us with an abundance of knowledge to challenge, refine, reshape and validate our clinical practice, but it cannot provide all of the information needed in any individual patient encounter; it does not paint the whole picture of the patient. In order to effectively treat patients, therapists need to have well-organized knowledge including propositional (knowledge ratified by research trials), non-propositional (professional craft or 'knowing how' knowledge) and personal (knowledge gained from personal experiences (Jones & Rivett 2004).

> Understanding and successfully managing patients' problems requires a rich organization of all three types of knowledge. Propositional knowledge provides us with theory and levels of substantiation by which the patient's clinical presentation can be considered against research-validated theory and practice. Non-propositional professional craft knowledge allows us the means to use that theory in the clinic while providing additional, often cutting-edge (albeit with unproven generality) clinically derived evidence. Personal knowledge allows a deeper understanding of the clinical problem to be gained within the context of the patient's particular situation and enabling us to practice in a holistic and caring way.
>
> (Jones & Rivett 2004)

Personal and craft knowledge cannot be learned from RCTs, mechanistic studies, basic physiology studies, or clinical prediction rules. Ultimately, it is the development of *clinical expertise* that creates optimal patient care. According to Ericsson & Smith (1991) expertise has been defined as 'having the ability to do the right thing at the right time'.

Clinical expertise has two components: skill acquisition (do the right thing) and clinical reasoning (at the right time) (Figure 7.5). Clinical reasoning skills facilitate the organization and integration of knowledge gained both in and out of the clinic, and the wise application of that knowledge for each individual patient.

Different classification systems provide us with a variety of perspectives to grow our knowledge base. However, hoping to find '*the* best classification system' to apply in every situation in clinical practice is like searching for the Holy Grail – it cannot be found. We are unique people trying to help other unique people. We need to re-evaluate how we value the 'levels of evidence' and the role of science in directing clinical practice, and develop a more balanced view that values the insight that is uniquely derived from clinical practice. The clinical 'lab' plays a key role in new knowledge generation through the development of innovative techniques for assessment and treatment, which can then be tested by science. Knowledge gained from clinical experience

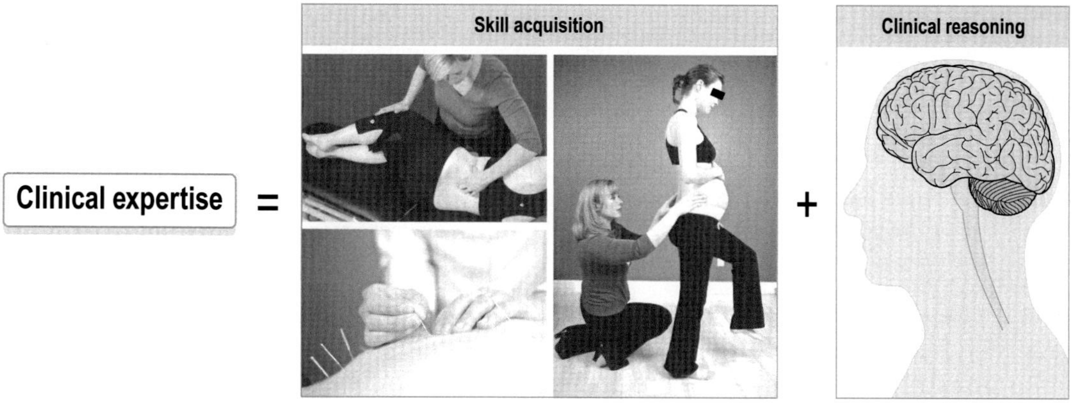

Figure 7.5 • Clinical expertise comprises two components: skill acquisition (the ability to do the right thing) and clinical reasoning (at the right time)

is not more important than science, but it certainly is no less important. Overall, maintaining an open mind and broad perspective will assist both scientists and clinicians to discover how best to work together and learn from each other in the common goal of providing best care for our patients.

It's about more than pain – Integrated systems for optimal health

While pain is important, it is also recognized that simply relieving a patient's pain does not necessarily result in a full return to all functional activities. Furthermore, there are subgroups of patients, such as high-level athletes, whose functional goals and measures (race time, power delivery in a stroke for example) are just as, if not *more*, meaningful to them than the relief of pain. Indeed, there is an increasing market in helping people *without pain* to optimize performance as well as prevent injury by facilitating strategies for better posture and movement. Pain is not a problem for these people, but an inability to meet their functional goals is. Non-painful impairments are also recognized as a potential contributor to the development of pain, both in sites distal to the impaired area and in the area itself. Furthermore, if we take the broader view that 'pain is an opinion on the organism's state of health rather than a mere reflexive response to injury' (Ramachandran in Doidge 2007), we need to alter our focus and consider what it means to be 'in health' and not only what it means to be 'in pain'. The World Health Assembly has defined health as 'a state of complete physical, mental, and social well-being and not merely the absence of disease or infirmity' (WHO Constitution). Speaking at the 1985 annual conference of the American Medical Association (Seattle, USA), Dr. Paul Brenner defined health even more broadly as 'the full acceptance and appreciation of life'. Restoring health is about more than removing disease; creating optimal strategies for function and performance is about more than removing pain.

What it means to be 'in health' is individually defined. Therefore, changing our focus from removing pain to restoring optimal health and optimal strategies for function and performance is intrinsically linked to the patient's values and goals. Our role as clinicians is to best facilitate and empower patients on their journey to achieve their personal optimal health and function. To do this effectively, we need not only to understand their pain, but also to understand to them as a person. Jones & Rivett (2004) refer to this as 'understanding both the problem and the person':

> To understand and manage patients and their problems successfully, manual therapists must consider not only the physical diagnostic possibilities (including the structures involved and the associated pathobiology) but also the full range of factors that can contribute to a person's health, particularly the effects these problems may have on patients' lives, and the understanding patients (and significant others) have of these problems and their management.
>
> (Jones & Rivett 2004)

This paradigm requires that clinicians broaden their perspectives and skill sets, and also opens up a wider range of potential and possibility for effecting change.

The Integrated Model of Function was developed from anatomical and biomechanical studies of the pelvis, as well as from the clinical experience of treating patients with lumbopelvic pain (Lee DG & Vleeming 1998, 2004, 2007, Lee DG 2004, Lee DG & Lee LJ 2008). From its inception, the Integrated Model of Function focused on the evaluation of the function of the pelvis, and how the pelvis effectively transfers loads across tasks with varying characteristics. The model addresses *why* the pelvis is painful by identifying the underlying impairments in four specific components: form closure, force closure, motor control and emotions. This is in opposition to pathoanatomical models that seek only to identify pain-generating structures. This model has continued to evolve with the publication of anatomical, biomechanical and neurophysiological research as well as the clinical expertise gained through collaborative efforts worldwide, and remains a useful framework to understand the pelvis in function and in dysfunction.

The Integrated Systems Model for disability and pain (Lee LJ & Lee DG 2011a) evolved from working with the Integrated Model of Function and was first introduced in 2007 as the System-Based Classification for Failed Load Transfer (Lee DG & Lee LJ 2007, Lee DG et al. 2008). We have since recognized that using the word 'classification' is limiting for this model because its primary purpose is not to place patients into homogeneous subgroups. In contrast, it is a framework to understand and interpret the unique picture of each individual patient in the clinical context to facilitate decision-making and treatment planning. The model provides a context to organize all the different types of knowledge needed (scientific, theoretical, professional craft, procedural, and personal) and provides for the development and testing of multiple hypotheses as the multidimensional picture of the patient emerges. A multimodal treatment plan can then be designed based on the complete picture of the person and their presenting problem(s).

The Integrated Systems Model for disability and pain allows clinicians to characterize all the components that contribute to what Melzack terms the 'message that represents the whole body' as a 'flow of awareness' (Melzack 2005). It is an integrated, evidence-based model that considers disability and pain as defined and directed by the patient's values and goals. The model relates impairments found in systems, underlying pain mechanisms, and the impact of these impairments on their current whole-body strategies for function and performance. Thus the model analyses the patient's current whole-body strategies, determines the underlying reasons for those strategies, and relates these to current knowledge about the necessary state required in all systems to provide optimal strategies for function and performance and, ultimately, for health. As a systems-based model, it has inherent flexibility to evaluate and integrate new evidence from research and innovative clinical approaches as they emerge. As a patient-centred model, it can continually adapt to changing goals and values of the patient. As the model applies to the whole person, rather than to a specific type of pain presentation or body region, it can be used across pain and disease populations and is not only applied to patients with pelvic pain. In the context of the lumbopelvic–hip (LPH) complex, the Integrated Model of Function fits within, and is encompassed by, The Integrated Systems Model for disability and pain. The Integrated Model of Function provides a way to subgroup patients with failed load transfer (FLT) in the LPH complex, i.e. those with a primary form closure, force closure, motor control or emotional deficits. The broader Integrated Systems Model for disability and pain also allows for subgrouping according to the primary system impairment but includes the role of the *rest of the body, multiple system types, and all brain/mind states* to the observed FLT in the LPH complex (considers more systems and causes both intrinsic and extrinsic to the pelvis). For example, is the primary impairment causing the FLT intrinsic to the pelvis itself (SIJ laxity → pelvic-driven pelvic pain) or extrinsic to the pelvis (thorax-driven or foot-driven pelvic pain) or due to a negative cognitive or emotional state. The Integrated Systems Model also considers the interaction and contribution of multiple systems (articular, myofascial, neural, visceral, hormonal, neuroendocrine, etc.). Several cases that highlight this approach can be found in the fourth edition of the *Pelvic Girdle* (Lee DG & Lee LJ 2011a).

Therefore, while The Integrated Systems Model is based on the identification of the multisystem impairments that are the key drivers behind the problems facing the whole person, which could then be used to subgroup patients, the primary purpose of the model is to provide a framework for building a unique tapestry that tells the patient's story. It also facilitates clinical reasoning 'on the fly' as the patient's story unfolds and the clinician begins to understand the significant pieces of their tapestry. When used reflectively, it is our goal that The Integrated Systems Model will facilitate, foster and promote the development of clinical expertise.

The Integrated Systems Model for disability and pain: A framework for understanding the whole person and their problem

Underlying constructs of the model

Before we can describe the components of The Integrated Systems Model, it is important to define its underlying constructs. These include the definitions of key terms and are as follows:

1. The terms *body, function/functioning, disability, impairment* and *health condition* are taken from the International Classification of Functioning, Disability and Health (ICF) definitions (2001, pp. 189–190):
   a. *Body functions* are the physiological functions of body systems, including psychological functions. 'Body' refers to the human organism as a whole, and thus includes the brain. Hence, mental (or psychological) functions are subsumed under body functions.
   b. *Body structures* are the structural or anatomical parts of the body such as organs, limbs and their components classified according to body systems.
   c. *Functioning* is an umbrella term for body functions, body structures, activities and participation. It denotes the positive aspects of the interaction between an individual (with a health condition/(perceived problem(s))) and that individual's contextual factors (environmental and personal factors).
   d. *Disability* is an umbrella term for impairments, activity limitations and participation restrictions. It denotes the negative aspects of the interaction between an individual (with a health condition) and that individual's contextual factors (environmental and personal factors).
   e. *Impairment* is a loss or abnormality in body structure or physiological function (including mental functions).
   f. *Health condition* is an umbrella term for disease, disorder, injury or trauma. A health condition may also include other circumstances such as pregnancy, ageing, stress, congenital abnormality or genetic predisposition.
2. A *body system* is a group of organs/structures with co-ordinated activities, achieving the same general function in the body. A *system* shares common characteristics, including:
   a. *Structure*, defined by parts and their composition;
   b. *Behaviour*, which involves inputs, processing and outputs of material, energy or information;
   c. *Interconnectivity*, the various parts of a system have functional as well as structural relationships between each other (Wikipedia).
3. In a state of optimal health, an individual will have the option to choose from a wide variety of strategies that provide for optimal function and performance during any meaningful task (movement, activity, or role in a desired context and environment). Determining whether a task is meaningful requires understanding the person and their values and goals.
4. By definition, optimal function and performance occurs in a state of health, and will be a state free from undesired pain experiences. Given the definitions of health above, optimal function and performance is individually defined, and attainable in the presence of any health condition, although it may be influenced by specific features of the health condition.
5. Pain is not the only reason that people become disabled. Disability, or the inability to do what the person wants to do, can exist without pain.
6. Optimal function and performance for any task requires the synergistic, integrated operation of multiple systems in the body. 'Synergy' is defined as a 'combined or cooperative action or force' (Webster's New World College Dictionary) and, 'simply defined, it means that the whole is greater than the sum of its parts' (Wikipedia). To 'integrate' is to 'form, coordinate, or blend into functioning or unified whole' (Merriam-Webster's Online Dictionary). Synergy and integration require that each system, and thus the components of each system down to the cellular level, is functioning, and that the many complex feedback and feedforward mechanisms that control each system are working optimally. Then, the systems must work together to produce desired outputs in the body.

Congruence of information received from feedback and sensory systems is also important. Not all the underlying mechanisms that produce the integrated, synergistic operation of body systems are fully understood, although science is continuing to reveal the connectedness and interdependence of body systems. Melzack's concept of the body-self neuromatrix (see Figure 7.10) highlights this need for synergy and integration.

7. Impairment(s) in any one or combination of systems can give rise to undesired outputs in one or more systems. These outputs include painful states, non-optimal posture and movement (inefficient, loss of desired performance or output), loss of function, overactive and/or sustained stress response, and negative emotional states.
8. Designing and implementing the most effective treatment plan for restoring health depends on identifying the relevant impairments in the key systems that are barriers to healing and that need to be addressed in order to restore function and health. The relevance of each impairment is determined through a clinical reasoning process that uses a combination of different types of reasoning. Each impairment is evaluated in the context of meaningful tasks to determine how much the impairment contributes to the non-optimal strategies for function and performance, and the pain experience. The impairments/systems/regions with high contribution values are called the key 'driver(s)' in this model. The term 'pain driver' is used to refer to the underlying cause(s) of the pain experience, which could be the pain mechanism itself or a multitude of combined impairments that collectively increase physical and psychological stress and perpetuate the pain experience by exceeding the adaptive/coping mechanisms of specific tissues and the person as a whole. Note that, since the human body is dynamic, i.e. a *changing* entity, the key drivers for disability and/or pain at different points in time can change. Furthermore, the driver(s) of disability may be different than the driver(s) of pain.
9. The Integrated Systems Model is applicable to disability and/or pain of any duration; i.e., from acute onset to chronic, persistent or recurrent problems.
10. Every person is unique genetically, emotionally, cognitively, culturally and socially; the activities and roles that have meaning for them and their pain experience will be uniquely their own. In this way, the specific combination of impairments and systems that contribute to output experiences will be different for each patient. However, taken together, science and clinical expertise provide us with the necessary information to allow us to identify common patterns and parameters for normal and abnormal functioning of systems, as well as how subgroups of patients with certain common features (determined in research by inclusion and exclusion criteria of the study) respond to different treatment approaches. This information is invaluable and indispensable, and the continued pursuit of furthering our knowledge base (both propositional and non-propositional knowledge) in research and in the clinic creates a continually refined understanding of what allows us to enjoy health. However, knowledge gained from either the clinic or the research lab has limitations. Clinicians must constantly examine their emerging hypotheses for multiple types of bias. While clinical practice guidelines derived from research can be helpful and provide new insight, they may also be inappropriate and incorrect for certain patients. Therefore, caution is always necessary when developing general treatment protocols based on 'homogeneous populations' since homogeneous populations are an illusion and do not truly exist outside of research constructs.
11. Each person is a dynamic entity and can change from moment to moment and day to day. Science continues to find more evidence of this. Clinically, this implies that continual reassessment is essential for revising hypotheses about the drivers of the patient's problem.

Components of the model: The Clinical Puzzle – A tool for clinical reasoning and developing clinical expertise

The Clinical Puzzle (Figure 7.6) is a graphic that conceptualizes The Integrated Systems Model for disability and pain. It represents the person and their problem(s), and the systems that support optimal

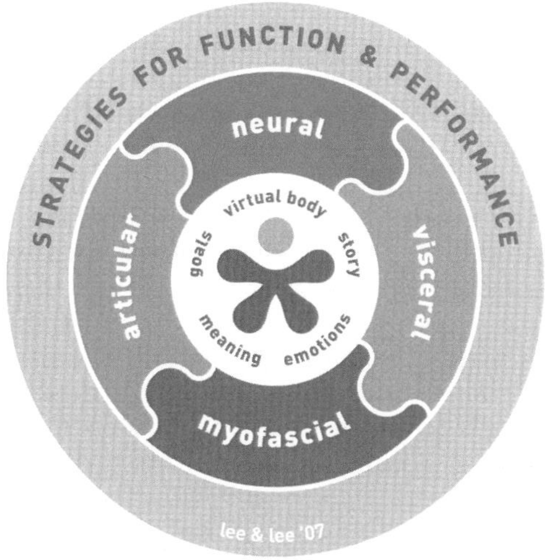

Figure 7.6 • The Clinical Puzzle conceptualizes The Integrated Systems Model for disability and pain. The outer circle of the puzzle represents the strategies for function and performance that the patient currently uses for meaningful tasks (e.g. forward bending, one leg standing, step forward, sit, squat, etc.). The meaningful tasks chosen for analysis are determined from listening to the patient's story. Failed load transfer (FLT; non-optimal alignment, biomechanics, and/or control required for the given task) may be due to one or more impairment(s) in any piece(s) and can 'drive' non-optimal strategies for function and performance. Conversely, non-optimal strategies can 'drive' impairments in any system(s). The centrepiece of the puzzle represents several systems that relate to the person and the sensorial (sensations, perceptions), cognitive (beliefs, attitudes, motivations) and emotional (fears, anger, anxiety) dimensions of their current experience. It also includes systemic systems (such as endocrine balance, immune function) and genetic factors. It is the place where primary symptoms, goals and barriers to recovery are noted. The four other pieces of the puzzle represent the various systems in which impairments are assessed and noted during the clinical examination. During this process, the therapist also considers and reflects upon the relationship of these impairments to the person in the middle of the puzzle (e.g. the meaning these impairments may or may not have, how they relate to health conditions or genetic factors, how they relate to the pain experience, etc.) and the relevance these impairments may have to the non-optimal strategies for function and performance during meaningful tasks. All clinical puzzles are unique since no two individuals have the same life experiences and this graphic is a useful tool for organizing the key information gained through the examination process and for reflection and interpretive reasoning of the findings

strategies for function and performance. The puzzle is used clinically and in teaching as a tool for clinical reasoning and decision-making.

The person in the middle of the puzzle

At the centre of the model is the patient, the person in the middle of the Clinical Puzzle. Seeking to understand the unique makeup of the person (the colour, shape and content of their tapestry), without judgement, is the goal of listening to the patient's story. It is essential that during the subjective examination the therapist create a supportive, compassionate environment that allows the patient to tell their story freely. Open-ended questions, such as 'What can I do for you today?' or 'Please tell me your story' create an invitation for the patient to share the things about their current experience that are most meaningful and relevant to them, along with their goals and values. This is in contrast to the therapist who has a checklist of questions to obtain answers to, and who strongly directs the subjective examination along a path that the therapist deems (in their wisdom) to be the best. This checklist format of subjective examination is more likely to miss out on essential information from the patient.

Understanding the person in the middle of the Clinical Puzzle also incorporates information about the sensorial, cognitive and emotional dimensions to their experience of their problem(s). Problems may be disability and/or pain. The sensorial dimension includes the location and behaviour of the problem(s), the cognitive dimension includes their beliefs and attitudes about their current experience, and the emotional dimension encompasses both positive and negative feelings about the experience. Problems such as incontinence (stress and/or urge), symptoms of pelvic organ prolapse (vaginal bulge or pressure), difficulty with breathing, and effortful movement, are all examples of problems that the patient may not talk about if they are only asked about their pain/symptoms, but that are important to identify when present. From these multiple dimensions, the therapist can glean potential barriers to, and potential facilitators of, recovery.

How the patient perceives their body, and their current experience of their body, constitutes the current state of their *virtual body*. The virtual body is made up of both conscious and unconscious components. As the objective examination proceeds, discrepancies between the actual body and the virtual body will become evident. An example of this would be when a patient perceives that they are standing with equal weight bearing on both feet, but postural examination reveals that the centre of mass is shifted to load one extremity to a greater degree than the other.

Meaningful tasks are postures and/or activities that are determined by aggravating activities, relieving activities, activities associated with negative beliefs and emotions (e.g. movements the patient is fearful of), activities in specific environments or contexts, and the patient's goals (e.g. 'What would you really like to do that you are not currently able to do due to this problem?'). All characteristics of meaningful tasks, including biomechanical requirements, environmental, social and emotional context must be considered during the objective examination in order to most accurately analyse the strategies used by the patient during the meaningful task analysis.

The centre of the puzzle (the person in the middle of the Clinical Puzzle) also represents the patient's genetic makeup and systemic health status, including the nutritional, neuroendocrine, autonomic and homeostatic/stress/immune systems. Past experiences, social background and other psychosocial features are also a part of the centre of the puzzle. The experienced clinician will start to link information in the patient's story and form initial hypotheses that direct the priorities of the objective examination to follow.

Strategies for function and performance

The meaningful tasks identified from the patient's story direct the tasks chosen for analysis of strategies for function and performance, and are noted in the outside ring of the puzzle. These tasks, or the relevant component movements of the task, must be assessed to determine if the patient is using an *optimal* or *non-optimal* strategy for the meaningful task. Since the strategies that people use for whole-body function are a result of, and depend on, the integrated function of all systems in the body, including all the systems represented by the person in the middle of the puzzle, the 'strategies ring' encircles the entire puzzle. If a non-optimal strategy is observed, the objective findings characterizing how the strategy is non-optimal are written beside the task listed in the outer circle of the puzzle.

Articular, myofascial, neural, visceral systems

The four other pieces of the puzzle represent the systems that are assessed during the clinical examination. Specific impairments, as well as information gained from diagnostic tests (e.g. X-rays, MRI, etc.) and other sources, are charted within the relevant system in the puzzle. The therapist also considers and reflects upon the relationship of these impairments to the person in the middle of the puzzle (e.g. sensorial, cognitive and emotional dimensions of the problem(s)) and the relationship these impairments have to the non-optimal strategies for function and performance during meaningful tasks.

As the examination proceeds, the therapist evaluates whether or not the observed non-optimal strategies for function and performance for each meaningful task are *appropriate* or *inappropriate* given all the information available (beliefs about the task, state of tissue healing/integrity of tissue, characteristics of the task and the task context including load requirements, mobility requirements, level of predictability, threat value, availability of accurate proprioceptive input). Note that, for some tasks, the patient may have appropriate strategies (side bent lumbar spine posture due to acute radicular pain), while for other tasks the patient may have inappropriate strategies (fear of moving in any direction in the lumbar spine due to pain that only occurs in one direction of movement). If the therapist has reason to believe that a strategy is inappropriate, determining the reasons a patient chooses a particular strategy is essential for identifying the driver(s) of the problem and planning the most effective treatment programme.

Specific impairments in the *articular, myofascial, neural* and *visceral* systems are listed in Box 7.1. The articular system includes the bones and joints (passive structures) in the musculoskeletal system. The myofascial system includes muscle, tendinous and fascial connections, as well as the multiple layers of fascia throughout the body. The neural system includes all components of the central and peripheral nervous system. It also includes the neural drive to muscles, which is reflected in the resting tone and activity or control of the muscle system. The visceral system includes all the viscera of the body.

An impairment in any piece(s) of the puzzle within the outer circle (the 'systems'), or loss of congruence and synergy between the pieces of the puzzle, can 'drive' non-optimal strategies for function and performance. Conversely, non-optimal strategies for function and performance can drive or create impairments within any of the systems inside the puzzle (the person in the middle of the puzzle, the neural, myofascial, articular and visceral systems). Thus, the entire puzzle is connected, linked and interdependent and visually represents the integrated systems required for optimal

Box 7.1

The conditions associated with the four systems of the Clinical Puzzle

Articular

- Capsular sprain or tear
- Ligament sprain or tear (grades I–III)
- Labral or intra-articular meniscal tear
- Intervertebral disc strain/tear/herniation/prolapse
- Fracture
- Joint subluxation or dislocation
- Periosteal contusion
- Stress fracture, osteitis, periostitis, apophysitis
- Osteochondral/chondral fractures, minor osteochondral injury
- Chondropathy (softening, fibrillation, fissuring, chondromalacia)
- Synovitis
- Apophysitis
- Fibrosis/osteophytosis of the zygapophyseal and intervertebral joints, sacroiliac joint, hip joint

Myofascial

- Intramuscular strain/tear (grades I–III)
- Muscle contusion
- Musculotendinous strain/tear
- Complete or partial tendon rupture or tear
- Fascial strain/tear
- Tendon pathology – tendon rupture, partial tendon tears, tendinopathy (acute or chronic), paratendinopathy, pantendinopathy
- Skin lacerations/abrasions/puncture wounds
- Bursa – bursitis
- Muscular or fascial scarring or adhesions
- Loss of fascial integrity of the anterior abdominal wall including:
  - Diastasis rectus abdominis
  - Sports hernia (tear of transversalis fascia)
  - Hockey hernia (tear of the external oblique)
  - Inguinal hernia
  - Loss of fascial integrity of the endopelvic fascia leading to cystocele, enterocele and/or rectocele

Neural

- Peripheral nerve trunk or nerve injury (neuropraxia, neurotemesis, axonotemesis)
- Central nervous system injury
- Altered motor control
- Absence of recruitment, inappropriate timing (early or late) of muscle recruitment
- Inappropriate amount (increased or decreased) of muscle activity (all relative to demands of task)
- Hypertonicity or hypotonicity of muscles at rest
- Altered neurodynamics
- Sensitization of the peripheral or central nervous system, altered central nervous system processing

Visceral

- Inflammatory organ disease or pathology (e.g. appendicitis, cystitis, acute ulcerative gastritis, pleuritis, endometriosis)
- Infective disorders of the pelvic organs
- Organ disease

health. All clinical puzzles are unique since no two individuals have the same life experiences.

If one considers all of the possible combinations of impairments and the associated findings that can lead to disability and/or pain, the pelvis can seem complicated. In reality, when reflective critical thinking and a thorough examination are used, the primary cause and initial treatment plan emerges. The Clinical Puzzle for The Integrated Systems Model is a useful tool for understanding the whole person and their problem(s). It allows for organization of key information gained through the examination process, comparing and contrasting this information to current propositional knowledge and personal knowledge of the clinician, and for reflection and interpretive reasoning of the findings. This facilitates the formation of hypotheses to explain the relationships between physical impairments, pain mechanisms, psychosocial features, disability, health conditions, and the patient's values and goals. The goal of the clinical reasoning process, facilitated by the puzzle, is to determine which hypothesis provides the 'most likely and most lovely' (Kerry et al. 2008) explanation of the patient's whole experience, from which an integrated multimodal treatment plan is formulated and implemented. As treatment evolves over several sessions, the focus often changes as the patient's journey towards function and better health occurs.

What follows is a case study of a woman with peripartum pelvic pain. This case will illustrate how clinical reasoning and The Integrated Systems Model is used to establish a prescriptive treatment plan for the management of one clinical puzzle. All of the assessment tests described in the case below are fully described in Chapter 8 of the fourth edition of *The Pelvic Girdle* (Lee DG & Lee LJ 2011b).

Case study 7.1

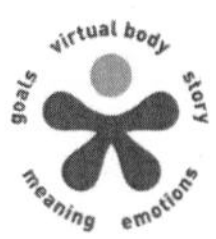

Kristi's story

Kristi was a 31-year-old mother who presented with pelvic pain (central sacral and pubic symphysis) at 31.5 weeks of her second pregnancy. Her first child was delivered vaginally 3 years prior and she felt that she had fully recovered from this pregnancy and delivery prior to conceiving her second child; she reported having no symptoms nor any difficulty performing any tasks prior to this time. Walking aggravated her symptoms, especially if she carried her son. She had no complaints of incontinence or difficulties breathing.

Strategies for function and performance

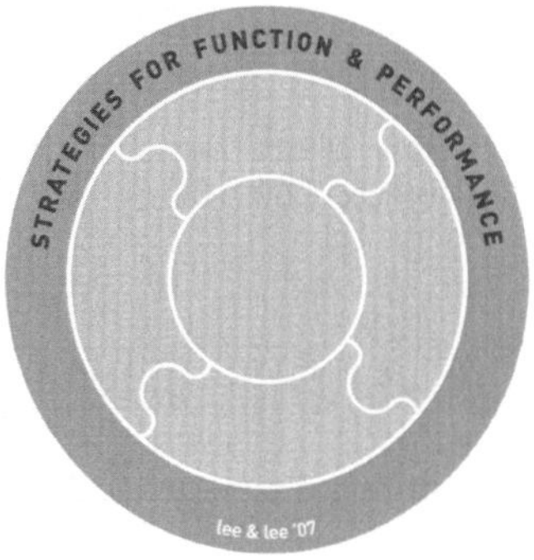

Standing posture

Kristi's stood with a left lateral shift of her thorax relative to her pelvis (Figure 7.7) and the strategy she used to support her abdomen was non-optimal in that there was excessive use of the external obliques (EOs) bilaterally and insufficient use of transversus abdominis (TrA) (confirmed via ultrasound imaging). (Note: while we recognize that it is possible that there was a very small activation of TrA that is below the threshold for detection with ultrasound (Hodges et al. 2003a), clinical experience suggests that if no architectural change in TrA is seen on ultrasound imaging, then there is insufficient activation for functional tasks.)

One leg standing

Kristi found it more difficult to stand on the right leg and flex the left hip (right one leg standing, ROLS). With respect to intrapelvic mobility during this task, asymmetry of motion was noted between the left and right sides of the pelvis; the right side posteriorly rotated less during LOLS than the left side did in ROLS. In addition, there was failure to control motion at the right sacroiliac joint (SIJ) during ROLS (the right innominate rotated anteriorly relative to the sacrum).

Active straight leg raise

During the active straight leg raise (ASLR) test (Mens et al. 1999), Kristi did not note any difference in the effort required to lift her right or left leg; however, she did note that the effort to perform this task was reduced when her pelvis was compressed at the anterior aspect at the level of the anterior superior iliac spines (ASIS).

Curl-up task

Two things of concern occurred during a short head and neck curl-up task:

1. The infrasternal angle narrowed, which is reflective of excessive activation of the EOs;
2. The midline of the abdomen 'domed', which is suggestive of insufficient activation of the TrAs and this was confirmed via ultrasound imaging.

Clinical reasoning at this point

Kristi was using non-optimal strategies to support her growing abdomen for all tasks evaluated. Her inability to control motion of the right side of her pelvis during right single leg loading could explain both her low back and pelvic pain since repetitive anterior rotation of the right innominate during single leg loading during walking could be provocative to the articular and myofascial tissues of the lumbosacral junction, right SIJ and the pubic symphysis (peripherally mediated pain). Further tests are required to determine *why* Kristi was using non-optimal strategies, which at this point were characterized by excessive activation of the EOs and insufficient activation of the TrAs across all tasks. The fact that anterior compression of her pelvis made the ASLR task easier is consistent with the finding that there is insufficient activation of the TrAs. Taken together, the findings from strategy analysis support a hypothesis that a non-optimal pattern of abdominal wall recruitment (imbalance between the EO and the TrA) is contributing to FLT of the right side of the pelvis during multiple functional tasks, as well as contributing to overload of

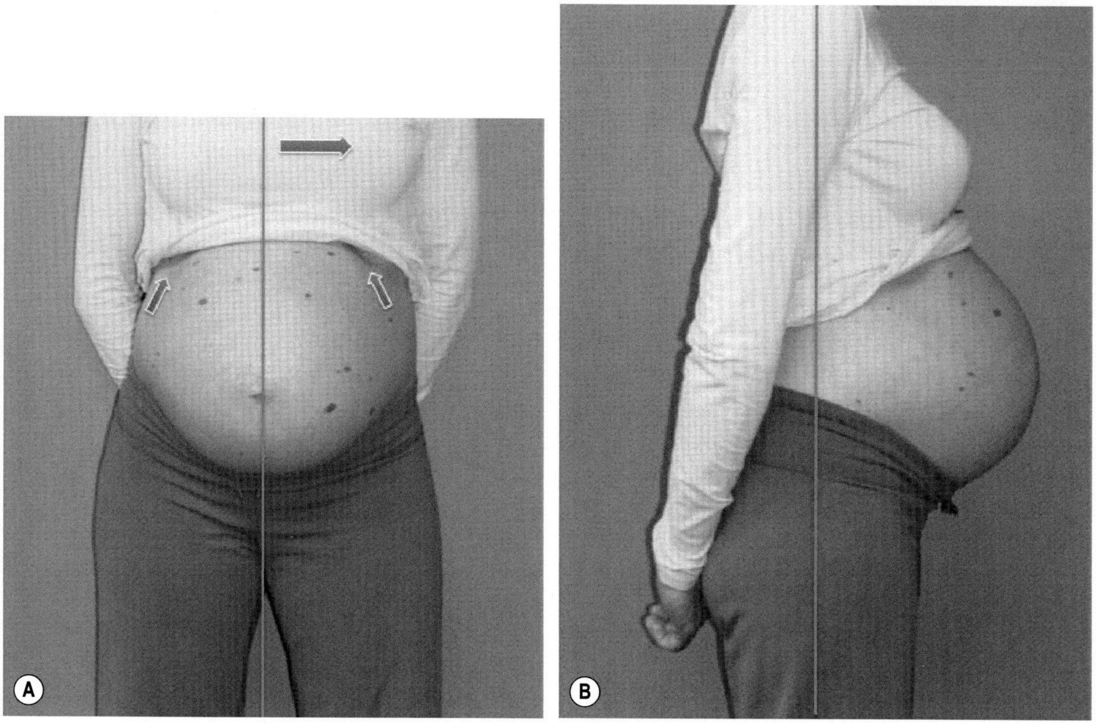

Figure 7.7 • Standing posture at 31.5 weeks pregnant. (A) Note the left lateral shift of her thorax relative to her pelvis in the coronal plane (large arrow). Also note the indentations of the upper abdomen bilaterally (small arrows). This indentation is often seen when there is excessive activation of the external oblique in the strategy used for standing. (B) In this view, the orientation of her thorax over her pelvis looks acceptable; however, the strategy that she is using to maintain this alignment is non-optimal in that there is excessive use of the external oblique bilaterally (see Video 1)

structures driving peripherally mediated pain. Further tests are needed to confirm or negate this hypothesis.

Articular system analysis

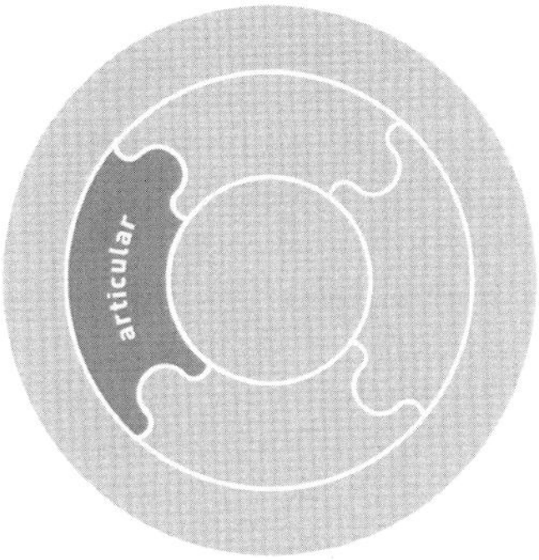

This system requires analysis whenever there is failure to control articular motion during any functional task. Given the location of Kristi's pain, both the SIJs and pubic symphysis required analysis for mobility and integrity of the passive system restraints. The pubic symphysis was dynamically controlled and pain-free on stress testing, and there was no loss of integrity of the passive system. The mobility of the SIJs was symmetric when tested passively (compared to asymmetric when tested actively; see OLS above) and the passive restraints to articular motion were intact (i.e. no motion of the joint was palpable when the joint was tested in the close-packed position). These findings indicate that the articular system is *not* the cause of her lack of motion control during right single leg loading.

Neural system analysis

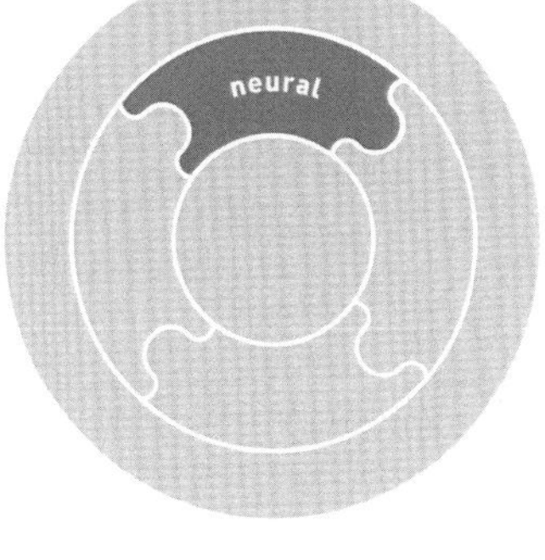

When Kristi was given a verbal cue intended to isolate a co-contraction of the deep system (TrA, pelvic floor) from the superficial muscle system, an asymmetrical response to the bilateral cue occurred between the left and right TrA; the left TrA responded (and was isolated from the superficial muscles) whereas the right did not respond at all. This finding was confirmed via ultrasound imaging. In addition, an asymmetrical response occurred between the left and the right IO; the right IO responded whereas the left did not. These findings support the hypothesis that Kristi's current pattern of deep and superficial abdominal muscle recruitment was providing insufficient support to the anterior pelvis during the ASLR and other tasks. This indicates that the neural system needs to be trained in order to restore optimal load transfer through the right side of the pelvis. However, given that 66% of women present with a diastasis of the rectus abdominis in the third trimester (Boissonault & Blaschak 1988), the myofascial system warrants examination (and follow-up) in every pregnant woman attending for treatment (Lee DG 2011). One of the mechanisms by which TrA provides support to the lumbopelvis is via increasing fascial tension (Hodges et al. 2003b); if there are impairments in the myofascial system of the abdominal wall (midline abdominal fascia and linea alba), TrA may not be able to provide support to the pelvis regardless of whether optimal control by the neural system is restored. Thus, further tests are required to determine if Kristi's inability to transfer load through the right side of her pelvis is primarily driven by a neural impairment, or a combination of both a neural and a myofascial impairment.

Myofascial system analysis

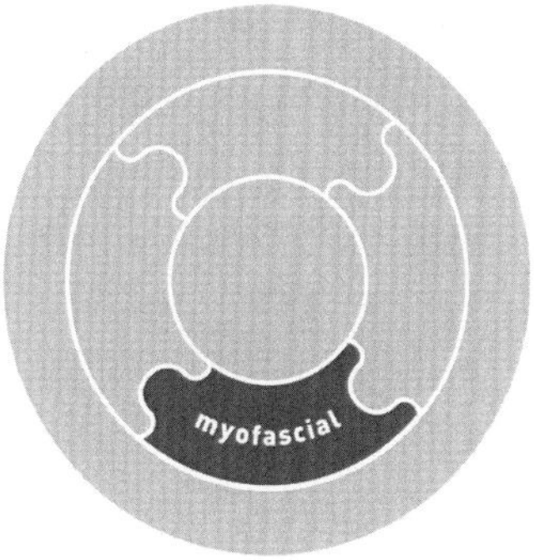

In individuals less than 45 years of age, the distance between the left and right rectus abdominis (i.e. the inter-recti distance) is considered to be 'normal' if it is no greater than 1 cm at a midway point between the pubic symphysis and the umbilicus (PU point), 2.7 cm just above the umbilicus (U point) and 0.9 cm at a midway point between the umbilicus and the xyphoid (UX point) (Rath et al. 1996). At 31.5 weeks gestation, Kristi was within these normal limits at the PU point (0.82 cm) and greater than this at both the U point (>width of probe at rest and 3.46 cm during a curl-up) and UX point (3.52 cm at rest and 3.03 cm during a curl-up) (Table 7.2, Figure 7.8). It was again noted that Kristi was using a non-optimal strategy for the curl-up task (insufficient and asymmetric activation of TrA and excessive activation of the EO). Palpation of the linea alba between the left and right rectus abdominis suggested it was intact; however, the ability of linea alba to transfer forces could not be assessed at this time since Kristi was unable to contract TrA optimally (neural impairment, see above). That is, since Kristi was unable to recruit an optimal isolated contraction of the deep system, the impact of a precontraction of the deep system on the inter-recti distance and the shape of the linea alba could not be assessed at this time.

Clinical impression derived from hypothesis development, reflection and interpretive reasoning

From this initial assessment, the primary hypothesis was that Kristi's pain experience was primarily peripherally mediated and, according to The Integrated Systems Model the impairment that needed to be addressed first was in the neural system (see Kristi's clinical puzzle, Figure 7.9). The passive restraints of the pubic symphysis and the right and left sacroiliac joints were intact (no articular impairment). The neural system assessment revealed deficits in the activation of both the deep and superficial systems; asymmetric responses were noted in both the TrAs and the internal obliques (IOs) in response to a verbal cue intended to isolate a symmetric response of the deep system. While the inter-recti distances at both the U and UX points of the linea alba (myofascial tests) were wider than normal values according to Rath et al. (1996), there appeared to be sufficient tension in this midline structure to effectively force close and control motion of the joints of the pelvis *if* the deep system (i.e. TrA and PF) was functioning optimally. This hypothesis would have to be tested after the neural system deficits were addressed.

Table 7.2 Inter-recti distance measured via ultrasound imaging both at rest and during a short head/neck curl-up task at 31.5 weeks gestation and 6 weeks postpartum. The rest measures are also provided at 14 weeks postpartum

	At rest			Curl-up		Curl-up with precontraction of the deep system	
	31.5 weeks gestation	6 weeks postpartum	14 weeks postpartum	31.5 weeks gestation	6 weeks postpartum	31.5 weeks gestation	6 weeks postpartum
Inter-recti distance half way between pubic symphysis and umbilicus (PU)	0.82 cm	0.96 cm	0.52 cm	1.14 cm	0.60	Unable to contract TrA well therefore unable to test	0.54 cm
Inter-recti distance just above the umbilicus	Unable to measure since distance was greater than width of probe	3.60 cm (Figure 7.15A)	2.62 cm	3.46 cm	2.14 cm with 'sagging' linea alba (Figure 7.15B)	Unable to contract TrA well therefore unable to test	2.12 cm with less sag in the linea alba (Figure 7.15C)
Inter-recti distance half way between umbilicus and xyphoid	3.52 cm	1.42 cm	2.34 cm	3.03 cm	1.61 cm	Unable to contract TrA well therefore unable to test	1.64 cm

The findings from this examination were explained to Kristi and a treatment session followed to teach her a better strategy for supporting her abdomen and for transferring loads through her trunk and pelvis. This involved releasing (relaxing) the left and right EOs and then 'waking up' the right TrA and facilitating its co-contraction with the other muscles of the deep system. She was able to feel a 'lightening of load' on her pubic symphysis with this better strategy and was also able to stand on her right leg without losing control of the right side of her pelvis. Kristi was encouraged to practice this co-activation of the deep system (pelvic floor and TrA) frequently (three sets of ten contractions held for 10 seconds) over the remaining weeks of her pregnancy and a post-delivery home visit was advised (Lee LJ & Lee DG 2011b).

Two days postpartum

Kristi had an uneventful home delivery and incurred a small tear in her perineum requiring two stitches in the 'muscular layer' and one stitch in her skin. She reported that, during the final weeks of her pregnancy, she was able to control her pelvic pain when she engaged her deep system. Currently, her pelvic pain had re-curred and additionally she was now experiencing pain in her perineum and occasional urinary incontinence.

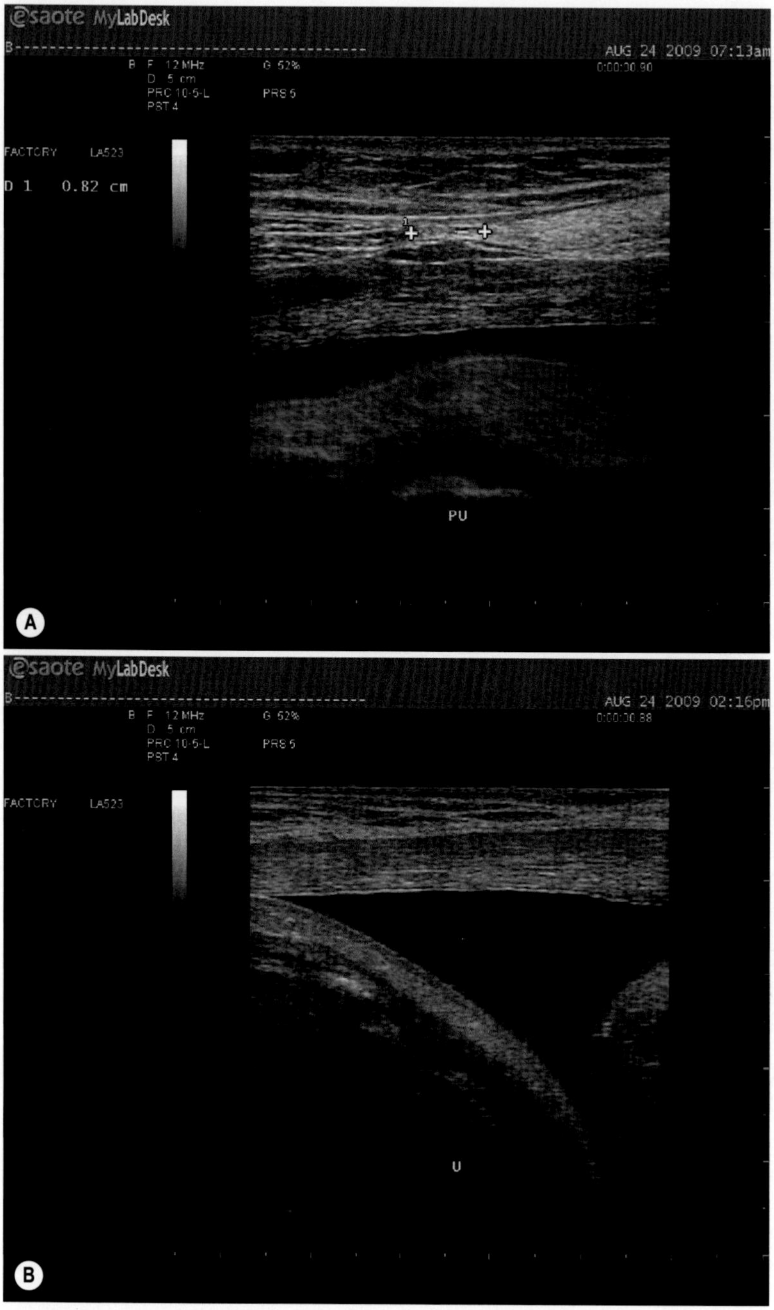

Figure 7.8 • Inter-recti distance measured via ultrasound imaging. (A) PU point = 0.82 cm. (B) The medial borders of the rectus abdominis cannot be imaged and the distance between them is wider than the ultrasound probe (i.e. >4.66 cm) *(Continued)*

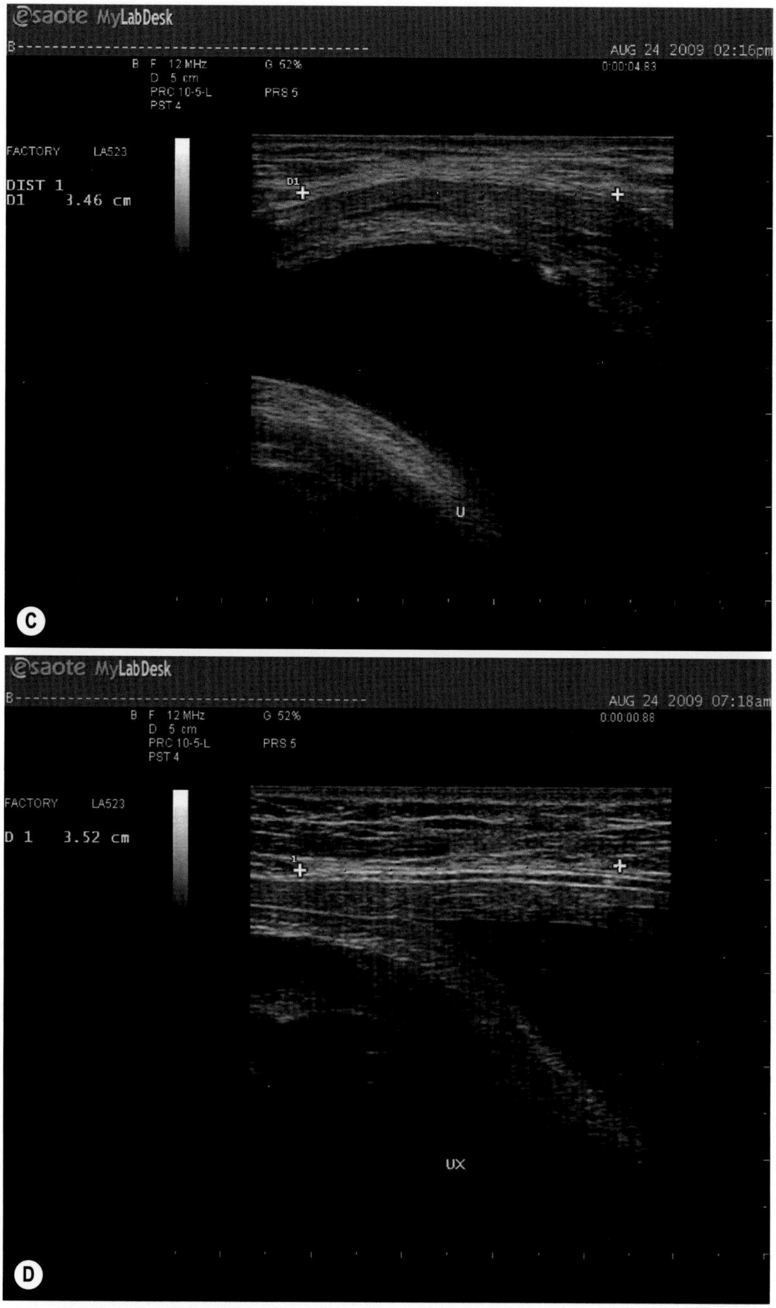

Figure 7.8—Cont'd (C) U point during a curl-up. As the midline of the abdomen 'domes' and tension increases in the linea alba, the inter-recti distance narrowed to 3.46 cm. (D) UX point = 3.52 cm

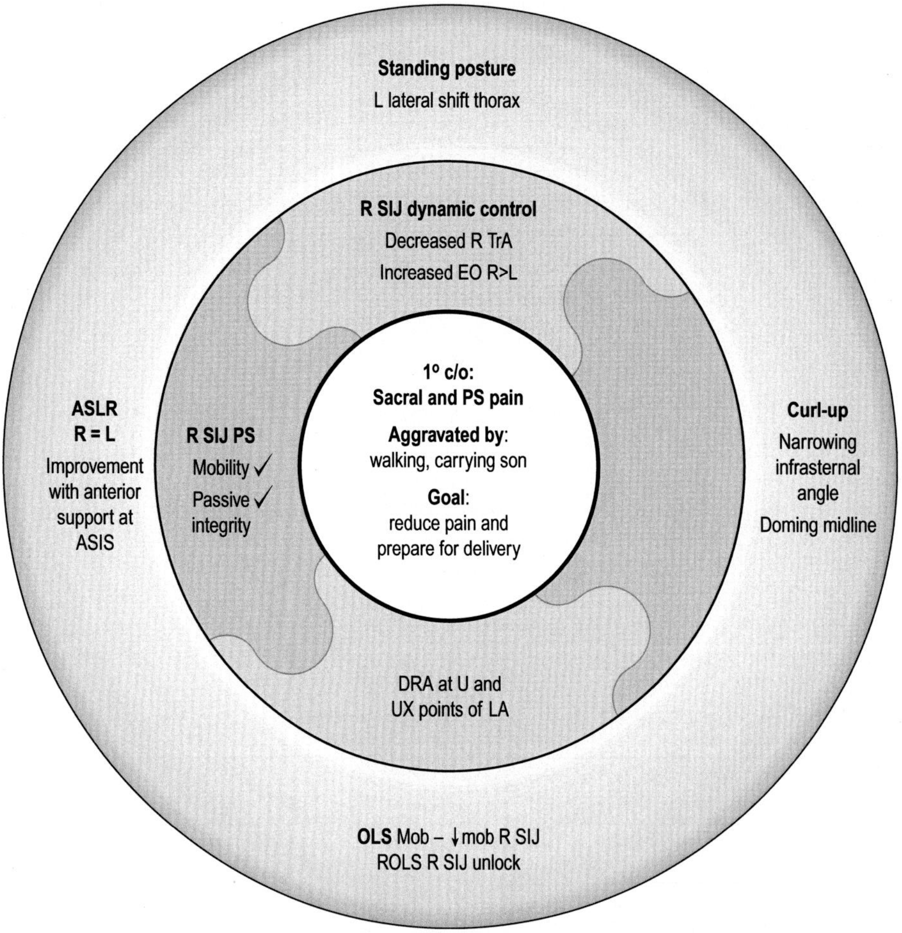

Figure 7.9 • Kristi's clinical puzzle at 31.5 weeks gestation. 1° c/o, primary complaints; L, left; R, right; PS, pubic symphysis; SIJ, sacroiliac joint; OLS, one leg standing; mob, mobility; ASLR, active straight leg raise; R = L, right and left leg equally hard to lift; ASIS, anterior superior iliac spine; ✓, OK; EO, external oblique; TrA, transversus abdominis; DRA, diastasis rectus abdominis; LA, linea alba

Strategies for function and performance, myofascial and neural system analysis

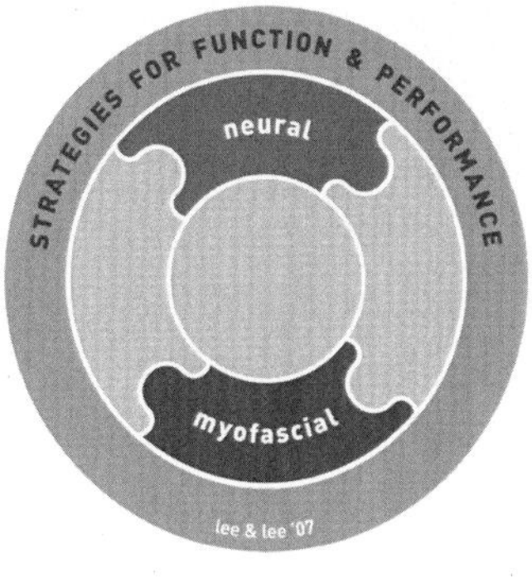

Standing posture

Kristi's standing posture was quite different from that noted at 31.5 weeks gestation (Figure 7.10). She stood with an anterior pelvic sway and a posterior pelvic tilt, a flattened lumbar lordosis, and increased extension of the upper lumbar spine and lower thorax.

One leg standing, active straight leg raise and curl-up tasks

Kristi was unable to control motion of either the left or right side of her pelvis during single leg loading; both legs were difficult to lift and the effort to do so was reduced when her pelvis was compressed anteriorly during the ASLR task. Significant doming of the midline of her abdomen was noted during a

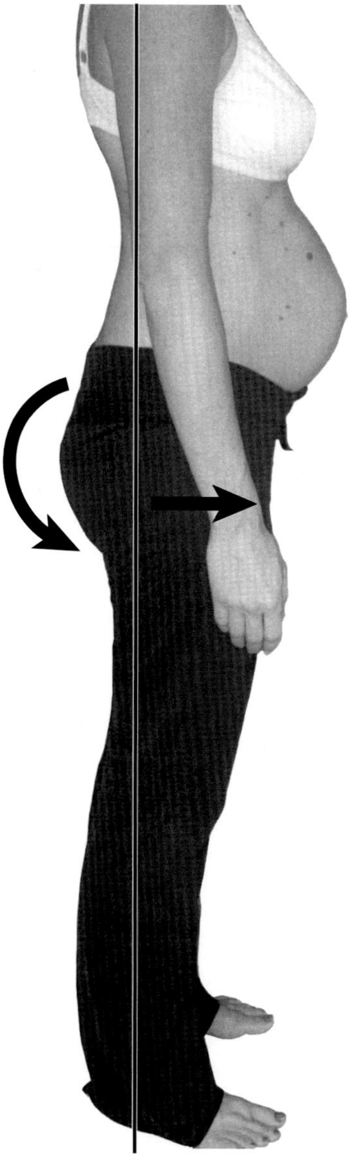

Figure 7.10 • Standing posture – 2 days postpartum. Note the anterior pelvic sway (horizontal arrow) and posterior pelvic tilt (curved arrow). The low lumbar spine is flexed (flattened) and the lumbar lordosis has shifted to the upper lumbar spine and lower thorax. This is a non-optimal standing posture for load transfer through the bones and joints of her lumbopelvis and associated organs. The lateral divots of the upper abdomen suggest that Kristi is still using the EOs excessively

curl-up task (Figure 7.11). There was minimal palpable tension in the linea alba during the curl-up task when no attempt was made to precontract the transversus abdominis (myofascial system analysis). There was a significant diastasis of the rectus abdominis (DRA) from the U to UX points (>3 finger widths).

Since Kristi had continued to practice an isolated contraction of her deep system in the final weeks of her pregnancy, it was not a surprise that she was still able to perform this task well even at 2 days postpartum. A symmetric activation of the left and right TrA, isolated from the EOs and IOs, occurred when she was given a cue to gently connect her ASISs together (neural system analysis). When she contracted the TrAs and then sustained the contraction as she performed the curl-up task, more tension was palpable in the linea alba and the doming was reduced. When cues were given to contract her pelvic floor, Kristi reported an increase in her perineal pain.

See Figure 7.12 for Kristi's current clinical puzzle, reflect on the findings, and make a hypothesis as to what her management should be prior to reading the next section.

Clinical reasoning and early postpartum management

At this very early postpartum stage, Kristi was doing quite well. She had sustained some trauma to her pelvic floor as a consequence of her vaginal delivery and this would need to be further assessed once her wounds had healed. In the meantime, she was given postural advice regarding her standing, sitting and nursing positions and advised to wear an abdominal binder to help support her pelvis as healing occurred (Figure 7.13). The binder would also help to 'remind her brain' as to the way her lower abdomen should be supported by the deep muscle system. She was also advised to apply ice to her perineum and to slowly increase the activation of her pelvic floor as her pain subsided. A subsequent in-office visit was recommended at 6 weeks postpartum.

Six weeks postpartum

Kristi reported that she was now pain-free and no longer incontinent and was keen to return to her kickboxing class. She was managing all her homecare responsibilities with ease and was eager to 'get fit' once again. However, even though she was asymptomatic, several things of potential concern were noted on her follow-up examination.

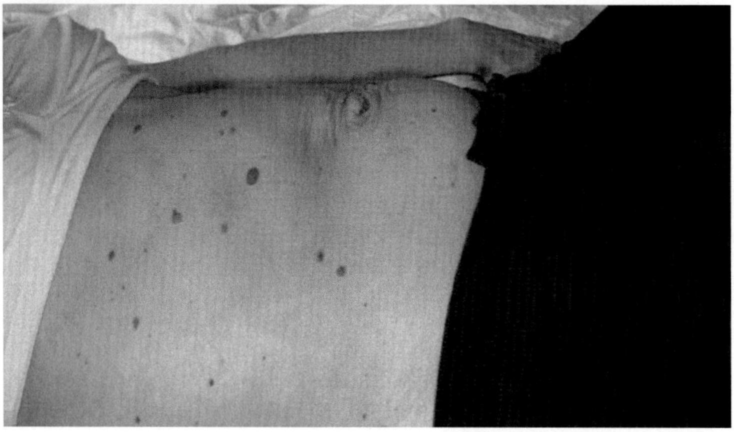

Figure 7.11 • Curl-up task 2 days postpartum. Note the doming in the midline of the abdomen. This is reflective of either imbalance of the deep and superficial abdominal muscles with insufficient activation of the deep system during this task or an inability of the midline fascia to transfer load. Further tests are necessary to differentiate the cause of the doming

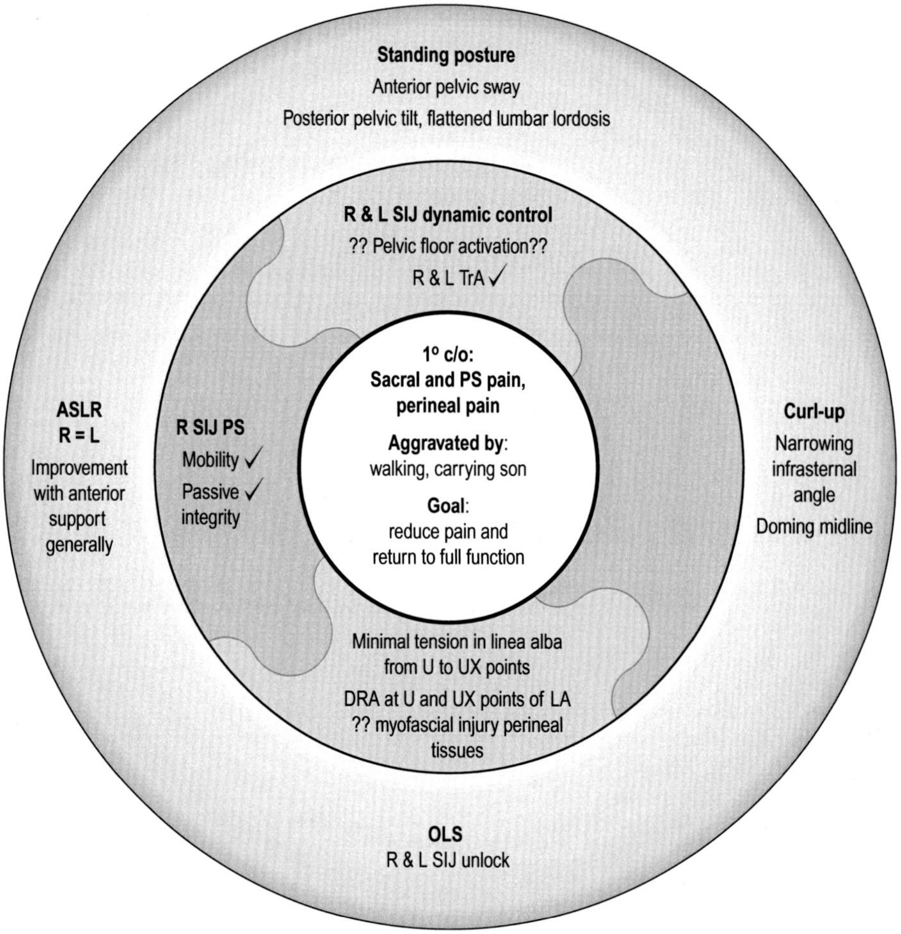

Figure 7.12 • Kristi's clinical puzzle at 2 days postpartum. 1° c/o, primary complaints; L, left; R, right; PS, pubic symphysis; SIJ, sacroiliac joint; OLS, one leg standing; ASLR, active straight leg raise; R = L, right and left leg equally hard to lift; ✓, OK; TrA, transversus abdominis; DRA, diastasis rectus abdominis; U point, just above the umbilicus; UX, point halfway between the umbilicus and the xyphoid; LA, linea alba

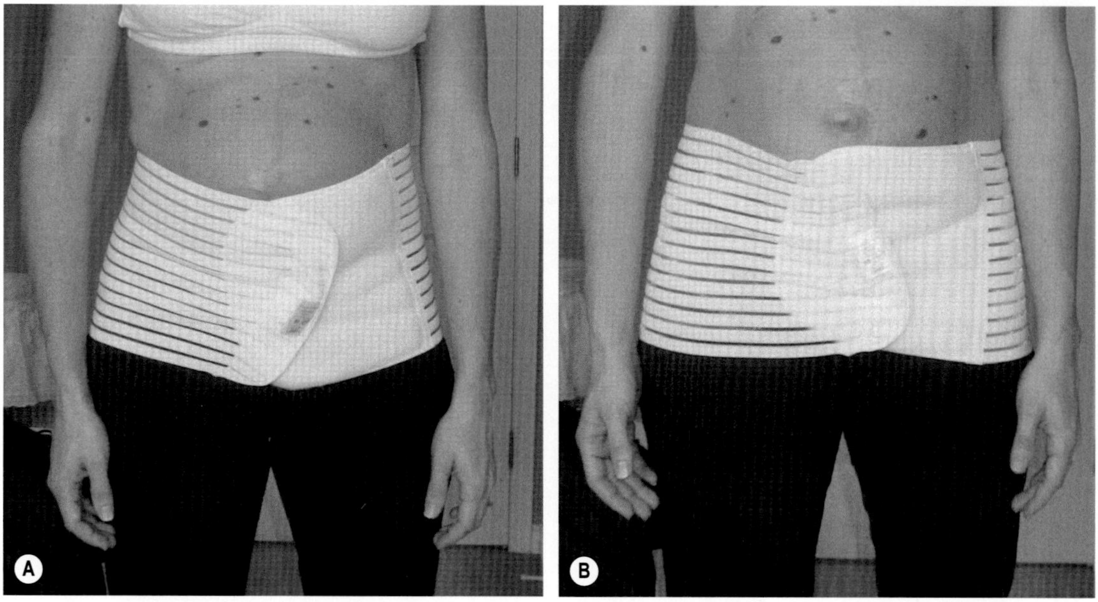

Figure 7.13 • Postpartum abdominal binder. (A) This is the wrong way to wear a postpartum abdominal binder (i.e. tighter at the top). (B) This is the correct way to wear the binder, with more support at the inferior part thereby supporting the abdomen from 'bottom up'

Strategies for function and performance

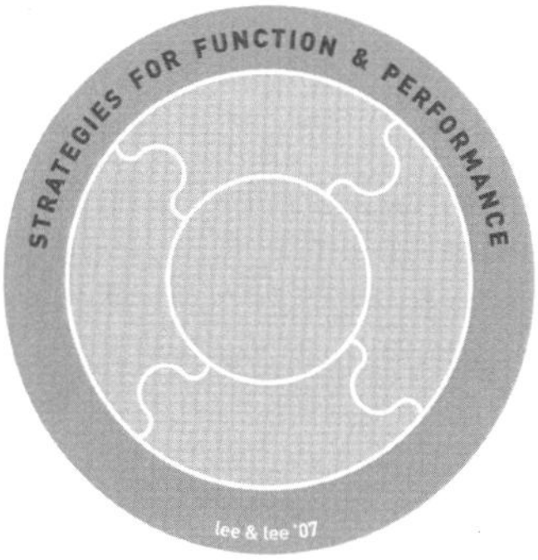

Standing posture

Kristi was able to find a much better standing posture (Figure. 7.14A) although she still had a tendency to sway her pelvis anteriorly especially when she carried her newborn (Figure 7.14B). A better strategy for standing was reviewed (Figure 7.14C).

One leg standing and active straight leg raise tasks

Kristi found it more difficult to stand on the right leg and flex the left hip (ROLS). With respect to intrapelvic mobility during this task, asymmetry of motion was noted between the left and right sides of the pelvis; the *left* side posteriorly rotated less during ROLS than the right did during LOLS. This is an opposite mobility finding to her initial assessment. In addition, there was failure to control motion of *both* SIJs (initially it was just the right) with the left side unlocking (i.e. innominate anteriorly rotating) earlier in the task than the right. During the ASLR task, Kristi noted that the left leg was harder to lift and that the effort required to perform this task was reduced when compression was applied to the inferior part of her pelvis (level of the ischii and pubic symphysis).

Articular and neural system analysis

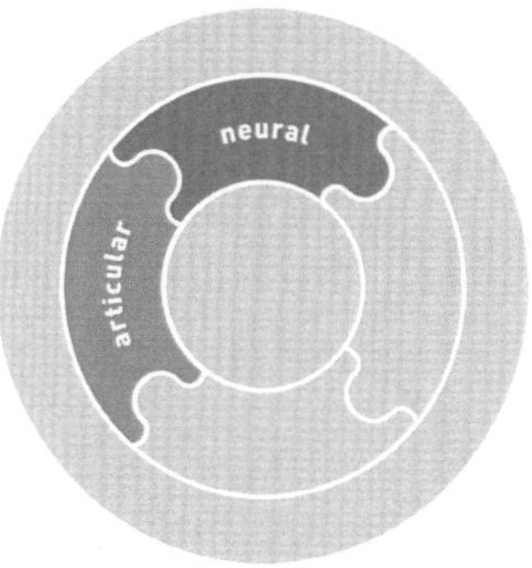

The passive mobility of the SIJs was symmetric and the integrity of the passive system restraints was intact, therefore the articular system was not hypothesized to be the cause of the unlocking noted during single leg loading. With respect to the deep muscle system,

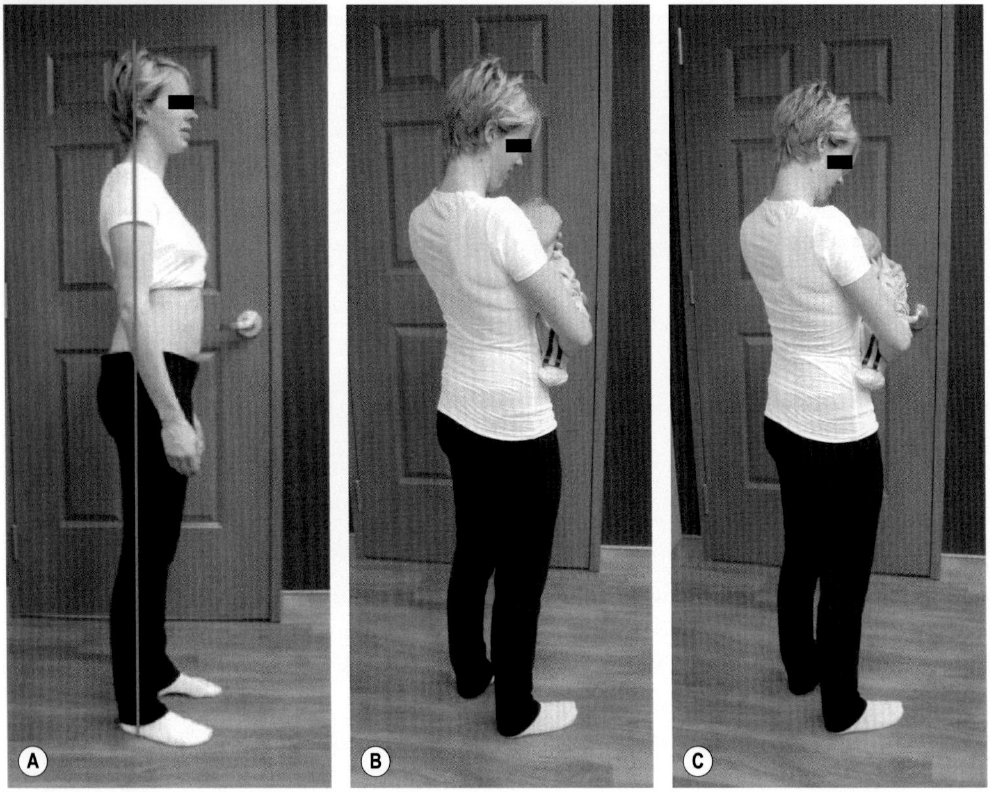

Figure 7.14 • Standing posture 6 weeks postpartum. (A) Slight anterior pelvic sway, which (B) increased when she held her baby. (C) Here, Kristi is standing with a better strategy while holding her baby

an isolated, symmetric response of the TrAs occurred with a cue to contract the pelvic floor; however, no response of the pelvic floor was seen via ultrasound imaging (both perineal and transabdominal approach) in response to any verbal cue (Lee DG & Lee LJ 2011b). Video 12A shows an optimal response of the pelvic floor to a cue to contract; note the cranioventral lift of the anorectal angle towards the neck of the bladder. This contrasts significantly with the lift seen in Video 12B, which contains perineal ultrasound imaging of her attempt to recruit her pelvic floor.

Curl-up task and myofascial system analysis

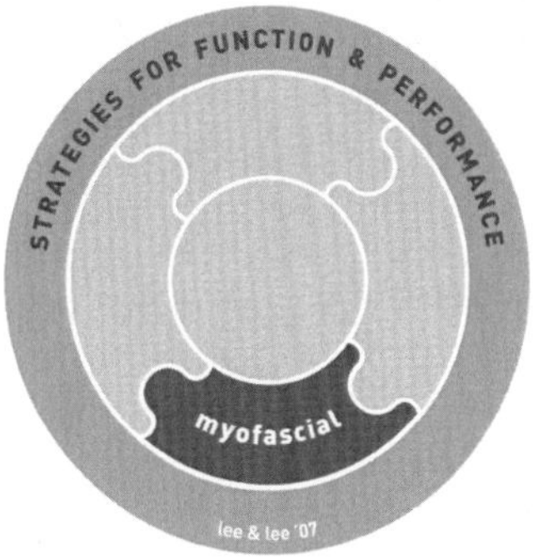

During a curl-up task, doming of the midline of the abdomen occurred and minimal tension was palpable in the linea alba, particularly just above the umbilicus; however, the infrasternal angle did not narrow (i.e. there didn't appear to be excessive activation of the EOs during this task). At rest, the inter-recti distance was within normal limits at the PU point (0.96 cm), and still wider than normal at both the U (3.60 cm) and UX (1.42 cm) points (Table 7.2, Figure 7.15A). Just above the umbilicus, this distance narrowed to 2.14 cm during a curl up, which is within normal limits; however, the strategy that produced this narrowing was non-optimal in that insufficient tension was generated in the linea alba (note the sagging of the linea alba in Figure 7.15B). When Kristi activated the TrAs prior to doing the curl-up, the inter-recti distance at the U point was 2.12 cm (essentially no change); however, the strategy was better in that there was no doming of the midline abdomen and more tension could be seen, and felt, in the linea alba (Figure 7.15C, Video 13). Kristi also noted that it took less effort to curl when she activated the TrAs first. Coldron et al. (2008) have measured the inter-recti distance

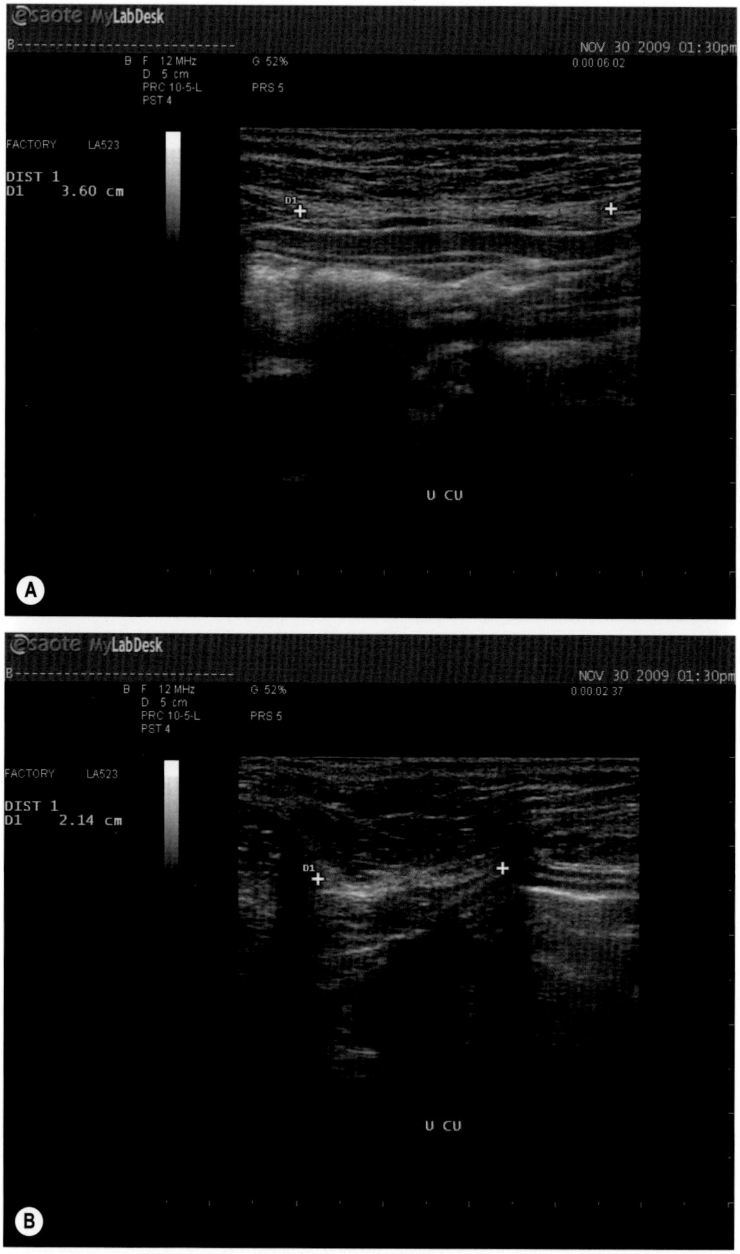

Figure 7.15 • Ultrasound images of the linea alba and response during a curl-up task. (A) This is the inter-recti distance at the U point at rest – 3.60 cm which is wider than normal values according to Rath et al. (1996) (2.70 cm). (B) During a curl-up with no precontraction of the deep system, Kristi's strategy resulted in narrowing of the inter-recti distance (2.14 cm); however, note the 'sagging', which is reflective of minimal, if any, tension in the linea alba

(Continued)

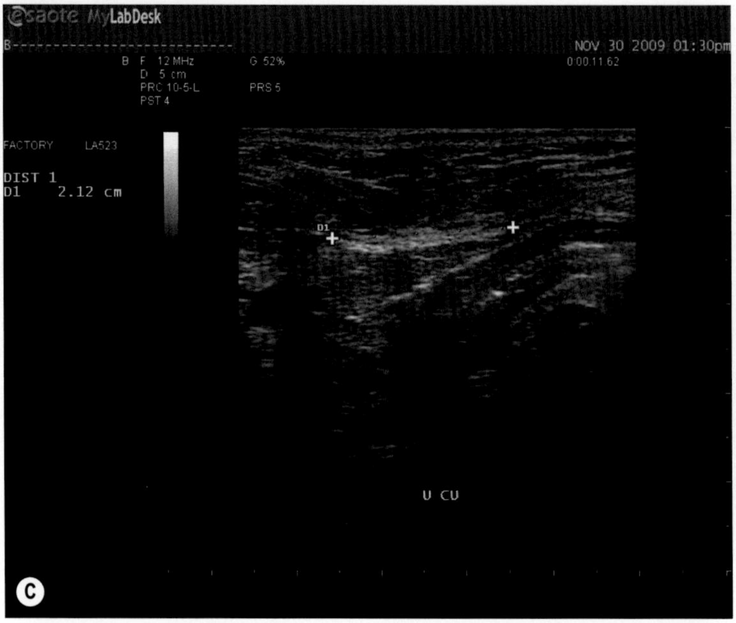

Figure 7.15—cont'd (C) When the deep system was activated prior to the curl-up task, the inter-recti distance at the U point also narrowed; however, the strategy chosen to curl-up was better in that the linea alba was tensed and sagged less

from 1 day to 1 year postpartum and note that the distance decreases markedly from day 1 to 8 weeks, and that without any intervention (e.g. exercise training or other physiotherapy) there was no further closure at the end of the first year. Whether training has any effect on the inter-recti distance has not been studied nor do we definitively know if closure is necessary for restoration of function in all women.

See Figure 7.16 for Kristi's current clinical puzzle and reflect on the findings to determine what her management should be prior to reading the next section. Would you allow her to return to kickboxing at this time?

Clinical reasoning and management

Kristi was surprised to discover that her 'Kegel' exercises were not effectively producing a contraction of her pelvic floor. Bump et al. (1991) reported that 50% of women cannot effectively activate the pelvic floor in response to a verbal cue and either an internal or ultrasound imaging examination is needed to ensure that a response is occurring. Although she was not experiencing incontinence of urine, stool or gas, the OLS and ASLR tests as well as the results of her neural system evaluation support a specific training programme to 'wake up' and integrate her pelvic floor with the other muscles of the deep system. It is possible that this deficit was responsible for the 'unlocking' of both sides of her pelvis in single leg loading tasks and while she was disappointed at not being able to attend her kickboxing class immediately, she did understand the reasons why it was necessary to address the neural deficit and train her deep muscle system before increasing the loads through her pelvis.

Kristi was given the Pelvic Floor Educator™ (www.neenhealth.com) (Figure 7.17), which is a useful biofeedback tool for training the pelvic floor. She was instructed on how to use this tool to ensure proper activation of her pelvic floor and once she was able to do this, she was advised to integrate the contraction with her TrA cue such that the deep muscle system was trained together.

Twelve weeks postpartum

Kristi reported that she was now painfree and no longer incontinent of urine in any task. However, she had been unable to obtain an optimal response from the Pelvic Floor Educator™; she could not make

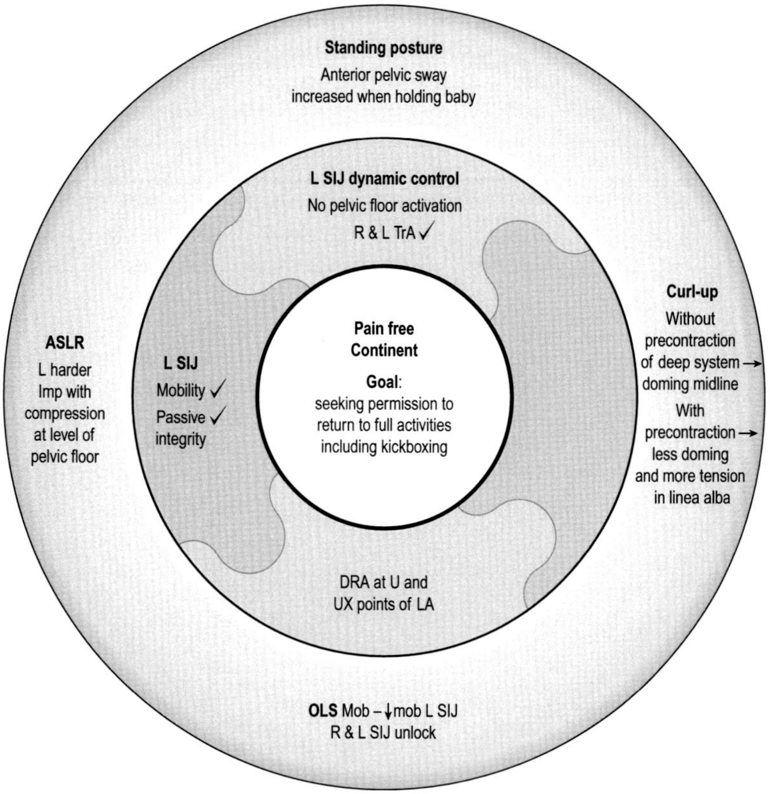

Figure 7.16 • Kristi's clinical puzzle at six weeks postpartum. Imp, improves. See Figure 7.12 for further abbreviations

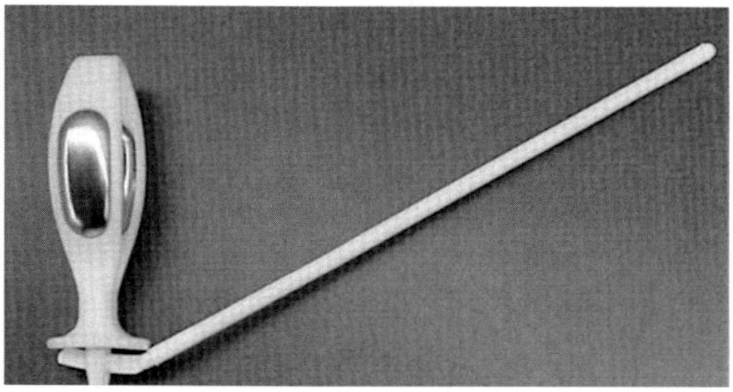

Figure 7.17 • The Pelvic Floor Educator™ (www.neenhealth.com) is a useful biofeedback tool for 'waking' up and training the pelvic floor

the stick go down with her pelvic floor contraction. On objective examination, she was still unable to control motion of the left SIJ, which continued to unlock during left single leg loading. When her pelvic floor was imaged via ultrasound imaging there was still no apparent activation with any cue given. She was then scheduled to see Johanne Sabourin who is a physiotherapist specializing in the assessment and treatment of the pelvic floor.

From her assessment (which included an intravaginal examination), Johanne noted the following:

1. Hyperaesthesia (pain) in the deep posterolateral vaginal wall;
2. A low cervix (and uterus) (0.5 cm above the hymen) which was likely interfering with the trajectory of lift from the pelvic floor contraction;
3. Hypertonicity of the levator ani with decreased ability to relax; and
4. Restricted mobility of the right obturator nerve and the nerves of both the pelvic and coccygeal plexus.

The nerve plexi were released/mobilized with internal techniques; after these techniques a much better contraction and relaxation of the levator ani was palpable. She was advised to perform her pelvic floor exercises in the inverted position (modified child's prayer pose) and to avoid abdominal curl-up exercises (crunches). She was also advised to continue using the Pelvic Floor Educator™ for biofeedback training at home.

Fourteen weeks postpartum

Kristi reported that her pelvic floor contractions 'felt much different' after her session with Johanne and that she was now able to move the stick of the Pelvic Floor Educator™ properly. She had returned to a fairly high level of physical activity and was not experiencing any pain, symptoms of loss of pelvic organ support or incontinence of urine.

Strategies for function and performance

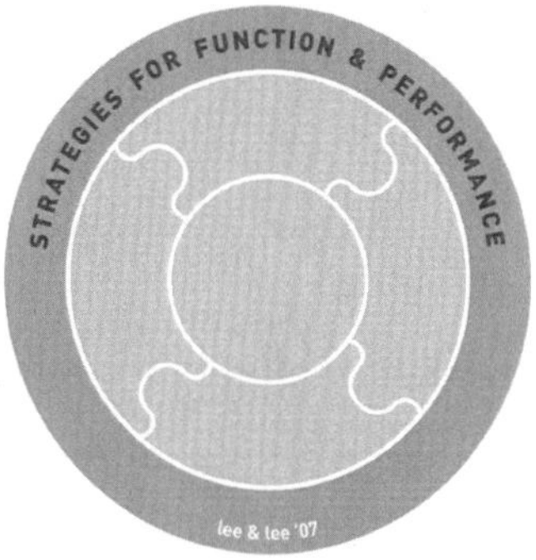

One leg standing and active straight leg raise

Kristi's intrapelvic mobility was now symmetric (noted via the OLS task) and she was able to control motion of the left SIJ *when she precontracted her deep system*. Her automatic strategy (without a conscious precontraction of the deep system) did not provide control of this joint. During the ASLR task, Kristi did not report any effort difference to lift either leg and there was no change in the effort required to perform this task when compression was applied anywhere to her pelvis.

Curl-up task and myofascial system analysis

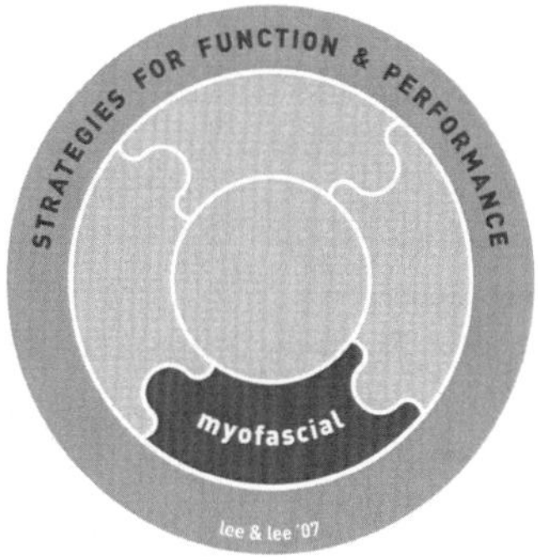

During a curl-up task, there was no doming of the midline of the abdomen and lovely tension was now palpable in the linea alba. The infrasternal angle, however, was now widening suggesting an imbalance of activation between the IOs and EOs during this task (with net vector from internal oblique). This was a change in strategy for this task from that used in the final trimester of her pregnancy. At rest, the inter-recti distance at the PU point was now 0.52 cm (reduced from 0.96 cm at 6/52 postpartum), at the U point was 2.62 cm (reduced from 3.60 cm at 6/52 postpartum) and at the UX point was 2.34 cm (an *increase* from 1.42 cm at 6/52 postpartum) (see Table 7.2). The widening of the upper portion of the linea alba is reflective of the non-optimal strategy she was using to do her curl-up exercises.

Neural system analysis

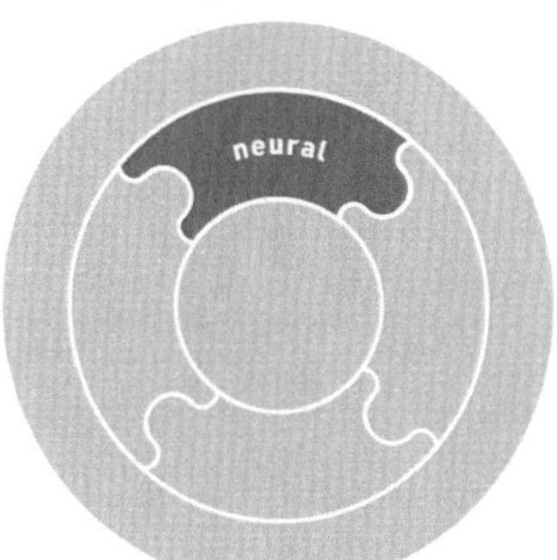

An isolated, symmetric response of the TrAs continued to occur with a cue to contract the pelvic floor and a small cranioventral lift could now be seen via ultrasound imaging of the pelvic floor (perineal approach). Her pelvic organs appeared to be well supported when she performed a valsalva manoeuvre.

Clinical reasoning and management

The widening of the upper portion of the linea alba can be explained by the over-activation of the IOs (or underactivation of the EOs) during the multiple curl-ups Kristi was doing to 'get back in shape'. She was advised on how to correct this strategy (Video 15) to prevent further widening of the linea alba and perhaps to facilitate its closure. The treatment provided by Johanne Sabourin for Kristi's pelvic floor had certainly 'released and woken up' the levator ani, yet more improvement was needed if effective load transfer and pelvic organ support were to be ensured throughout her lifetime. Kristi was advised to continue with the training programme provided and to work on integrating these new strategies into her activities of daily living and other physical activities (i.e. kickboxing) (Lee LJ 2011). She was also advised to return for a follow-up examination in 6 months time.

Case conclusion

This case illustrates the need to screen all postpartum women within the first 8 weeks of delivery since impairments in function do exist in the absence of pain and/or symptoms of pelvic organ prolapse/incontinence. More studies are needed to determine if these impairments would indeed lead to pain and disability and which impairments specifically predict future problems.

Summary

According to the definition of Sackett et al. (2000), we believe that The Integrated Systems Model is an evidence-based approach in that it considers the patient's values (thoughts, feelings, expectations) and integrates the practitioner's expertise (clinical reasoning and skills) and the available research evidence into decision-making for appropriate therapeutic interventions. In our experience, there are no recipes, prediction rules or guidelines for patients presenting with chronic pelvic disability with or without pain and it is likely that a multimodel approach will always be more effective for long-term success. While temporary improvement in function and/or pain may be gained by using one component of the therapeutic intervention (release or align or connect or move), it is the long-term solution that is sought by the patient. We strive to empower our patients to understand what is driving their disability or pain experience, to be aware of the contexts or situations that facilitate their poor strategies and to learn how they can change those strategies and move towards ones that are more optimal for their bodies and health (Empower through Knowledge, Movement and Awareness). In this way, we hope that they can Move better, Feel better, and Be better! More information on The Integrated Systems Model approach can be found in the fourth edition of *The Pelvic Girdle* and online at www.discoverphysio.ca.

This chapter has illustrated the myriad of factors the clinician may need to take into account when assessing and developing a treatment plan for the patient with CPP. The next chapter describes the multidisciplinary and multispeciality approach to the management of CPP, from a pain specialist (Chapter 8.1) and from a physiotherapeutic perspective (Chapter 8.2).

References

Beattie, P., Nelson, R., 2006. Clinical prediction rules: what are they and what do they tell us? Aust. J. Physiother. 52 (3), 157.

Bernard, T.N., Kirkaldy-Willis, W.H., 1987. Recognizing specific characteristics of nonspecific low back pain. Clin. Orthop. 217, 266.

Boissonault, J.S., Blaschak, M.J., 1988. Incidence of diastasis recti abdominis during the childbearing year. Phys. Ther. 68 (7), 1082.

Bonica, J.J., 1953. The management of pain. Lea & Febiger, Philadelphia.

Brukner, P., Khan, K., 2007. Clinical sports medicine, second ed. McGraw-Hill, Sydney, Australia.

Bump, R.C., Hurt, G.W., Fantl, J.A., et al., 1991. Assessment of Kegal pelvic muscle exercise performance after brief verbal instruction. Am. J. Obstet. Gynecol. 165, 322.

Butler, D.S., 2000. The sensitive nervous system. NOI Group Publications, Adelaide, Australia.

Cochrane, A.L., 1972. Effectiveness and Efficiency: Random Reflections on Health Services. Nuffield Provincial Hospitals Trust, London. Reprinted in 1989 in association with the BMJ; Reprinted in 1999 for Nuffield Trust by the Royal Society of Medicine Press, London.

Coldron, Y., Stokes, M.J., Newham, D.J., et al., 2008. Postpartum characteristics of rectus abdominis on ultrasound imaging. Man. Ther. 13, 112.

Cook, C., 2008. Potential pitfalls of clinical prediction rules. J. Man. Manip. Ther. 16 (2), 69.

Coste, J., Paolaggi, J.B., Spira, A., 1992. Classification of nonspecific low back pain, I: psychological involvement in low back pain. Spine 17, 1028.

Delitto, A., Erhard, R.E., Bowling, R.W., 1995. A treatment-based classification approach to low back syndrome: identifying and staging patients for conservative treatment. Phys. Ther. 75, 470.

Doidge, N., 2007. The brain that changes itself. Stories of personal triumph from the frontiers of brain science. Penguin Books, New York.

Ericsson, K.A., Smith, 1991. Towards a general theory of expertise: prospects and limits. Cambridge University Press, New York.

Fisher, J.P., Hassan, D.T., O'Connor, N., 1995. Minerva. BMJ 310, 70.

Fritz, J.M., 2009. Clinical prediction rules in physical therapy: coming of age? J. Orthop. Sports Phys. Ther. 39 (3), 159.

Fritz, J.M., Cleland, J.A., Childs, J.D., 2007. Subgrouping patients with low back pain: evolution of a classification approach to physical therapy. J. Orthop. Sports Phys. Ther. 37 (6), 290.

Gifford, L., 1998. Pain, the tissues and the nervous system: a conceptual model. Physiotherapy 84 (1), 27.

Gombatto, S.P., Collins, D.R., Sahrmann, S.A., Engsberg, J.R., Van Dillen, L.R., 2007. Patterns of lumbar region movement during trunk lateral bending in 2 subgroups of people with low back pain. Phys. Ther. 87 (4), 441.

Guyatt, G., Cairns, J., Churchill, D., et al., [Evidence-Based Medicine Working Group], 1992. Evidence-based medicine. A new approach to teaching the practice of medicine. J. Am. Med. Assoc. 268, 2420.

Higgs, J., 2004. Educational theory and principles related to learning clinical reasoning. In: Jones, M.A., Rivett, D.A. (Eds.), Clinical reasoning for manual therapists. Elsevier, Edinburgh.

Higgs, J., Titchen, A., 1995. Propositional, professional and personal knowledge in clinical reasoning. In: Higgs, J., Jones, M. (Eds.), Clinical reasoning in the health professions. second ed. Butterworth-Heinemann, Oxford, p. 129.

Hodges, P.W., Kaigle Holm, A., et al., 2003a. Intervertebral stiffness of the spine is increased by evoked contraction of transversus abdominis and the diaphragm: in vivo porcine studies. Spine 28 (23), 2594.

Hodges, P.W., Pengel, L.H.M., Herbert, R.D., Gandevia, S.C., 2003b. Measurement of muscle contraction with ultrasound imaging. Muscle Nerve 27, 682.

Jensen, G.M., Gwyer, J., Hack, L.M., Shepard, K.F., 2007. Expertise in Physical Therapy Practice, second ed. Saunders.

Jones, M.A., Rivett, D., 2004. Introduction to clinical reasoning. In: Jones, M.A., Rivett, D.A. (Eds.), Clinical reasoning for manual therapists. Elsevier, Edinburgh, p. 3.

Kerry, R., Maddocks, M., Mumford, S., 2008. Philosophy of science and physiotherapy: an insight into practice. Physiother. Theory Pract. 24 (6), 1.

Kirkaldy-Willis, W.H. (Ed.), 1983. Managing low back pain. Churchill Livingstone, New York.

Kirkaldy-Willis, W.H., Hill, R.J., 1979. A more precise diagnosis for low back pain. Spine 4, 102.

Kirkaldy-Willis, W.H., Wedge, J.H., Yong-Hing, K., et al., 1978. Pathology and pathogenesis of lumbar spondylosis and stenosis. Spine 3, 319.

Laslett, M., Williams, W., 1994. The reliability of selected pain provocation tests for sacroiliac joint pathology. Spine 19 (11), 1243.

Laslett, M., Aprill, C.H., McDonald, B., et al., 2005. Diagnosis of sacroiliac joint pain: validity of individual provocation tests and composites of tests. Man. Ther. 10, 207.

Leboeuf-Yde, C., Lauritsen, J.M., Lauritzen, T., 1997. Why has the search for causes of low back pain largely been inconclusive? Spine 22 (8), 877.

Lee, D.G., 2004. The pelvic girdle. third ed. Churchill Livingstone, Edinburgh.

Lee, D.G., 2011. Pregnancy and its potential complications. Ch. 6. In: Lee, D.G. (Ed.), The Pelvic Girdle. fourth ed. Churchill Livingstone, Edinburgh (at press).

Lee, D.G., Lee, L.J., 2007. Bridging the gap: the role of the pelvic floor in musculoskeletal and urogynecological function. In: Proceedings of the World Physical Therapy Conference. Vancouver, Canada.

Lee, D.G., Lee, L.J., 2008. Integrated, multimodal approach to the treatment of pelvic girdle pain and dysfunction. In: Magee, D.J., Zachazewski, J.E., Quillen, W.S. (Eds.), Pathology and intervention in musculoskeletal rehabilitation. Saunders, Elsevier, p. 473.

Lee, D.G., Lee, L.J., 2011a. Clinical reasoning, treatment planning and case reports. Ch. 9. In: Lee, D.G. (Ed.), The Pelvic Girdle. fourth ed. Churchill Livingstone, Edinburgh (at press).

Lee, D.G., Lee, L.J., 2011b. Techniques and tools for assessing the lumbopelvic-hip complex. Ch. 8. In: Lee, D.G. (Ed.), The Pelvic Girdle. fourth ed. Churchill Livingstone, Edinburgh (at press).

Lee, D.G., Vleeming, A., 1998. Impaired load transfer through the pelvic girdle – a new model of altered neutral zone function. In: Proceedings from the 3rd interdisciplinary world congress on low back and pelvic pain. Vienna, Austria.

Lee, D.G., Vleeming, A., 2004. The management of pelvic joint pain and dysfunction. In: Boyling, J.D., Jull, G. (Eds.), Grieve's modern manual therapy. The vertebral column. third ed. Churchill Livingstone, Elsevier, p. 495.

Lee, D.G., Vleeming, A., 2007. An integrated therapeutic approach to the treatment of pelvic girdle pain. In: Vleeming, A., Mooney, V., Stoeckart, R. (Eds.), Movement, stability & lumbopelvic pain. second ed. Elsevier, p. 621.

Lee, D.G., Lee, L.J., McLaughlin, L.M., 2008. Stability, continence and breathing: The role of fascia following pregnancy and delivery. J. Bodyw. Mov. Ther. 12, 333.

Lee, L.J., 2011. Training new strategies for posture and movement. Ch. 12. In: Lee, D.G. (Ed.), The Pelvic Girdle. fourth ed. Churchill Livingstone, Edinburgh.

Lee, L.J., Lee, D.G., 2011a. Clinical practice – the reality for clinicians. Ch. 7. In: Lee, D.G. (Ed.), The Pelvic Girdle. fourth ed. Churchill Livingstone, Edinburgh.

Lee, L.J., Lee, D.G., 2011b. Tools and techniques for 'waking up' and coordinating the deep and superficial muscle systems. Ch. 11. In: Lee, D.G. (Ed.), The Pelvic Girdle. fourth ed. Churchill Livingstone, Edinburgh.

MacNab, I., 1977. Backache. Williams & Wilkins, Baltimore.

Magee, D.J., Zachazewski, J.E., Quillen, W.S., 2007. Scientific foundations and principles of practice in musculoskeletal rehabilitation. Saunders Elsevier, St Louis.

McKenzie, R.A., 1981. The lumbar spine: mechanical diagnosis and therapy. Spinal Publications, New Zealand, Wellington.

Melzack, R., 2001. Pain and the neuromatrix in the brain. J. Dent. Educ. 65 (12), 1378.

Melzack, R., 2005. Evolution of the neuromatrix theory of pain. The Prithvi Raj Lecture: Presented at the third World Congress of World Institute of Pain, Barcelona 2004. Pain Pract. 5 (2), 85.

Melzack, R., Wall, P.D., 1965. Pain mechanisms: a new theory. Science 150, 971.

Mens, J.M.A., Vleeming, A., Snijders, C.J., Stam, H.J., Ginai, A.Z., 1999. The active straight leg raising test and mobility of the pelvic joints. Eur. Spine J. 8, 468.

Merskey, H., Bogduk, N., 1994. Classification of chronic pain: descriptions of chronic pain syndromes and definitions of pain terms, second ed. Prepared by the Task Force on Taxonomy of the International Association for the Study of Pain. IASP Press, Seattle, USA.

Moseley, G.L., 2007. Reconceptualising pain according to modern pain science. Phy. Ther. Rev. 12, 169.

Nachemson, A., 1999. Back pain; delimiting the problem in the next millennium. Int. J. Law Psychiatry 22 (5–6), 473.

O'Sullivan, P., 2005. Diagnosis and classification of chronic low back pain disorders: maladaptive movement and motor control impairments as underlying mechanism. Man. Ther. 10 (4), 242.

O'Sullivan, P., Beales, D., 2007. Diagnosis and classification of pelvic girdle pain disorders – Part 1: a mechanism based approach within a biopsychosocial framework. Man. Ther. 12, 86.

Pengel, L.H.M., Herbert, R.D., Maher, C.G., Refshauge, K.M., 2003. Acute low back pain: systematic review of its prognosis. Br. Med. J. 323–327.

Rath, A.M., Attali, P., Dumas, J.L., et al., 1996. The abdominal linea alba: an anatomo-radiologic and biomechanical study. Surg. Radiol. Anat. 18, 281.

Reeves, N.P., Cholewicki, J., Milner, T.E., 2005. Muscle reflex classification of low-back pain. J. Electromyogr. Kinesiol. 15 (1), 53.

Riddle, D.L., 1998. Classification and Low Back Pain: A Review of the Literature and Critical Analysis of Selected Systems. Phys. Ther. 78, 708.

Rivett, D.A., Jones, M.A., 2004. Improving clinical reasoning in manual therapy. In: Jones, M.A., Rivett, D. (Eds.), Clinical reasoning for manual therapists. Elsevier, Edinburgh, p. 403.

Sackett, D.L., Straus, S., Richardson, W.S., Rosenberg, Haynes, R.B., 2000. Evidence-based medicine. How to practice & teach EBM. Elsevier Science, New York.

Sahrmann, S.A., 1988. Diagnosis by the physical therapist: a prerequisite for treatment. Phys. Ther. 68 (11), 1703.

Sahrmann, S., 2001. Diagnosis and treatment of movement impaired syndromes. Mosby, St Louis.

Waddell, G., 2004. The back pain revolution, second ed. Churchill Livingstone, Edinburgh.

Wright, A., 2002. Neurophysiology of pain and pain modulation. In: Strong, J., Unruh, A.M., Wright, A., Baxter, G.D. (Eds.), Pain, a textbook for therapists. Churchill Livingstone, Edinburgh.

Multispeciality and multidisciplinary practice: A UK pain medicine perspective

8.1

Andrew Paul Baranowski

CHAPTER CONTENTS

As discussed in Chapters 1 and 3, several groups have tried to tackle the issue of defining chronic pelvic pain (CPP), and the Pain of Urogenital Origin (PUGO) Special Interest Group of The International Association for the Study of Pain (IASP) are currently proposing the following:

> **Chronic Pelvic Pain Syndrome (CPPS)** is a sub-division of CPP and is the occurrence of CPP where there is no proven infection or other obvious local pathology that may account for the pain. It is often associated with negative cognitive, behavioural, sexual and emotional consequences as well as with symptoms suggestive of lower urinary tract, sexual, bowel or gynaecological dysfunction.

The implications of the above for clinical management are huge. Essentially pain perceived to be both chronic and sited within the pelvis is associated with a wide range of causes and associated symptoms that must be investigated and managed in their own right. For this to occur, patients with CPP must have access to the appropriate resources through multispeciality (e.g. urology, urogynaecology, gynaecology, neurology and pain medicine) and multidisciplinary (e.g. medical doctor, nurse, psychology and physiotherapy) teams (Baranowski et al. 2008).

Multispeciality and multidisciplinary practice (Baranowski et al. 2008)

In this chapter the term *speciality* refers to the team and the term *discipline* to the training and background of the individuals within the team. What has to be recognized is that individuals of a discipline working within different specialities will have different skills and experience.

Patients with chronic pain will have to go through two processes:

1. Diagnostic and treatment of specific diseases (Fall et al. 2008);
2. Identification and management of symptoms that are ongoing (Baranowski et al. 2008, Fall et al. 2008).

This chapter focuses primarily on those conditions where we are looking at the second stage: identification of troublesome symptoms and their management. However, it is worthwhile to emphasize the negative prognostic aspect of multiple investigations and inappropriate treatment supposedly aimed at diagnostic and treatment of spurious specific diseases (Abrams et al. 2006).

The medical teams

Very little work has been undertaken looking at the phenotypes of those patients with no specific disease process presenting to different teams because of where the symptoms are perceived/focused. However, it is suggested that there is much overlap in the patient characteristics in those patients seen, for example, by a urologist as compared to a gynaecologist.

At the end of the day many patients will end up in the chronic pain management centre where the medical doctors are experienced in the management of ongoing, persistent pain. The more complex CPP patients may be referred to a specific pelvic pain/urogenital pain management centre.

In our urogenital pain management centre, all patients are initially assessed by a chronic pain consultant with a primary interest in urogenital pain as well as by a clinical nurse specialist. The initial consultation takes the form of a structured history, a range of health questionnaires (psychological and disability based, such as BPI, PSEQ, self-efficacy, DAPOS), clinical examination and review of past investigations. Following an in-depth explanation the patient is triaged to one or more of the following: psychology, physiotherapy or a specific multispeciality clinic as well as receiving medical management.

The multispeciality clinic

Whereas the pain consultant is best able to manage the pain symptoms, input from other specialists, such as urologists (Fall et al. 2008), urogynaecologists, gynaecologists, neurologists, colorectal physicians (Emmanuel & Chatoor 2009), is important for other symptoms.

These joint clinics are invaluable for team education which helps us to manage the simpler non-pain problems and also to identify those issues that may require a more complex work-up and management plan from the joint clinic.

The multidisciplinary team and clinic

Within our pain management centre we have a specific team of urogenital physiotherapists, psychologists, nurses and clinicians. We have regular meetings to discuss our patients as well as access to multidisciplinary clinics where several members of the team may meet up with an individual patient and their significant others. Such an approach ensures a consistent message and reduces the chance of misunderstanding within the team.

The exact role of a team member in managing the patient will depend upon training and experience. Inevitably there will be some overlap.

The role of the pain medicine consultant

1. Diagnosis:
   a. To ensure specific disease processes have been identified and managed as appropriate. The medical consultant may consider onward referral if further investigation and medical management appear necessary.
   b. Identify the pain mechanisms that are present (Vecchiet et al. 1992, Giamberardino 2005, Baranowski & Curran 2008). Most information will be achieved from a good history and full examination. However, there may be a role for specialist techniques such as differential neural blockade, intravenous drug challenges, imaging, muscle electromyographs and nerve conduction studies.
2. Triage to other team members.
3. Medical management of pain mechanisms (Baranowski et al. 2008):
   a. *Specialist drugs* (Chong & Hester 2008): neuropathic analgesics (e.g. tricyclics and other antidepressants, anticonvulsants, sodium channel blockade, N-methyl-D-aspartate (NMDA) antagonists, α-blockade). Many of these drugs have a limited evidence base for the management of pelvic pain and as such these drugs should only be initiated in pelvic pain by an experienced practitioner in the field.
      i. The mainstream simple analgesics are usually prescribed prior to the patient presenting at the pain management centre. These drugs will include simple analgesics such as paracetamol (acetaminophen), the non-steroidal anti-inflammatory drugs and simple opioids such as codeine. The evidence base for these in CPP is limited, though the role of non-steroidal anti-inflammatory drugs in dysmenorrhoea is well established.

ii. Antidepressant drugs, especially the tricyclic antidepressant amitriptyline, have a long history of use for neuropathic pain. Amitriptyline has a number needed to treat in the range of 2–3. That is one patient in two or three will have a 30–50% reduction in pain depending upon the study. It has been shown to be superior to placebo for neuropathic pain of diabetic painful neuropathy and postherpetic neuralgia and it is thought that would be the case for all neuropathic pains. As you might expect, the drug may produce significant benefit for an individual, but be of no help for many others. The fact that drugs are not cures but often only take the edge off the pain, needs to be emphasized. Selective serotonin reuptake inhibitors are thought not to be as effective as the tricyclics but may be considered when side effects from the tricyclics are a problem. Citalopram may be a consideration if there is anxiety. The selective noradrenaline reuptake inhibitor duloxetine is said to be effective for neuropathic pain and is gaining widespread acceptance in various guidelines. As it may have a role in stress incontinence it may also be useful for pelvic pain with a significant bladder irritability. However, duloxetine is an example of the difficulties we may face with prescribing complex drugs. Duloxetine has National Institute for Health and Clinical Excellence, England, UK (NICE) guidelines approval for diabetic neuropathic pain and formulary approval for stress urinary incontinence (SUI) in Europe and Canada. It did not gain FDA approval for SUI because of concerns about suicidal thoughts as well as lack of concerns about efficacy. Suicidal ideation has been associated with other drugs as well (Patorno et al. 2010).

iii. Antiepileptic drugs. Gabapentin and pregabalin are the two most commonly prescribed for pelvic pain, though oxycarbazepine, carbamazepine, topiramate and phenytoin may be considered. The dose of gabapentin in one study was 3.6 g a day, well above the recommendation within the British National Formulary. Whether pregabalin has any advantage over gabapentin is debated. However, it is often prescribed as a trial if side effects are seen with gabapentin. See above with respect to suicidal ideation.

iv. Strong opioids. There is a big move towards using stronger opioids in chronic pain conditions. However, the risks of doing so are still not fully evaluated. There are certain rules that must be adhered to and these can be found at several websites such as the British Pain Society http://www.britishpainsociety.org/book_opioid_patient.pdf. The salient features are that:
- Opioid prescription should involve two professionals, usually a pain medicine consultant and the patient's family doctor.
- The drugs should only come from one source, usually the family doctor supported by the specialist.
- Slow- or modified-release preparations should be used in preference to rapid-onset of action drugs as the slow or modified drugs are less likely to be associated with addiction (though dependence will always be an issue). Slow-release morphine is the gold standard, though this has been debated and some specialists prefer oxycodone or fentanyl.
- A contract should be drawn up with the patient and if the patient exhibits evidence of drug-seeking behaviour consideration to discontinuing the prescription or involving the advice of a drug dependency team should be given. Pseudo addiction is where the patient exhibits addictive behaviour because of a lack of analgesic effect and this must be considered.
- The prescription must be reviewed on a regular basis and it is considered prudent to consider a therapeutic trial of effect (possibly an intravenous drug trial) before considering long-term prescription.

v. Other drugs that may be considered in a pain management centre: NMDA antagonists (ketamine and amantadine), cannabinoids (Sativex) and sodium channel blockade (intravenous lidocaine, mexiletine). Intravenous phentolamine may be considered as a trial of sympathetic blockade.

b. *Injection type therapy* (Dickson & Humphrey 2008): somatic and autonomic nerve blockade. Rarely if ever is there justification for neurolytic blockade. Injection therapy appears to be best when combined with a holistic approach involving physiotherapy and psychology. Somatic nerves that may be blocked include those supplying the anterior part of the pelvis (ilioinguinal, iliohypgastric and genitofemoral) and those arising in the posterior pelvis (pudendal, perineal branches of the posterior femoral and cluneal nerves). These may be blocked at multiple sites from their source in the spine to the peripheral branches. Appropriate imaging and neurotracing technology should be considered. National Institute of Health and Clinical Excellence (NICE) guidelines suggest that ultrasound guidance should be used for peripheral blocks where appropriate. Otherwise fluoroscopy/X-ray guidance and in certain cases computed tomography should be considered. The evidence base that injections cure is limited; however, injections can reverse certain pathologies (such as local inflammation or reduce scar tissue). They can have a role in the management of muscle trigger points. Here, as with any hands-on treatment, maintenance of the positive effect can be an issue. It has been suggested that botulinum toxin may prolong the effect. Similarly, peripheral injections may transiently reduce central sensitization, and a technique of pulsed radiofrequency neuromodulation may prolong the effect. (For further details see Chapter 8.2.)

c. *Neuromodulation* such as the use of implanted neurostimulators (British Pain Society 2005). NICE has published guidelines on the use of spinal cord stimulation for neuropathic pain: http://www.nice.org.uk/nicemedia/pdf/TA159Guidance.pdf. The problem with conventional spinal cord stimulation and CPP is successfully stimulating the right area so that the neuromodulation stimulus is perceived in the painful area. One way to achieve this is by retrograde stimulation where the stimulating electrode is passed in a retrograde direction from the entry point. Usually spinal cord stimulation is said to have its effect by stimulation of the dorsal horn, the retrograde electrode being adjacent to the preganglionic roots. The effect of this difference is not known. What is known is that transforaminal sacral root stimulation (usually S3) can have an effect on bladder and bowel function. S3 stimulation is recommended by NICE for both faecal and urinary incontinence under specific circumstances: http://www.nice.org.uk/nicemedia/pdf/ip/IPG099guidance.pdf; http://www.nice.org.uk/nicemedia/pdf/ip/IPG064guidance.pdf. Sacral root stimulation probably acts at the dorsal root ganglion level or possibly on the peripheral nerve. Work in patients with pelvic functional disorders and coincidental pain suggests that S3 neuromodulation may reduce the pain. A trial of peripheral nerve evaluation is easy to undertake with a simple unipolar electrode being available for S3 stimulation. This is our unit's preferred way of exploring neuromodulation in a patient and then considering either a full S3 implant with a tined lead (a lead with flanges to reduce the chance of movement and 4 electrodes to allow maximum chance of maintaining stimulation) or going on to the more complex retrograde trial and possibly full implant with that technology. The systems are essentially like a pacemaker with the electrode being attached to an internalized pulse generator. The more sophisticated pulse generators can be programmed by an external hand-held device and some may even be recharged externally. (Refer to Chapter 8.2 for further information regarding neuromodulation.)

d. *Explanation and support*. Often the patient will have been given a lot of misinformation and the most influential person in the team who can address this is the medical consultant.

The role of the psychologist

As with any discipline, psychologists may have different training. Pain management psychologists have specific training in the management of those aspects of psychology most likely to require attention in a pain patient. A urogenital pain psychologist, as well as dealing with mood and other emotional disorders associated with pain such as anger and catastrophizing (Rabin et al. 2000, Sullivan et al. 2006, Nickel et al. 2008), will manage sexual disorders (Binik & Bergeron 2001) and help with socializing, work issues and functional problems (Drossman et al. 2003). They may refer on for specific problems such as post-traumatic stress associated with rape or torture. A referral to a psychiatrist may be necessary. The main emphasis is on quality of life rather than pain reduction – simplified, the patient may either be in pain and distressed or in pain and have fewer emotional problems and an increased quality of life. There is no doubt that access to psychology must be a priority for the complex pelvic pain patient (see Chapter 4).

The role of the clinical nurse specialist or nurse consultant (Cambitzi & Baranowski 2009)

Senior nursing staff play a key role in co-ordinating care as well as running their own specialist clinics (e.g. TENS, neuromodulation programming and follow-up, sleep hygiene, education, drug reduction). They are often the cornerstone of any pain clinic team.

The role of the physiotherapist

Different physiotherapy approaches include: hands-on manipulation including patient self-management (Weiss 2001), stretching, pacing and exercise programmes (with and without pelvic floor electromyography) (Hetrick et al. 2006). Physiotherapists have an important role in the behavioural aspects of management (Hetrick et al. 2003, Nederhand et al. 2006). Much of this will be covered in Chapters 9, 11, 12 and 13.

The pain management programme

A cognitive-behavioural approach to pain management has some of the strongest evidence base for improving quality of life but less of an effect on pain (Eccleston et al. 2009). This approach is usually run by physiotherapy and psychology practitioners with contributions from nursing and medical doctors. There is little evidence to suggest whether individual or group programmes are better; however, the latter are more cost-effective. Similarly, there is little evidence to support a specific group urogenital programme as being better than a generic programme but that would be logical and is what we run at our centre. In general, pain management programmes appear to be the most helpful for those patients for whom physical treatment options have been tried and little progress made. As a consequence, traditionally the role of the chronic pain physiotherapist and psychologist has been to manage those patients who are no longer receiving medical interventions. However, it is generally accepted that earlier intervention by these specialists may help to prevent many of the problems associated with the chronicity that the chronic pain patient has to face. It has therefore been the main aim of our group to introduce patients at an early stage to our psychologists and chronic pain physiotherapists to provide individualized one-to-one programmes where possible.

Summary

Urogenital pain is associated with a range of sensory and functional abnormalities that affect multiple systems. For certain complex cases a multidisciplinary, multispeciality approach is thus necessary. A close working relationship between different speciality teams such as urology, pain management, urogynaecology, gynaecology and the colorectal team is essential. Each of these teams will be composed of individuals from multiple disciplines all of whom will provide a small component to improving the health and well-being of the patient with CPP.

References

Abrams, P., Baranowski, A.P., Berger, R.E., et al., 2006. A new classification is needed for pelvic pain syndromes - are existing terminologies of spurious diagnostic authority bad for patients? J. Urol. 175 (6), 1989–1990.

Baranowski, A.P., Curran, N.C., 2008. Pharmacological diagnostic tests. In: Rice, A., Howard, R., Justins, D., Miaskowski, C., Newton-John, T. (Eds.), Clinical Pain Management - Practice and Procedures, Principles of Measurement and Diagnosis. OUP, London.

Baranowski, A.P., Abrams, P., Berger, R.E., et al., 2008. Urogenital pain–time to accept a new approach to phenotyping and, as a consequence, management. Eur. Urol. 53, 33–36.

Baranowski, A.P., Abrams, P., Fall, M., 2008. Urogenital Pain in Clinical Practice. Informa Healthcare, New York.

Binik, I., Bergeron, S., 2001. Chronic vulvar pain and sexual functioning. In: National Vulvodynia Association News Spring 2001, 5–7.

British Pain Society, 2005. Spinal cord stimulation for the management of pain. http://www.britishpainsociety.org/pub_professional.htm#spinalcord.

Cambitzi, J., Baranowski, A.P., 2009. Urogenital multidisciplinary pain management. Defining a nurse's role. European Association of Urology Nurses. Eur. Urol. Today.

Chong, M.S., Hester, J., 2008. Pharmacotherapy for neuropathic pain with special reference to urogenital pain. In: Baranowski, A.P., Abrams, P., Fall, M. (Eds.), Urogenital Pain in Clinical Practice. Informa Healthcare, New York, pp. 427–439.

Dickson, D., Humphrey, V.R., 2008. Nerve blocks in urogenital pain. In: Baranowski, A.P., Abrams, P., Fall, M. (Eds.), Urogenital Pain in Clinical Practice. Informa Healthcare, New York, pp. 441–449.

Drossman, D.A., Toner, B.B., Whitehead, W.E., et al., 2003. Cognitive-behavioural therapy versus education and desipramine versus placebo for moderate to severe functional bowel disorders. Gastroenterology 125, 19–31.

Eccleston, C., Williams, A.C., Morley, S., 2009. Psychological therapies for the management of chronic pain (excluding headache) in adults. Cochrane Database Syst. Rev. 15 (2): CD007407.

Emmanuel, A., Chatoor, D., 2009. Proctology and pelvic disorders. Best Pract. Res. Clin. Gastroenterol. 23 (4), 461.

Fall, M., Baranowski, A.P., Elneil, S., et al., 2008. 2008 members of the European Association of Urology (EAU) Guidelines Office. Guidelines on Chronic Pelvic Pain. In: EAU Guidelines, edition presented at the 23rd EAU Annual Congress Milan 978-90-70244-91-0.http://www.uroweb.org/nc/professional-resources/guidelines/online/.

Giamberardino, M.A., 2005. Visceral pain. Pain: Clinical Updates XIII (6), 1–6.

Hetrick, D.C., Ciol, M.A., Rothman, I., et al., 2003. Musculoskeletal dysfunction in men with chronic pelvic pain syndrome type III: a case–control study. J. Urol. 170 (3), 828–831.

Hetrick, D.C., Glazer, H., Liu, Y.-W., et al., 2006. Pelvic floor electromyography in men with chronic pelvic pain syndrome: a case-control study. Neurology and Urodynamics 25 (1), 46–49.

Nederhand, M.J., Hermens, H.J., Ijzerman, M.J., et al., 2006. The effect of fear of movement on muscle activation in posttraumatic neck pain disability. Clin. J. Pain 22 (6), 519–525.

Nickel, J.C., Tripp, D.A., Chuai, S., et al., the NIH-CPCRN Study Group, 2008. Psychosocial parameters impact quality of life in men diagnosed with chronic prostatitis/chronic pelvic pain syndrome (CP/CPPS). Br. J. Urol. 101 (1), 59–64.

Patorno, E., Bohn, R.L., Wahl, P.M., 2010. Anticonvulsant medications and the risk of suicide, attempted suicide, or violent death. JAMA 303 (14), 1401–1409.

Rabin, C., O'Leary, A., Neighbors, C., et al., 2000. Pain and depression experienced by women with interstitial cystitis. Women Health 31, 67–81.

Sullivan, M.J.L., Martel, M., Tripp, D., et al., 2006. The relation between catastrophizing and the communication of pain experience. Pain 122, 282–288.

Vecchiet, L., Giamberardino, M.A., de Bigontina, P., 1992. Referred pain from viscera: when the symptom persists despite the extinction of the visceral focus. Adv. Pain Res. Ther. 20, 101–110 12.

Weiss, J.M., 2001. Pelvic floor myofascial trigger points: manual therapy for interstitial cystitis and the urgency-frequency syndrome. J. Urol. 166, 2226–2231.

Interdisciplinary management of chronic pelvic pain: A US physical medicine perspective

8.2

Stephanie A. Prendergast   Elizabeth H. Rummer

CHAPTER CONTENTS

Introduction

As discussed in Chapter 8.1, historically, medical management of chronic pelvic pain (CPP) has frustrated both patients and providers, leading to the evolution of multimodal therapeutic strategies. Specialists are now viewing CPP as a polymorphic syndrome that may include organic pathology, musculoskeletal dysfunction, neuropathology and psychosocial impairments. Medical practice utilizing interdisciplinary, co-ordinated interventions is resulting in more successful treatment outcomes (Montenegro 2008).

Patients with pelvic pain seek help from multiple medical disciplines due to the wide variations in symptoms:

- In addition to genital, anal, coccygeal, perineal, buttock and abdominal pain, CPP can include urinary symptoms such as dysuria, urinary urgency, frequency, hesitancy and poor stream strength.
- Bowel complaints include constipation, difficulty with evacuation, dyschezia and 'pencil stool' or varied, abnormal shapes of stool.
- Sexually, patients may experience anorgasmia or difficulty achieving orgasm, genital hyperarousal disorder, post-orgasmic pain, pain during or after intercourse, erectile dysfunction and/or excessive or lack of vaginal discharge in women.

Due to the varied symptoms, patients may seek the help of primary care physicians, gynaecologists, urologists, colorectal surgeons, orthopedists, neurologists and/or psychiatrists. It is reported that 85–90% of patients with CPP have musculoskeletal dysfunction (Tu et al. 2006, Butrick 2009) that has been identified as either a primary cause of pain and dysfunction or a secondary consequence of vulvodynia, painful bladder syndrome/interstitial cystitis, chronic pelvic pain syndrome/non-bacterial chronic prostatitis, irritable bowel syndrome, pudendal neuralgia and endometriosis (Tu et al. 2006, Butrick 2009).

Furthermore, 30% of patients seen in primary care settings, and 85% in dedicated pain centres, are diagnosed with myofascial pain syndrome, demonstrating the importance of including musculoskeletal investigation early in the assessment of a patient with CPP (Butrick 2009). Ideally such investigation would be undertaken as part of a team approach to the condition.

Team management

As in the UK, physicians, physical therapists and mental health providers in the US commonly form interdisciplinary teams working with chronic pain in general and CPP in particular (see Figure 8.2.1). Surgical interventions and invasive procedures run the risk of symptom exacerbation in patients with CPP, therefore conservative therapies such as manual physical therapy techniques, psychotherapies and pharmaceuticals are often utilized first to modulate pain. Simultaneously, organic pathology needs to be addressed if identified. Interventional medicine strategies have shown efficacy in treatment of CPP and should be utilized if conservative measures fail (Simons et al. 1999, Zhang et al. 2004, Maria et al. 2005, Amir et al. 2006). Numerous treatment options exist, and more than one medical professional may be able to treat particular pathophysiological features, whereas certain treatments may only be available from one team member. Treatment of CPP should be considered as a dynamic process with many possible effective treatment combinations. Certain treatments will be more or less important than others as a patient's presentation changes.

As CPP is a syndrome associated with numerous pathophysiological features (see Box 8.2.1), extensive patient education and excellent interdisciplinary communication is imperative. Commonly, the treatment of a single impairment does not translate into the dramatic change the patient may expect. For example, if a patient with a 5-year history of severe vaginal burning is given an anticonvulsant and the pain is reduced, but not eradicated, the patient reports 'disappointment', and may think 'it is not working'. In actuality, studies cited later in this chapter show anticonvulsants are effective for treating the central processing dysfunction this patient likely has. However, this patient may also present with pelvic floor myofascial trigger points and pudendal nerve inflammation, and until these impairments are also addressed, the overall syndrome is likely to persist. Through examinations, re-examinations, differential diagnoses and communication, the team can manage patient expectations more effectively.

Box 8.2.1

Pathophysiological features associated with CPP

- Muscle hypertonus
- Myofascial trigger points
- Altered neurodynamics
- Connective tissue restrictions
- Biomechanical/structural abnormalities
- Sleep deprivation
- Malnutrition
- Depression
- Anxiety
- Central sensitization

The interventions listed in this text are effective treatments for the pathophysiological features listed in Box 8.2.1. The multimodal algorithm (see Figure 8.2.1) helps explain how to turn the complex problem of CPP into a sum of more manageable parts, expanding on the decision-making process to determine when and how to use different modalities. Clinical examples will be used to demonstrate the utility of the interdisciplinary approach.

Organic pathology intervention

Organic pathologies associated with CPP may include: yeast and bacterial infections, urinary tract, bladder and prostate infections, irritable bowel syndrome, endometriosis, colitis, Crohn's disease, gastritis and sexually transmitted diseases. Symptoms of these pathologies mimic the symptoms of CPP and appropriate treatment protocols for the pathology should be followed (Butrick 2009).

Cognitive behavioural therapy

Cognitive behavioural therapy (CBT) should be considered an important component in a comprehensive treatment plan for patients with CPP. Behavioural interventions for chronic pain have become commonly available alternatives to medical and rehabilitative therapies (Campbell & Mitchell 1996, Gatchel & Turk 1996). CBT has been shown to be an effective treatment for chronic pain patients, by helping to develop self-management skills to improve their personal control of their condition, reduce pain, distress, and pain behaviour, and improve daily functioning (Turk et al. 1983, Eccleston et al. 2009). Treatment that focuses on decreasing negative thinking, emotional responses to pain, and perceptions of disability, while increasing orientation toward self-management, are predictive of favourable treatment outcomes (Morely et al. 1999, McCracken & Turk 2002).

CBT has been shown to be efficacious for the treatment of vulvodynia in two uncontrolled studies (Abramov et al. 1994, Weijmar et al. 1996) and in one well-controlled, randomized study (Bergeron et al. 2008). Masheb et al. conducted a randomized trial to test the relative efficacy of CBT and supportive psychotherapy (SPT) in women with vulvodynia. The results suggest that psychosocial treatments for vulvodynia are well tolerated and produce clinically meaningful improvements in pain. They observed that CBT, relative to SPT, resulted in significantly greater improvements in pain severity and sexual function. Additionally, participants in the CBT condition reported significantly greater treatment improvement, satisfaction and credibility than in the SPT condition (Masheb et al. 2009).

Manual physical therapy intervention

The musculoskeletal impairments that may cause pelvic pain and dysfunction are connective tissue restrictions, muscle hypertonus with or without myofascial trigger points (including muscles of the pelvic floor, trunk and lower extremities), altered neurodynamics of peripheral nerves and pelvic girdle and biomechanical abnormalities. After a thorough history, an extensive physical examination is performed. The entire surface areas of the abdomen, trunk, thighs, pelvis (up to the base of the clitoris and penis including the labia and scrotum) should be examined for connective tissue restrictions (Fitzgerald 2009).

Conservative medical management starts with manual therapy to eradicate or modify the impairments, which may in turn, decrease pain. In 2009, the Urological Pelvic Pain Collaborative Research Network (UPPCRN) concluded that somatic abnormalities, including myofascial trigger points and connective tissue restrictions, were found to be very common in women and men with IC/PBS and chronic prostatitis/chronic pelvic pain syndrome, respectively (Fitzgerald et al. 2009).

Somatic abnormalities may be the primary abnormality in at least some patients and secondary in others, but in either situation they should be identified and treated. The UPPCRN also published the outcomes of their feasibility trial comparing connective tissue manipulation (CTM) and myofascial physical therapy, versus global therapeutic massage, in patients with CPP. The group receiving skilled CTM and myofascial therapy had a significantly higher response rate than the group receiving massage alone (Fitzgerald et al. 2009). See Chapter 11.2 for a summary of CTM methodology.

Altered neurodynamics

Peripheral nerves commonly involved in myofascial pelvic pain syndromes include the dorsal, perineal and inferior rectal branch of the pudendal nerve, the ilioinguinal, iliohypergastric, genitofemoral, obturator, femoral, sciatic and posterior femoral cutaneous nerves.

Compromised blood supply and/or neurobiomechanics of peripheral nerves may cause altered neurodynamics, thereby contributing to pelvic pain and dysfunction (Butler 2004). Connective tissue restrictions, muscle hypertonus and faulty joint mechanics can affect the dynamic protective mechanisms of peripheral nerves and lead to burning, stabbing, shooting pain in the territory of the nerve (Butler 2004).

For example, consider a patient with severe pelvic floor hypertonus. This patient may have inflammation around the pudendal nerve, secondary to compression by the muscles. Each time this patient attempts to have a bowel movement he is forced to strain, and several attempts are made before he succeeds at evacuating the stool. In addition to static compression causing inflammation, the muscles can fixate a normally mobile nerve as the patient forcefully lengthens the pelvic floor during straining. This can cause further neural irritation. The patient may experience shooting, stabbing rectal pain, either during or after the bowel movement, reflective of this neural irritation (Prendergast & Rummer 2008).

Treatment of altered neurodynamics involves removing the aggravating stimuli and restoring mobility. Myofascial treatment of connective tissue restrictions and muscle hypertonus may reduce aggravating neural input. Neural mobilization techniques to restore mobility along the path of the nerve have also shown efficacy (Ellis & Hing 2008).

Chapters 2, 9, 11, 12, 13 and 14 discuss the evaluation and treatment of the pelvic floor muscles, myofascial trigger points, biomechanics and the pelvic girdle at length.

Lifestyle modifications and home exercise programmes

All members of the interdisciplinary team can help the patient make temporary lifestyle modifications to improve function while the patient is being treated. Techniques to promote autonomic nervous system quieting, improve sleep hygiene, decrease stress, and improve diet and nutrition are all helpful, if not imperative, to the treatment process. Examples include the use of cushions, posture and/or breathing education, workstation, home and car modifications, clothing and footwear recommendations, and advice on exercise programme development (Prendergast & Rummer 2008).

Pharmacological therapy

The approach to pharmacological therapy for CPP in the USA is very similar to that in the UK. See Chapter 8.1.

Simple analgesics

Acetaminophen has both analgesic and antipyretic activity and has been used in acute and chronic painful conditions (Bannwarth & Pehourcq 2003); however, there is little evidence about its role in CPP. There is also very little evidence for the use of non-steroidal anti-inflammatory drugs (NSAIDs) in the treatment of CPP and even less for cyclooxygenase 2 (COX-2) selective drugs.

Neuropathic analgesics

Tricylic antidepressants are widely used for other chronic pain conditions such as fibromyalgia, chronic headaches, interstitial cystitis and irritable bowel syndrome. They have been studied for several pain disorders and have consistently shown benefit (Ohghena & Van Houdenhove 1992). The benefit of tricyclics is not generated by decreasing depression. If depression is present, it should be treated separately. Amitriptyline is the most commonly studied and has been shown to be an effective treatment for neuropathic pain, but side effects often limit its clinical use (Max 1994, Richeimer et al. 1997). A few studies have compared the use of amitriptyline versus placebo in patients with pelvic pain (McKay 1993). Some authors recommend it as the treatment of choice, whereas others have reported disappointing results (Richeimer et al. 1997, Rose & Kam 2002). Mixed reuptake inhibitors have been shown to be more effective than selective serotonin reuptake inhibitors in the treatment of chronic pain (Fishbain et al. 2000, Yokogawa et al. 2002).

Anticonvulsants

Anticonvulsants have been used in pain management for many years. Gabapentin has been reported to be well tolerated and an effective treatment in various pain conditions, particularly in neuropathic pain (Beydoun et al. 1995, Rosenberg et al. 1997). Gabapentin failed to show effectiveness in genitourinary tract pain in some studies, but has shown success in the treatment of diabetic neuropathy, post-herpetic neuropathy, neuropathic pain associated with carcinoma, multiple sclerosis, genitourinary tract pain and vulvodynia in others (Ben & Friedman 1999, Sasaki et al. 2001). Sator-Katzenschlager et al. reported that after 6, 12 and 24 months, pain relief was significantly greater in patients receiving gabapentin either alone or in combination with amitriptyline than in patients on amitriptyline alone. In this study gabapentin was more effective than amitriptyline in improving neuropathic burning or spontaneous, paroxysmal pain (Sator-Katzenschlager et al. 2005). Pregabalin (Lyrica) is a relatively new drug that has been found to be very beneficial for patients with myofascial pain disorder and neuropathic symptoms, such as in fibromyalgia (Butrick 2009).

N-methyl-D-aspartate antagonists

The N-methyl-D-aspartate (NMDA) receptor channel complex is known to be an important channel for the development and maintenance of chronic pain. NMDA antagonists have been useful in the management of neuropathic pain (Hewitt 2000). Ketamine has been beneficial in several chronic pain conditions including peripheral neuropathies, but its long-term role remains unclear (Visser & Schug 2006). Challenging pelvic pain conditions may be helped by ketamine if there is nerve injury or central sensitization.

Opioids

Opioids have a role in the management of chronic non-malignant pain, however, opioids in pelvic pain are poorly defined (McQuay 1999). The following guidelines for the use of opioids in chronic/non-acute urogenitial pain are (Fall et al. 2008):

- All other treatments must have been tried and failed;
- An appropriately trained specialist should consult with another physician when instigating opioid therapy;
- With a history or suspicion of drug abuse, psychological consultation is imperative;
- Patient should undergo a trial of opioids;
- Patient should be made aware of the rules and regulations of opioid use as well as the risk of addiction and dependency;
- Morphine is the first-line drug, unless there are contraindications to morphine or special indications for another drug.

Trigger point injection therapy

As described in Chapters 11 and 15, myofascial trigger points (MTrPs) are a nodular and hyperirritable area within a taut band of skeletal muscle. They can cause characteristic referred pain, local tenderness, autonomic phenomena, motor dysfunction and/or weakness and proprioceptive disturbances (Simons et al. 1999). Trigger points can be successfully treated with several approaches, one of which is trigger point injections. The most accepted theory hypothesizes that the mechanical disruption of the skeletal muscle fibres by an anaesthetic injection inactivates the trigger point (Simons 1999). Another possible mechanism is that the fluid injection may dilute nerve-sensitive substances that are present. Therefore, the injection may cause muscle fibre trauma releasing intracellular potassium, which can cause depolarization and block nerve fibres. A study looked at 18 women with pelvic pain for at least 6 months. All the women were found to have three to five trigger points in the pelvic floor muscles upon vaginal examination. Post trigger point injections, there was a significant decrease in a visual analogue scale, and improved patient global satisfaction and patient global cure visual scales (Langford et al. 2007). Trigger point injection therapy appears to be a viable treatment option for MTrPs in patients with CPP and should be considered when developing a comprehensive treatment plan.

Nerve blocks

Nerve blocks can be utilized for therapeutic and/or diagnostic purposes, however, interpreting a diagnostic block can be challenging given the many mechanisms by which a block acts. These mechanisms must be thoroughly understood as local anaesthetic agents are often utilized in nerve blocks. They primarily act by blocking sodium channels and can be effectively used for pain modulation at low doses that do not completely block nerve impulse propagation (Zhang et al. 2004, Amir et al. 2006). When managing neuropathic pain, sodium channels accumulate in the area of neural damage and develop abnormal discharge patterns at the periphery, and in the region of the dorsal root ganglia. Both the periphery and the dorsal root ganglia are sensitive to lidocaine (Ramer et al. 1999, Zhang et al. 2004, Amir et al. 2006). When neuropathic pain has become chronic, the mechanisms change over time resulting in several central and peripheral neural changes (Zhang et al. 2004). The reversal of these peripheral and central sensitizations or up-regulations would require the central nervous system to return to a more normal state, thus reducing pain (Abdi et al. 1998). It has been hypothesized that sodium channel blockade over an extended period can achieve this (Abdi et al. 1998). In addition to local anaesthetic, corticosteroids have also been used in the symptomatic relief of CPP (Antolak & Antolak 2009). The specifics on the techniques used, risks associated with, and the individual specialists performing neural blockades are available in various texts and will not be described here. The effectiveness of neural blockades for the treatment of the CPP population will be reviewed.

- Serial multilevel nerve blocks, including a caudal epidural, pudendal nerve block, and vestibular infiltration of local anaesthetic agents, may be an effective treatment for vulvar vestibulitis (Rapkin et al. 2008).
- A trans-sacrococcygeal approach to a ganglion impar block, for the management of chronic perineal pain may be an effective treatment (Toshniwal et al. 2007).
- Pudendal nerve blocks may be an effective tool for both diagnostic and therapeutic purposes in the management of pudendal-nerve-related pain and

pelvic floor muscle hypertonus (Calvillo et al. 2000, McDonald & Spigos 2000, Kovacs et al. 2001, Hough et al. 2003).

- Peripheral nerve blocks, such as ilioinguinal/iliohypogastric/genitofemoral, may be an effective treatment for the management of neuropathic pain associated with nerve damage (Kennedy et al. 1994).

Botulinum toxin therapy

Botulinum toxin A (BTX/A) has been successfully used with myofascial pain and pain associated with chronic muscle spasm (Acquardo & Borodic 1994, Cheshire et al. 1994, Yue 1995, Porta et al. 1997). Initially it was thought that the mechanism of pain relief involved muscle relaxation induced by blockade of the release of acetylcholine at the neuromuscular junction. Now it is also thought to involve the direct antinociceptive activity of blocking the release of local neurotransmitters involved in pain signalling as well as maintaining stimulation of local inflammatory mediators. This decrease in peripheral sensitization results in a secondary decrease in central sensitization by a direct reduction in neurotransmitter release in the dorsal horn (Aoki 2003). Additionally, there is a reduction in the release of substance P and glutamate within the dorsal horn (Porta 2000). It has been postulated that the relaxation of affected muscles by BTX/A should decompress entrapped nerves in patients with myofascial pain syndrome or pain from chronic muscle spasm and should facilitate physical therapy (Filippi et al. 1993, Rosalis et al. 1996). Physical therapy is imperative if maximum benefits are to be achieved with BTX/A. The effects of BTX/A are typically evident within 3–10 days and last for approximately 3 months (Porta 2000). The potential use of BTX/A in the treatment of CPP has been recognized for more than 10 years (Brin & Vapnek 1997). The literature presents recent evidence for utilizing BTX/A in successfully treating CPP conditions:

- BTX/A has been used with benefit for many pelvic floor hypertonic dysfunctions including vulvodynia, CPP, vaginismus, obstructed defecation, voiding dysfunction, urinary retention, perianal pain disorders and anal fissures (Maria et al. 2005).
- Ghazizadeh and Nikzad showed that 150–400 units of BTX/A resulted in a 75% response rate in women with vaginismus with no recurrence and a mean follow-up of 12 months (Ghazizadeh & Nikzad 2004).
- A double-blind randomized, placebo-controlled trial of BTX/A (80 units) versus physical therapy for CPP caused by levator spasm showed a statistically significant decrease in dyspareunia and non-menstral pain (Abbot et al. 2006).
- In a pilot study, Dykstra and Presthus showed a significant decrease in mean pain score, medication use and improved quality of life in women with provoked vestibulodynia with the use of BTX/A (35 units) (Dykstra & Presthus 2006).
- In 2007 Yoon et al. reported a marked improvement in subjective pain score following treatment with BTX/A (20–40 units) in a group of seven women with intractable genital pain (Yoon et al. 2007).
- A pilot study of 12 women with CPP for more than 2 years were treated with 40 units of BTX/A into the puborectalis and pubococcygeus. The authors reported significant decreases in dyspareunia and dysmenorrhoea. Quality of life and sexual activity were also significantly improved (Jarvis et al. 2004).
- Bertolasi et al. treated 67 women with either lifelong vaginismus or secondary dyspareunia complicated by vulvar vestibulitis with 20 units of BTX/A. They documented 46–76% symptom reduction and a 'cure' rate of 20–46% (Bertolasi et al. 2006).

Pulsed radiofrequency

There are two types of radiofrequency used clinically: continuous radiofrequency (CRF) and pulsed radiofrequency (PRF). CRF ablation has been in use for over 25 years. It uses a constant output of high-frequency current and produces temperatures greater than 45°C, which is neuroablative (Racz & Ruiz-Lopez 2006). PRF, on the other hand, uses brief pulses of high-voltage electric current which pauses between pulses to allow heat to dissipate. This causes less nerve destruction since the temperature does not usually exceed 42°C (Racz & Ruiz-Lopez 2006). The exact mechanism of PRF is unknown (Sluijter et al. 1998), but the current hypothesis proposes that PRF acts by modulating pain perception rather than directly destroying neural tissue (Cahana et al. 2006). Current evidence suggests that PRF may be useful in treating refractory neuropathic conditions (Hammer & Menesse 1998, Robert et al. 1998, Munglani 1999, Mikeladeze et al. 2003, Shah & Racz 2003, Van Zundert et al. 2003a,b, 2007, Cahana et al. 2006, Abejon et al. 2007, Martin et al. 2007, Wu & Groner 2007). There has been one reported case study of successfully using PRF on the pudendal nerve for CPP (Rhame et al. 2009). See Chapter 16.

Neuromodulation

Neuromodulation is technology that acts directly upon nerves by altering, or modulating, nerve activity by delivering electrical or pharmaceutical agents directly to a target area.

Sacral neuromodulation

The pelvic floor is controlled by a complex set of neural reflexes that can be modified through neuroplasticity. Neuroplasticity is necessary for activities such as toilet training, but it can result in a disruption of neural reflexes that can cause pelvic floor dysfunction. Neuromodulation, typically of the sacral nerves, can correct this disruption of neural reflexes in approximately 60–75% of patients with urinary retention, urge incontinence and urinary frequency (Chartier-Kastler et al. 2008). Using sacral neuromodulation to treat voiding dysfunction has been studied for many years (Schmidt et al. 1979, Baskin & Tanagho 1992). Neuromodulation has also been used to successfully treat chronic pain conditions such as migraine headaches, back pain and idiopathic angina pectoris (Alo & Holsheimer 2002). Even though it is not typically indicated for pelvic pain, there have been reports of up to 50% resolution of CPP and 85% improvement in pain and quality of life for patients with interstitial cystitis (Peters 2002, Mayer & Howard 2008). The exact mechanism of pain relief by neuromodulation is not known. The treatment is partly based upon the gate control theory. This implies that activity in the large-diameter Aβ fibres inhibit transmission of pain signals to the brain (Alo & Holsheimer 2002). Specific examples in the literature show evidence of sacral neuromodulation as a treatment for pelvic pain:

- Maher et al. reported a significant reduction of pain scores in 15 patients with interstitial cystitis (Maher et al. 2001).
- Siegel et al. reported a 60% significant improvement in pelvic pain in ten patients at a median follow-up of 19 months (Siegel et al. 2001).
- Peters and Konstandt implanted 21 patients with interstitial cystitis and reported a marked to moderate improvement in pain after 15 months in 20 patients. They also noted a corresponding significant reduction in narcotic medication use for control of their pain (Peters & Konstandt 2004).
- Zabihi et al. used bilateral S2–S4 caudal epidural sacral neuromodulation for the treatment of CPP, painful bladder syndrome and interstitial cystitis. They reported that 42% reported more than 50% improvement in their urinary symptoms and their visual analogue pain score improved by 40% (Zabihi et al. 2008).

Posterior tibial nerve stimulation

Percutaneous posterior tibial nerve stimulation (PTNS) (intermittent stimulation of the S3 nerve) developed as a less-expensive alternative to sacral nerve root stimulation. The goal is to stimulate the tibial nerve via a fine needle electrode inserted into the lower, inner aspect of the leg, slightly cephalad to the medial malleolus. The needle electrode is then connected to an external pulse generator which delivers an adjustable electrical pulse that travels to the sacral plexus via the tibial nerve. Percutaneous tibial nerve stimulation is currently used to treat lower urinary tract dysfunction such as urge incontinence, urgency/frequency and non-obstructive retention (Stoller 1999, Klingler et al. 2000, Govier et al. 2001, van Balken et al. 2001). Until recently there were few studies that showed improvement in the CPP population with PTNS. Most recently, Kabay et al. conducted a randomized controlled prospective clinical trial to evaluate the clinical effect of PTNS in patients with chronic prostatitis/chronic pelvic pain syndrome. They reported that after 12 weeks of treatment, the VAS (visual analogue scale) score for pain and the National Institutes of Health Chronic Prostatitis Symptom Index significantly improved (Kabay et al. 2009). Kim et al. showed that after 12 weeks of PTNS an objective response occurred in 60% of patients with CPP and 30% had an improvement of 25–50% in the VAS score for pain (Kim et al. 2007). Another study showed PTNS had a positive effect in 39% of 33 pelvic pain patients (van Balken et al. 2003).

Chronic/continuous pudendal nerve stimulation

Another alternative approach to nerve stimulation is chronic or continuous pudendal nerve stimulation (CPNS). Instead of placing the leads at the sacral nerve root, the lead is placed at the pudendal nerve using neurophysiological guidance (Peters et al. 2009). There are few published studies that report outcomes of CPNS. Peters et al. looked at 84 patients who had interstitial cystitis/painful bladder syndrome or overactive bladder. Most of these patients had previously failed sacral neuromodulation. They reported a positive response, ≥50% improvement being achieved in 71.4% (Peters et al. 2009). Electrotherapy and hydrotherapy in the treatment of CPP are discussed further in Chapter 16.

Multimodal treatment algorithm (Figure 8.2.1)

Patients with CPP present with a wide range of symptoms, impairments, disability and syndrome chronicity. Unfortunately, in many cases the patient is also suffering from the neuropathological and psychological consequences of having chronic pain. Thorough evaluations will lead to the initiation of appropriate, individualized treatments. This collection of individual, impairment-based treatments will comprehensively form an effective treatment plan. Once a pelvic pain syndrome has been diagnosed, a multimodal treatment algorithm can be a useful tool to organize the different therapies, re-formulate treatments after re-evaluations, and provide alternatives for ineffectual or intolerable therapies (Figure 8.2.1).

The process starts with the identification of CPP, treating organ pathologies (if present), and introducing the patient to the interdisciplinary team concept. (Fig 8.2.1: top two boxes). The interdisciplinary team (Fig 8.2.1: centre circles) may consist of many providers in four general therapeutic domains: physical therapy, interventional pain management, pharmaceuticals and psychosocial services. As the relevant literature and this chapter describe, the patient will benefit from a physical therapy evaluation to identify somatic dysfunction. The severity and chronicity of the patient's case will dictate which other therapies are initiated. If a provider suspects central sensitization, anxiety, depression, nutritional, diet and/or sleep issues, simultaneous referrals to the psychosocial domain and for pharmacotherapy management may be indicated and beneficial. Patients are often evaluated over several appointments to identify all pain generators, dysfunction and limiting factors to treatment plans.

The multidirectional arrows of the algorithm stress the interdependent relationships between the providers, treatments and desired therapeutic outcomes. Once a treatment plan has been initiated, each provider needs to think critically about the efficacy of the intended individual treatment for the impairment in question (Fig 8.2.1: upper boxes). When two patients have the same diagnosis under the umbrella of pelvic pain (i.e. vulvodynia, painful bladder syndrome, etc.), it is almost certain their objective findings and treatment plans will be quite different. For example, as mentioned in this text, BTX/A has shown efficacy for decreasing pelvic floor hypertonus, which is known to cause pelvic pain. Often ineffectually, practitioners have administered BOX/A to treat 'CPP'. However, a patient may have pelvic pain and not necessarily pelvic floor hypertonus. Therefore, BTX/A is likely ineffectual for this patient. Conversely, myofascial trigger points in the adductors, rectus abdominis and gluteal muscles can also cause CPP. The introduction of manual therapy, dry needling or trigger point injections, to the involved muscles, is reasonable and may be helpful. BTX/A may decrease hypertonus and MTrP therapy may eradicate MTrPs. Since the diagnosis of 'pelvic pain' does not explain the source of the problem it is more practical to think of interventions as tools for impairments rather than treatments for 'pelvic pain'. In other areas of medicine, batteries of tests and a history and physical lead to a diagnosis. The diagnosis then dictates treatment. As Figure 8.2.1 depicts, multiple impairments are causal of CPP. The algorithm demonstrates that it is not appropriate to apply a linear therapeutic approach to complex syndromes such as CPP.

The overall treatment plan comprises the sum of individual therapeutic modalities as seen in the algorithm. Providers need to think globally about the function of the patient, but also locally about the intended intervention. Examples of individual treatments include connective tissue manipulation to restricted tissues, manual trigger point therapy to myofascial trigger points, prescribing of a sleep aid, talk therapy for a patient to decrease anxiety or use of hypnosis for pain management (Fig 8.2.1: upper boxes).

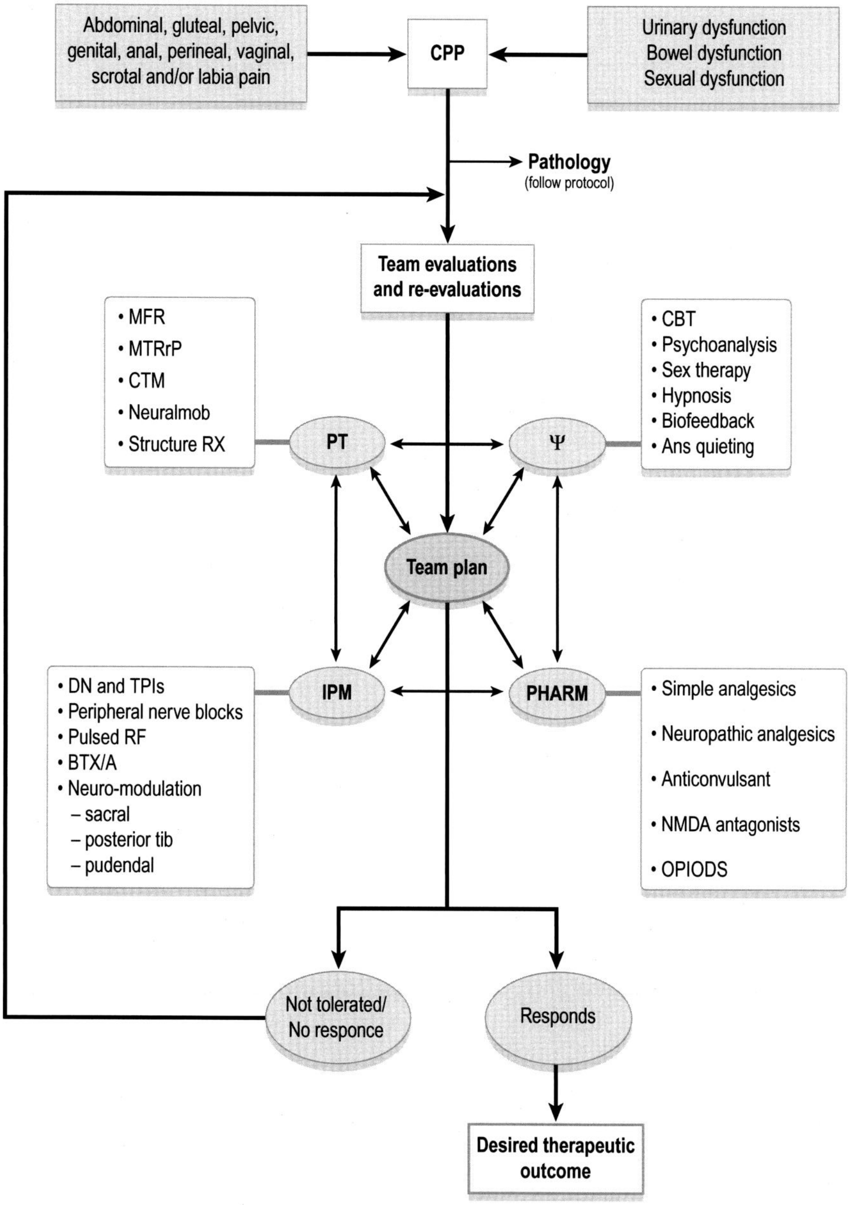

Figure 8.2.1 • Multimodal treatment algorithm, ψ; PT, physical therapy; IPM, interventional pain management; RF, radiofrequency; ANS, autonomic nervous system. See text for further abbreviations

Once a treatment is initiated, patients will either respond, not tolerate the intervention, tolerate the intervention but have no response (i.e. a decrease in or elimination of the impairments, not necessarily an immediate change in the pain and/or functional status of the patient), or they may tolerate the treatment but generally not comply with the treatment plan (missed appointments, failure to take or tolerate medications, non-compliance with necessary lifestyle modifications, etc.) (Fig 8.2.1: lowest circles).

Reasons for poor treatment tolerance

There are numerous reasons why patients do not tolerate certain treatments. Patients may not tolerate medications because of side effects. Other drugs or another class of drugs could be tried. As the algorithm shows, other treatments in different domains could be substituted or employed in concert. Pharmaceuticals may help neuropathic components of pain; however, eradicating somatic dysfunction can also provide pain relief if medications are not tolerated. Manual therapy techniques and interventional medicine may also be used to eliminate primary or secondary sources of pain if medication is not tolerated.

Conversely, painful manual therapy techniques may be augmented by pain medications. CBT therapies may be used to help patients cope with the pain while they are being treated. If a patient with a hypertonic pelvic floor has a history of sexual abuse, he or she may not be able to tolerate internal manual pelvic floor therapy until psychosocial services are effectively utilized. Even then, this method of therapy may not be appropriate for this particular patient and perhaps BTX/A injections to the pelvic floor muscles under anaesthesia should be considered. In general, the individual treatments may need to be modified due to pain from the treatment, side effects, psychosocial distress with the treatment, belonephobia or personal choices and/or religious beliefs regarding particular therapies. The team has the ability to present the patient with choices so that collectively a tolerable and effective treatment plan can be developed.

Modifying manual treatment

Commonly, manual therapy techniques to impaired tissues cause pain both during and after treatment. For example, a patient with an obturator internus myofascial trigger point may also have pudendal nerve irritation if the trigger point is close to Alcock's canal. Internal manual therapy to the trigger point may further aggravate the nerve and the patient may not be able to tolerate internal trigger point work due to hyperpathic reactions. This is another example where a patient could perceive the plan as 'not working'. In actuality, the patient is not tolerating a single treatment and is experiencing a transient increase in pain. Even though it is certainly less than ideal, the reality of treating chronic pain is that certain treatments may temporarily create more pain before relief is achieved. The therapist could change the plan and attempt to externally release the trigger point or utilize dry needling. It may also be reasonable to consider a pudendal nerve block, which may decrease neural irritation and pain and allow the patient to tolerate internal trigger point therapy. Numerous therapeutic strategies, combined with interdisciplinary communication and patient education will help move patients out of treatments they cannot tolerate and into plans they can.

Non-responding symptoms

It is also possible that patients can, in fact, tolerate a treatment; however, they are 'not responding'. It is crucial to differentiate between an impairment not changing versus the patient's overall functional status not changing as a result of a sole treatment. Rarely does a sole intervention translate into what a patient desires and deems as 'success'. For example, a patient is tolerating neural mobilizations to the pudendal nerve; however, the nerve continues to be exquisitely tender to palpation and their pain levels are not changing. If the neural mobility is *not* improving and pain persists it is advisable to change the technique or progress to more invasive procedures to facilitate impairment improvement. If the neural mobility *is* improving objectively but the subjective complaints persist, it is advisable to continue the current plan as well as re-evaluate to determine what other impairments are pain generators and implement treatment. Trigger point treatment can be used as a second example. Consider an accurate trigger point injection to a coccygeus trigger point. After the injection, the patient reports no change in their coccygeal pain. Upon examination, the trigger point is gone. The treatment was successful, now the team needs to address other impairments such as the sacrococcygeal joint, sacroiliac joint or pelvic floor muscles could be contributing to the coccygeal pain. It appears that the coccygeal trigger point was not relevant to the syndrome, though a reasonable thought, and now the team can move on to other treatments in the algorithm.

In the past, linear treatment approaches for CPP have yielded limited success. Current views of CPP as a multipathological syndrome have led to comprehensive interdisciplinary treatment strategies that recognize management of provider and patient expectations, while modulating pain and dysfunction, as hallmarks of the syndrome and its solution. With an evidenced-based team approach, excellent interdisciplinary communication, and appropriate patient education, providers and patients are progressing towards greater treatment efficacy and achieving desired therapeutic outcomes.

These chapters have emphasized the requirement to develop a team approach in the management of the patient with CPP, reminding the reader of the treatment paradigm 'cure sometimes, help always'. No one person or speciality can fix everything, but that does not mean that help cannot be offered, even if it just means referring the patient to the appropriate speciality.

References

Abbot, J.A., Jarvis, S.K., Lyons, S.D., et al., 2006. Botulinum toxin type A for chronic painand pelvic floor spasm in women: a randomized controlled trial. Obstet. Gynecol. 108 (4), 915–923.

Abdi, S., Lee, D.H., Chung, J.M., et al., 1998. The anti-allodynic effects of amitriptyline, gabapentic, and lidocaine in a rat model of neuropathic pain. Anesth. Analg. 87, 1360–1366.

Abejon, D., Garcia-del-Valle, S., Fuentes, M.L., et al., 2007. Pulsed radiofrequency in lumbar radicular pain: Clinical effects in various etiological groups. Pain Pract. 7, 21–26.

Abramov, L., Wolman, I., David, M.P., et al., 1994. Vaginismus: an important factor in the evaluation and management of vulvar vestibulitis syndrome. Gynecol. Obstet. Invest. 38 (3), 194–197.

Acquardo, M., Borodic, G., 1994. Treatmetn of myofascial pain with botulinum A toxin. Anesthesiology 80, 705–706.

Alo, K.M., Holsheimer, J., 2002. New trends in neuromodulation for the management of neuropathic pain. Neurosurgery 50, 690–703.

Amir, R., Argoff, C.E., Bennett, G.J., et al., 2006. The role of sodium channels in chronic inflammatory and neuropathic pain. J. Pain 7, S1–S29.

Antolak, S.J., Antolak, C.M., 2009. Therapeutic pudendal nerve blocks using corticosteroids cure pelvic pain after failure of sacral neurmodulation. Pain Med. (10), 186–189.

Aoki, K.R., 2003. Evidence for antinociceptive activity of botulinum toxin type A in pain management. Headache 43 (Suppl. 1), S9–S15.

Bannwarth, B., Pehourcq, F., 2003. Pharmacologic basis for using paracetamol: pharmacokinetic and pharmacodynamic issues. Drugs 63S (2), 5–13 [French].

Baskin, L.S., Tanagho, E.A., 1992. Pelvic pain without pelvic organs. J. Urol. 147, 683–686.

Ben, D.B., Friedman, M., 1999. Gabapentin therapy for vulvodynia. Anesth. Analg. 89, 1459–1460.

Bergeron, S., Khalife, S., Glazer, H.I., et al., 2008. Surgical and behavioral treatments for vestibulodynia: two-and-one-half year follow-up and predictors of outcome. Obstet. Gynecol. 111 (1), 159–166.

Bertolasi, L., Bottanelli, M., Graziottin, A., et al., 2006. Dyspareunia, vaginismus, hyperactivity of the pelvic floor and botulin toxin: the neurologists role. G. Ital. Ostet. Ginecol. 28, 264–268.

Beydoun, A., Uthman, B.M., Sackellares, J.C., et al., 1995. Gabapentin: pharmacokinetics, efficacy, and safety. Clin. Neuropharmacol. 14, 469–481.

Brin, M.F., Vapnek, J.M., 1997. Treatment of vaginismus with botulinum injections. Lancet 349, 252–253.

Butler, D., 2004. Mobilization of the Nervous System. Churchill Livingstone, NY.

Butrick, C.W., 2009. Pelvic Floor Hypertonic Disorders: Identification and Management. Obstet. Gynecol. Clin. North Am. 36, 707–722.

Cahana, A., Van Zundert, J., Macrea, L., et al., 2006. Pulsed radiofrequency: Current clinical and biological literature available. Pain Med. 7, 411–423.

Calvillo, O., Skaribas, I.M., Rockett, C., et al., 2000. Computed tomography-guided pudendal nerve block. A new diagnostic approach to long-term anoperineal pain: a report of two cases. Reg. Anesth. Pain Med. 25 (4), 420–423.

Campbell, J.N., Mitchell, M.J., 1996. Pain treatment centers at a crossroads: A practical and conceptual reappraisal. IASP Press, Seattle, WA.

Chartier-Kastler, E., 2008. Sacral neuromodulation for treating the symptoms of overactive bladder syndrome and non-obstructive urinary retention: >10 years of clinical experience. BJU Int. 101 (4), 417–423.

Cheshire, W.P., Abashian, S.W., Mann, J.D., et al., 1994. Botulinum toxin in the treatment of myofascial pain syndrome. Pain 59, 65–69.

Dykstra, K.K., Presthus, J., 2006. Botulinum toxin type A for the treatment of provoked vestibulodynia. J. Reprod. Med. 51, 467–470.

Eccleston, C., Williams, A., Morely, S., 2009. Psychological therapies for the management of chronic pain (excluding headache) in adults. Cochrane Database Syst. Rev. 15 (2), CD007407.

Ellis, R.F., Hing, W.A., et al., 2008. Neural mobilizations: a systematic review of randomized controlled trials with an anaylsis of therapetic efficacy. J. Man. Manip. Ther. 16 (1), 8–22.

Fall, M., et al., 2008. EAU Guidelines on Chronic Pelvic Pain. Eur. Urol. Aug 31 [Epub].

Filippi, G.M., et al., 1993. Botulinum A toxin effects on rat jaw muscle spindles. Acta Oto-laryngol. (Stockh) 113, 400–404.

Fishbain, D.A., Cutler, R., Rosomoff, H.L., et al., 2000. Evidence-based data from animal and human experimental studies on pain relief with antidepressants: a structured review. Pain Med. 1 (4), 310–316.

Fitzgerald, M.P., Anderson, R.U., Potts, J., et al., 2009. Randomized feasibility trial of myofascial physical therapy for the treatment of urologic chronic pelvic pain syndromes. J. Urol. 182, 570–580.

Gatchel, R.J., Turk, D.C., 1996. Psychological treatments for pain. A practitioners handbook. Guilford Press, New York.

Ghazizadeh, S., Nikzad, M., 2004. Botulinum toxin in the treatment of refractory vaginismus. Obstet. Gynecol. 104 (5 Pt 1), 922–925.

Govier, F.E., Litwiller, S., Nitti, V., et al., 2001. Percutaneous afferent neuromodulation for the refractory overactive bladder: results of a multicenter study. J. Urol. 165 (3), 1193–1198.

Hammer, M., Menesse, W., 1998. Principles and practice of radiofrequency neurolysis. Curr. Rev. Pain 2, 267–278.

Hewitt, D.J., 2000. The use of NMDA-receptor antagonists in the treatment of chronic pain. Clin. J. Pain 16 (Suppl. 2), S73–S79.

Hough, D.M., Wittenberg, K.H., Pawlina, W., et al., 2003. Chronic perineal pain caused by pudendal nerve entrapment: anatomy and CT-guided perineural injection technique. AJR Am. J. Roentgenol. 181 (2), 561–567.

Jarvis, S., Abbott, J.A., Lenart, M.B., et al., 2004. Pilot study of botulinum toxin type A in the treatment of chronic pelvic pain associated with spasm of the levator ani muscles. Aust. N.Z. J. Obstet. Gynaecol. 44, 46–50.

Kabay, S., Kabay, S.C., Yucel, M., et al., 2009. Efficiency of posterior tibial nerve stimulation in category IIIB chronic prostatitis/chronic pelvic pain: a sham-controlled comparative study. Urol. Int. 83, 33–38.

Kennedy, E.M., Harms, B.A., Starling, J.R., et al., 1994. Absence of maladaptive neuronal plasticity after genitofemoral ilioinguinal neurectomy. Surgery 116 (4), 665–670.

Kim, S.W., Paick, J.S., Ku, J.H., et al., 2007. Percutaneous posterior tibial nerve stimulation in patients with chronic pelvic pain: a preliminary study. Urol. Int. 78, 58–62.

Klingler, H.C., Pycha, A., Schmidbauer, J., et al., 2000. Use of peripheral neuromodulation of the S3 region for treatment of detrusor overactivity: a urodynamic-based study. Urology 56 (5), 766–771.

Kotarinos, R., 2009. International Continence Society Annual Meeting. Myofascial findings in patients with chronic urologic pain syndromes.

Kovacs, P., Gruber, H., Piegger, J., et al., 2001. New, simple, ultrasound-guided infiltration of the pudendal nerve: ultrasonographic technique. Dis. Colon Rectum. 44 (9), 1381–1385.

Langford, C., Udvari Nagy, S., Ghoniem, G.M., 2007. Levator ani trigger point injections: an underutilized treatment for chronic pelvic pain. Neurourol. Urodyn. 26, 59–62.

Maher, C.F., Carey, M.P., Dwyer, P.L., et al., 2001. Percutaneous sacral nerve root neuromodulation for intractable interstitial cystitis. J. Urol. 884–886.

Maria, G., Cadeddu, F., Brisinda, D., et al., 2005. Management of bladder, prostatic and pelvic floor disorders with botulinum neurotoxin. Curr. Med. Chem. 12 (3), 247–265.

Martin, D.C., Willis, M.L., Mullinax, L.A., et al., 2007. Pulsed radiofrequency application in the treatment of chronic pain. Pain Pract. 7, 21–25.

Masheb, R.M., Kerns, R.D., Lozano, C., et al., 2009. A randomized clinical trial for women with vulvodynia: cognitive-behavioral therapy vs. supportive psychotherapy. Pain 141 (1–2), 8–9.

Max, M.B., 1994. Antidepressants as analgesics. In: Fields, H.I., Liebeskind, J.C. (Eds.), Progress in brain research and management. IASP, Seattle, pp. 229–246.

Mayer, R.D., Howard, F.M., 2008. Sacral nerve stimulation: neuromodulation for voiding dysfunction and pain. Neurotherapeutics 5 (1), 107–113.

McCracken, L., Turk, D., 2002. Behavioral and cognitive-behavioral treatment for chronic pain: outcome, predictors of outcome, and treatment process. Spine 27 (22), 2564–2573.

McDonald, J.S., Spigos, D.G., 2000. Computed tomography-guided pudendal block for treatment of pelvic pain due to pudendal neuropathy. Obstet. Gynecol. 95 (2), 306–309.

McKay, M., 1993. Dysesthetic ("essential") vulvodynia treatment with amitriptyline. J. Reprod. Med. 38, 9–13.

McQuay, H., 1999. Opioids in pain management. Lancet 353 (9171), 2229–2232.

Mikeladeze, G., Espinal, R., Finnegan, R., et al., 2003. Pulsed radiofrequency application in treatment of chronic zygapophyseal joint pain. Spine J. 3, 360–362.

Montenegro, M.L., 2008. Physical therapy in the management of women with chronic pelvic pain. Int. J. Clin. Pract. 62 (2), 263–269.

Morely, S., Eccleston, C., Williams, A., 1999. Systematic review and meta-analysis of randomized controlled trials of cognitive behavior therapy and behaviour therapy for chronic pain in adults, excluding headaches. Pain 80, 1–13.

Munglani, R., 1999. The longer term effect of pulsed radiofrequency for neuropathic pain. Pain 80, 437–439.

Ohghena, P., Van Houdenhove, B., 1992. Antidepressant-induced analgesia in chronic non-malignant pain: a meta-analysis of 39 placebo-controlled studies. Pain 49 (2), 205–219.

Peters, K.M., 2002. Neuromodulation for the treatment of refractory interstitial cystitis. Rev. Urol. 4 (Suppl. 1), S36–S43.

Peters, K.M., Konstandt, D., 2004. Sacral neuromodulation decreases narcotic requirements in refractory interstitial cystitis. BJU Int. 93, 777–779.

Peters, K.M., Killinger, K.A., Boqsulawski, B.M., et al., 2009. Chronic pudendal neuromodulation: expanding available treatment option for refractory urologic symptoms. Neurourol. Urodyn. Sept 28 [Epub].

Porta, M., 2000. A comparative trial of botulinum toxin type A and methylprednisolone for the treatment of myofascial pain syndrome and pain from chronic muscle spasm. Pain 85 (1–2), 101–105.

Porta, M., et al., 1997. Compartment botulinum toxin injections for myofascial pain relief. Dolor 12 (Suppl. 1), 42.

Prendergast, S.A., Rummer, E.H., 2008. De-mystifying pudendal neuralgia. Current Directions in Women's Health, a division of the Canadian Physiotherapy Association. Fall.

Racz, G.B., Ruiz-Lopez, R., 2006. Radiofrequency procedures. Pain Pract. 6, 46–50.

Ramer, M.S., Thompson, S.W., McMahon, S.B., 1999. Causes and consequences of sympathetic basket formation in dorsal root ganglia. Pain (Suppl. 6), S111–S120.

Rapkin, A., McDonald, J.S., Morgan, M., et al., 2008. Multilevel local anesthetic nerve blockade for the treatment of vulvar vestibulitis syndrome. Am. J. Obstet. Gynecol. 198, 41.e1–41.e5.

Rhame, E., Levey, K.A., Gharibo, C.G., 2009. Successful treatment of refractory pudendal neuralgia with pulsed radiofrequency. Pain Physician 12, 633–638.

Richeimer, S.H., Bajwa, Z.H., Kahraman, S.S., et al., 1997. Utilization patterns of tricyclic antidepressants in a multidisciplinary pain clinic: a survey. Clin. J. Pain 13, 324–329.

Robert, R., Prat-Prada, I.D., Labatt, J.J., et al., 1998. Anatomic basis of chronic perineal pain: Role of the pudendal nerve. Surg. Radiol. Anat. 20, 93–98.

Rosales, R.L., Arimura, K., Takenaga, S., et al., 1996. Extrafusal and intrafusal muscle effects in experimental botulinum toxin-A injection. Muscle Nerve 19, 488–496.

Rose, M.A., Kam, P.C., 2002. Gabapentin: pharmacology and its use in pain management. Anaesthesia 57, 451–462.

Rosenberg, J.M., Harrell, C., Ristic, H., et al., 1997. The effect of gabapentin on neuropathic pain. Clin. J. Pain 13, 251–255.

Sasaki, K., Smith, C.P., Chuang, Y.C., et al., 2001. Oral gabapentin (neurontin) treatment of refractory genitourinary tract pain. Tech. Urol. 7, 47–49.

Sator-Katzenschlager, S.M., Scharbert, G., Kress, H.G., et al., 2005. Chronic pelvic pain treated with gabapentin and amitriptyline: A randomized controlled pilot study. Wien. Klin. Wochenschr. 117 (21–22), 761–768.

Schmidt, R.A., Bruschini, H., Tanagho, E.A., 1979. Urinary bladder and sphincter responses to stimulation of dorsal and ventral sacral roots. Invest. Urol. 16, 300–304.

Seigel, S., Paszkiewicz, E., Kirkpatrick, C., et al., 2001. Sacral nerve stimulation in patients with chronic intractable pelvic pain. J. Urol. 166, 1742–1745.

Shah, R.V., Racz, G.B., 2003. Pulsed radiofrequency lesioning of the suprascapular nerve for the treatment of chronic shoulder pain. Pain Physician 6, 503–506.

Simons, D.G., Travell, J.G., Simons, L.S., 1999. Travell and Simons' myofascial main and dysfunction: the trigger point manual, second ed, vol. 1. Lippincott William & Wilkins, Baltimore.

Sluijter, M.E., Cosman, E.R., Rittman II, W.B., et al., 1998. The effects of pulsed radiofrequency fields applied to dorsal root ganglion – a preliminary report. Pain Clin. 11, 109–117.

Stoller, M.L., 1999. Afferent nerve stimulation for pelvic floor dysfunction. Eur. Urol. 35 (Suppl. 2), 16.

Toshniwal, G.R., Dureja, G.P., Prashanth, S.M., 2007. Transsacrococcygeal approach to ganglion impar block for management of chronic perineal pain: a prospective observational study. Pain Physician 10 (6), 70–71.

Tu, F.F., As-Sanie, S., Steege, J.F., 2006. Prevalence of pelvic musculoskeletal disorders in a female chronic pelvic pain clinic. J. Reprod. Med. 51 (3), 185–189.

Turk, D.C., Meichenbaum, D., Genest, M., 1983. Pain and behavioral medicine: A cognitive-behavioral perspective. Guilford Press, New York.

Van Balken, M.R., Vandoninck, V., Gisolf, K.W., et al., 2001. Posterior tibial nerve stimulation as neuromodulative treatment of lower urinary tract dysfunction. J. Urol. 166, 914–918.

Van Balken, M.R., Vandoninck, V., Messelink, B.J., et al., 2003. Percutaneous tibial nerve stimulation as neuromodulative treatment of chronic pelvic pain. Eur. Urol. 43, 158–163.

Van Zundert, J., Lame, I., Jansen, J., et al., 2003a. Percutaneous pulsed radiofrequency treatment of the cervical dorsal root ganglion in the treatment of chronic cervical pain syndromes: A clinical audit. Neuromodulation 6, 6–14.

Van Zundert, J., Brabant, S., Van de Kelft, E., et al., 2003b. Pulsed radiofrequency treatment of the gasserian ganglion in patients with idiopathic trigeminal neuralgia. Pain 104, 449–452.

Van Zundert, J., Patijn, J., Kessels, A., et al., 2007. Pulsed radiofrequency adjacent to the cervical dorsal root ganglion in chronic cervical radicular pain: A double blind sham controlled randomized clinical trial. Pain 127, 173–182.

Visser, E., Schug, S.A., 2006. The role of ketamine in pain management. Biomed. Pharmacother. 60 (7), 341–348.

Weijmar Schultz, W.C., Gianotten, W.L., van der Meijden, W.I., et al., 1996. Behavioral approach with or without surgical intervention to the vulvar vestibulitis syndrome: a prospective randomized and non-randomized study. J. Psychosom. Obstet. Gynaecol. 17 (3), 143–148.

Wu, H., Groner, J., 2007. Pulsed radiofrequency treatment of articular branches of the obturator and femoral nerves for the management of hip joint pain. Pain Pract. 7, 341–344.

Yokogawa, F., Kiuchi, Y., Ishikawa, Y., et al., 2002. An investigation of monoamine receptors involved in antinociceptvie effects of antidepressants. Anesth. Analg. 95 (1), 163–168.

Yoon, H., Chung, W.S., Shim, B.S., 2007. Botulinum toxin A for the management of vulvodynia. Int. J. Impot. Res. 19, 84–87.

Yue, S.K., 1995. Initial experience in the use of botulinum toxin A for the treatment of myofascial related muscle dysfunctions (abstract). J. Musculoskelet. Pain 3 (Suppl. 1), 22.

Zabihi, N., Mourtzinos, A., Maher, M.G., et al., 2008. Short-term results of bilateral S2–S4 sacral neuromodulation for the treatment of refractory interstitial cystitis, painful bladder syndrome, and chronic pelvic pain. Int. Urogynecol. J. 19, 553–557.

Zhang, J.M., Li, H., Munir, M.A., 2004. Decreasing sympathetic sprouting in pathologic sensory ganglia: a new mechanism for treating neuropathic pain using lidocaine. Pain 109, 143–149.

Chronic pelvic pain and nutrition

8.3

Leon Chaitow

CHAPTER CONTENTS

Introduction

This brief summary section lists current evidence relating to the influence of nutritional features on pelvic pain in general, and a number of specific conditions in particular. Some of the evidence is clear, while much of it remains equivocal, with a mixture of conflicting research evidence, and anecdotal evidence, clouding the conclusions. Despite some uncertainty, there is evidence that inflammatory processes can safely be modulated by a variety of nutrients and dietary strategies that involve anti-inflammatory and antioxidant substances in the diet. Several preventative measures also appear to be fairly solidly established (involving the balance of lipid substances omega-3, omega-6, etc. in the diet). In general, two areas stand out: the influence of diet on inflammatory processes, and the influence of vitamin D deficiency on a number of pelvic floor disorders affecting women.

Inflammation

Butrick (2009) notes that when muscle fibre trauma occurs, inflammatory mediators (e.g. bradykinin, serotonin, prostaglandins, adenosine triphosphate, histamine) are released locally, resulting in sensitization of muscle nociceptors, reducing their mechanical threshold. This results in muscle hyperalgesia and mechanical allodynia in which innocuous pressure may be perceived as painful. If prolonged, this peripheral sensitization leads to central sensitization, via a series of neuroplastic changes that occur in the central nervous system. These processes are described in greater detail in Chapter 3.

While pharmacological control of inflammation is clearly an option, there are also well-founded strategies for modulating this process, via dietary manipulation.

Dietary anti-inflammatory strategies

- Herbs such as turmeric can suppress expression of cyclo-oxygenase-2 (COX-2); and nutmeg inhibits release of tumour necrosis factor (TNF-α) (Sanders & Sanders-Gendreau 2007).

- Lopez-Miranda et al. (2010) report that phenolic compounds in olive oil have antioxidant and anti-inflammatory properties, prevent lipoperoxidation, induce favourable changes of lipid profile, improve endothelial function and have antithrombotic properties. Oleocanthal, a compound in olive oil retards the production of pro-inflammatory enzymes cyclo-oxygenase-1 (COX-1) and COX-2.
- A study by Beauchamp et al. (2005) suggests that 50 ml or 3.5 tablespoons of olive oil has the same effect as a 200-mg tablet of ibuprofen. Note however that consumption of 50 ml olive oil as an anti-inflammatory intervention requires caution, as this volume of olive oil contains in excess of 400 calories. This is of importance in chronic pelvic pain (CPP), since studies (Greer et al. 2008) have noted that weight loss leads to significant improvements in pelvic floor disorder symptoms.
- Moschen et al. (2010) confirmed that weight loss is an effective anti-inflammatory strategy, achieving its effects by decreasing expression of TNF-α and interleukin (IL)-6 as well as by increasing anti-inflammatory adipokines such as adiponectin.

Antioxidants and anti-inflammatory nutrients

Mier-Cabrera et al. (2009) and Kamencic & Thiel (2008) have demonstrated that, in endometriosis, oxidative stress may be improved by use of antioxidant compounds. Antioxidant nutrients have been shown to protect against cell-damaging free radicals, and to reduce activity of COX-2, a major cause of inflammation (Nijveldt 2001, Kim et al. 2004). Closely tied to anti-inflammatory strategies are nutritional approaches that emphasize enhanced intake of antioxidant foods containing phytochemicals such as carotenoids, flavonoids, limonene, indole, ellagic acid, allicin (from garlic) and sulphoraphane.

Examples include:

- Resveratrol, a polyphenolic found in the skins of red fruits, including grapes, is an antioxidant and is also found in wine. It has antichemotactic activities, as well as being a regulator of aspecific leukocyte activation (Jang et al. 1997, Bertelli et al. 1999, Szewczuk et al. 2004, Indraccoloa & Barbieri 2010).
- Resveratrol has been found to be a more potent anti-inflammatory agent than aspirin or ibuprofen (Takada et al. 2004)
- Carvacrol (derived from the essential oils of oregano and thyme) efficiently suppresses COX-2 expression (Baser 2008, Hotta et al. 2010)
- Antioxidant anthocyanins from pomegranate (POMx), and blueberry extract (*Vaccinium corymalosum*) which is also rich in anthocyanins, have been shown to have active antioxidant and antinociceptive properties (Torri et al. 2007).
- POMx inhibited inflammation associated with activated human mast cells, involved in disease processes associated with connective tissues (Zafar et al. 2009).
- Mixtures of antioxidants – resveratol, green tea extract, α-tocopherol, vitamin C, omega-3 polyunsaturated fatty acids (PUFAs), tomato extract – were found, in a placebo-controlled study, to modulate inflammation in overweight males.
- Bromelain, an aqueous extract obtained from both the stem and fruit of the pineapple plant, contains a number of proteolytic enzymes with anti-inflammatory and analgesic properties (Maurer 2001, Brien et al. 2004).
- Catechins and epicatechins, found in red wine and tea (particularly green tea), are polyphenolic antioxidant plant metabolites that quench free radicals and provide protection against oxidative damage to cells (Hara 1997, Yang et al. 2001, Sutherland et al. 2006, Kim et al. 2008).
- In a 14-day, prospective randomized study, involving a total of 284 patients affected by chronic bacterial prostatitis (CBP; NIH class II prostatitis), Cai et al. (2009) evaluated the therapeutic antioxidant effects of extracts from the plants *Serenoa repens* and *Urtica dioica* (ProstaMEV®) and curcumin, as well as the antioxidant plant-derived nutrient quercitin (FlogMEV®) extracts, compared with prulifloxacin. One month after treatment, 89.6% of patients who had received prulifloxacin as well as ProstaMEV® and FlogMEV® (Group A) reported no symptoms related to CBP, whilst only 27% of patients who received antibiotic therapy alone (Group B) were recurrence-free ($P < 0.0001$). Six months after treatment, no patients in Group A had recurrence of disease whilst two patients in Group B did.

Anti-inflammatory effects of omega-3 and -6 oils

Eicosanoids – biologically active substances including prostaglandins, prostacyclins, thromboxanes and leukotrienes – are derived from either omega-3 or omega-6 fatty acids. Since essential fatty acids cannot be synthesized by the body and must be supplied through dietary intake, the type of fatty acid that predominates in the diet can promote or oppose the inflammatory response. Metabolism of saturated fats and omega-6 fatty acids (e.g. arachidonic acid) leads to the biosynthesis of inflammatory prostaglandins, prostacyclins, thromboxanes, leukotrienes and lipoxins.

Omega-3 fatty acids are essential nutrients, which means that humans cannot manufacture their own, and so must be found in the diet. The main food sources are flaxseed oil, walnut oil and oily fish. Omega-3 oils reduce inflammation, by competing with arachidonic acid in the cell membrane, reducing the available amount; they also compete with cyclo-oxygenase and lipo-oxygenase enzymes which are up-regulated in the inflammatory process (Obata et al. 1999, Ringbom et al. 2001).

The ratio of omega-6:omega-3 fatty acids appears to be critical (Simopoulos 2002). Although the optimal ratio remains under review, it is suggested that approximately four parts omega-6 to one part omega-3 essential fatty acids should be the target for optimum balance (Yehuda et al. 2000, 2005). A ratio of 3:1, and lower, is also recommended by some authorities (Chrysohoou et al. 2004).

Simopoulos (2002) has observed that the ratio of omega-6 to omega-3 is clinically variable:

> A ratio of 2–3/1 suppressed inflammation in patients with rheumatoid arthritis, and a ratio of 5/1 had a beneficial effect on patients with asthma, whereas a ratio of 10/1 had adverse consequences. These studies indicate that the optimal ratio may vary with the disease under consideration. This is consistent with the fact that chronic diseases are multigenic and multifactorial. Therefore, it is quite possible that the therapeutic dose of omega-3 fatty acids will depend on the degree of severity of disease resulting from genetic predisposition. A lower ratio of omega-6/omega-3 fatty acids is more desirable in reducing the risk of many of the chronic diseases of high prevalence in Western societies.

This emphasizes the need for careful assessment and testing of fatty-acid status prior to prescription of changes in patient's omega 6:3 ratio. As a generalization, a nutritionist would test fatty acid status, and make recommendations ranging from 4:1 through to a 1:1 ratio based on the test results, although the 4:1 ratio is the 'ideal' for someone who is optimally healthy.

- Short-chain omega-3 fatty acids oppose inflammation through decreased production of inflammatory prostaglandins, leukotrienes and arachidonic acid. Food sources include flaxseed, hempseed, walnuts, canola and rapeseed oils, as well as dark green leafy vegetables, pumpkin seeds and oily fish (Saldeen & Saldeen 2004).
- Long-chain omega-3 fatty acids are found in the following food sources and should be widely integrated into the anti-inflammatory diet: oily fish from cold northern waters such as salmon and mackerel; sardines, herring, black cod (sablefish or butterfish); fish oil, algae and eggs rich in DHA (docosahexaenoic acid).
- PUFAs, and especially total omega-3 fatty acids, were independently associated with lower levels of proinflammatory markers (IL-6, IL-1ra, TNF, C-reactive protein) and higher levels of anti-inflammatory markers (soluble IL-6r, IL-10, TGF) independent of confounders. Ferrucci et al. (2006) suggest that these findings support omega-3 fatty acids as being beneficial in patients affected with diseases characterized by active inflammation.

Vitamin D and pelvic floor disorders in women

Using 2005–2006 National Health and Nutrition Examination Survey data, Badalian & Rosenbaum (2010) reported on the prevalence of vitamin D deficiency in women with pelvic floor disorders, and the possible associations between vitamin D levels and pelvic floor disorders. Analysis of results collected from 1881 non-pregnant women, over the age of 20 were that:

- One or more pelvic floor disorders were reported by 23% of women;
- Mean vitamin D levels were significantly lower for women reporting at least one pelvic floor disorder and for those with urinary incontinence, irrespective of age;
- In adjusted logistic regression models, it was observed that there was a significantly decreased risk of one or more pelvic floor disorders with increasing vitamin D levels in all women aged 20 or older, and in the subset of women 50 years and older;
- The likelihood of urinary incontinence was significantly reduced in women 50 and older with vitamin D levels 30 ng/ml or higher.

The conclusion was that higher vitamin D levels are associated with a decreased risk of pelvic floor disorders in women.

CPP/endometriosis and diet

There is limited evidence – from animal studies – that dietary strategies such as a high fruit and vegetable, and low meat intake, may be useful in preventing endometriosis (Parazzini et al. 2004).

A 12-year prospective study has linked trans fats with increased risk of endometriosis. The study reported that:

> During the 586,153 person-years of follow-up, 1199 cases of laparoscopically confirmed endometriosis were reported. Although total fat consumption was not associated with endometriosis risk, those women in the highest fifth of long-chain omega-3 fatty acid consumption were 22% less likely to be diagnosed with endometriosis compared with those with the lowest fifth of intake [95% confidence interval (CI) = 0.62–0.99; P-value, test for linear trend (Pt) = 0.03]. In addition, those in the highest quintile of trans-unsaturated fat intake were 48% more likely to be diagnosed with endometriosis (95% CI = 1.17–1.88; Pt = 0.001).
>
> (Missmer et al. 2010)

Britton et al. (2000) investigated the relation between diet and benign ovarian tumours (BOT) in a case–control study involving 673 women with BOT, of whom 280 had endometrioid tumours. It was noted that an intake of vegetable fat was positively associated with endometrioid tumours in a dose–response manner. Specifically, there was an elevated risk for intake of polyunsaturated fat.

A review of the literature on diet and endometriosis (Fjerbæk & Knudsen 2007) noted that evidence (at that time) was sparse. In some instances, dietary modifications, including the intake of fish oils (see discussion of inflammation above), have been shown to beneficially influence dysmenorrhoea.

Dysmenorrhoea: Studies and meta-analyses

For example, a number of studies have shown that a correlation exists between increased risk of more intense dysmenorrhoea and:

- Low fibre intake (Nagata et al 2005);
- Low fruit, fish and egg intake, and increased alcohol intake (Balbi et al. 2000);
- Low intake of total fat, saturated fat, omega-3 fatty acids, vitamins D and B12 (Deutsch et al. 2000);
- Barnard et al. (2000) demonstrated that during phases of a 'low-fat vegetarian diet, compared to the normal diet phase, sex-hormone binding globulin concentration was significantly higher, and dysmenorrhoea duration and pain intensity fell';
- In a randomized controlled study Harel (2002) observed a significant reduction in menstrual symptoms, together with a reduction in use of analgesic medication, in adolescents after intake of fish oil;
- Evidence from these studies suggests that coffee and soy intake have no effect on the symptoms of dysmenorrhoea;
- In a Cochrane Collaboration review, Proctor & Murphy (2001) report that there is evidence that vitamin B1 (100 mg daily) and magnesium (no dosage recommended because of conflicting reports) help reduce pain of dysmenorrhoea;
- They also report that omega-3 fatty acids were more effective than placebo for pain relief.

Painful bladder syndrome

- Ward & Haoula (2008), in a review of current literature, suggest that while there is no evidence to link diet with painful bladder syndrome, elimination of substances that are considered to either irritate the bladder or may contribute to bladder inflammation, may help some patients. These substances include caffeine, alcohol, tomatoes, spices, chocolate, citrus and high-acid foods or beverages.

Vulvar vestibulitis syndrome and interstitial cystitis

- Farage & Galask (2005) observe that urinary excretion of oxalates (found naturally in many foods, including spinach and other green leafy vegetables, most nuts, legumes, berries, wheat, and high in vitamin C supplements – and also manufactured by the body) have been proposed as contributing to vulvar vestibulitis syndrome (VVS), based initially on a single case report (Solomons et al. 1991). In that case, symptoms of burning and itching of the urethra, were apparently associated with hyperoxaluria.

- Reports by Fitzpatrick et al. (1993), Stewart & Berger (1997) and Tarr et al. (2003) have all suggested a possible shared pathogenesis for VVS and interstitial cystitis, involving high-oxalate presence. This hypothesis has however not been confirmed in a study of a low-oxalate diet involving 130 patients and 23 controls (Baggish et al. 1997).

Irritable bowel syndrome and diet

Rapin & Wiernsperger (2010) note that increased intestinal permeability is a common feature of irritable bowel syndrome (IBS). Management of increased gut permeability, and associated food intolerances, has been shown to be improved by careful nutritional strategies, including use of probiotics (Mennigen & Bruewer 2009, also see below) and glutamine (Li & Neu 2009).

In a comprehensive review of IBS, Heizer et al. (2009) suggest that dietary changes are commonly a useful strategy. It is recommended that dietary restrictions should be introduced one at a time, beginning with any food or food group that appears to cause symptoms based on a careful patient history or review of a patient's food diary. The most effective duration for dietary trials has not been well studied, although 2–3 weeks is commonly suggested.

A modified exclusion diet, followed by stepwise reintroduction of foods is likely to be more effective in identifying the irritating substance, but is more time-consuming (Parker et al. 1995). Any improvement in symptoms after an unblinded dietary change could be a placebo effect, and may not persist.

General dietary recommendations for patients with IBS, based on clinical experience and anecdotal reports (Heizer et al. 2009) include:

- Avoiding large meals;
- Reducing lactose (eliminate milk, ice cream and yogurt);
- Reducing fat to no more than 40–50 g/day;
- Reducing sorbitol, mannitol, xylitol (mainly 'sugarless' gum, read labels);
- Reducing fructose in all forms, including high-fructose corn syrup (read labels), honey, and high-fructose fruits (e.g. dates, oranges, cherries, apples and pears);
- Reducing gas-producing foods (e.g. beans, peas, broccoli, cabbage and bran);
- Eliminating all wheat and wheat-containing products;
- A diet low in fermentable oligo-, di-, and monosaccharides and polyols, i.e. sugar alcohols such as sorbitol (Shepherd & Gibson 2006);
- Eliminate wheat, banana, corn, potato, milk, eggs, peas and coffee.

Peppermint oil

Many studies suggest that use of peppermint oil is likely to be of benefit in symptomatic treatment of relatively mild cases of IBS (Grigoleit & Grigoleit 2005, Cappello et al. 2007).

Turmeric (curcumin)

While some mainly pilot studies have shown potential benefit for use of turmeric (a member of the ginger family of plants) in treatment, no placebo-controlled studies have as yet been conducted (Bundy et al. 2004, Heizer et al. 2009).

Probiotics

Two meta-analyses (McFarland & Dublin 2008, Nikfar et al. 2008) and two comprehensive narrative reviews (Spiller 2008, Wilhelm et al. 2008) were published in 2008 on the use of probiotics in the treatment of IBS. All concluded that probiotics may be useful but that there are many variables affecting the results such as the type, dose and formulation of bacteria comprising the probiotic preparation, the outcome measured as well as size and characteristics of the IBS population studied.

The conclusions of a review of the evidence for use of probiotics in both IBS and inflammatory bowel disease are cautiously positive (Iannitti & Palmieri 2010):

> Probiotics seem to play an important role in the lumen of the gut elaborating antibacterial molecules such as bacteriocins. Moreover they seem to be able to enhance the mucosal barrier increasing the production of innate immune molecules, including goblet cell derived mucins and trefoil factors and defensins produced by intestinal Paneth cells. Some strains promote adaptive immune responses (secretory immune globulin A, regulatory T cells, IL-10). Some probiotics have the capacity to activate receptors in the enteric nervous system, which could be used to promote pain relief in the setting of visceral hyperalgesia (Sherman et al. 2009). Moreover probiotics exert an important action improving the abnormalities of both the colonic flora and the intestinal microflora. They

could be effective for treating various pathologies preventing the dysbiosis which characterizes or is associated with these conditions. Further future clinical trials, involving large numbers of patients, will be mandatory to achieve definite evidence of the preventive and curative role of probiotics in medical practice.

Acknowledgement

The editors thank Louise Nicholson FdSc, Dip ION of NutriProVita (www.nutriprovita.com) for her valuable assistance in the review of the nutritional literature presented in this section.

This brief chapter has summarized current understanding of nutritional influences on CPP, both in preventive and in therapeutic contexts. While general dietary advice can safely be offered by healthcare providers, it is suggested that skilled and well-trained nutritional experts should be involved before any major dietary modifications are suggested to patients. The next chapter describes the connections between respiratory dysfunction and pelvic pain, as well as means of restoring enhanced breathing function.

References

Badalian, S.S., Rosenbaum, P.F., 2010. Vitamin D and pelvic floor disorders in women: results from the National Health and Nutrition Examination Survey. Obstet. Gynecol. 115 (4), 795–803.

Baggish, M.S., Sze, E.H., Johnson, R., 1997. Urinary oxalate excretion and its role in vulvar pain syndrome. Am. J. Obstet. Gynecol. 177 (3), 507–511.

Balbi, C., Musone, R., Menditto, A., et al., 2000. Influence of menstrual factors and dietary habits on menstrual pain in adolescence age. Eur. J. Obstet. Gynecol. Reprod. Biol. 91 (2), 143–148.

Barnard, N.D., Scialli, A.R., Hurlock, D., Bertron, P., 2000. Diet and sex-hormone binding globulin, dysmenorrhea, and premenstrual symptoms. Obstet. Gynecol. 95 (2), 245–250.

Baser, K.H., 2008. Biological and pharmacological activities of carvacrol and carvacrol bearing essential oils. Curr. Pharm. Des. 14, 3106–3109.

Beauchamp, G.K., Keast, R., Morel, D., et al., 2005. Phytochemistry: Ibuprofen-like activity in extra-virgin olive oil. Nature 437, 45–46.

Bertelli, A., Ferrara, F., Diana, G., et al., 1999. Resveratrol, a natural stilbene in grapes and wine, enhances intraphagocytosis in human promonocytes: a co-factor in inflammatory and anticancer chemopreventive activity. Int. J. Tissue React. 21, 93–104.

Brien, S., Lewith, G., Walker, A., et al., 2004. Bromelain as a treatment for osteoarthritis: a review of clinical studies. Evid. Based Complement. Alternat. Med. 1, 251–257.

Britton, J.A., Westhoff, C., Howe, G., et al., 2000. Diet and benign ovarian tumors (United States). Cancer Causes Control 11 (5), 389–401.

Bundy, R., Walker, A.F., Middleton, R., et al., 2004. Turmeric extract may improve irritable bowel syndrome symptomology in otherwise healthy adults: A pilot study. J. Altern. Complement. Med. 10, 1015–1018.

Butrick, C., 2009. Pathophysiology of Pelvic Floor Hypertonic Disorders. Obstet. Gynecol. Clin. North Am. 36 (3), 699–705.

Cai, T., Mazzoli, S., Bechi, A., et al., 2009. Serenoa repens associated with Urtica dioica (ProstaMEV®) and curcumin and quercitin (FlogMEV®) extracts are able to improve the efficacy of prulifloxacin in bacterial prostatitis patients: results from a prospective randomised study. Int. J. Antimicrob. Agents 33 (6), 549–553.

Cappello, G., Spezzaferro, M., Grossi, L., et al., 2007. Peppermint oil (Mintoil) in the treatment of irritable bowel syndrome: A prospective double blind placebo-controlled randomized trial. Dig. Liver Dis. 39, 530–536.

Chrysohoou, C., Panagiotakos, B., Pitsavos, C., et al., 2004. Adherence to the Mediterranean diet attenuates inflammation and coagulation process in healthy adults: The ATTICA Study. J. Am. Coll. Cardiol. 44, 152–158.

Deutsch, B., Jorgensen, E.B., Hansen, J.C., 2000. Menstrual discomfort in Danish women reduced by dietary supplements of omega-3 PUFA and B12 (fish oil or seal oil capsules). Nutr. Res. 20 (5), 621–631.

Farage, M., Galask, R., 2005. Vulvar vestibulitis syndrome: A review. Eur. J. Obstet. Gynecol. Reprod. Biol. 123, 9–16.

Ferrucci, L., Cherubini, A., Bandinelli, S., et al., 2006. Relationship of plasma polyunsaturated fatty acids to circulating inflammatory markers. J. Clin. Endocrinol. Metab. 91 (2), 439–446.

Fitzpatrick, C.C., DeLancey, J.O., Elkins, T.E., et al., 1993. Vulvar vestibulitis and interstitial cystitis: a disorder of urogenital sinus-derived epithelium? Obstet. Gynecol. 81 (5 Pt. 2), 860–862.

Fjerbæk, A., Knudsen, B., 2007. Endometriosis, dysmenorrhea and diet—What is the evidence? Eur. J. Obstet. Gynecol. Reprod. Biol. 132, 140–147.

Greer, W., Richter, H., Bertolucci, A., et al., 2008. Obesity and pelvic floor disorders: a systematic review. Obstet. Gynecol. 112 (2 Pt 1), 341–349.

Grigoleit, H.G., Grigoleit, P., 2005. Peppermint oil in irritable bowel syndrome. Phytomedicine 12, 601–606.

Hara, Y., 1997. Influence of tea catechins on the digestive tract. J. Cell. Biochem. Suppl. 27, 52–58.

Harel, Z., 2002. A contemporary approach to dysmenorrhea in adolescents. Paediatr. Drugs 4 (12), 797–805.

Heizer, W., Southern, S., McGovern, S., 2009. Role of diet in symptoms of irritable bowel syndrome in adults: a narrative review. J. Am. Diet. Assoc. 109 (7), 1204–1214.

Hotta, M., Nakata, R., Katsukawa, M., et al., 2010. Carvacrol, a component of thyme oil, activates PPARalpha and gamma and suppresses COX-2 expression. J. Lipid Res. 51, 132–139.

Iannitti, T., Palmieri, B., 2010. Therapeutical use of probiotic formulations in clinical practice. Clin. Nutr. In Press, Corrected Proof, Available online 23 June 2010.

Indraccoloa, U., Barbieri, F., 2010. Effect of palmitoylethanolamide–polydatin combination on chronic pelvic pain associated with endometriosis: Preliminary observations. Eur. J. Obstet. Gynecol. Reprod. Biol. 150 (1), 76–79.

Jang, M., Cai, L., Udeani, G.O., et al., 1997. Cancer chemopreventive activity of resveratrol, a natural product derived from grapes. Science 275, 218–220.

Kamencic, H., Thiel, J., 2008. Pentoxifylline after conservative surgery for endometriosis: a randomized, controlled trial. J. Minim. Invasive Gynecol. 15, 62–66.

Kim, H., Kun, H., et al., 2004. Anti-inflammatory plant flavonoids and cellular action mechanisms. J. Pharm. Sci. 96 (3), 229–245.

Kim, H.R., Rajaiah, R., Wu, Q.L., et al., 2008. Green tea protects rats against autoimmune arthritis by modulating disease-related immune events. J. Nutr. 138 (11), 2111–2116.

Li, N., Neu, J., 2009. Glutamine deprivation alters intestinal tight junctions via a PI3-K/Akt mediated pathway in Caco-2 cells. J. Nutr. 139, 710–714.

Lopez-Miranda, J., Perez-Jimenez, F., Ros, E., et al., 2010. Olive oil and health: Summary of the II international conference on olive oil and health consensus report. Nutr. Metab. Cardiovasc. Dis. 20 (4), 284–294.

Maurer, H., 2001. Bromelain: biochemistry, pharmacology and medical use. Cell. Mol. Life Sci. 58, 1234–1245.

McFarland, L.V., Dublin, S., 2008. Meta-analysis of probiotics for the treatment of irritable bowel syndrome. World J. Gastroenterol. 14, 2650–2661.

Mennigen, R., Bruewer, M., 2009. Effect of probiotics on intestinal barrier function. Ann. N. Y. Acad. Sci. 1165, 183–189.

Mier-Cabrera, J., Aburto-Soto, T., Burrola-Méndez, S., et al., 2009. Women with endometriosis improved their peripheral antioxidant markers after the application of a high antioxidant diet. Reprod. Biol. Endocrinol. 7, 54.

Missmer, S.A., Chavarro, J.E., Malspeis, S., et al., 2010. A prospective study of dietary fat consumption and endometriosis risk. Hum. Reprod. 25, 1528–1535.

Moschen, R.A., Molnar, C., Geiger, S., et al., 2010. Anti-inflammatory effects of excessive weight loss: potent suppression of adipose interleukin 6 and tumour necrosis factor α expression. Gut 10, 1136.

Nagata, C., Hirokawa, K., Shimizu, N., et al., 2005. Associations of menstrual pain with intakes of soy, fat and dietary fiber in Japanese women. Eur. J. Clin. Nutr. 59 (1), 88–92.

Nijveldt, R., 2001. Flavonoids: a review of probable mechanisms of action and potential applications. Am. J. Clin. Nutr. 74, 418–425.

Nikfar, S., Rahimi, R., Rahimi, F., et al., 2008. Efficacy of probiotics in irritable bowel syndrome: A meta-analysis of randomized, controlled trials. Dis. Colon Rectum 51, 1775–1780.

Obata, T., Nagakura, T., Masaki, T., et al., 1999. Eicosapentaenoic acid inhibits prostaglandin D2 generation by inhibiting cyclo-oxygenase-2 in cultured human mast cells. Clin. Exp. Allergy 29, 1129–1135.

Parazzini, F., Chiaffarino, F., Surace, M., et al., 2004. Selected food intake and risk of endometriosis. Hum. Reprod. 19 (8), 1755–1759.

Parker, T.J., Naylor, S.J., Riordan, A., et al., 1995. Management of patients with food intolerance in irritable bowel syndrome: The development and use of an exclusion diet. J. Hum. Nutr. Diet. 8, 159–166.

Proctor, M., Murphy, P., 2001. Herbal and dietary therapies for primary and secondary dysmenorrhoea. Cochrane Database Syst. Rev. (3) Art. No.: CD002124. DOI:10.1002/14651858.CD002124.

Rapin, J.R., Wiernsperger, N., 2010. Possible links between intestinal permeability and food processing: a potential therapeutic niche for glutamine. Clinics 65, 1590.

Ringbom, T., Huss, U., Stenhold, A., et al., 2001. Cox-2 inhibitory effects of naturally occurring and modified fatty acids. J. Nat. Prod. 64, 745–749.

Saldeen, P., Saldeen, T., 2004. Women and omega-3 fatty acids. Obstet. Gynecol. Surv. 59 (10), 722–730.

Sanders, K., Sanders-Gendreau, K., 2007. The college student and the anti-inflammatory diet. Explore 3, 410–412.

Shepherd, S.J., Gibson, P.R., 2006. Fructose malabsorption and symptoms of irritable bowel syndrome: Guidelines for effective dietary management. J. Am. Diet. Assoc. 106, 1631–1639.

Sherman, P., Ossa, J., Johnson-Henry, K., 2009. Unraveling mechanisms of action of probiotics. Nutr. Clin. Pract. 1, 24.

Simopoulos, A.P., 2002. The importance of the ratio of omega-6/omega-3 essential fatty acids. Biomed. Pharmacother. 56, 365–379.

Solomons, C.C., Melmed, M.H., Heitler, S.M., 1991. Calcium citrate for vulvar vestibulitis: a case report. J. Reprod. Med. 36 (12), 879–882.

Spiller, R., 2008. Probiotics and prebiotics in irritable bowel syndrome. Aliment. Pharmacol. Ther. 28, 385–396.

Stewart, E.G., Berger, B.M., 1997. Parallel pathologies? Vulvar vestibulitis and interstitial cystitis. J. Reprod. Med. 42 (3), 131–134.

Sutherland, B., Rahman, R., Appleton, I., 2006. Mechanisms of action of green tea catechins with a focus on ischemia-induced neurodegeneration. J. Nutr. Biochem. 17, 291–306.

Szewczuk, L.M., Forti, L., Stivala, L.A., et al., 2004. Resveratrol is a peroxidase-mediated inactivator of COX-1 but not COX-2: a mechanistic approach to the design of COX-1-selective agents. J. Biol. Chem. 279, 22727–22737.

Takada, Y., Bhardwaj, A., Potdar, P., Aggarwal, B.B., 2004. Nonsteroidal anti-inflammatory agents differ in their ability to suppress NF-kappaB activation, inhibition of expression of cyclooxygenase-2 and cyclin D1, and abrogation of tumor cell proliferation. Oncogene 23, 9247–9258.

Tarr, G., Selo-Ojeme, D.O., Onwude, J.L., 2003. Coexistence of vulvar vestibulitis and interstitial cystitis. Acta Obstet. Gynecol. Scand. 82 (10), 969.

Torri, E., Lemos, M., Caliari, V., et al., 2007. Anti-inflammatory and antinociceptive properties of blueberry extract (Vaccinium corymbosum). J. Pharm. Pharmacol. 59, 591–596.

Ward, S., Haoula, Z., 2008. Painful bladder in women. Obstet. Gynaecol. Reprod. Med. 19 (4), 112–114.

Wilhelm, S.M., Brubaker, C.M., Varcak, E., et al., 2008. Effectiveness of probiotics in the treatment of irritable bowel syndrome. Pharmacotherapy 28, 496–505.

Yang, F., Oz Helieh, S., Barve, et al., 2001. The green tea polyphenol (−)-epigallocatechin-3-gallate blocks nuclear factor-κB activation by inhibiting IκB kinase activity in the intestinal epithelial cell line IEC-6. Mol. Pharmacol. 60, 528–533.

Yehuda, S., Rabinovitz, S., Carasso, R.L., Mostofsky, D.I., 2000. Fatty acid mixture counters stress changes in cortisol, cholesterol, and impair learning. Int. J. Neurosci. 101 (1–4), 73–87.

Yehuda, S., Rabinovitz, S., Mostofsky, D.I., 2005. Essential fatty acids and the brain: From infancy to aging. Neurobiol. Aging 26 (Suppl. 1), 98–102.

Zafar, R., Akhtar, N., Anbahagan, A., et al., 2009. Polyphenol-rich pomegranate fruit extract (POMx) suppresses PMACI-induced expression of pro-inflammatory cytokines by inhibiting the activation of MAP kinases and NF-κB in human KU812 cells. J. Inflamm. 6, 1.

Breathing and chronic pelvic pain: Connections and rehabilitation features

9

Leon Chaitow Chris Gilbert Ruth Lovegrove Jones

CHAPTER CONTENTS

Introduction

This chapter's initial aims are to clarify, and emphasize, the intimate structural connections between the pelvic floor and the respiratory diaphragm. The hope is that a wider understanding of these myriad muscular and fascial associations will lead to greater clinical focus on the two-way traffic of influences that exist between breathing patterns, pelvic (dys)function and their aetiological origins.

In addition to the interacting features of pelvic and respiratory structure and function, the overarching influences of posture and behaviour patterns are discussed in relation to chronic pelvic pain (CPP). Within that discussion psychological and emotional factors can be seen to contribute to both respiratory, pelvic pain and dysfunction.

A variety of therapeutic and rehabilitation approaches – some associated with physical medicine, and others more to do with stress management and psychologically oriented interventions – will be seen to emerge organically from this background.

The lumbopelvic cylinder: Functional and structural connections

The pelvic floor and the respiratory diaphragm are structurally and functionally bound together by fascial and muscular connections (Figure 9.1). The abdominal canister has been described as a functional unit that involves the diaphragm, including its crura; psoas; obturator internus; deep abdominal wall and its associated fascial connections; deep fibres of multifidus; intercostals; quadratus lumborum; thoracolumbar vertebral column (T6–T12 and associated ribs, L1–L5) and osseous components of the pelvic girdle (Jones 2001, Gibbons 2001, Newell 2005, Lee et al. 2008). Gibbons (2001) has described the anatomical link between the diaphragm, psoas and the pelvic floor: 'The diaphragm's medial arcuate ligament is a tendinous arch in the fascia of the psoas major. Distally, the psoas fascia is continuous with the PF fascia, especially the pubococcygeus'. See Box 9.1 for detailed anatomy of the diaphragm.

Newell (2005) has further detailed the relationship between psoas and quadratus lumborum, with the diaphragm and thoracic structures, observing that the posterior edge of the diaphragm crosses the psoas muscles medially, forming the medial arcuate ligaments, and the quadratus lumborum muscles laterally, forming the lateral arcuate ligaments.

- The skeletal attachments of the lateral arcuate ligaments are the first lumbar transverse process and the midpoint of the 12th rib. The costal origins include the lower six ribs and costal cartilages, the fibres of the diaphragm interdigitating with those of transversus abdominis.
- The medial arcuate ligament is continuous medially with the lateral margin of the crus, and is attached to the side of the body of the first or second lumbar vertebra. Laterally, it is fixed to the front of the transverse process of T12, and arches over the psoas muscle. Abnormal tensions in this ligament may irritate psoas, resulting in pain and

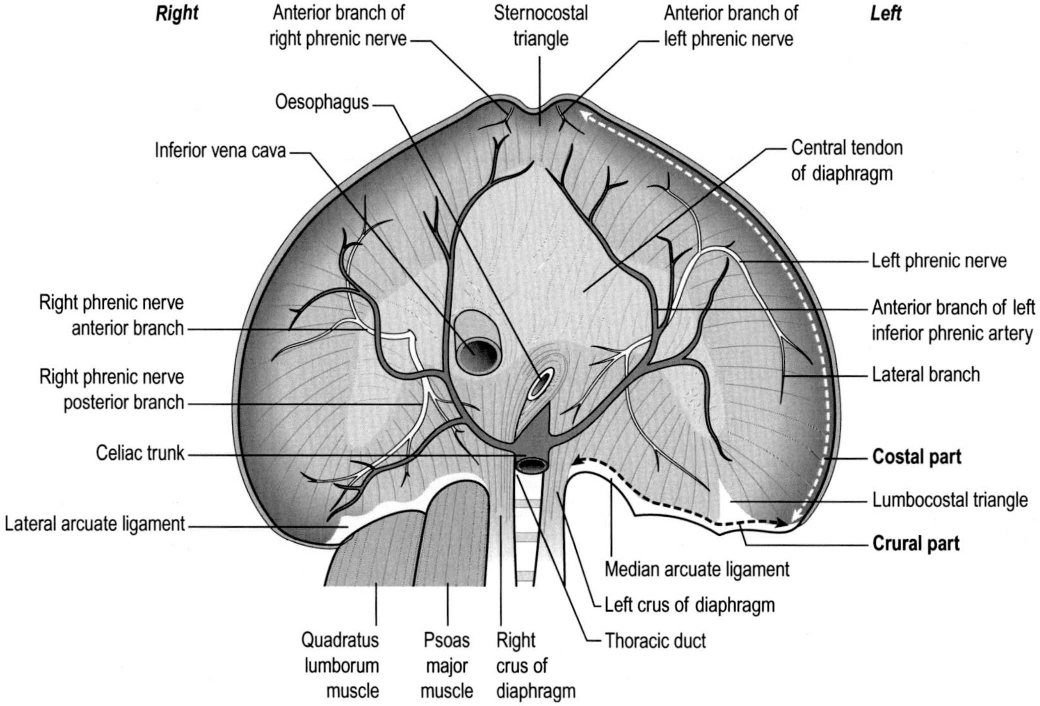

Figure 9.1 • Diaphragm seen from the abdomen

Box 9.1

Anatomy of the diaphragm

Leon Chaitow

The elliptical cylindroid-shaped diaphragm is a dome-shaped, musculotendinous structure with a non-contractile central tendon. Diaphragmatic fibres radiate peripherally to attach to all margins of the lower thorax, representing the inferior aspect of the pleural cavity, as well as a superior arch that covers the abdominal cavity (Pacia & Aldrich 1998). Its structures comprise both striated skeletal muscle and tendinous elements. When the diaphragm contracts, it increases the vertical, transverse and anteroposterior diameter of the internal thorax (Kapandji 1974).

The lumbar, costal and sternal muscular components (Schumpelick & Steinau 2000) (see Figures 9.1 and 9.2)

The muscular segments of the diaphragm originate from the entire circumference of the lower thoracic aperture: from the lumbar spine, ribs and sternum. There are three components, which are typically separated from each other by muscle-free gaps, the lumbar costal and sternal sections. These muscular diaphragmatic components insert at the central tendon, which is considered the central aponeurosis. In good health the diaphragm comprises type I, slow-twitch, fatigue-resistant muscle fibres as well as type II, fast-twitch, fatiguing muscle fibres. Fibre-type modifies in response to chronic obstructive pulmonary disease and to diaphragmatic inactivity (Anraku & Shargall 2009).

Lumbar (crural) part

The lumbar section is located bilaterally beside the lumbar spine, where it forms right and left crura (pillars), which arise from the anterior surface of the lumbar vertebrae (the right from L1–L4 and the left from L1–L2 and sometimes L3), the intervertebral disks, and the anterior longitudinal ligament. This is the most powerful part of the diaphragm. The posterior muscular part of the diaphragm arises from the crura and the lumbocostal arches (medial and lateral arcuate ligaments). According to the arrangement of the muscular origins, the right and left crura are subdivided into three additional portions:

1. Medial, which is tendinous in nature and lies in the fascia covering psoas major. Medially it is continuous with the corresponding medial crus and also attaches to the body of L1 or L2. Laterally it attaches to the transverse process of L1. The medial arcuate ligament is continuous medially with the lateral margin of the crus and is attached to the side of the body of the first or second lumbar vertebra. Laterally, it is fixed to the front of the transverse process of T12 and arches over the psoas muscle. Abnormal tensions in this ligament may irritate the psoas muscle, resulting in pain and spasm. Conversely psoas spasm may influence diaphragmatic mechanics (Burkill & Healy 2000, Carriero 2003, Carriere 2006).
2. Intermedial.
3. The lateral arm, which is formed from a thick fascial covering that arches over the upper aspect of quadratus lumborum, to attach medially to the anterior aspect of the transverse process of L1, and laterally to the inferior margin of the 12th rib.

Carriero (2003) notes that the lateral arcuate ligament is a thickened band of fascia extending from the anterior aspect of the transverse process of the first lumbar vertebra to the lower margin of the 12th rib near its midpoint. It arches across the upper part of the quadratus lumborum muscle. Besides affecting respiratory excursion, dysfunction of the 12th rib may affect the lateral arcuate ligament, resulting in irritation of the iliohypogastric or ilioinguinal nerves that pass under it; 'this may present as paresthesias or radiating pain over the anterior aspect of the thigh and groin with running activities'.

With attachments at the entire circumference of the thorax, ribs, xyphoid, costal cartilage, spine, discs and major muscles, the various components of the diaphragm form a central tendon with apertures for the vena cava, aorta, thoracic duct and oesophagus. When all these connections are considered, the direct influence on respiratory function of the lumbar spine and ribs, as well as psoas and quadratus lumborum, becomes apparent.

Costal part

Alternating with the dentations of the transverse abdominis muscle (Standring 2008), the costal part originates from the six caudal ribs, radiating into the central non-contractile tendon. In most cases, a triangle lacking muscle fibres, the lumbocostal triangle, exists between the lumbar and costal parts of the diaphragm, more commonly on the left side. In these weak areas, the gaps are usually closed only by means of pleura, peritoneum and fascia (i.e. fascia transversalis and fascia phrenicopleuralis).

Sternal part

The sternal part originates with small dentations from the posterior layer of the rectus sheath, and from the back of the xyphoid process, inserting at the central tendon. Bilaterally between the sternal and costal parts, narrow gaps (right and left sternocostal triangle, or Morgagni's and Larrey's gaps) are closed with connective tissue. The superior epigastric and lymphatic vessels pass through these gaps.

Tendinous part

Schumpelick & Steinau (2000) note that the tendinous part (i.e. the central tendon) has 'almost the shape of a cloverleaf (one anterior and two lateral leaves), with its

Continued

Box 9.1

Anatomy of the diaphragm—cont'd

largest expansion in the transverse plane'. The inferior vena cava, firmly anchored by connective tissue, passes through a foramen located to the right of the midline. The pericardium is also firmly attached to the cranial surface of the central tendon.

The left and right domes of the diaphragm arise lateral to the heart.

The right dome is commonly slightly higher than the left.

The location of the diaphragm is considered to be 'variable' (Schumpelick & Steinau 2000) depending on variables such as age, gender, posture and the extent of inhalation and exhalation, as well as on intestinal status. Any changes in the volume in the pleural or peritoneal cavity are likely to influence altered shape and position of the diaphragm.

The position of the dome of the diaphragm modifies according to the phase of respiration – with the right dome at the level of the fourth intercostal space (mammillary line), when at rest, while the left dome is marginally lower.

Following full inhalation, the right dome of the diaphragm is situated close to the level of the cartilage–bone transition of the sixth rib, while the left dome is approximately one intercostal space lower (Tondury & Tillman 1998).

Innervation of the diaphragm

The phrenic nerves (C3–5) supply motor innervation while lower 6–7 intercostal nerves are the origin of sensory supply (Gray's Anatomy 2008).

Schumpelick & Steinau (2000) observes that the peripheral parts of the diaphragm also receive motor innervation via the lower six intercostal nerves.

The phrenic nerve is located between the pericardium and mediastinal pleura.

Blood supply to the diaphragm

The major blood supply is from the pericardiophrenic, musculophrenic (from the internal thoracic artery), superior phrenic (from the thoracic aorta), and inferior phrenic (from the abdominal aorta) arteries (Anraku & Shargall 2009).

---

spasm. Conversely psoas spasm may influence diaphragmatic mechanics (Burkill & Healy 2000, Carriere 2006).

The retroperitoneal space

Lying between the posterior parietal peritoneum and the transversalis fascia is the retroperitoneal space, an anatomical region seldom discussed in relationship to CPP (Burkill & Healy 2000). This space houses (in whole or in part): the adrenal glands, kidneys, ureters, bladder, aorta, inferior vena cava, oesophagus (part), superior two-thirds of the rectum; as well as parts of the pancreas, duodenum and colon (Ryan et al. 2004). This area involves vital connections that intimately bind pelvic and thoracic structures. The anterior pararenal space extends superiorly to the dome of the diaphragm, and hence to the mediastinum. Inferiorly it communicates with the pelvis and below the inferior renal cone with the posterior pararenal space. The posterior pararenal opens inferiorly towards the pelvis but fuses superiorly with the posterior perirenal fascia the fascia of the quadratus lumborum (QL) and psoas muscles (Burkill & Healy 2000).

With structural and functional continuity between the diaphragm, pelvis, pelvic floor muscles (PFM), quadratus lumborum, psoas and organs of the retroperitoneal space it suggests that structures of the abdominal canister require assessment and, if appropriate, treatment, in relation to pelvic dysfunction.

Grewar & McLean (2008) indicate that respiratory dysfunctions are commonly seen in patients with low back pain, pelvic floor dysfunction and poor posture. Additional evidence exists connecting diaphragmatic and breathing pattern disorders, with various forms of pelvic girdle dysfunction (including sacroiliac pain) (O'Sullivan et al. 2002, O'Sullivan & Beales 2007) as well as with CPP and associated symptoms, such as stress incontinence (Hodges et al. 2007). Similarly Carriere (2006) noted that disrupted function of either the diaphragm or the PFM may alter the normal mechanisms for regulating intra-abdominal pressure (IAP).

The presence of dysfunctional breathing patterns which influence pelvic function (McLaughlin 2009) and pelvic dysfunction which influences breathing patterns (Hodges et al. 2007) therefore suggests that rehabilitation of the thorax, pelvic girdle and pelvic floor will be enhanced by more normal physiological breathing patterns. This can be achieved through exercise, breathing retraining, postural reeducation, manual therapy and other means (Chaitow 2007, O'Sullivan & Beales 2007, McLaughlin 2009).

Interaction of CPP, pelvic girdle pain and breathing pattern disorders aetiological features

- Aetiologically, pregnancy or trauma may result in pelvic girdle problems and pain, via skeletal malalignment, such as separation of the symphysis pubis or sacroiliac dysfunction (Shuler & Gruen 1996).
- Additionally, the development of low back pain during pregnancy increases the odds of developing pelvic floor disorder complaints (Pool-Goudzwaard et al. 2004).
- The combined prevalence of lumbopelvic pain, incontinence and breathing disorders has suggest that pelvic floor dysfunction is related to altered breathing patterns or disorders of breathing (Smith et al 2006, 2007, O'Sullivan & Beales 2007).
- Hodges et al. (2007) observe that there is a clear connection between sacroiliac joint (SIJ) stability and respiratory and pelvic floor function, particularly in women. They suggest that if the PFM are dysfunctional, spinal support may be compromised, increasing obliquus externus activity, which in turn may alter PFM activity.
- It is suggested that any part of the structural unit, involving the respiratory diaphragm and the pelvic floor ('pelvic diaphragm'), that fails to operate efficiently, will necessarily influence the function of other aspects of the complex.

Postural and breathing patterns as aetiological features

In a study involving 40 women with CPP, 20 received standard gynaecological attention, while the 20 women in the experimental group received the same attention, together with somatocognitive therapy, comprising postural, movement, gait and breathing assessment, re-education and rehabilitation. Haugstad et al. (2006a) observed that in the experimental group, women with CPP 'typically' displayed upper chest breathing patterns, with almost no movement of the thorax or the abdominal area. Haugstad et al. (2006a) were also able to confirm 'a characteristic pattern of standing, sitting, and walking, as well as lack of coordination and irregular high costal respiration'. Of interest in relation to diaphragmatic function was their finding that: 'the highest density, and the highest degree of elastic stiffness, [was] found in the iliopsoas muscles'.

Key (2010) suggests that clinicians should keep in mind: 'the continuous, largely internal three dimensional myofascial web, providing a scaffold of tensile inner support and stability [...] contributing to a structural and functional bridge between the lower torso and legs'. Key also notes that: 'This includes the obvious contractile elements for which there is accumulating evidence of deficient function in subjects with low back and/or pelvic pain – the transversus abdominis (Hodges & Richardson 1996, 1998, 1999), multifidus (Hides et al. 1996), the diaphragm and PFM'.

Impressions from clinical practice suggest attention should also be given to the obturators, iliacus, psoas, and all their related and interconnecting fascial sheaths. Sound activity within this myofascial 'inner stocking' sustains many functional roles: providing deep anterior support to the lower half of the spinal column; with the spinal intrinsic muscles it contributes to lumbopelvic control (Hodges 2004); while also contributing to the generation of IAP (Cresswell et al. 1994), continence and respiration (Figure 9.2).

The lack of normal diaphragmatic movement in individuals with breathing pattern disorders (BPD) deprives the viscera and abdominal cavity of rhythmic stimulation (internal 'massage') which may be important for maintaining normal pelvic circulation. Pelvic pain and congestion have been correlated with chronic muscle tension, chronic hypoxia, as well as accumulation of metabolites such as lactic acid and potassium (Kuligowska et al. 2005).

Jones (2001) has summarized the integrated structural and functional thoracopelvic unit as follows:

> The PFMs are part of a multi-structural unit forming the bottom of a lumbopelvic cylinder, with the respiratory diaphragm forming its top, and transversus abdominis, the sides. The spinal column is part of this cylinder and runs through the middle, supported posteriorly by segmental attachments of lumbar multifidus and anteriorly by segmental attachments of psoas to the abdominal muscles.

With psoas fibres (and those of QL) merging with the diaphragm, and the pelvic floor, any degree of inappropriate stiffness in these muscles is likely to impact on the ability of either of the diaphragms to function normally.

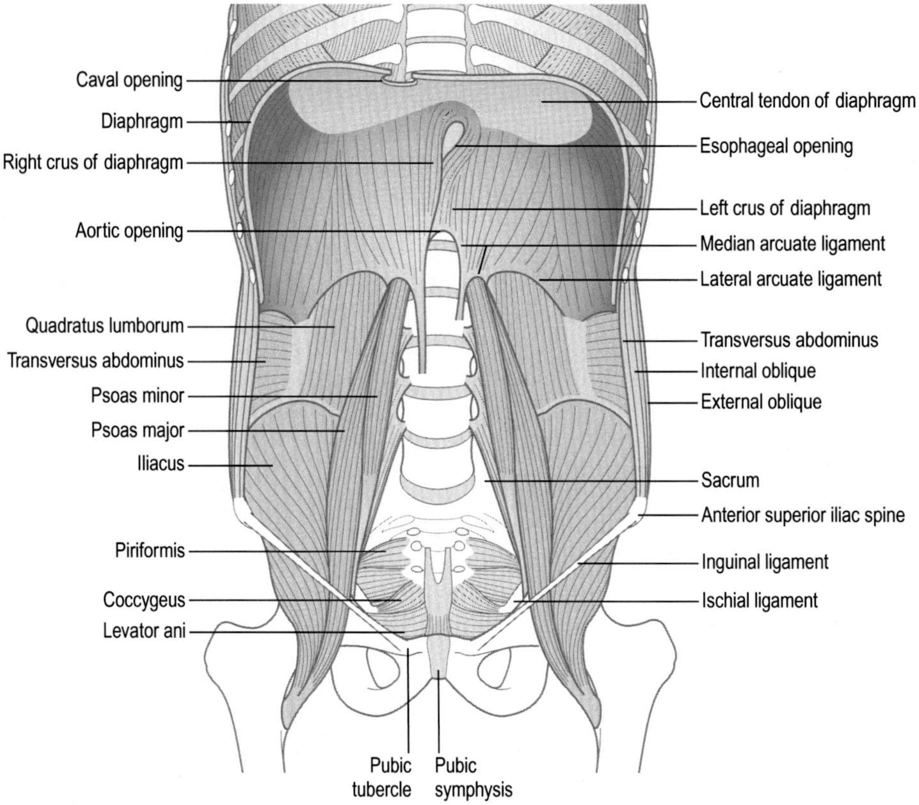

Figure 9.2 • The myofascial 'inner stocking' (or envelope) which involves a prevertebral and intrapelvic myofascial web of support. Reproduced from Key (2010) J. Bodyw. Mov. Ther. 14, 299–301.

Pelvic girdle pain: Respiratory connections

As discussed in Chapter 2, stabilization of the SIJs is enhanced by a combination of self-bracing and self-locking mechanisms, which have colloquially been described as 'form closure' (Vleeming et al. 1990a) and 'force closure' (Snijders et al. 1997, Hu et al. 2010) (Figure 9.3).

Cusi (2010) has suggested that shear is prevented by a combination of the specific anatomical features (form closure) and the compression generated by muscles and ligaments (force closure) that can accommodate to specific loading situations. Force closure has been defined as the effect of changing joint reaction forces generated by tension in ligaments, fasciae, and muscles and ground reaction force (Vleeming et al. 1990a, 1990b).

A significant part of this process involves increases in muscular, ligamentous and fascial stiffness, including that of the thoracolumbar fascia, and the multifidus and transversus abdominis, i.e. the major local stabilizers of the lumbar spine and the pelvis (Mens et al. 2001).

Additionally, and important to this discussion, using cadaveric studies the PFM have been shown to be capable of enhancing stiffness in the lumbar-pelvic region of women (Pool-Goudzwaard et al. 2004).

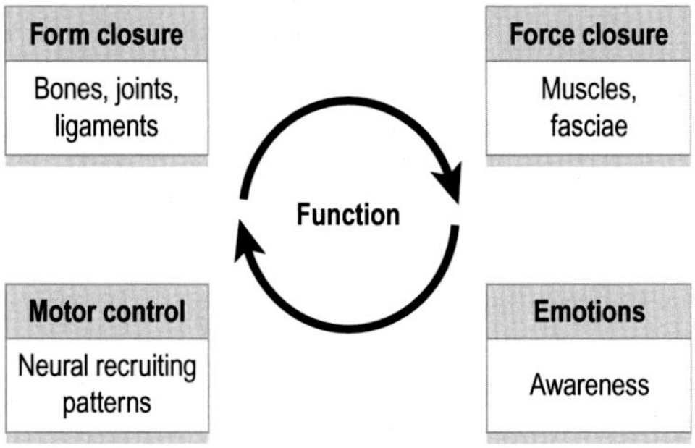

Figure 9.3 • Integrated model of function of the SIJ

By performing biomechanical analysis of SIJ stability, Pel et al. (2008) have demonstrated that the training of transversus abdominis and the PFM helps to relieve SIJ related pelvic pain, via reduction of vertical shear forces. In rehabilitation of sacroiliac dysfunction, related to force closure, Cusi (2010) notes that a successful exercise programme needs to be specific, targeted and progressive. The initial demands of such a programme require the individual to develop the ability to recruit transversus abdominis, deep multifidus and the muscles of the pelvic floor.

Hodges et al. (2001) have demonstrated that, after approximately 60 seconds of over-breathing (hyperventilation), the postural (tonic) and phasic functions of both the diaphragm and transversus abdominis are reduced or absent, with major implications for spinal and sacroiliac stability. As major hip flexors the psoas muscles have the potential to influence pelvic girdle position and function. They should therefore attract therapeutic attention (along with the accessory breathing muscles) in any attempt to rehabilitate respiratory or pelvic function.

Gut connections to CPP and to respiration

Various studies of pelvic pain patients have shown irritable bowel syndrome (IBS) to be a common co-morbid condition (Zondervan et al. 1999, Whitehead et al. 2002). IBS, defined as pain more than once a month, associated with bloating and altered bowel habit (Moore & Kennedy 2000), is common in women with CPP. For example in one study, among 798 women referred to a gynaecology clinic, the incidence of IBS was 37%, compared to 28% among women attending ENT or dermatology clinics. Among those with chronic pain symptoms (including dyspareunia or dysmenorrhoea), the incidence was 50% (Prior et al. 1989).

Ford et al. (1995) have reported on the high incidence of increased colonic tone and dysfunction in hyperventilating individuals. Hypocapnic hyperventilation (low CO_2 blood levels) produces an increase in colonic tone and phasic contractility in the transverse and sigmoid regions. These findings are consistent with either inhibition of sympathetic innervation to the colon, or the direct effects of hypocapnia on colonic smooth muscle contractility, or both.

It has also been observed – based on rectal and anal sphincter recordings – that during defecation the respiratory diaphragm and abdominal wall contract together, which results in an increase in IAP and rectal pressure (Olsen & Rao 2001).

Additionally pelvic floor contraction during exhalation allows for synergy between the pelvic and respiratory diaphragms (Prather et al. 2009), suggesting that when normal, respiratory function and the pelvic floor can be seen to synchronize intimately.

In the study by Prior et al. (1989), the authors did not seek to address whether IBS was the *cause* of the pelvic pain, but in a similar study, patients with symptoms of IBS were found to be less likely to receive a positive gynaecological diagnosis, and more likely to be still in pain, one year later, than patients without IBS symptoms (Whitehead et al. 2002). Rosenbaum & Owens (2008) note that gastroenterological conditions, such as coeliac disease and IBS, affect sexual function/comfort (Fass et al. 1998).

The anatomical location and innervation of both bladder and colon mean that they share similar vital functions, so that malfunction of one organ may result in a functional disturbance in the other. Furthermore the concepts of organ cross-talk, and organ cross-sensitization, between the bladder and the colon are important in the understanding of complex CPP syndromes (Watier 2009).

An integrated system

The concept of an integrated continence system (Grewar & McLean 2008) allows some coherence to be identified in apparently random presence of pain and dysfunction, in the pelvic region. Grewar & McLean suggest that the foundational mechanisms that support continence are relatively impervious to manual therapy when dysfunctional. However, there are also 'external' features that exert influence over these structural components – which are potentially modifiable.

These comprise:

- Motor control factors – including postural and movement dysfunction, BPD, pelvic floor dysfunction and low back and pelvic girdle dysfunction;
- Musculoskeletal features – including altered muscle strength, length and range of motion;
- Behavioural factors – such as physical inactivity, psychosocial issues, abnormal IAP and dysfunctional bowel and bladder habits.

There is evidence that respiration also has an influence on motor control (Butler 2000, Chaitow

2004) – emphasizing its importance amongst those factors to be considered in rehabilitation of continence dysfunction.

Within this complex, the focus of this chapter emerges: BPD, their influence on pelvic dysfunction, and the factors that lead to these, and how they might beneficially be modified therapeutically.

Varieties of breathing pattern disorder

Courtney et al. (2008) and Courtney & Greenwood (2009) suggest a distinction can be made between those BPD that appear to have a predominately biomechanical nature – where the patient may have a 'perception of inappropriate, or restricted, breathing', as distinguished from BPDs where a chemoreceptor aetiology may exist, for example linked to reported sensations such as there being a 'lack of air'. Courtney et al. (2008) note that the sensory quality of 'air hunger' or 'urge to breathe' is most strongly linked to changes in blood gases, such as CO_2, or changes in the respiratory drive deriving from central and peripheral afferent input. These sensations may be distinguishable from breathing sensations related to the effort of breathing, which are biomechanical in nature (Simon et al. 1989, Banzett et al. 1990, Lansing 2000, Chaitow et al. 2002).

Questionnaires exist for assessment of these BPD variations, with the Nijmegen Questionnaire (NQ) (van Dixhoorn & Duivenvoorden 1985) having greater relevance for hyperventilation, and the Self-Evaluation Breathing Questionnaire (SEBQ) (Courtney et al. 2009) discriminating between the chemoreceptor and the biomechanical variations of BPD (see Appendix).

Irrespective of the major aetiological features (see above and listed below in Box 9.2), chronic BPD results in altered function and, in time, structure of accessory and obligatory respiratory muscles. It is suggested that these should attract therapeutic attention in any attempt to normalize breathing, or the distant effects of BPD, on pelvic function (Chaitow 2004).

Breathing pattern disorders – The postural connection

Carriere (2006) has reported that respiratory dysfunction is commonly observed in patients with low back pain and pelvic floor dysfunction.

Key et al. (2007) have observed and catalogued a number of variations within the patterns of compensation/adaptation associated with chronic postural realignment involved in crossed-syndromes commonly associated with pelvic deviation.

In Figure 9.4A the major features include:

- Trunk extensors shortened;
- Thoracolumbar region hyperstabilized in extension;
- Poor pelvic control;
- Decreased hip extension;
- Abnormal axial rotation.

Box 9.2

Aetiological features in BPD

Beyond these distinctions – which have implications in rehabilitation choices – a variety of factors may lead to individuals experiencing changes in their breathing patterns:

- *Acidosis*: Hyperventilation may represent a homeostatic response to acidosis. Chaulier et al. (2007) note that acidosis may result from iatrogenic sources, major hypoxaemia, cardiovascular collapse or sepsis.
- *Atmosphere/altitude*: 'During expeditions ... mountaineers have extremely low values of arterial oxygen saturation (SaO_2), similar to those of patients with severe respiratory failure'. Hyperventilation would be the physiological response to this (Botella De Maglia et al. 2008). Altitude implications are not confined to mountaineers. Travellers to, for example, Johannesburg, Mexico City or Denver, would find themselves at altitude and potentially hyperventilating for some days, or weeks, before acclimatizing.
- *Allergies/intolerances*: Haahtela et al. (2009) report that airway inflammation commonly affects swimmers, ice hockey players, and cross-country skiers, which suggests multifactorial features in which both allergic and irritant mechanisms play a role in resultant over-breathing.
- *Deconditioning influences*:
  1. Nixon & Andrews (1996) suggest that deconditioned individuals utilize anaerobic glycolysis to generate energy, resulting in relative lowering of pH, and consequent homeostatic hyperventilation. In effect, lower pH due to deconditioning would trigger hyperventilation, which would further encourage deconditioning.

2. Troosters et al. (1999) suggest that research indicates that physical deconditioning may be more a consequence, than a cause, of the response to exercise, possibly explained by a psychological conditioning process. They report that: 'A psychological conditioning process generated by, or linked to exercise, might be the origin of the many symptoms [reported], i.e. the high anxiety level and a peculiar breathing pattern. The symptoms, when marked, result in a tendency to hyperventilate during and following exercise, with production of new symptoms (paresthesias, dizziness). The learned response is then reinforced by every new trial to exercise. Finally, the occurrence of symptoms with the slightest exertion leads to a reduction of physical activity and an ensuing deterioration of exercise tolerance.' Deconditioning would be the outcome.

- *Diabetic ketoacidosis* (DKA): Patients with DKA generally present with classic clinical findings of hyperventilation, altered mental status, weakness, dehydration, vomiting and polyuria (Bernardon et al. 2009; see also Kitabchi et al. 2006).
- *Emotional states*:
  1. Stress or fear can 'completely overwhelm' the reflex centres causing an increase in ventilation (Levitsky 2003).
  2. A wide range of symptoms have been shown to be related to stress-induced hyperventilation (Schleifer et al. 2002) frequently leading to: 'disruption in the acid-base equilibrium triggers a chain of systemic physiological reactions that have adverse implications for musculoskeletal health, including increased muscle tension, muscle spasm, amplified response to catecholamines, and muscle ischemia and hypoxia'.
- *Functional somatic syndrome* (FSS): Tak & Rosmalen (2010) describe disturbed stress response systems, in relation to functional somatic syndromes – such as irritable bowel syndrome – as representing 'multifactorial interplay between psychological, biological, and social factors'. Beales (2004) describes FSS as having multiple contributory factors in which too much sustained stress leads to the loss of internal balance, reduced performance, and a mind–body system in overdrive, ultimately leading to breathing pattern disorders, as a consequence of the perceived threat to survival eliciting fight, flight or freeze reactions.
- *Habit*:
  1. According to Brashear (1983), the causes of hyperventilation are (1) organic and physiological and (2) psychogenic (emotional/habit), and that hyperventilation and respiratory alkalosis, accompanied by various signs and symptoms, occurs in about 6–11% of the general patient population.
  2. Lum (1984) discussed the reasons for people becoming hyperventilators: 'Neurological considerations leave little doubt that habitually unstable breathing is the prime cause of symptoms. Why people breathe in this way must be a matter for speculation, but manifestly the salient characteristics are pure habit.'
- *Hormonal – progesterone, oestradiol*: Slatkovska et al. (2006) demonstrated that phasic menstrual cycle changes in Pa_{CO2} may be partially due to stimulatory effects of progesterone and oestradiol on ventilatory drive. See also Damas-Mora et al. (1980).
- *Pregnancy*: Jensen et al. (2008) suggest that hyperventilation and attendant hypocapnia/alkalosis during pregnancy result from an interaction of pregnancy-induced changes in central chemoreflex drives to breathe and wakefulness, acid–base balance, metabolic rate and cerebral blood flow.
- *Pseudo-asthma*: A high proportion of individuals diagnosed as asthmatics have been shown to in fact be hyperventilators.
  1. Weinberger & Abu-Hasan (2007) note that the perception of dyspnoea is a prominent symptom of hyperventilation attacks, that can occur in those with or without asthma, and that patients with asthma may not readily be able to distinguish the perceived dyspnoea of a hyperventilation attack from asthma.
  2. Ternesten-Hasséus et al. (2008) report that exercise-induced dyspnoea may be associated with hypocapnia, resulting from hyperventilation, and that the diagnosis of exercise-induced asthma should be questioned when there are no signs of bronchoconstriction.
- *Pain:*
  1. Kapreli et al. (2008) suggested that the connection between neck pain and respiratory function could impact on patient assessment, rehabilitation and pharmacological prescription.
  2. Nishino et al. (1999) found that pain intensifies dyspnoeic sensation (commonly linked with BPD) presumably by increasing the respiratory drive.
  3. Perri & Halford (2004), in a survey of a convenience sample of 111 consecutive patients attending a chiropractic clinic, reported that neck pain had a significant relationship with dysfunctional breathing patterns.
- *Sleep disorders*: There is an direct temporal, and possibly aetiological, connection, between sleep disorders and overbreathing, including sleep apnoea and cardiorespiratory fitness (Vanhecke et al. 2008).

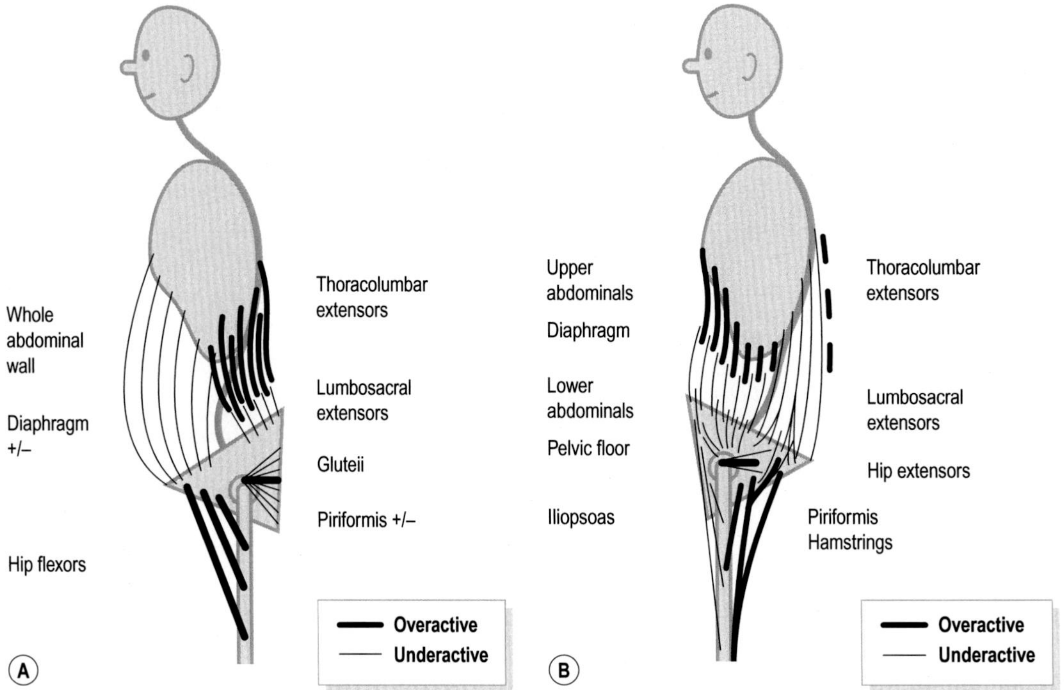

Figure 9.4 • Schematic views of (A) posterior (B) anterior pelvic crossed syndrome. Reproduced from Key (2010) J. Bodyw. Mov. Ther. M. 14, 299–301.

The likely outcome of such postural distress, Key et al. suggest, would include dysfunctional breathing patterns and pelvic floor dysfunction.

In Figure 9.4B the major features include:

- Flexors tend to dominate;
- Loss of extension throughout spine;
- Thoracolumbar junction hyperstabilized in flexion.

The likely outcome of such postural distress, Key et al. suggest, would include dysfunctional breathing patterns and pelvic floor dysfunction.

For example Key et al. report that, in relation to what they term the posterior pelvic crossed syndrome, characterized by 'a posterior [pelvic] shift with increased anterior sagittal rotation or tilt', together with an anterior shunt/translation of the thorax, among many other stressful modifications, there will inevitably be poor diaphragmatic control and altered PFM function.

Examples

These postural examples are not uncommon, as evidenced by the descriptions offered below that demonstrate postural and/or respiratory links with pelvic floor dysfunction. In such cases it is difficult to envision anything other than short-term symptomatic improvement without a degree of structural, postural and respiratory assessment, and where appropriate, rehabilitation.

For example:

1. Haugstad et al. (2006a) evaluated 60 women with CPP, compared to healthy controls. They reported that in the standing posture, the area of support was minimal, with the feet being posed close together, the pelvic area pushed forward, and the shoulders and upper parts of the back pulled backwards. Compare this description with Figure 9.4B. In addition they identified a common pattern of high costal respiration with almost no movement in the thorax or in the abdominal area.
2. Psoas involvement has been identified in men with CPP. In a case-control series Hetrick et al (2003) noted that: 'controls and patients with pain showed a significant difference in muscle spasm, increased muscle tone, pain with internal transrectal palpation of the pelvic muscles, and increased tension and pain with palpation of the levator ani and coccygeus muscles ($P < 0.001$), as

well as significantly greater pain and tension with palpation of the psoas muscles and groin'.

Repercussions of breathing pattern disorders

BPD has been shown to potentially have multiple, body-wide, influences which are summarized below.

Nixon & Andrews (1996) vividly summarize a common situation applying to the individual with BPD tendencies: 'Muscular aching at low levels of effort; restlessness and heightened sympathetic activity; increased neuronal sensitivity; and, constriction of smooth muscle tubes (e.g. the vascular, respiratory and gastrointestinal) can accompany the basic symptom of inability to make and sustain normal levels of effort'.

Breathing pattern disorders (with hyperventilation as the extreme of this) may influence health by:

- Altering blood pH, creating respiratory alkalosis (Pryor & Prasad 2002, Celotto et al. 2008);
- Inducing increased sympathetic arousal, altering neuronal function – including motor control (Dempsey et al. 2002, Brotto et al. 2009);
- Encouraging a sense of apprehension, anxiety, affecting balance, muscle tone and motor control (Rhudy & Meagher 2000, Balaban & Thayer 2001, Van Dieën et al. 2003);
- Depleting Ca and Mg ions, enhancing sensitization, encouraging reduced pain threshold and the evolution of myofascial trigger points (Gardner 1996, Cimino et al. 2000, Schleifer et al. 2002, Simons et al. 1999);
- Triggering smooth muscle cell constriction, leading to vasoconstriction and/or spasm – including colon spasm (Ford et al. 1995, Yokoyama et al. 2008, Debreczeni et al. 2009) or pseudo-angina (Evans et al. 1980, Wilke et al. 1999);
- Reducing oxygen release to cells, tissues, brain (Bohr effect) so encouraging ischaemia, fatigue, pain and the evolution of myofascial trigger points (Freeman & Nixon 1985, Suwa 1995);
- Creating biomechanical overuse stresses and compromising core stability and posture (Lewit 1980, 1999, Haugstad et al. 2006b, Hodges et al. 2007).

BPD and hyperventilation: Physical features – Implications for rehabilitation

Deep and rapid breathing (hyperpnoea) results in progressive muscular fatigue and increasing sensations of distress, to the point of breathlessness. For example, Renggli et al. (2008) report that during normocapnic hyperpnoea (involving partial rebreathing of CO_2), contractile fatigue of the diaphragm and abdominal muscles develops, long before task failure, triggering an increased recruitment of rib cage muscles. Since the diaphragm and abdominal muscles are key features of low back and pelvic stability, the implications for core instability of chronic, habitual, overbreathing – where normocapnic hyperpnoea would be unlikely – are clear. Respiratory alkalosis, and its numerous effects as described earlier in this chapter, would then accompany reduced pelvic and low back stability.

- The implication is that methods to help avoidance of hyperpnoea should be a feature of breathing retraining.

Hudson et al. (2007) observe that human scalenes are *obligatory* inspiratory muscles that have a greater mechanical advantage than sternocleidomastoid (SCM) muscles, which are *accessory* respiratory muscles. They found that irrespective of respiratory tasks these muscles are recruited in the order of their mechanical advantages – with scalenes starting to operate earlier than SCM, involving what they term to be an 'efficient, fail-safe, system of neural control'.

- The implication in breathing rehabilitation is to ensure that these muscles receive focused attention as to their functionality.

Schleifer et al. (2002) recapitulate the known effects of overbreathing which they have identified as occurring in stress-related work settings:

> Hyperventilation (overbreathing) refers to a drop in arterial CO_2, caused by ventilation that exceeds metabolic demands for O_2. Excessive loss of CO_2 that results from hyperventilation produces a rise in blood pH (i.e. respiratory alkalosis). This disruption in the acid-base equilibrium triggers a chain of systemic physiological reactions that have adverse implications for musculoskeletal health, including increased muscle tension, muscle spasm, amplified response to catecholamines, and muscle ischemia and hypoxia. Hyperventilation is often characterized by a shift from a diaphragmatic to a thoracic breathing pattern, which imposes biomechanical stress on the neck/shoulder region

due to the ancillary recruitment of sternocleidomastoid, scalene, and trapezius muscles in support of thoracic breathing.

- The implications suggest that these changes: 'provide a unique rationale for coping with job stress and musculoskeletal discomfort through breathing training, light physical exercise, and rest breaks'.

Masubuchi et al. (2001) used fine-wire electrodes inserted into muscles, and high-resolution ultrasound, to identify the activity of three muscle groups, in response to various respiratory and postural manoeuvres. They concluded that the scalenes are the most active, and trapezius the least active, cervical accessory inspiratory muscles, while SCM is intermediate.

- This confirms what has long been suspected by observation and palpation – that the scalenes are the most important respiratory muscle group lying superior to the thorax.

Scalene dysfunction and the presence of trigger points ('functional pathology') were identified in excess of 50% of individuals, in a series of 46 hospitalized patients who demonstrated paradoxical patterns of respiration. A combination of Muscle Energy Technique ('post-isometric relaxation') and self-stretching of the scalenes, was used during rehabilitation (Pleidelová et al. 2002).

- The implication is that these key respiratory muscles require focused attention via palpation and appropriate therapeutic interventions, as part of breathing rehabilitation.

Renggli et al. (2008) showed (see above) that the progressive fatigue of the diaphragm and abdominal muscles, during overbreathing, results in recruitment of the muscles of the rib cage (intercostals).

Han et al. (1993) described the action, and interaction, of these rib cage muscles, during ventilation, noting that the parasternal intercostal muscles, act in concert with the scalenes to expand the upper rib cage, and/or to prevent it from being drawn inward by the action of the diaphragm, during quiet breathing. The respiratory activity of the external intercostals however appear to constitute a reserve system, only to be recruited when increased expansion of the rib cage is required.

- The implications of this information point to the need for attention to the often-neglected intercostal muscles, during breathing rehabilitation.

Earlier in this chapter the relationship between the psoas and quadratus lumborum muscles, and the retroperineal space, the pelvic floor, the pelvic girdle and respiratory function have been summarized (see Burkill & Healy 2000, Hetrick et al. 2003, Haugstad et al. 2006a, Key et al. 2007, Lee et al. 2008).

Viscerosomatic effects

Prather et al. (2009) expand on these relationships in a review of the anatomy, evaluation and treatment of musculoskeletal pelvic floor pain in women. They note that persistent muscle contraction of the pelvic floor, related to noxious visceral stimulation, such as that deriving from endometriosis or IBS, can lead to splinting and pain, with reduction of normal PFM function. Specifically, they report that viscerosomatic reflex activity may be responsible for increased resting tone of the pelvic floor with reduced ability to fully relax the muscle group as a whole. As a result, they suggest, adaptation occurs via recruitment of global muscles in the region – e.g. psoas and iliacus – leading to symptoms such as posterior pelvic and low back pain.

As noted above, Prather et al. have pointed out that: 'proper breathing techniques, while performing exercises and activities, are essential for pelvic floor relaxation. Pelvic floor contraction during exhalation allows for synergy between the pelvic and respiratory diaphragms'.

Tu et al. (2008) compared the biomechanical features of the pelvic girdle, as well as the associated muscles in 20 CPP patients and 20 normal controls. Among their findings – relevant to this chapter – are the following:

1. Several tests of pelvic girdle instability were more common in CPP cases than in controls (asymmetric iliac crest and pubic symphysis heights and positive posterior pelvic provocation testing).
2. In addition, patients with CPP were more tender on palpation of the left oblique, right and left rectus and right psoas ($P > 0.05$). Previous evidence, described above, suggests that such changes would be likely to impair respiration; however, this feature was not a part of Tu et al.'s study.

The implication can be drawn that attention to possibly impaired breathing pattern function should form part of therapeutic focus in cases involving CPP, and that in doing so attention to key dysfunctional muscles (tender, asymmetrically hypertonic/shortened, with altered tissue texture and/or reduced range of motion) should play a part.

- Optimal rehabilitation of breathing function, requires appropriate attention to both psoas and QL status, as well as key accessory and obligatory respiratory muscles. Additionally, optimal rehabilitation of the pelvic floor requires attention to respiration and the multiple structures that influence it.

'Biologically unsustainable patterns' (Garland 1994)

Garland has summarized the structural modifications that are likely to inhibit successful breathing rehabilitation, as well as psychological intervention, until they are at least in part normalized.

He describes a series of changes including:

- Visceral stasis/pelvic floor weakness;
- Abdominal and erector spinae muscle imbalance;
- Fascial restrictions from the central tendon via the pericardial fascia to the basiocciput;
- Upper rib elevation with increased costal cartilage tension;
- Thoracic spine dysfunction and possible sympathetic disturbance;
- Accessory breathing muscle hypertonia and fibrosis;
- Evolution of myofascial trigger points in hypertonic and ischemic tissues;
- Promotion of rigidity in the cervical spine with possibility of fixed lordosis;
- Reduction in mobility of 2nd cervical segment and disturbance of vagal outflow.

These changes, Garland states: 'run physically and physiologically against biologically sustainable patterns, and in a vicious circle, promote abnormal function, which alters structure, which then disallows a return to normal function'.

Myofascial trigger points

Within the patterns of overuse and misuse that characterize postural and respiratory insults to the body as described above, the evolution of myofascial trigger points is a common feature (Lewit 1999, Travell & Simons 1999, Schleifer et al. 2002, Anderson et al. 2009, Key 2010). Greater detail regarding myofascial trigger points can be found in Chapter 14. One of the pioneers of manual approaches to CPP, Slocumb (1984) described how trigger points in the following areas can all produce virtually identical referred pelvic pain:

1. The lower abdominal wall;
2. In tissue overlying the pubic bone;
3. In levator ani;
4. Tissues lateral to the cervix;
5. Close to vaginal cuff scar tissue more than 3 months after hysterectomy;
6. The dorsal aspect of the sacrum.

Slocumb demonstrated, in a study involving 130 patients, that he was able to remove CPP in nearly 90% of cases by deactivating trigger points in these sites.

In addition, Weiss (2001), Anderson et al. (2009), Fitzgerald et al. (2009) and many others have unequivocally demonstrated that trigger points are the cause of serious levels of pelvic pain and dysfunction.

What remains unclear is trigger point causation, and the potential functionality in some circumstances (e.g. ligamentous laxity) of the effects of myofascial trigger points. Recently, the European Association of Urology has published guidelines suggesting that trigger points should be considered in the diagnosis of CPP (Fall et al. 2010).

Breathing rehabilitation assessment and interventions (Chaitow et al. 2002)

Earlier in this chapter the usefulness of questionnaires such as the Nijmegen instrument was discussed. In addition, a variety of evaluation and rehabilitation methods have evolved to manage BPD – with some focusing on psychological, behavioural, functional approaches, and others on more structural, biomechanical features of respiratory function.

For example, in relation to retraining, Mattsson et al. (2000) have reported altered patterns of posture, movement and respiration in a study of women with CPP. In the context of treating women with CPP who had a history of sexual abuse, using what is termed psychiatric physiotherapy to develop body awareness, Mattsson et al. (1997) note that 'Focusing on breathing ... mostly works indirectly by practicing to become more aware of one's breathing in different situations'.

Breathing retraining appears to require a combination of elements for best results:

1. Understanding the processes – a cognitive, intellectual, awareness of the mechanisms and issues involved in BPDs;

2. Retraining exercises that include aspects that operate subcortically, allowing replacement of currently habituated patterns with more appropriate ones;
3. Biomechanical structural modifications that remove obstacles to desirable and necessary functional changes;
4. Time for these elements to merge and become incorporated into moment-to-moment use patterns.

Box 9.3 offers a summary of physical medicine approaches as utilized by one of this chapter's authors (L.C.).

Functional examination: Identifying the locus of motion

An initial assessment is required to determine whether the breathing pattern is paradoxical, upper chest or diaphragmatic/abdominal (Lewit 1980). Two validated methods are described below – the so-called HiLo test (Bradley 1998, Courtney et al. 2009), and the MARM (manual assessment of respiratory motion) method (Courtney 2008, Courtney & Greenwood 2009).

Box 9.3

Phases of breathing intervention (modified from McLaughlin 2009)

Assessment

- Identify symptoms related to poor breathing chemistry and biomechanics
- Observe breathing pattern, e.g. paradoxical pattern/upper chest (Courtney et al. 2008, 2009)
- Observe posture, particularly crossed patterns (Key et al. 2007)
- Assess spinal, rib mobility/restriction, form/force closure (active straight leg raise test), shortness and/or weakness of key muscles, as well as assessing for active trigger points (Lee & Lee 2004, Lee 2007, Lee et al. 2008)
- Identify BPD triggers (pain, stress, situations, thoughts, emotions, etc.)
- Identify faulty breathing behaviours (upper chest, no pause between breaths, etc.)
- Utilize questionnaires (Nijmegen, SEBQ; see Appendix)
- Utilize palpation assessments such as HiLo and manual assessment of breathing pattern (see text)
- Use capnography if available, to monitor end-tidal CO_2

Education

- Inform as to role altered breathing can play in symptom production
- Discuss assessment findings
- Teach elements of appropriate breathing
- Discuss symptoms of breathing pattern disorders
- Help with understanding of external situations and internal states (thoughts, emotions) that may trigger altered breathing

Retraining

- Teach smooth and rhythmic breathing methods in which ratio of inhalation to exhalation is roughly 1:2 (i.e. exhale should take longer). A key to changing breathing behaviour is to focus on long, slow exhalation, informing patient that, if this is adequate, 'inhalation takes care of itself'
- Consider home use of a capnograph designed for biofeedback can help skill acquisition

Behaviour modification

- Modify poor breathing in response to subtler and subtler cues through increased awareness of the symptoms and mechanics of both poor and good breathing
- Teach basic strategies to inhibit habitual overuse of accessory breathing muscles on inhalation (see below)
- Encourage daily practice, morning and evening, of breathing exercises, to reinforce new learning

Manual therapy

- If restrictions are identified in the articular or myofascial tissues of the trunk or cervical spine, use manual therapy to free the tightness and provide extensibility, particularly of key muscles: psoas, QL, scalenes, intercostals, diaphragm attachment region. See examples later in this chapter and in Chapter 14
- If pelvic girdle structures are restricted, these should be mobilized. See Chapter 16 for examples
- If poor motor control is identified in the trunk or cervical spine add an appropriate exercise programme
- Postural correction may be required to optimize ventilation mechanics

Time

- Depending on chronicity, evidence suggests 6 weeks to 6 months may be required to normalize breathing habits (Lum 1996)

HiLo test

Courtney & Greenwood (2009) note that: 'The HiLo test can be used to assess the motion of the upper rib cage and lower rib cage/abdomen and determine aspects of breathing such as rate, rhythm, relative motion and phase relation of upper and lower breathing compartments' (Figure 9.5).

The patient is requested to place one hand on the sternum, and one hand on the upper abdomen. The practitioner/observer stands in front and to one side of the patient, so that a clear view is possible of the patient's abdomen, thorax and hands. By observing the direction, and degree, of hand movement, the observer determines whether thoracic or abdominal motion is dominant, during inhalation, or whether it is balanced.

If the abdomen moves in a direction opposite to the direction of movement of the thorax, during inhalation or exhalation, this is regarded as a paradoxical pattern (for example, if during inhalation the abdomen moves toward the spine, and/or if during exhalation the abdomen moves in an outward direction, paradoxical breathing is taking place). Assessment of upper rib status can usefully be performed at this time.

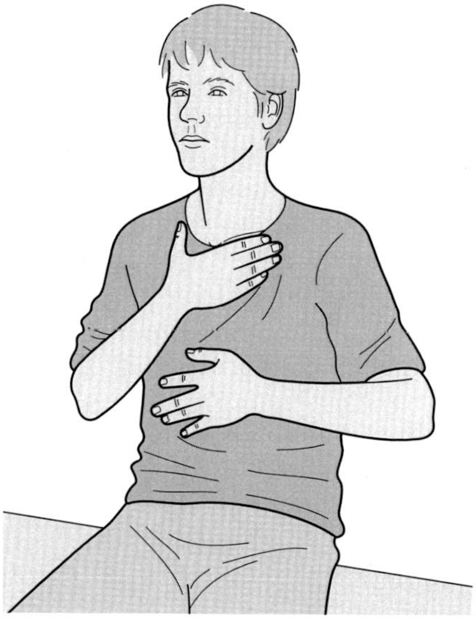

Figure 9.5 • HiLo test for rapid assessment of current breathing pattern

Manual assessment of respiratory motion (Figure 9.6)

The examiner sits behind the subject with hands resting lightly on the lower lateral rib cage, so as not to inhibit breathing motion. The hands should be placed so that the little fingers are oriented horizontally, with the thumbs more or less vertical. The lower fingers should be inferior to the lower ribs to allow assessment of abdominal expansion (Figure 9.6).

An attempt should be made to assess the overall vertical motion relative to the overall lateral motion. Judgement is exercised as to the degree that motion is taking place predominantly in the upper rib cage or the lower rib cage/abdomen.

Charting is possible by means of two lines being drawn relative to a horizontal line representing the lumbodorsal junction (see line C on Figure 9.7). The upper line (A) represents the degree of vertical and upper thoracic motion, while the lower line (B) represents the degree of lower rib and abdominal motion. Calculations are made for thoracic diaphragm 'balance' and percentage of rib cage motion.

Current thoracic excursion

For the purpose of subsequent reassessment, a record of the current excursion at various levels of the thorax should be recorded. Pryor & Prasad (2002) report that normal total lateral rib excursion in the lower thorax is between 3 and 5 cm – ideally with

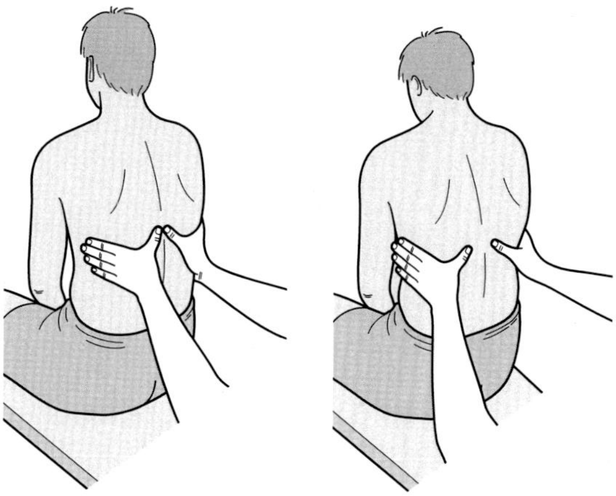

Figure 9.6 • Hand positions for assessment of rib movement

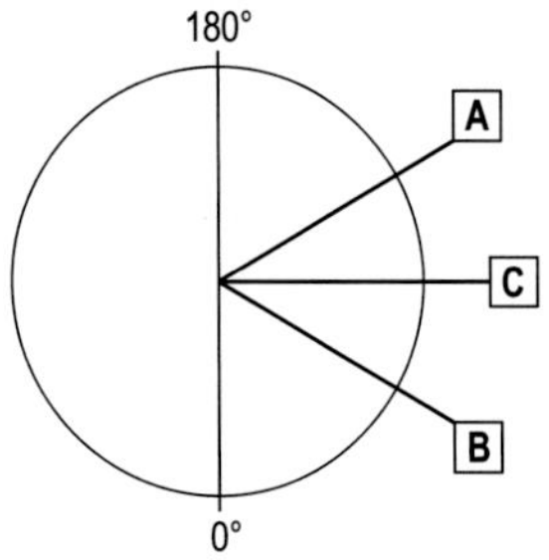

Variable	Description	Calculation
Area of breathing	Angle formed between upper line and lower line	Angle **AB**
Balance	Difference between angle made by horizontal axis (**C**) and upper line (**A**) and horizontal line (**C**) and lower line (**B**)	**AC–CB**
Percent rib cage motion	Area above horizontal/ total area between upper line and lower line x100	**AC/AB** x100

Variables calculated from MARM graphic notation

Figure 9.7 • Chart used to identify areas, balance and percentage of rib movement

an equal excursion bilaterally. Assessment is accurately achieved by means of a cloth tape measure.

The reliability of measuring thoracic excursion has been established, ideally using a standard cloth tape measure (taken at 5th and 10th thoracic levels). It is suggested that upper thoracic excursion measurements should be taken at the level of the fifth thoracic spinous process and the third intercostal space at the mid-clavicular line. Lower thoracic excursion measurements should be taken at the level of the 10th thoracic spinous process and the xiphoid process. (Bockenhauer et al. 2007).

Breath-holding tests

There is no agreed 'normal' breath-holding time, but it can be a useful clinical point of reference. Gardner (1996) reports that patients with hyperventilation syndrome seldom breath hold beyond 10–12 seconds. In the Buteyko (1990) system, a control pause is practised regularly to encourage increased CO_2 tolerance.

- Control pause: normal exhalation is held until 'a need to breathe again' is experienced. 'Normal' is between 25 and 30 seconds. Less than 15 seconds, it is suggested, represents low tolerance to CO_2.

Courtney et al. (2011) have suggested that two breath-holding tests may usefully be performed:

1. The participant exhales and holds the breath until experiencing a definite sensation of discomfort or recognizable difficulty in holding the breath (BHT-DD).
2. The time may be measured until the first involuntary movement of respiratory muscles (BHT-IRM).

Courtney et al. (2011) found that where MARM assessment demonstrated thoracic dominance, this correlated with diminished breath-holding time until first involuntary movement (BHT-IRM). They hypothesized that this may be because both measures reflect respiratory drive, with increased respiratory drive increasing the extent of thoracic breathing and decreasing breath-holding time.

Teaching control of breathing

Learning to modify and regulate breathing may at first seem unrelated to the problem of pelvic pain, but there are several ways that it can help to alleviate CPP, as well as pain in other sites. Breathing has special significance for the pelvic region, because it is a constantly occurring event that physically affects the pelvic muscles, tissues and circulatory systems. Various modes of biofeedback can be used to facilitate learning breathing control (see Chapter 13).

Advantages of controlled breathing include:

1. Promotes general calming, reduction of emotional arousal, and feeling of control.
2. Ensures that level of CO_2 in bloodstream is optimal, so that pH stays in normal range, muscle tension and myofascial trigger points are not stimulated, smooth muscle is less likely to constrict, and cerebral circulation remains stable.
3. Abdominal circulation of both the blood and the lymph is stimulated by regular diaphragm action.
4. Pelvic floor muscles are 'entrained' by diaphragmatic action and participate in the rhythmic contraction and relaxation.

5. Heart rate variability is enhanced by breathing at a particular frequency. This also helps stabilize the autonomic nervous system (ANS).
6. The parasympathetic nervous system (PNS) becomes stronger relative to the sympathetic nervous system (SNS) because of prolonged exhalation. Imbalance of SNS relative to PNS is minimized.

Teaching individuals to alter their breathing patterns is more complicated if the goal goes beyond producing a temporary change to revising faulty breathing habits. Some suggestions for this procedure, using generally accepted guidelines from physiotherapy, respiratory therapy and psychology, are presented below.

These are brief instructions and practice procedures for teaching relaxed breathing, first for quick intervention with full consciousness, and eventually for forming habits of better breathing. Fuller coverage of breathing improvement can be found in Dinah Bradley's *The Hyperventilation Syndrome*, Ley & Timmons *Behavioral and Psychological Approaches to Breathing Disorders*, and the work of J. van Dixhoorn.

In breathing training (some say 'retraining') the goal is to simulate natural, optimal breathing, which would occur in most individuals under ideal conditions of calm, low stress and no pain. Distressed breathing deviates from this ideal pattern toward either an action-preparation or 'freeze' mode which includes upper-chest breathing rather than abdominal, a faster, usually shallower breathing rate; irregular rhythm from one breath to the next with more frequent sighs or gasps; and breathing through the mouth.

Natural relaxed breathing, when at rest physically and emotionally, will normally be more abdominal, with the external abdominal muscles relaxed and able to expand; more diaphragmatic movement; lips closed; minimal chest expansion; slower rate; regular rate (usually 12–14), fewer sighs, and sometimes prolonged exhalation. Unless using pursed lips to slow the exhale, breathing should be done through the nose, both in and out. Simulating the breathing style of a relaxed person will begin to create the desired state, to a degree, with some or all of the benefits listed above (see pursed lip breathing instructions below).

Dinah Bradley, a New Zealand physiotherapist and co-author of *Self-Help for Hyperventilation Syndrome* (2001), recommends to patients the phrase 'low and slow' to encapsulate good breathing. This means breathing low down in the upper body, expanding the abdomen during inhalation, and reducing the breathing rate.

A more detailed approach might list specific goals and encourage practice of each control procedure separately:

1. Practice slowing the breathing rate to 20–30% below whatever it is at that moment. Tidal volume should automatically enlarge to compensate for the reduced rate. If that goes well, try for even slower, down to six breaths per minute without straining or gasping.
2. Practice abdominal breathing, including lateral expansion of lower ribs. Stand before a mirror or use your hands to note where the body is expanding. This will usually help regain a natural breathing style and relieve overuse of chest and neck accessory breathing muscles.
3. Practice shifting between abdominal and 'paradoxical breathing' – meaning drawing in the abdomen and expanding the chest on the inhale. Alternating between one and the other, and comparing the two, accentuates the contrast between the two styles and strengthens the ability to shift into abdominal breathing.
4. Prolong the exhale to a maximum of twice as long as the inhale. This can be done either with diaphragm control or with pursed lips exhalation.
5. Imagine breathing as an internal downward expansion, feel the sensations of this action, and imagine the abdominal and pelvic organs being gently massaged by this breathing.

Each of the steps above can be expanded in sensory and motor detail and practised so that they are available when needed during pain flares. With practice, relaxed breathing becomes more the default, easier to access and easier to sustain when needed. See Boxes 9.4 and 9.5 for additional breathing rehabilitation methods.

Box 9.4

Example of breathing rehabilitation exercise (morning and evening, 30–40 cycles each session)

Pursed lip breathing, combined with diaphragmatic breathing, enhances pulmonary efficiency (Tiep et al. 1986, Faling 1995). One study (Hochstetter et al. 2005) found that pursed lip breathing has the potential to help the individual control breathing and improve functional activity, during episodes of breathlessness associated with BPD as well as chronic obstructive lung disease.

In addition both anxiety and pain should reduce (Cappo & Holmes 1984, Grossman et al. 1985).

Continued

Box 9.4

Example of breathing rehabilitation exercise (morning and evening, 30–40 cycles each session)—cont'd

- The patient is seated or supine with dominant hand on the abdomen and the other hand on the chest.
- The patient is asked to breathe in through the nose, and out through the mouth, with pursed lips, ensuring diaphragmatic involvement by means of movement of the abdomen against the hand, on inhalation.
- Exhalation through the pursed lips is performed slowly, and has been shown to relieve dyspnoea, to slow the respiratory rate, increase tidal volume, and to help restore diaphragmatic function (Tiep et al, 1986, Faling 1995).
- The patient is asked to imagine blowing a thin stream of air at a candle flame about 6 inches from the mouth. Exhalation should be slow and continuous.
- After exhaling fully, *without strain*, a pause for a count of 'one' is introduced, followed by inhalation through the nose.
- Without pausing to hold the breath after inhalation, the patient is asked to again exhale slowly and fully, through pursed lips, blowing the air in a thin stream, and to then pause for a count of one.
- The inhalation and exhalation should be repeated for not less than 30 cycles.
- After some weeks of daily practice an inhalation phase which lasts 2–3 seconds, and an exhalation phase of 6–7 seconds should be achieved, without strain.
- The patient is asked to practise twice daily, and to repeat the exercise for a few minutes (6 cycles takes about a minute) every hour if anxious, or when stress levels increase.

Box 9.5

Instructions to patient to minimize overuse of accessory breathing muscles during retraining, using Brugger's Relief Position (Lewit 1999, Brugger 2000, Liebenson 2006) (see Figure 9.8)

1. Perch on chair edge, arms hanging down, feet below knees, slightly apart and turned outward.
2. Let arms hang loose, so that palms face forward.
3. Roll pelvis forward to produce *slight* low back arching.
4. Ease sternum *slightly* forward and up.
5. Tuck chin in.
6. Practise slow, pursed lip breathing, turning arms further outward until thumbs face slightly back, *on inhalation*.
7. Relax arms to neutral, *on exhalation*.

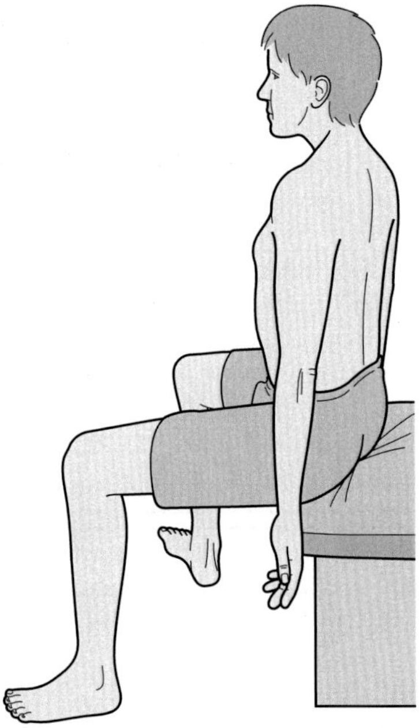

Figure 9.8 • Brugger's position for enhanced diaphragmatic function during inhalation phase of breathing exercises. Individual is seated as shown, palm facing forward. On inhalation external rotation of the arm (thumbs tend to then point backwards) inhibits activity of accessory respiratory muscles. On exhalation the arms return to neutral (palms forward)

CO_2 regulation study

McLaughlin & Goldsmith (2007) and McLaughlin (2009) described a case series of 24 patients with either chronic pelvic or lower back pain. They were included because they were either not improved from manual therapy and exercise, or their improvement had plateaued. These patients were first assessed with capnometry (Box 9.6) for level of baseline (resting) end-tidal CO_2 and evidence of hyperventilation. Initially, all had lower than normal CO_2 levels. They were then helped to improve their breathing pattern (more abdominal breathing, avoiding lower back bracing, nose rather than mouth breathing, lowering the breathing rate, practising breathing with capnometer feedback). Treatment was individualized to address individual aberrations from optimal breathing and to maximize the chance of generalization outside of the therapy context. The number of individual training sessions varied; the mean number was six.

The results showed success in raising the resting CO_2 to normal (a mean of 7 mmHg rise; only one patient could not rise to within normal CO_2 range).

Box 9.6

Assessment by capnography

Monitoring end-tidal CO_2 is a simple process, used either as spot assessment for hyperventilation or as continuous biofeedback procedure to help optimize breathing and keep pCO_2 within normal limits. No mask is needed, only a nasal cannula or nostril sampling tube. Under normal circumstances end-tidal CO_2 correlates very well with arterial CO_2. Instrumentation is available in several forms: small and portable, desktop size, and integrated into computer via software.

The first type usually offers a small display of the breathing waveform plus respiration rate, end-tidal CO_2 of each breath, and usually memory and data upload functions. Desktop models include in addition a larger display and sometimes a built-in printer. A computer-integrated model offers a variety of displays, printing and biofeedback training modes, is lightweight and transferable to other computers. All three types can include an oximetry option.

The website capnography.com has basic and advanced information about monitoring CO_2.

Two-thirds of the patients reported clinically meaningful reductions in their pain. Functional improvements were evident in approximately half of the patients. Many also reported reduced anxiety and fewer breathing difficulties.

- Such widespread improvement from simply developing a more normal breathing pattern can be understood with reference to the effect of low CO_2 (hypocapnia) on various body systems. Low CO_2 alters the pH of the blood, making it more alkaline (respiratory alkalosis). Smooth muscle is stimulated to constrict, including blood vessels, viscera and bronchial airways. (Cardiologists use brief hyperventilation to test for susceptibility to vasospastic angina (Hirano et al. 2001).). Skeletal muscle becomes hypertonic, contraction thresholds drop, and muscle may twitch. The nervous system in general becomes hyperexcitable and oxygen delivery is reduced (haemoglobin retains O_2 under alkaline conditions; see West (2008) or pulmonology texts for details).
- Mehling et al. (2005) also demonstrated the value of breathing rehabilitation in cases of chronic low back pain, when this approach was compared to standard physical therapy in a randomized, controlled study. At 6 months follow-up, patients in both groups maintained statistically significant improvements in the main outcome measures, pain reduction and functional ability.

The Mensendieck approach

The Mensendieck therapeutic approach combines elements of physical therapy (postural adjustment, breathing regulation, movement patterns) and elements of psychology, particularly self-perception and body awareness. The procedure is a learning and training sequence which includes developing new motor patterns (posture, breathing, moving) in conjunction with full attention to the experience of being in one's own body while learning new motor patterns for performing common activities. The goal is to improve use through improved body awareness in combination with new habits of movement and breathing.

CPP of obscure origin can be effectively treated by addressing muscle tension, body attitude, patterns of movement and dysfunctional breathing. Practitioners of the Mensendieck technique, as practised mostly in Europe and Scandinavia, use a comprehensive assessment which rates movement, gait, posture, self-awareness of body sensations, variables related to breathing, and emotional status, including depression and anxiety. This allows a thorough evaluation of status before, during, and after the training.

This technique proceeds through three stages:

1. The 'cognitive' phase: attending more closely to body sensations – visual, tactile, kinesthetic and others – in essence providing a richer basis for change by maximizing attention to the feedback signalling system while focusing on more ideal sensation patterns;
2. The 'associative' phase: developing awareness of new or enhanced body sensations in comparison with the ideal patterns;
3. The 'automatized' phase – where the person uses more efficient or functional motor patterns with less or no conscious intention, and new motor and behavioural patterns are integrated into activities of daily life.

An important feature of the Mensendieck approach is its emphasis on improving poor body awareness. Practitioners have found that women with CPP are deficient in the ability to integrate proprioceptive and other interoceptive impressions with concurrent thoughts and feelings. They describe a pattern in many patients of loss of contact with parts of the body, in this case the pelvic region. This characteristic is compared to alexithymia (relative lack of ability to feel or express emotions); the parallel term 'alexisomia' was suggested to describe a type of dissociative process in which body awareness is suppressed. Nijenhuis (2004) surveyed the evidence and made the case for what is called 'somatic dissociation'. This disconnection from normal somatic feedback leads to poor regulation of muscle tension, breathing, movement, and posture. Mensendieck practitioners note that CPP patients typically cannot contract their PFMs in isolation, and when asked to do so, may contract adjacent muscles instead.

In a systematic comparison of clinical characteristics of 60 women with CPP with 15 controls, several differences were apparent that may be implicated in the creation and maintenance of the pain (Haugstad et al. 2006a). The method of examination used was the Standardized Mensendieck Test, a set of prescribed movements to be observed in order to assess several features of posture, movement, gait, sitting posture and respiration. The protocol was individually administered, and movements were rated by how much they deviated from optimal performance.

Among the many differences observed between the pelvic pain patients and the controls, those with chronic pain had obvious deficits in breathing, including a primarily upper-chest breathing pattern with little movement in thorax or abdomen, and more irregular rhythm. Reflex respiratory responses to certain induced movements were sub-optimal: for instance, breathing response to lifting the pelvis in supine position should be a deeper breath to restore normal rhythm. Also, general muscle tension in several muscles near the pelvic area was higher in both density and stiffness, as measured by palpation. The authors observed that 'Clinical examination revealed a characteristic pattern of standing, sitting, and walking, as well as lack of coordination and irregular high costal respiration'.

Because of this linkage between the pelvis and breathing activity, the authors postulate a 'vicious circle' typically present in women with CPP: tight, inflexible muscles around the pelvis maintain a guarding pattern, and the breathing displays avoidance of abdominal expansion.

In the main Mensendieck-specific study to date (Haugstad et al. 2006b) a group of 40 women with CPP were divided into two groups: both groups first received standard gynaecological treatment, including hormones, non-opioid analgesics, general education, dietary and sexual advice. Participants with major psychiatric problems were excluded. The experimental group also participated in the Mensendieck somatocognitive protocol, training in body awareness through ten individual sessions. Six months later, the symptomatic improvement in group 1 was near zero, and changes in the Mensendieck scores (posture, movement, breathing) were not evident upon retesting. The improvement in the experimental group included a near 50% reduction in pain scores, plus clear improvements in posture, movement and breathing. Breathing variables showed the most improvement.

Although the experimental design included a control group, it was not double-blinded and group 1 received less therapeutic attention than group 2. So conclusions about efficacy therefore must be tempered by these limits to the research design. However, the improvements held, and were stable at follow-up testing 1 year later. The improvements in experienced pain, psychological distress, natural movement and breathing all were maintained or increased beyond what was noted at the 90-day point (Haugstad et al. 2008) and the breathing pattern was especially improved. Natural diaphragmatic movement and abdominal expansion were generally restored.

The authors propose that normalizing breathing, among other benefits, increases pelvic circulation, and that lymphatic drainage and blood circulation in the lower pelvic region may be improved by rhythmic abdominal breathing when done habitually. This idea fits with other research on congestion as one cause of pelvic pain.

Breathing pattern is not simply a mechanical function, but is influenced by psychological factors. For instance, Fry et al. (1997) studied social–psychological correlates of pelvic venous congestion in a series of women seeking help for CPP. Detailed interviews and questionnaires assessed social and psychological variables, present and past family background, illness history, hostility, parenting patterns and childhood sexual abuse. Compared with women having CPP but without venous congestion, those with congestion had more history of childhood sexual abuse and differences in parenting patterns. The father's parenting style seemed influential, and presence of hostility in childhood seemed suspect as increasing the development of chronic congestion. Breathing patterns were not assessed in Fry's study, but given the more stressful backgrounds in those with pelvic congestion, breathing may be the missing variable mediating between social stress, deficient pelvic circulation and pain. Myofascial trigger points could also emerge from the restricted movements of breathing.

Smith et al. (2006) studied reports of symptoms correlated with or predicting back pain in over 38 000 women, using data from the Australian Longitudinal Study on Women's Health. Complaints of breathing difficulties and incontinence were consistently associated with back pain, while the more traditional factors of obesity and degree of physical activity were not as predictive. The authors speculate that the involvement of the diaphragm, transversus abdominis, and PFMs in both trunk stabilization and breathing make back pain more likely if PFMs or diaphragm are weak. This would be the case if poor breathing habits (shallow chest breathing) distort the usual interactions among these muscles. Hodges et al. (2007) provided evidence about the muscle–function interrelationships among breathing, continence and spinal stabilization.

So it is plausible that long-term psychological factors contribute to a suboptimal breathing pattern, which in turn disrupts the abdominal–muscle balance and makes both back pain and pelvic pain more likely, with the added risk of pelvic venous congestion. More research could confirm or disconfirm these connections; intervention studies in which breathing pattern is normalized might show favourable consequences for many cases of both pelvic pain and back pain.

Research on breathing as a pain intervention

Many studies of pain control are performed with experimentally induced pain, on normal subjects. This temporary, induced pain differs from natural chronic pain in that is introduced to a non-compromised nervous system; research subjects are usually screened out if they have a chronic pain condition. In such cases, phenomena such as central and peripheral sensitization, kindling, wind-up, hyperalgesia and allodynia typically develop, amplifying and complicating the pain sensations. All this constitutes malfunction of the pain-detection system, and studies using acute, experimental pain do not address the extra factors that chronic pain presents.

Heart rate variability (HRV) is an emerging variable in the study of pain. It is a measure of cardiac activity sensitive to balance between sympathetic and parasympathetic influence, and can also be used as a biofeedback signal to help the patient regulate and balance the ANS by altering breathing. ANS imbalance is implicated in IBS (Mazur et al. 2007). There are no studies available for pelvic pain and HRV training, but a study by Appelhans & Luecken (2008), using an applied thermal pain stimulus and frequency-domain based spectral analysis with 59 normal subjects, found an inverse relationship between greater low-frequency HRV and pain intensity, including unpleasantness ratings. The low-frequency band (0.04–0.15 Hz) increases with both regular breathing and emotional calmness, and generally correlates with ANS balance and cardiovascular health.

An experimental pain stimulus such as heat or intramuscular hypertonic saline infusions can be adjusted and administered in order to measure pain thresholds. For example, (Chalaye et al. 2009) to study variability of pain tolerance and thresholds, the researchers applied thermal pain stimuli to subjects under two breathing conditions: distraction and feedback of heart rate (HRV). Compared to a 16/min breathing rate, slow deep breathing at a rate of 6/min resulted in better pain tolerance and higher pain thresholds. Increase in HRV correlates with increased vagal tone and general lowering of arousal.

Tan et al. (2009), using data from US war veterans suffering from chronic pain and other injuries, used a time-domain analysis of HRV. A –0.46 correlation was found between HRV (in this case SDNN, a time measure of variability) and presence of pain. So, in these two samples, a variable associated with breathing quality was also associated with presence of pain or sensitivity to pain. This is significant because HRV is a widely used biofeedback modality, and learning to raise low-frequency HRV by regulating breathing may have favourable effects on pain and homeostasis in general.

A study of experienced Zen meditators found that breathing pattern correlated with a significantly higher pain threshold to an applied heat stimulus. Better control over pain sensitivity was attributed to both attentional regulation and breathing regulation. The breathing pattern, being subject to disruptions in calmness and predictability, may be a good general index of peace of mind, which raises the threshold for pain of any sort. Zautra et al. (2010), comparing fibromyalgia patients to healthy controls, assigned slow breathing to volunteers subjected to controlled thermal stimuli. 'Slow breathing' was defined as breathing at one-half their normal rate. In general, slow breathing reduced pain intensity and unpleasantness more than normal breathing. The authors cited these results as support for Zen meditation and yogic breathing as a way to combat pain.

Pain may seem like a simple unitary sensation, but it has several facets, some mainly psychological. Using a brief intervention, Downey & Zun (2009) instructed patients in an emergency department to handle their pain by slow deep breathing. By self-report, no significant reduction in pain resulted, but the patients reported significant improvements in rapport with treating physicians, greater willingness to follow the medical recommendations, and conclusions that the intervention was useful.

Another study (Flink et al. 2009) of back pain patients showed that the effect of practising breathing exercises for 3 weeks was not so much on reducing pain levels as lowering catastrophizing and pain-related distress, along with greater acceptance of the pain condition.

Stress and breathing

Under stress of many sorts, the breathing pattern is likely to be disrupted. Breath-holding may occur as part of a state of suspense, becoming extra-vigilant, as in trying to detect a slight movement or sound. Gasping and sighing are more likely to occur during emotional instability, intense emotion, or preparation for exertion. Mouth-breathing can also be part of the preparation for heavy effort, since a larger volume of air can be inhaled quickly. Rate of breathing is sensitive to mental confusion or conflict, because thoughts and feelings carry various emotional loads which put conflicting demands on the respiratory system: freeze and remain concealed, get ready to run, prepare for attack, express anger, etc. Rapid breathing is common in anticipatory anxiety. Breathing changes may function like facial expressions, displaying emotional states to those nearby. In the same way that a scowl can be intimidating to humans or primates, breathing that shows aggression or preparation for action can convey it to others so they can act accordingly.

The human capacity for imagination allows us to create any scenario at any time, often in enough detail to initiate body responses as if the scene were real. Simply thinking about situations that require concealment, action, vigilance or emotional expression is likely to cause corresponding changes in the breathing pattern.

Another aspect of the interaction between breathing and emotion is the location of breathing in the body. Optimal breathing most often involves the diaphragm flattening on inhalation and the lower rib cage expanding outward, with the abdomen also expanding forward and laterally. Chest breathing, by contrast, minimizes the diaphragm action and substitutes pectoral, scalene, trapezius, SCM and upper intercostal muscles. This latter type of breathing is more prevalent during emotional stress and preparation for action. Thoracic breathing actually produces increases in cardiac output and heart rate (Hurwitz 1981). During emergency action, this kind of breathing would provide an advantage. The diaphragm also contributes to spinal stabilization, so during action preparation it is likely to be diverted from breathing duties.

Conditioned breathing responses

Breathing can be disrupted not only by current situations, but also by conditioned associations. A disturbing experience, whether traumatic or less so, can affect the breathing pattern in one of the ways described above. But unconscious memory processes link the experience with the body response in a way that preserves it, in case the experience, or something resembling it, occurs again. Reminders of the experience can be sufficient to re-enact the original physiological responses: for instance, the screech of brakes or a car horn reminding someone of an automobile crash.

This associative mechanism is activated not only for negative, disturbing experiences; recalling a pleasant, satisfying experience will activate the corresponding breathing pattern, in this case toward lower arousal and emotional calm. Using controlled breathing to calm down, take time out to think, and restore emotional balance is a fairly universal human strategy, and takes advantage of the conditioned link between, for example, visiting a peaceful lake and feeling the breathing become slow and full. If instructing someone in the details of breathing more abdominally (reducing the rate, keeping it more regular, breathing through the nose, etc.) seems too difficult, suggesting recall of a pleasant relaxing scene from the individual's personal past may do as well.

In the case of pelvic pain, positive changes in breathing and emotion interact with pelvic physiology and can affect pain mechanisms in both general and specific ways (inhibiting pain through descending inhibitory tracts, raising endorphins and dopamine, interrupting cycles of worry and suffering, lowering CCK and adrenaline, reducing sympathetic output to trigger points, and resuming rhythmic stimulation of viscera and PFMs) (Scott et al. 2007, Wager et al. 2007, Zubieta & Stohler 2009).

A linear, sequential conception of CPP in relation to poor breathing is difficult because of the interactions of several factors. But a basic sketch is as follows: breathing that is primarily thoracic deprives the viscera and abdominal cavity of rhythmic stimulation, normally provided by the push–pull vertical movement of the pulmonary diaphragm. In addition, excessive breathing in relation to oxygen demand excretes more CO_2 from the body than is being replaced, creating hypocapnic, high pH conditions. The systemic effect of the combined low CO_2 and alkalinity is to interfere with circulation throughout the body, constricting critical blood vessels. In addition, visceral and pelvic smooth muscle suffers from the same constriction. The Bohr effect reduces oxygen available to tissues. The skeletal muscles of the pelvic floor are subject to the same tension increase as other muscles, plus they are deprived of the rhythmic diaphragm movement which may stimulate circulation. In this impoverished environment trigger points may develop, becoming another source of pain.

Pelvic and abdominal pain from trigger points or other pain sources can be aggravated by full abdominal breathing, so downward expansion may be avoided, consciously or not. Shallow thoracic breathing is substituted, but this compounds the problem. The thoracic breathing is consistent with excessive emotional arousal, which may further the dysfunctional breathing pattern. Lewit (1999, described in Carrière 2006) describes how trigger points in either the diaphragm or the pelvic floor can make full abdominal breathing painful, and also that manually releasing trigger points in one region can relieve them in the other.

Psychology is very relevant to breathing pattern problems. The original source of thoracic breathing and chronic hyperventilation could be in early experience, trauma or chronic abuse, or an insecure environment fostering hypervigilance (Conway et al. 1988, Gilbert 1998). A transient breathing reaction can persist for years and become the default breathing style, even if the formative context has changed; breathing habits can be embedded through repetition. Lum (1975) observed that regardless of the source of hyperventilation, it could become habitual, persistent but amenable to reversal through breathing retraining with therapeutic guidance.

The improvements in pelvic pain noted by the authors cited above were specifically linked to improved breathing patterns, along with associated increases in somatic self-awareness. Changing the emotional and psychological context maintaining the thoracic breathing pattern may seem like a large task, but assessments of mood and psychological comfort usually show improvement as the breathing pattern changes and pain diminishes. So there may be a synergy among the factors involved.

Manual treatment of selected key structures associated with respiration

Therapeutically, it is suggested that rehabilitation of the pelvic girdle and pelvic floor will be enhanced by more normal physiological breathing patterns, while enhancing these patterns will be aided by pelvic functionality, whether achieved through exercise, breathing retraining, manual therapy or other means (Chaitow 2007, Mehling et al. 2005, McLaughlin 2009) (see Box 9.7).

Newell (2005), Gibbons (2001), Prather et al. (2009), Pleidelová et al. (2002), Cox & Bakkum (2005), Lewit (1999), Janda et al. (2007), Fitzgerald et al. (2009), and many others, have implicated (in particular) psoas, iliacus, quadratus lumborum, piriformis, the adductors, rectus abdominis, abdominal obliques and scalenes intercostals.

The muscles associated with respiratory function can be grouped as either inspiratory or expiratory, and are either primary in that capacity or provide accessory support. It should be kept in mind that

Box 9.7

Trigger points, BPD and pelvic pain

Trigger points in cervical, shoulder-girdle, thoracic, or lumbar muscles strongly influence and can be strongly influenced by:

- Disturbances of ventilation mechanics
- Disturbances of posture
- Disturbances of the functional dynamics of the neck, shoulder girdle and lumbar spine
- Paradoxical respiration is a critical link in many such pathogenetic chain reactions (Travell & Simons 1999).

Anderson (2002) has described palpation and treatment protocols for locating myofascial trigger points (TrPs) associated with prostatitis symptoms.

Anderson et al. (2009) have identified the most common location of TrPs related to pelvic pain as follows:

- Pubococcygeus (90%)
- External oblique (80%)
- Rectus abdominis (75%)
- Hip adductors (19%)
- Gluteus medius (18%).

Other relevant muscles in which TrPs also contribute to CPP are levator ani, iliopsoas, quadratus lumborum, gluteus maximus and thoracolumbar extensor muscle (Travell & Simons 1999, FitzGerald & Kotarinos 2003a, Chaitow 2007a, Montenegro et al. 2008, Anderson et al. 2009).

the role which these muscles might play in inhibiting respiratory function (due to trigger points, ischaemia, etc.) has not yet been clearly established and that their overload, due to dysfunctional breathing patterns, is likely to impact on cervical, shoulder, lower back and other body regions.

- The primary inspirational muscles are the diaphragm, the more lateral external intercostals, parasternal internal intercostals, scalene group and the levator costarum, with the diaphragm providing 70–80% of the inhalation force (Simons et al. 1999).
- These muscles are supported by the accessory muscles during increased demand (or dysfunctional breathing patterns): SCM, upper trapezius, pectoralis major and minor, serratus anterior, latissimus dorsi, serratus posterior superior, iliocostalis thoracis, subclavius and omohyoid (Kapandji 1974, Simons et al. 1999) (see Box 9.7).

Connective tissue manipulation

In 2009, the Urological Pelvic Pain Collaborative Research Network (UPPCRN) concluded that somatic abnormalities, including myofascial trigger points and connective tissue restrictions, were found to be very common in women and men with IC (interstitial cystitis)/painful bladder syndrome and chronic prostatitis/CPP syndrome, respectively (Fitzgerald et al 2009).

It appears that somatic abnormalities may be the primary abnormality in at least some patients and secondary in others, but in either situation it is suggested that they should be identified and treated.

In a study to assess the value of combined connective tissue manipulation (CTM) and trigger point deactivation, in cases of urologic CPP, Fitzgerald et al. (2009) report:

> Patients randomized to the treatment group underwent CTM to all body wall tissues of the abdominal wall, back, buttocks and thighs that clinically were found to contain connective tissue abnormalities and/or painful myofascial trigger points. CTM was applied bilaterally to the patient in the prone position, posteriorly from inferior thoracic level 10 to the popliteal crease. This was done until a texture change was noted in the treated tissue layer. Manual techniques such as trigger point barrier release, with or without active contraction or reciprocal inhibition, manual stretching of the trigger point region, and myofascial release, were used on the identified trigger points.

The group receiving skilled CTM and myofascial therapy had a significantly higher response rate than the group receiving massage.

Trigger point deactivation and slow stretching (Travell & Simons 1999, Cox 2005)

Travell & Simons described (1983, 1999) variations on their basic trigger point release approach:

- Ischaemic compression (1983): Pressure is applied to the point lying in a fully lengthened muscle. The pressure should be sufficient to maintain pain at a level of between 5 and 7 – where 10 is the maximum that can be tolerated, until pain eases by around 50–75% – or until 90 seconds have passed.
- Trigger point release (1999): In this version the muscle is partially lengthened and pressure is to the first perception of a tissue barrier, ideally with no sign of discomfort. Pressure is maintained until a sense of a release of the characteristic taut band is noted, or until 90 seconds have passed.
- Other versions exist including pulsed ischaemic compression (Chaitow 1994) in which a trigger point in a partially lengthened muscle received 5 seconds of compression, sufficient to induce pain at level 7 (numerical pain rating scale) – followed by 2 seconds of no pressure – repeated for up to 90 seconds or until local or referred pain changes are reported or palpated.

In these, and all other variants, it is considered essential to stretch the muscle housing the trigger point towards or to its normal resting length, subsequent to the pressure deactivation.

Diaphragm

Two manual methods to encourage release of excessive tone in the diaphragm are described here; one is based on neuromuscular technique (NMT) methodology and the other on positional release (PRT) methods.

NMT for diaphragm (Chaitow 2007, Chaitow & DeLany 2008)

- The patient is supine with the knees flexed and feet resting flat on the table. This position will relax the overlying abdominal fibres and allow better access to the diaphragm attachments.

- It is suggested that the upper rectus abdominis fibres should be treated before the diaphragm.
- This treatment of the diaphragm is contraindicated for patients with liver and gallbladder disease or if the area is significantly tender or swollen.
- The practitioner stands at the level of the abdomen contralateral to the side being treated.
- The fingers, thumbs or a combination of thumb of one hand and fingers of the other may be used to extremely gently insinuate contact beneath the lower border of the rib cage, directed partly cephalad and obliquely laterally, until a barrier is noted.
- As the patient exhales, the fingers penetrate further.
- As the patient inhales the diaphragm attachments press against the treating digit(s), forcing these caudally, unless this pressure is resisted – which it should be.
- When penetration appears to be as far as possible, the finger (thumb) tips are directed toward the inner surface of the ribs where static pressure or gentle friction is applied to the diaphragm's attachment.
- The treatment may be applied on full exhalation or at half-breath and is repeated to as much of the internal costal margins as can be reached.
- While it is uncertain as to the degree to which diaphragm's fibres can be reached by this exercise, the connective tissue associated with its costal attachment is probably influenced.
- Simons et al. (1999) describe a similar procedure, which ends in an anterior lifting of the rib cage (instead of friction or static pressure) to stretch the fibres of the diaphragm.

PRT for diaphragm

- The patient is supine and the practitioner stands at waist level facing cephalad and places the hands over the lower thoracic structures with the fingers along the lower rib shafts.
- Treating the structure being palpated as a cylinder, the hands test the preference this cylinder has to rotate around its central axis, one way and then the other. 'Does the lower thorax rotate more easily to the right or the left?'
- Once the rotational preference has been established, with the lower thorax held in its preferred rotation direction, the preference to sidebend one way or the other is evaluated. 'Does the lower thorax sideflex more easily to the right or the left?'
- Once these two pieces of information have been established, the combined positions of ease (rotation and side-flexion), are introduced, and maintained for between 30 and 90 seconds, before slowly restoring the structures to neutral.
- Re-evaluation should demonstrate a marked change in previously restricted motion.

Intercostals

There are many manual therapy approaches to release of excessive tone in the intercostal muscles. One, based on neuromuscular technique methodology, is described here.

NMT for the intercostal muscles

Fingertip or thumb glides, as described below, are applied to the intercostal spaces of the posterior, lateral and anterior thorax for initial examination as to tenderness and rib alignment. On the anterior thorax, all breast tissue (including the nipple area on men) is avoided with the intercostal treatment.

- The intercostal areas are commonly extremely sensitive and care must be taken not to distress the patient by using inappropriate pressure.
- In most instances the intercostal spaces on the contralateral side will be treated using the finger stroke.
- The (well-trimmed) thumb tip or a finger tip should be run along both surfaces of the rib margins, as well as along the muscle tissue itself.
- In this way the fibres of the internal and external intercostal muscles will receive adequate assessment contacts.
- When there is over-approximation of the ribs, a simple stroke along the intercostal space may be all that is possible until a degree of rib and thoracic normalization has taken place, allowing greater access.
- The tip of a finger (supported by a neighbouring digit) is placed in one intercostal space at a time, close to the mid-axillary line (patient prone or supine), and gently but firmly brought around the curve of the trunk toward the midline, combing for signs of dysfunction.
- The probing digit feels for contracted or congested tissues, in which trigger points might be located.
- When an area of contraction is noted, firm pressure toward the centre of the body is applied

to elicit a response from the patient ('Does it hurt? Does it radiate or refer? If so, to where?').
- Trigger points noted during the assessment may be treated using standard manual protocols.
- Caution: Dry needling or acupuncture to deactivate trigger points in the intercostal spaces is not recommended due to high risk of penetration of the lungs.

Psoas

Strategies for reducing excessive tone, and deactivating trigger points, in psoas are to be found in Chapter 14. There are a variety of alternative measures, and one, a muscle energy procedure, is described here.

MET for psoas (Grieve 1994, Chaitow 2006)

- The patient is supine with the buttocks at the very end of the table, non-treated leg fully flexed at hip and knee, and either held in that state by the patient or by the practitioner.
- The practitioner stands at the foot of the table and the leg on the affected side (shortened/hypertonic psoas) is placed so that the medioplantar aspect of the foot rests on the practitioner's knee or shin (Figure 9.9).

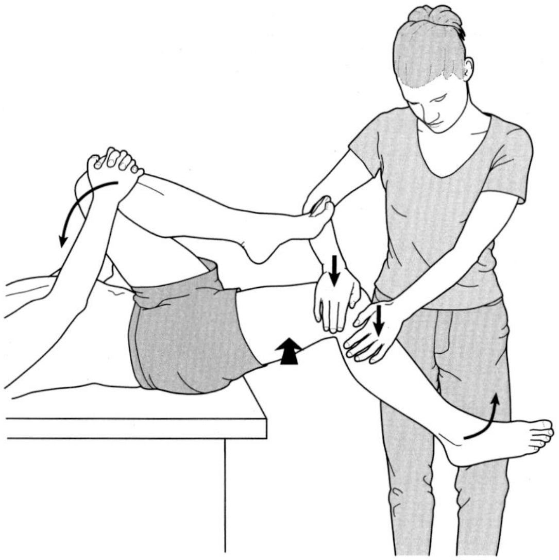

Figure 9.9 • Grieve's position during application of muscle energy technique prior to stretching psoas. (See text for full description)

- The leg should be placed so that the hip flexors, including psoas, are in a mid-range position, not at their barrier.
- The practitioner should request the patient to use *a small degree of effort* to *externally rotate the leg* and, at the same time, *to flex the hip*.
- The practitioner resists both efforts and an isometric contraction of the psoas and associated muscles therefore takes place.
- After a ~7-second isometric contraction, and complete relaxation of effort, the thigh should, on an exhalation, be taken without force into slight stretch. This stretch position is held there for 30 seconds.
- Repeat once more.

Quadratus lumborum

Strategies for reducing excessive tone, and deactivating trigger points, in quadratus lumborum are to be found in Chapter 14.

A PRT procedure, is described here.

PRT for quadratus lumborum

- The patient is prone and the practitioner stands on the side contralateral to that being treated.
- The tender points for quadratus lie close to the transverse processes of L1–5. Medial pressure (toward the spine) is usually required to access the tender points, which should be pressed lightly as pain in the area is often exquisite.
- Once the most sensitive tender point has been identified this should be lightly compressed and the patient asked to register the discomfort as a '10'.
- While the practitioner maintains the monitoring contact on the tender point, the patient is asked to externally rotate, abduct and flex the hip on the side being treated to a position that reduces the 'score' significantly.
- The limb, flexed at hip and knee, should lie supported on the treatment table
- The patient turns his head ipsilaterally and slides his ipsilateral hand beneath the flexed thigh, easing the hand very slowly toward the foot of the treatment table, until a further reduction in the pain score is noted.
- This combination of hip flexion/abduction/ rotation and arm movement effectively laterally

flexes the lumbar spine, so slackening quadratus fibres.

- If further reduction is required in the pain score (i.e. if it is not already at '3' or less), the practitioner's caudad hand should apply gentle cephalad pressure from the ipsilateral ischial tuberosity.
- This final compressive force usually reduces the score to '0'. This position should be held for at least 30, and ideally up to 90, seconds before a slow return to the starting position.

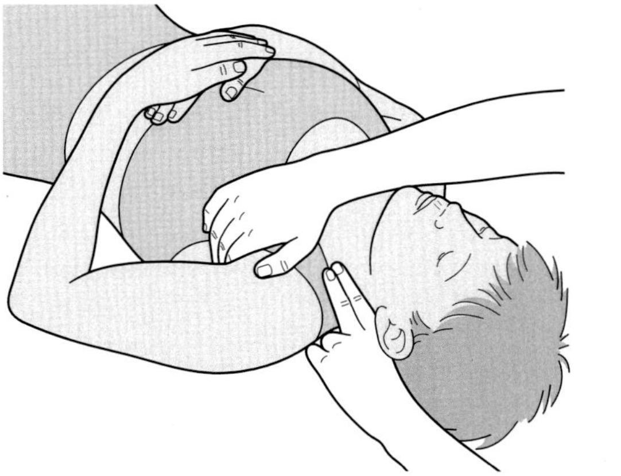

Figure 9.10 • Positional release of scalenes. Therapist's left hand monitors area of tenderness in scalenes as right hand crowds the tissues in cephalad direction, until sensitivity drops by at least 70%. This is 'ease' position and is held for up to 90 seconds. (See text for fuller description)

Scalenes (and other upper fixators of the shoulder/accessory breathing muscles)

The scalene and other upper fixators of the shoulder/accessory breathing muscles (e.g. levator scapula, upper trapezius, sternocleidomastoid, pectorals) are amenable to soft tissue manipulation methods. PRT methods are described here. Muscle energy release methods are also recommended; see video illustrations of "MET release of scalenes" and "MET release of pectoralis major".

PRT for scalenes

The tender points relating to the scalene muscles lie on the transverse processes (sometimes on the very tips of these) of C2–6.

- The patient lies supine and the practitioner sits at the head of the table, palpating a tender point with sufficient pressure to allow the discomfort to be ascribed a value of no more than 7/10 (where 10 is extreme pain on a VAS).
- The patient is then told, for the purpose of the technique, to change this value to '10'.
- For the anterior and medial scalene, the head and neck are flexed and side-flexed toward the affected side.
- For the posterior scalene a neutral position may be employed.
- The head and neck may be supported on a small cushion or rolled towel.
- The non-palpating hand engages the 2nd and 3rd ribs close to the axilla and eases them cephalad, until the reported discomfort reduces from '10' to '3' or less (Figure 9.10)
- This is held for 30–90 seconds, after which a slow release of the tissues being held is allowed.

Thoracic and costal mobilization

A wide range of mobilization and manipulation approaches exist by means of which restricted thoracic spine and rib structures can be encouraged towards more normal function.

These include high-velocity, low-amplitude thrust techniques, MET, PRT and general mobilization methods.

An effective MET procedure for mobilizing the thoracic spine is described below (Lenehan et al. 2003).

MET for thoracic spine

- The patient is seated on a treatment table, with arms folded, hands on shoulders, elbows forward.
- The practitioner stands behind and to the side, one hand cupping the patient's elbows, and the other palpating or stabilizing the thoracic spine.
- The ability of the trunk to rotate left and right is assessed.
- It is then taken into rotation, to its *easy end of range*, in the direction of greatest restriction.
- In that position the patient is asked to attempt, using no more than 20% of available strength, to side flex (either direction) for 5 seconds while the practitioner prevents any movement.

- Following this isometric contraction the patient should be taken into a new easy end of range of rotation – commonly (Lenehan et al. 2003) around 10% further than previously.
- This process is repeated once more, in the same direction, and is then performed with the trunk rotated in the opposite direction.

Scar tissue release

- Kobesova et al. (2007) suggest that scars may develop adhesive properties that compromise tissue tensioning, altering proprioceptive input, behaving in much the same way as active myofascial trigger points. It is suggested that faulty afferent input can result in disturbed efferent output leading to, for example, protective postural patterns, increased neurovascular activity and pain syndromes. The term *active* scar is designated to describe the ongoing additional neural activity associated with adhesive scar formations.
- Lewit & Olsanska (2004) reported a series of 51 such cases in which postsurgical scar tissue was found to be the primary pain generator for a multitude of locomotor system pain syndromes. On palpation (light stretching) of dysfunctional tissues the patient commonly reports sensations of 'burning, prickling, or lightning-like jabs of pain'.
- Valouchova & Lewit (2009) report that active scars in the abdomen and pelvis commonly restrict back flexion, which the patient feels as low back pain.
- Treatment methods are simple, involving 'mini-myofascial release' methods – where skin alongside scars is treated initially, with subsequent attention to deeper layers. Treatment involves 'engaging the pathologic barrier and waiting; after a short delay, a release gradually occurs until the normal barrier is restored'.

Myofascial release (myofascial induction)

King (2010) notes that myofascial release (MFR) is 'a system of diagnosis and treatment first described by A.T. Still, and his early students, which involves continual palpatory feedback to achieve release of myofascial tissues'.

- Direct MFR: a myofascial tissue restrictive barrier is engaged for the myofascial tissues and the tissue is loaded with constant force, until tissue release occurs.
- Indirect MFR: the dysfunctional tissues are guided along the path of least resistance, until free movement is achieved (Educational Council on Osteopathic Principles 2009).

Myofascial induction is a simultaneous evaluation and treatment process using tri-dimensional movements of sustained pressures, applied to myofascial structures in order to release restrictions. The term 'induction' is preferred because clinicians do not passively stretch the system but only apply an initial tension or compression force and follow the facilitating movement. The aim of the process is the recovery of motion amplitude, force and coordination (Pilat 2009).

Study

- Weiss (2001) used MFR in patients with CPP and found that 70% had marked or moderate improvement in symptoms after treatment. He found that pelvic floor therapy decreased neurogenic triggers, decreased central nervous system sensitivity, and alleviated pain.

Conclusions

This chapter has offered a wide-ranging description of the intersection of breathing and pelvic pain, with therapeutic suggestions in the areas of manual therapy and breathing training. Both approaches work with structure in an attempt to improve function. In the physical realm, configurations of muscles, joints, bones, fascia and circulation comprise 'structure' and are influenced by genetics, disease and injury. The 'function' part includes how well body structures can carry out the demand for patterns of use, misuse and disuse. Improving function therapeutically can feed back into structure, to a degree (muscle strengthening, improving breathing and movement patterns, etc.).

The body of course is animated by a mind that determines how the body is used, and in this realm we can discern a roughly parallel division into structure and function.

- 'Structure' would include temperament and enduring personality traits whether genetically based or formed early in life: chronic depression, anxiety, anger, tendency to take risks, or predisposition to ignore body warnings.
- 'Function' denotes the behaviour following from habits and personality traits: examples are the persistent slump of depression, the tense rigid body and clenched jaw of anger, and the hyperventilation of one prone to panic.

Priorities and choices about body use and misuse, especially outside the parameters of what the structure permits, will ultimately lead to behaviour that undoes what any therapeutic strategy can do, unless some attention is paid to psychological and behavioural factors.

Chapter 12 examines the research and techniques of biofeedback as a way to improve function by providing precise information about body changes, allowing the person to expand self-influence.

Chapter 4 covers the area of psychophysiology and pelvic pain in some detail.

This chapter has described the structural connections between the pelvic floor and the respiratory diaphragm and proposed that disorders of breathing need to be addressed in the patient with CPP. The correction of breathing patterns can be seen to influence physical, psychological and emotional factors that may be contributing to the chronic pain state. The next chapter explores in further detail how pain can be modulated by specific chemical and neurological changes, demonstrating the effect of various biofeedback systems to modulate the pain response.

References

Anderson, R., 2002. Management of chronic prostatitis – chronic pelvic pain syndrome. Urol. Clin. North Am. 29 (1), 235–239.

Anderson, R.U., Sawyer, T., Wise, D., et al., 2009. Painful myofascial trigger points and pain sites in men with chronic prostatitis/chronic pelvic pain syndrome. J. Urol. 182 (6), 2753–2758.

Anraku, M., Shargall, Y., 2009. Surgical conditions of the diaphragm: anatomy and physiology. Thorac. Surg. Clin. 19, 419–429.

Appelhans, B.M., Luecken, L.J., 2008. Heart rate variability and pain: associations of two interrelated homeostatic processes. Biol. Psychol. 77 (2), 174–182.

Balaban, C., Thayer, J., 2001. Neurological bases for balance–anxiety links. J. Anxiety Disord. 15 (1–2), 53–79.

Banzett, R.B., Lanzing, R.W., Brown, R., Topulos, G.P., Yagar, D., Steel, S.M., 1990. Air hunger' from increased PCO_2 persists after complete neuromuscular block in humans. Respir. Physiol. 81, 1–17.

Beales, D., 2004. "I've got this pain ..." Hum. Givens J. 11 (4), 16–18.

Bernardon, M., Limone, A., Businelli, C., 2009. Diabetic ketoacidosis in pregnancy. Gazz. Med. Ital. Arch. Sci. Med. 168 (1), 45–49.

Bockenhauer, S., Chen, H., Julliard, K., et al., 2007. Measuring thoracic excursion: reliability of the cloth tape measure technique. J. Am. Osteopath. Assoc. 107, 191–196.

Botella De Maglia, J., Real Soriano, R., Compte Torrero, L., 2008. Arterial oxygen saturation during ascent of a mountain higher than 8,000 meters. Med. Intensiva 32 (6), 277–281.

Bradley, D., 1998. Hyperventilation Syndrome/Breathing Pattern Disorders. Tandem Press, Auckland, NZ.

Bradley, D., 2001. Self-help for hyperventilation syndrome. Hunter House, Alameda, CA, p. 70.

Brashear, R., 1983. Hyperventilation syndrome. Lung 161 (1), 257–273.

Brotto, L., Klein, C., Gorzalka, B., 2009. Laboratory induced hyperventilation differentiates female sexual arousal disorder subtypes. Arch. Sex. Behav. 38 (4), 463–475.

Brugger, A., 2000. Lehrbuch der Funktionellen Storungen des Bewegungssystems. Brugger-Verlag, Zollikon Benglen.

Burkill, G., Healy, J., 2000. Anatomy of the retroperitoneum. Imaging 12 (1), 10–20.

Buteyko, K., 1990. Buteyko Method : Experience of Application in Medical Practice. Patriot, Moscow.

Butler, D., 2000. The Sensitive Nervous System. Noigroup Publications, Adelaide, p. 89.

Cappo, B., Holmes, D., 1984. Utility of prolonged respiratory exhalation for reducing physiological and psychological arousal in non-threatening and threatening situations. J. Psychosom. Res. 28 (4), 265–273.

Carriere, B., 2006. Interdependence of posture and the pelvic floor. In: Carriere, B., Markel Feldt, C. (Eds.), The pelvic floor. Thieme, New York, p. 68, 76.

Carriero, J., 2003. An osteopathic approach to children. Churchill Livingstone, Edinburgh.

Celotto, A.C., Capellini, V.K., Baldo, C.F., 2008. Effects of acid-base imbalance on vascular reactivity. Braz. J. Med. Biol. Res. 41 (6), 439–445.

Chaitow, L., 1994. INIT in treatment of pain and trigger points. Br. J. Osteopathy XIII, 17–21.

Chaitow, L., 2004. Breathing pattern disorders, motor control, and low back pain. J. Osteopath. Med. 7 (1), 34–41.

Chaitow, L., 2006. Muscle Energy Techniques, third ed. Churchill Livingstone, Edinburgh.

Chaitow, L., 2007. Chronic pelvic pain: Pelvic floor problems, sacroiliac dysfunction and the trigger point connections. J. Bodyw. Mov. Ther. 11 (4), 327–339.

Chaitow, L., DeLany, J., 2008. Clinical Application of Neuromuscular Techniques. vol 1. second ed. The Upper Body, Churchill Livingstone, Edinburgh.

Chaitow, L., Bradley, D., Gilbert, C., 2002. Multidisciplinary Approaches to Breathing Pattern Disorders. Churchill Livingstone, Edinburgh.

Chalaye, P., Goffaux, P., Lafrenaye, S., Marchand, S., 2009. Respiratory effects on experimental heat pain and cardiac activity. Pain Med. 10 (8), 1334–1340.

Chaulier, K., Chalumeau, S., Ber, C.E., 2007. Metabolic acidosis in a context of acute severe asthma. Ann. Fr. Anesth. Reanim. 26 (4), 352–355.

Cimino, R., Farella, M., Michelotti, A., 2000. Does the ovarian cycle influence the pressure-pain threshold of the masticatory muscles in symptom-free women? J. Orofac. Pain 14 (2), 105–111.

Conway, A.V., Freeman, L.J., Nixon, P.G.F., 1988. Hypnotic examination of trigger factors in the hyperventilation syndrome. Am. J. Clin. Hypn. 30, 296–304.

Courtney, R., Greenwood, K.M., 2009. Preliminary investigation of a measure of dysfunctional breathing symptoms: the Self Evaluation of Breathing Questionnaire (SEBQ). Int. J. Osteopath. Med. 12, 121–127.

Courtney, R., van Dixhoorn, J., et al., 2008. Evaluation of breathing pattern: comparison of a manual assessment of respiratory motion (MARM) and respiratory induction plethysmography. Appl. Psychophysiol. Biofeedback 33, 91–100.

Courtney, R., Cohen, M., Reece, J., 2009. Comparison of the Manual Assessment of Respiratory Motion (MARM) and the Hi Lo Breathing Assessment in determining a simulated breathing pattern. Int. J. Osteopath. Med. 12 (2009), 86–91.

Courtney, R., Greenwood, K.M., Cohen, M., 2011. Relationship between measures of breathing functionality and dimensions of dysfunctional breathing. J. Bodyw. Mov. Ther. 15 (1), 24–34.

Cox, J., Bakkum, B., 2005. Possible generators of retrotrochanteric gluteal and thigh pain: the gemelli-obturator internus complex. J. Manipulative Physiol. Ther. 28, 534–538.

Cresswell, A.G., Oddsson, L., Thorstensson, A., 1994. The influence of sudden perturbations on trunk muscle activity and intra-abdominal pressure while standing. Exp. Brain Res. 98, 336–341.

Cusi, M., 2010. Paradigm for assessment and treatment of SIJ mechanical dysfunction. J. Bodyw. Mov. Ther. 14 (2), 152–161.

Damas-Mora, J., Davies, L., Taylor, W., et al., 1980. Menstrual respiratory changes and symptoms. Br. J. Psychiatry 136, 492–497.

Debreczeni, R., Amrein, I., Kamondi, A., et al., 2009. Hypocapnia induced by involuntary hyperventilation during mental arithmetic reduces cerebral blood flow velocity. Tohoku J. Exp. Med. 217 (2), 147–154.

Dempsey, J., Sheel, A., St. Croix, C., 2002. Respiratory influences on sympathetic vasomotor outflow in humans. Respir. Physiol. Neurobiol. 130 (1), 3–20.

Downey, L.V., Zun, L.S., 2009. The effects of deep breathing training on pain management in the emergency department. South Med. J. 102 (7), 688–692.

Educational Council on Osteopathic Principles (ECOP), 2009. Glossary of Osteopathic Terminology. American Association of Colleges of Osteopathic Medicine, Washington, DC.

Evans, D., Lum, L., Dart, A., 1980. Chest pain with normal coronary arteries. Lancet 315 (8163), 311.

Faling, L., 1995. Controlled breathing techniques and chest physical therapy in chronic obstructive pulmonary disease. In: Casabur, R. (Ed.), Principles and Practices of Pulmonary Therapy. WB Saunders, Philadelphia.

Fall, M., Baranowski, A.P., Elneil, S., et al., 2010. Guidelines on Chronic Pelvic Pain. European Association of Urology. Eur. Urol. 57, 35–48.

Fass, R., Fullerton, S., Naliboff, B., et al., 1998. Sexual dysfunction in patients with irritable bowel syndrome and non-ulcer dyspepsia. Digestion 59, 79–85.

FitzGerald, M.P., Kotarinos, R., 2003. Rehabilitation of the short pelvic floor. II: Treatment of the patient with the short pelvic floor. Int. Urogynecol. J. Pelvic Floor Dysfunction 14 (4), 269–275.

FitzGerald, M.P., Anderson, R.U., Potts, J., et al., 2009. Randomised multicenter feasibility trial of myofascial physical therapy for the treatment of urological chronic pelvic pain syndromes. J. Urol. 182, 570–580.

Flink, I.K., Nicholas, M.K., Boersma, K., Linton, S.J., 2009. Reducing the threat value of chronic pain: A preliminary replicated single-case study of interoceptive exposure versus distraction in six individuals with chronic back pain. Behav. Res. Ther. 47 (8), 721–728.

Ford, M., Camilleri, M., Hanson, R., 1995. Hyperventilation, central autonomic control, and colonic tone in humans. Gut 37, 499–504.

Freeman, L.J., Nixon, P., 1985. Chest pain and the hyperventilation syndrome - Some aetiological considerations. Postgrad. Med. J. 61 (721), 957–961.

Fry, R.P., Beard, R.W., Crisp, A.H., McGuigan, S., 1997. Sociopsychological factors in women with chronic pelvic pain with and without pelvic venous congestion. J. Psychosom. Res. 42 (1), 71–85.

Gardner, W., 1996. The pathophysiology of hyperventilation disorders. Chest 109, 516–534.

Garland, W., 1994. Somatic changes in hyperventilating subject. Presentation at International Society for the Advancement of Respiratory Psychophysiology Congress, Paris.

Gibbons, S.G.T., 2001. The model of psoas major stability function. In: Proceedings of 1st International Conference on Movement Dysfunction, Sept 21–23, Edinburgh, Scotland.

Gilbert, C., 1998. Emotional sources of dysfunctional breathing. J. Bodyw. Mov. Ther. 2, 224–230.

Grewar, H., McLean, L., 2008. The integrated continence system: A manual therapy approach to the treatment of stress urinary incontinence. Man. Ther. 13, 375–386.

Grieve, G., 1994. The masqueraders. In: Boyling, J.D., Palastanga, N. (Eds.). Grieve's modern manual therapy. second ed. Churchill Livingstone, Edinburgh.

Grossman, P., De Swart, J.C.G., Defares, P.B., 1985. A controlled study of breathing therapy for treatment of hyperventilation syndrome. J. Psychosom. Res. 29 (1), 49–58.

Haahtela, T., Tamminen, K., Kava, T., et al., 2009. Thirteen-year follow-up of early intervention with an inhaled corticosteroid in patients with asthma. J. Allergy Clin. Immunol. 124 (6), 1180.

Han, J., Gayan-Ramirez, G., Dekhuijzen, R., 1993. Respiratory function of the rib cage muscles. Eur. Respir. J. 6 (5), 722–728.

Haugstad, G.K., Haugstad, T.S., Kirste, U.M., 2006a. Posture, movement patterns, and body awareness in women with chronic pelvic pain. J. Psychosom. Res. 61 (5), 637–644.

Haugstad, G.K., Haugstad, T.S., Kirste, U.M., et al., 2006b. Mensendieck somatocognitive therapy as treatment approach to chronic pelvic pain: results of a randomized controlled intervention study. Am. J. Obstet. Gynecol. 194, 1303–1310.

Haugstad, G.K., Haugstad, T.S., Kirste, U.M., et al., 2008. Continuing improvement of chronic pelvic pain in women after short-term Mensendieck somatocognitive therapy: results of a 1-year follow-up study. Am. J. Obstet. Gynecol. 199, 615.e1–615.e8.

Hetrick, D., Ciol, M., Rothman, I., 2003. Musculoskeletal dysfunction in men with chronic pelvic pain syndrome type III: A case-control study. J. Urol. 170 (3), 828–831.

Hides, J.A., Richardson, C.A., Jull, G.A., 1996. Multifidus muscle recovery is not automatic following resolution of acute first episode low back pain. Spine 21, 2763–2769.

Hirano, Y., Ozasa, Y., Yamamoto, T., et al., 2001. Hyperventilation and cold-pressor stress echocardiography for noninvasive diagnosis of coronary artery spasm. J. Am. Soc. Echocardiogr. (6), 626–633.

Hochstetter, J., et al., 2005. An investigation into the immediate impact of breathlessness management on the breathless patient: randomised controlled trial. Physiotherapy 91, 178–185.

Hodges, P., 2004. Abdominal mechanism and support of the lumbar spine and pelvis. In: Richardson, C., Hodges, P., Hides, J. Therapeutic exercise for lumbopelvic stabilisation: A motor control approach for the treatment and prevention of low back pain. second ed. Churchill Livingstone, Edinburgh.

Hodges, P.W., Richardson, C.A., 1996. Inefficient muscular stabilisation of the lumbar spine associated with low back pain: a motor control evaluation of transversus abdominis. Spine 21 (22), 2640–2650.

Hodges, P.W., Richardson, C.A., 1998. Delayed postural contraction of transversus abdominis in low back pain associated with movement of the lower limb. J. Spinal Disorders 11 (1), 46–56.

Hodges, P.W., Richardson, C.A., 1999. Altered trunk muscle recruitment in people with low back pain with upper limb movements at different speeds. Arch. Phys. Med. Rehabil. 80 (9), 1005–1012.

Hodges, P., Sapsford, R., Pengel, L., 2007. Postural and respiratory functions of the PFMs. Neurourol. Urodyn. 26 (3), 362–371.

Hodges, P.W., Heinjnen, I., Gandevia, S.C., 2001. Postural activity of the diaphragm is reduced in humans when respiratory demand increases. J. Physiol. 537 (3), 999.

Hu, H., Meijer, O., van Dieën, J., 2010. Muscle activity during the active straight leg raise (ASLR), and the effects of a pelvic belt on the ASLR and on treadmill walking. J. Biomech. 43 (3), 532–539.

Hudson, A., Gandevia, S., Butler, J., 2007. The effect of lung volume on the co-ordinated recruitment of scalene and sternomastoid muscles in humans. J. Physiol. 584 (1), 261–270.

Hurwitz, B.E., 1981. The effect of inspiration and posture on cardiac rate and T-wave amplitude during apneic breathholding in man. Psychophysiology 18, 179–180 (abstract).

Janda, V., Frank, C., Liebenson, C., 2007. Evaluation of muscle imbalance. In: Liebenson, C. (Ed.). Rehabilitation of the Spine: A Practitioner's Manual, second ed. Lippincott/Williams & Wilkins, Baltimore.

Jensen, D., Duffin, J., Lam, Y.M., 2008. Physiological mechanisms of hyperventilation during human pregnancy. Respir. Physiol. Neurobiol. 161 (1), 76–86.

Jones, R., 2001. Pelvic floor muscle rehabilitation. Urol. News 5 (5), 2–4.

Kapandji, I.A., 1974. The physiology of the joints, vol. III: The trunk and the vertebral column, second ed. Churchill Livingstone, Edinburgh.

Kapreli, E., Vourazanis, E., Strimpakos, N., 2008. Neck pain causes respiratory dysfunction. Med. Hypotheses. 70 (5), 1009–1013.

Key, J., 2010. The pelvic crossed syndromes: A reflection of imbalanced function in the myofascial envelope; a further exploration of Janda's work. J. Bodyw. Mov. Ther. 14 (3), 299–301.

Key, J., et al., 2007. A model of movement dysfunction provides a classification system guiding diagnosis and therapeutic care in spinal pain and related musculo-skeletal syndromes: a paradigm shift. J. Bodyw. Mov. Ther. 12 (2), 105–120.

King, H., 2010. Osteopathic manipulative therapies and fascia. In: Chaitow, L., Findley, Huijing, Schleip, (Eds.), Fascia in Manual Therapy. Elsevier. In Press.

Kitabchi, A.E., Umpierrez, G.E., Murphy, M., et al., 2006. Hyperglycemic crises in adult patients with diabetes: a consensus statement from the American Diabetes Association. Diabetes Care 29 (12), 2739–2748.

Kobesova, A., et al., M 2007. Twenty-year-old pathogenic "active" postsurgical scar: a case study of a patient with persistent right lower quadrant pain. J. Manipulative Physiol. Ther. 30 (3), 234–238.

Kuligowska, E., Deeds 3rd, L., Lu 3rd, K., 2005. Pelvic pain: overlooked and underdiagnosed gynecologic conditions. Radiographics 25 (1), 3–20.

Lansing, R.W., 2000. The perception of respiratory work and effort can be independent of the perception of air hunger. Am. J. Respir. Crit. Care Med. 162, 1690–1696.

Lee, D., 2007. An integrated approach for the management of low back and pelvic girdle pain. In: Vleeming, A., Mooney, V., Stoekart, R. (Eds.), Movement stability & lumbopelvic pain. Churchill Livingstone/Elsevier, Edinburgh, pp. 593–620.

Lee, D., Lee, L., 2004. Stress urinary incontinence – a consequence of failed load transfer through the pelvis? Presented at the 5th World Interdisciplinary Congress on Low Back and Pelvic Pain, Melbourne, November 2004.

Lee, D., Lee, L.J., McLaughlin, L., 2008. Stability, continence and breathing: The role of fascia following pregnancy and delivery. J. Bodyw. Mov. Ther. 12, 333–348.

Lenehan, K., Fryer, G., McLaughlin, P., 2003. The effect of muscle energy technique on gross trunk range of motion. J. Osteopath. Med. 6 (1), 13–18.

Levitsky, M.G., 2003. Pulmonary Physiology, sixth ed. McGraw-Hill, Toronto, ON.

Lewit, K., 1980. Relationship of faulty respiration to posture, with clinical implications. J. Am. Osteopath. Assoc. 79, 525–528.

Lewit, K., 1999. Manipulative therapy in rehabilitation of the motor system, third ed. Butterworths, London.

Lewit, K., Olšanská, Š., 2004. Clinical importance of active scars as a cause of myofascial pain. J. Manipulative Physiol. Ther. 27 (6), 399–402.

Liebenson, C., 2006. J. Bodyw. Mov. Ther. 10, 65–70.

Lum, L., 1984. Editorial: Hyperventilation and anxiety states. J. R. Soc. Med. (January), 1–4.

Lum, L., 1996. Treatment difficulties and failures: causes and clinical management. Biol. Psychol. 43 (3), 24.

Lum, L.C., 1975. Hyperventilation: the tip and the iceberg. J. Psychosom. Res. 19 (5-6), 375–383.

Masubuchi, Y., Abe, T., Yokoba, M., 2001. Relation between neck accessory inspiratory muscle electromyographic activity and lung volume. Journal Japanese Respiratory Society 39 (4), 244–249.

Mattsson, M., Wikman, M., Dahlgren, L., et al., 1997. Body awareness therapy with sexually abused women Part 1: Description of a treatment modality. J. Bodyw. Mov. Ther. 1 (5), 280–288.

Mattsson, M., Wikman, M., Dahlgren, L., et al., 2000. Physiotherapy as empowerment – treating women with chronic pelvic pain. Advanced Physiotherapy 2, 125–143.

Mazur, M., Furgała, A., Jabłoński, K., et al., 2007. Dysfunction of the autonomic nervous system activity is responsible for gastric myoelectric disturbances in the irritable bowel syndrome patients. J. Physiol. Pharmacol. 58 (Suppl. 3), 131–139.

McLaughlin, L., 2009. Breathing evaluation and retraining in body work. J. Bodyw. Mov. Ther. 13 (3), 276–282.

McLaughlin, L., Goldsmith, C.H., 2007. Altered respiration in a case series of low back/pelvic pain patients. In: 6th Interdisciplinary World Congress on Low Back & Pelvic Pain, November 2007, Barcelona.

Mehling, W.E., Hamel, K.A., et al., 2005. Randomized, controlled trial of breath therapy for patients with chronic low-back pain. Altern. Ther. Health Med. 11 (4), 44–52.

Mens, J.M., Vleeming, A., Snijders, C.J., 2001. Reliability and validity of the active straight leg raise test in posterior pelvic pain since pregnancy. Spine 26 (10), 1167–1171.

Montenegro, M.L., Vasconcelos, E.C., Canidido Dos Reis, F.J., et al., 2008. Physical therapy in the management of women with chronic pelvic pain. Int. J. Clin. Pract. 62 (2), 174–175.

Moore, J., Kennedy, S., 2000. Causes of chronic pelvic pain. Baillieres Clin. Obstet. Gynaecol. 14 (3), 389–402.

Newell, R., 2005. Anatomy of the post-laryngeal airways, lungs and diaphragm. Surgery 23 (11), 393–397.

Nijenhuis, E.R.S., 2004. Somatoform dissociation: phenomena, measurement and theoretical issues. WW Norton & Company, NewYork.

Nishino, T., Shimoyama, N., Ide, T., et al., 1999. Experimental pain augments experimental dyspnea, but not vice versa in human volunteers. Anesthesiology 91 (6), 1633–1638.

Nixon, P., Andrews, J., 1996. A study of anaerobic threshold in chronic fatigue syndrome (CFS). Biol. Psychol. 43 (3), 264.

O'Sullivan, P., Beales, D., 2007. Changes in pelvic floor and diaphragm kinematics and respiratory patterns in subjects with sacroiliac joint pain following a motor learning intervention: A case series. Man. Ther. 12, 209–218.

O'Sullivan, P., Beales, D., Beetham, J., et al., 2002. Altered motor control strategies in subjects with sacroiliac joint pain during the active straight-leg-raise test. Spine 27 (1), E1–E8.

Olsen, A., Rao, S., 2001. Clinical neurophysiology and electrodiagnostic testing of the pelvic floor. Gastroenterol. Clin. North Am. 30, 33–54, v–vi.

Pacia, E.B., Aldrich, T.K., 1998. Assessment of diaphragm function. Chest Surg. Clin. North Am. 8 (2), 225–236.

Pel, J., Spoor, C., Pool-Goudzwaard, A., et al., 2008. Biomechanical analysis of reducing sacroiliac joint shear load by optimization of pelvic muscle and ligament forces. Ann. Biomed. Eng. 36 (3), 415–424.

Perri, M., Halford, E., 2004. Pain and faulty breathing: a pilot study. J. Bodyw. Mov. Ther. 8 (4), 297–306.

Pilat, A., 2009. Myofascial induction approaches for headache. In: Fernández-de-las- Peñas, C., Arendt-Nielsen, L., Gerwin, R.D. (Eds.), Tension Type and Cervicogenic Headache: pathophysiology, diagnosis and treatment. Jones & Bartlett Publishers, Boston.

Pleidelová, J., Balá!iová, M., Porubská, V., 2002. Frequency of scalenal muscle disorders. Rehabilitacia 35 (4), 203–207.

Pool-Goudzwaard, A., van Dijke, G., van Gurp, M., 2004. Contribution of PFMs to stiffness of the pelvic ring. Clin. Biomech. 19 (6), 564–571.

Prather, H., Dugan, S., Fitzgerald, C., et al., 2009. Review of anatomy, evaluation, and treatment of musculoskeletal pelvic floor pain in women. Phy. Med. Rehabil. 1 (4), 346–358.

Prior, A., Whorwell, P., Faragher, E., 1989. Irritable bowel syndrome in the gynaecological clinic. Survey of 798 new referrals. Dig. Dis. Sci. 34, 1820–1824.

Pryor, J.A., Prasad, S.A., 2002. Physiotherapy for respiratory and cardiac problems, third ed. Churchill Livingstone, Edinburgh, p. 81.

Renggli, A., Verges, S., Notter, D., 2008. Development of respiratory muscle contractile fatigue in the course of hyperpnoea. Respir. Physiol. Neurobiol. 164, 366–372.

Rhudy, J., Meagher, M., 2000. Fear and anxiety: divergent effects on human pain thresholds. Pain 84, 65–75.

Rosenbaum, T., Owens, A., 2008. The role of pelvic floor physical therapy in the treatment of pelvic and genital pain-related sexual dysfunction. J. Sex. Med. 5, 513–523.

Ryan, S., McNicholas, M., Eustace, S., 2004. Anatomy for Diagnostic Imaging. Saunders,Sydney, p. 191.

Schleifer, L., Ley, R., Spalding, T., 2002. A hyperventilation theory of job stress and musculoskeletal disorders. Am. J. Ind. Med. 41 (5), 420–432.

Schumpelick, V., Steinau, G., 2000. Surgical embryology and anatomy of the diaphragm with surgical applications. Surg. Clin. North Am. 80 (1), 213–239.

Scott, D.J., Stohler, C.S., Egnatuk, C.M., Wang, H., Koeppe, R.A., Zubieta, J.K., 2007. Individual differences in reward responding explain placebo-induced expectations and effects. Neuron 55 (2), 325–336.

Shuler, T., Gruen, G., 1996. Chronic postpartum pelvic pain treated by surgical stabilization. Orthopedics 19, 687–689.

Simon, P., Schwartzstein, M., Weiss, J., et al., 1989. Distinguishable sensations of breathlessness induced in normal volunteers. Am. Rev. Respir. Dis. 140, 1021–1027.

Simons, D., Travell, J., Simons, L., 1999. Myofascial pain and dysfunction: the trigger point manual. Upper Half of Body, vol. 1, second ed. Williams & Wilkins, Baltimore.

Slatkovska, L., Jensen, D., Davies, G., et al., 2006. Phasic menstrual cycle effects on the control of breathing in healthy women. Respir. Physiol. Neurobiol. 154 (3), 379–388.

Slocumb, J., 1984. Neurological factors in chronic pelvic pain: trigger points and the abdominal pelvic pain syndrome. Am. J. Obstet. Gynecol. 149 (5), 536–543.

Smith, M., Russell, A., Hodges, P., 2006. Disorders of breathing and continence have a stronger association with back pain than obesity and physical activity. Aust. J. Physiother. 21 (52), 11–16.

Smith, M., Russell, A., Hodges, P., 2007. Is there a relationship between parity, pregnancy, back pain and incontinence? Int. Urogynecol. J. Pelvic Floor Dysfunct. 19 (2), 205–211.

Snijders, C., Vleeming, A., Stoeckary, R., et al., 1997. Biomechanics of the interface between spine and pelvis in different poistures. In: Vleeming, A., Mooney, V., Dorman, T., Snijders, C.H., Stoeckart, R. (Eds.), Movement, Stability &Low Back Pain. The essential role of the pelvis. Churchill Livingstone, Edinburgh.

Suwa, K., 1995. Ischemia may be less detrimental than anemia for O_2 transport because of CO_2 transport: A model analysis. J. Anesth. 9 (1), 61–64.

Standring, S. (Ed.), 2008. Gray's Anatomy. The Anatomical Basis of Clinical Practice, 40th ed. Section 8 Abdomen & Pelvis. Elsevier Churchill Livingstone.

Tak, L., Rosmalen, J., 2010. Dysfunction of stress responsive systems as a risk factor for functional somatic syndromes. J. Psychosom. Res. 68 (5), 461–468.

Tan, G., Fink, B., Dao, T.K., et al., 2009. Associations among pain, PTSD, mTBI, and heart rate variability in veterans of Operation Enduring and Iraqi Freedom: a pilot study. Pain Med. 10 (7), 1237–1245.

Ternesten-Hasséus, E., Johansson, E.L., Bende, M., 2008. Dyspnea from exercise in cold air is not always asthma. J. Asthma 45 (8), 705–709.

Tiep, B., Burns, M., Kro, D., et al., 1986. Pursed lip breathing using ear oximetry. Chest 90, 218–221.

Tondury, G., Tillmann, B., 1998. Zwerchfell, Diaphragma. In: Leonhardt, H., Tillmann, B., Tondury, G. et al. (Eds.), Rauber/Kopsch: Anatomie des Menschen. vol. 1, second ed. Thieme, New York, pp. 303–307.

Travell, J., Simons, D., 1983. Myofascial pain and dysfunction, vol 1. Williams & Wilkins, Baltimore.

Troosters, T., Verstraete, A., Ramon, K., 1999. Physical performance of patients with numerous psychosomatic complaints suggestive of hyperventilation. Eur. Respir. J. 14 (6), 1314–1319.

Tu, F., Holt, J., Gonzales, J., et al., 2008. Physical therapy evaluation of patients with chronic pelvic pain: a controlled study. Am. J. Obstet. Gynecol. 198, 272e1–272e7.

Valouchová, P., Lewit, K., 2009. Surface electromyography of abdominal and back muscles in patients with active scars. J. Bodyw. Mov. Ther. 13, 262–267.

Van Dieën, J., Selen, L., Cholewicki, J., 2003. Trunk muscle activation in low-back pain patients, an analysis of the literature. J. Electromyogr. Kinesiol 13, 333–351.

Van Dixhoorn, J., Duivenvoorden, H.J., 1985. Efficacy of Nijmegen Questionnaire in recognition of the hyperventilation syndrome. J. Psychosom. Res. 29 (2), 199–206.

Vanhecke, T., Franklin, B., Ajluni, S., et al., 2008. Cardiorespiratory fitness and sleep-related breathing disorders. Expert Rev. Cardiovasc. Ther. 6 (5), 745–758.

Vleeming, A., Volkers, A.C.W., Snijders, C., Stoeckart, R., 1990a. Relation between form and function in the sacroiliac joint. Part I: Clinical anatomical aspects. Spine 15, 130–132.

Vleeming, A., Volkers, A.C.W., Snijders, C., Stoeckart, R., 1990b. Relation between form and function in the sacroiliac joint. Part 2. Biomechanical aspects. Spine 15 (2), 133–136.

Wager, T.D., Scott, D.J., Zubieta, J.K., 2007. Placebo effects on human mu-opioid activity during pain. Proc. Natl. Acad. Sci. U. S. A. 104 (26), 11056–11061.

Watier, A., 2009. Irritable bowel syndrome and bladder-sphincter dysfunction. Pelvi-perineologie 4 (2), 136–141.

Weinberger, M., Abu-Hasan, M., 2007. Pseudo-asthma: When cough, wheezing, and dyspnea are not asthma. Pediatrics 120 (4), 855–864.

Weiss, J., 2001. Pelvic floor myofascial trigger points: manual therapy for interstitial cystitis and the urgency-frequency syndrome. J. Urol. 166, 2226–2231.

West, J., 2008. Respiratory Physiology: The Essentials, eighth ed. Lippincott Williams & Wilkins, Baltimore, p. 78.

Whitehead, W., Palsson, O., Jones, K., 2002. Systematic review of the comorbidity of irritable bowel syndrome with other disorders: what are the causes and implications? Gastroenterology 122, 1140–1156.

Wilke, A., Noll, B., Maisch, B., 1999. Angina pectoris caused by extra-coronary diseases. Herz 24 (2), 132–139.

Yokoyama, I., Inoue, Y., Kinoshita, T., et al., 2008. Heart and brain circulation and CO_2 in healthy men. Acta Physiol. 193 (3), 202–330.

Zautra, A.J., Fasman, R., Davis, M.C., Craig, A.D., 2010. The effects of slow breathing on affective responses to pain stimuli: An experimental study. Pain (in press).

Zondervan, K., Yudkin, P., Vessey, M., et al., 1999. Patterns of diagnosis and referral in women consuiting for chronic pelvic pain in U.K. primary care. Br. J. Obstet. Gynaecol. 106, 1156–1161.

Zubieta, J.K., Stohler, C.S., 2009. Neurobiological mechanisms of placebo responses. Ann. N. Y. Acad. Sci. 1156, 198–210.

Biofeedback in the diagnosis and treatment of chronic essential pelvic pain disorders

10

Howard I. Glazer Christopher Gilbert

CHAPTER CONTENTS

Pain, relaxation and biofeedback

Changes in emotion and expectations have clear effects on level of pain. These underlying connections have been explored recently as part of research into the mechanism of the placebo effect (Wager et al. 2007, Zubieta & Stohler 2009). The conclusions go beyond mental constructs like distraction and endurance; pain intensity turns out to be modulated by specific chemical and neurological changes in a way resembling the gain control on an amplifier. Changes in synapses, in descending excitatory and inhibitory tracts, in specific brain site excitation and inhibition, in opioid receptor sensitivity, and positive and negative expectations about pain, all interact to enlarge or diminish the experience of pain. Evolution has apparently fine-tuned this set of mechanisms to maximize the chance of survival.

In the field of clinical biofeedback, chronic pain has been a frequent symptom of interest because it is common, distressing, and often seems unnecessary when the signal has little value for warning of body damage. Chronic pain seems to become detached from its origin, or spreads out so much (allodynia, spreading cortical representation; Flor 2002) that the mechanistically minded allopathic physician is without answers as to why something hurts so much. Medical imaging may offer little explanation as to pain sources, and blood tests may show nothing that would explain high pain levels not related or only loosely related to body use. Exercise sometimes improves and sometimes aggravates the pain. Decreased tolerance of the pain may be attributed to deconditioning, even though the original advent of the pain may have discouraged activity and thus led to deconditioning.

Biofeedback depends on providing continuous feedback of a signal to the person it is coming from. With pain, however, there is hardly any way to detect and feed back an actual 'pain signal'. The closest thing to this is the work done by de Charms et al. (2005) using fMRI for continuous monitoring and display of activity in a brain region known for correlating with experienced pain (anterior cingulate cortex (ACC)). Investigating both chronic pain patients and normal experimental subjects, these researchers found that displaying the moment-to-moment fluctuations in amplitude from the ACC provided an opportunity to influence the signal, which would mean influencing the brain area generating the signal and therefore voluntarily adjusting pain intensity. Whether this pain relief came about via emotional modulation, attentional shifts, or neurological–biochemical changes awaits further research, but the question challenges the mind–body distinction which has oversimplified so much research in this area. Subjects felt their pain intensity reduce, and they felt they were controlling it by doing something to manipulate the graphic display on a video screen. However, the subjects were sitting inside an fMRI device in a research lab, and this would be impractical for large-scale application.

Other than the MRI route, a biofeedback approach generally concentrates on altering a system considered responsible for the pain, or at least correlated with it. Thus we can provide biofeedback from voluntary muscles, feedback from the autonomic nervous system (ANS) variables such as skin temperature, skin conductance, heart rate, heart rate variability (RSA, see below), breathing (rate, rhythm, tidal volume, CO_2 level) and EEG, including cerebral blood flow and slow cortical potential. For biofeedback overviews see Schwartz & Andrasik (2003) and Basmajian (1989).

Sometimes a specific system is the source of pain: muscles and low back or repetitive strain, for example, or hand temperature for Raynaud's. But most often the pain, having turned chronic, becomes a distressing emotional experience regardless of its source, physical solutions have been exhausted, and long-term pain medication has become the solution. The usual pain patient rarely differentiates among these approaches and attributes to biofeedback a power to turn down pain by changing some correlate of it.

There is support (Arena 2002) for the non-specific use of biofeedback, however, and patients rarely question the lack of specificity. They may readily acknowledge that their pain seems responsive to variation in not only physical activity but emotional stress and depression. Thus the variables of effective or less effective coping, mood modulation in response to the pain, and the amount of co-occurring non-pain distress require consideration in pain management. It may seem that such complex emotional variables could not be detected and fed back via biofeedback devices. But emotions have biological correlates and teaching control over them amounts to gaining leverage over the feeling states themselves. And these feeling states (explored by the placebo researchers cited above) have neurochemical effects on pain intensity.

Pelvic floor biofeedback began with Arnold Kegel (1948), who designed a pressure perineometer to measure contractile force from inside the vagina, with pressure changes displayed on an external gauge. The intent was to improve strength of the pubococcygeus muscle, and it was usually successful. More modern use of biofeedback for pelvic pain usually relies on either manometric feedback (inflatable balloons with adjustable size, placed in the rectum) or surface electromyographic (SEMG) information gained via vaginal or rectal sensors. Information may also be gained from monitoring the external muscles of the lower abdomen, perineum, thighs, and buttocks. Pelvic pain can of course come from many sources, but if dysfunctional muscle activity is suspected, it is simple enough to feed back the continuous muscle amplitude to the patient, opening a channel for voluntary control.

Other approaches to pain in general and pelvic pain in particular are less specific than the EMG method, but capable of providing bodily information otherwise unavailable to consciousness. Below are descriptions of the main biofeedback instruments used in practice, followed by some applications of biofeedback to pelvic pain.

SEMG biofeedback

With adhesive surface electrodes and without skin penetration, this modality can measure muscle tension through skin just as EEG and EKG can, though the signal is attenuated compared with intramuscular electrodes. Monitoring small individual muscles is not very precise with SEMG, but for general muscle regions and groups such as the jaw, back of neck, upper shoulder, low back, or forearm flexors, this technique excels. Wider spacing of electrodes picks up a wider and deeper region of tissue.

Patients relate well to this variable because they can feel changes in muscle tension, and their perception can be validated by readings on a display or by audio feedback. For pelvic muscles, electrodes are in a special housing, but the electronics are the same as for external monitoring.

Skin temperature

A thermistor, usually a match-sized bimetallic junction encased in plastic, can be taped to the skin anywhere on the body to monitor local temperature. Biologically, what is monitored is a complex mix of cutaneous blood flow, blood vessel diameter, ambient temperature, gross shifts in regional allotment of circulation, and degree of emotional stress from moment to moment. Once the fight-or-flight response is triggered, blood is drawn away from the body surface, especially peripheral parts of the limbs, and as the blood vessels constrict, the skin temperature in that area drops. Pain is stressful, and this links skin temperature to pain and suffering via the emotional network and the sympathetic nervous system.

Hand temperature training has become a standard modality in biofeedback, regardless of where the pain is, because it tends to correlate with a reduction in perceived threat of some kind. Pain creates more distress at some times than others, and the state of distress can be reduced by focusing on hand-warming and peripheral circulatory increase in general, which by a kind of 'upstream' influence alters the ANS toward increased parasympathetic dominance.

Biofeedback thermometers are typically sensitive to at least 0.1°F, smaller than what the average person can perceive. As with muscle tension, tiny changes are amplified and displayed to the patient, who begins to feel some influence over this obscure body variable. Most uses of hand-temperature training for pain issues are non-specific, meaning the goal is general relaxation and shifting of autonomic dominance rather than warming of a specific body area. Hand-warming is often used for migraine prevention. Complex regional pain syndrome is sometimes approached from the self-regulation angle, especially when skin circulation is affected; the local area can be monitored and brought under temporary control via biofeedback principles.

Galvanic skin response

Galvanic skin response (GSR) is a variable that basically evaluates shifts in skin conductance, correlates well with sympathetic nervous system activity and can be used in a similar way to hand temperature, to lower the emotional stress related to pain. Two small electrodes are fastened to the palm or fingers and a tiny current passed between them samples the resistance of the skin. As eccrine sweat glands secrete more, skin resistance drops within seconds as part of the fight-or-flight response. Relaxation training can be enhanced by providing this indicator in either auditory or visual form. It is sensitive to various mental events such as surprise, apprehension, suffering or expectation of suffering, time urgency, confusion and recall of various stressors. GSR is less specific in pain treatment than hand temperature, but its value lies in fine-tuning the ability to self-calm and to reward emotional stability.

Breathing

Variables of breathing can be followed and fed back in several ways. Rate and rhythm can be monitored by a mechanical strain gauge around the torso, by changes in air temperature from the nostril, or by changes in tension of certain muscles in the neck and shoulders. Composition of exhaled air, primarily degree of CO_2, can be monitored and displayed by a capnograph. The relationship between breathing and pulse, often called RSA (respiratory-sinus arrhythmia), can be followed with a simple or complex analysis of how much the heart rate rises and falls with each breath.

Starting with yoga, breathing regulation has a long history in the field of voluntary self-regulation and every meditative tradition includes attention to breath regulation. Like the previous biofeedback variables, breathing is sensitive to the fight-or-flight reaction and is always subject to the central decision to accelerate breathing in order to prepare for exertion. Muscles need fuel in order to perform, and extra fuel must be delivered by the blood. When average individuals consciously attempt to reduce a state of alarm (perhaps responding to a general injunction 'Calm down!') they are not likely to think of keeping their limbs warm and their hands dry; they may attempt some muscle relaxation (fists, shoulders, face) but most likely they will try to control their breathing by means of one or more deep breaths. So the validity of breathing regulation is high for most people, though they may not see it as reversing their fight-or-flight reaction.

The five biofeedback-targeted variables of interest, then, in chronic pain treatment, are muscle tension, hand temperature, skin conductance, heart rate variability and breathing. These all in various ways reflect shifts in ANS activity, which is responsive to conscious and preconscious mental events related to current suffering and danger, as well as conditioned responses to cues associated with past or anticipated suffering and danger. Since pain is a prime signal of impending body damage, it is hard not to let pain perturb the nervous system toward emergency action even though the pain signal may not always be a valid warning.

Chronic pain creates a long-term 'orange alert' state which affects everyday functioning, including sleep quality, concentration, allotment of energy and resources, emotional stability, and resistance to depression and anxiety from other sources (Gatchel et al. 2007, Turk et al. 2008).

Research applications to pelvic pain problems

Hand temperature and pelvic pain

There is very little research using temperature biofeedback alone for pelvic pain problems. Hand temperature is a commonly used biofeedback modality, but is usually used in combination with others, for a variety of goals. But below is a study of hand temperature biofeedback and endometriosis.

In a small multiple baseline study (Hart et al. 1981) five women with pain from endometriosis were trained in hand-warming with individual sessions twice weekly over 2 months, with home practice in between sessions. The rationale was to reduce physiological arousal, and the intent was to have the skill generalize as a learned and perhaps automatic response to pain. All but one person learned to voluntarily increase hand temperature, and reports of pain relief were accompanied by decreases in life interference from pain, decrease in affective distress, and increase in 'life control'. One person could not learn the hand-warming skill; her pain remained the same and some indicators got worse.

Muscle biofeedback and pelvic pain

In chronic pelvic pain (CPP) there is usually an interaction among pelvic muscle activity, negative affect, pain thresholds, and nervous system factors modulating pain. The average pelvic pain patient knows nothing of this interaction and considers the pain a direct readout of tissue damage. Bracing, avoidance of activity, and an often passive despair are common responses.

There are several ways that excess muscle tension can cause pain: prolonged ischaemia, accumulation of metabolites such as lactic acid and potassium; reduced intramuscular circulation, release of bradykinin and serotonin, and various aggravators of inflammation (Mense 2000). In addition, pain intensity is mediated by co-occurring emotional factors. Brain sites such as the anterior cingulate cortex are responsive to allodynia and are also involved in conscious mediation of 'suffering' (Yoshino et al. 2009). Therefore, negative affect from any source is likely to make pain worse because at some level different kinds of distress are not differentiated. The most reliable predictors of hyperalgesia seem to be varieties of anxiety, fear of movement, fear of injury, and the tendency toward catastrophic thinking (Boersma & Linton 2006a, 2006b).

Muscle tension is often elevated in chronic pain patients as part of an attempt to brace and protect the body from damage. Muscular rigidity is a primary defensive response to threat, pain and trauma, and this response can be triggered by both relevant and irrelevant sensory and emotional stimuli. SEMG monitoring can detect and quantify the degree of inappropriate pelvic muscle hypertonicity and instability (White et al. 1997, Glazer et al. 1998). Many chronic pain syndromes besides pelvic pain are associated with increased muscle tension (Flor et al. 1992) and can be alleviated in part by better muscle control.

Granot et al. (2002) studied pain sensitivity in a group of women with vulvar vestibulitis using a heated bar on the skin. A matched control group without pain was used for comparison. The researchers collected anxiety measures and estimates of pain intensity and unpleasantness, and blood pressure was also recorded. The pain patients had significantly more state and trait anxiety before the procedure began; they gave higher estimates for pain magnitude, unpleasantness, and had higher systolic blood pressure. The authors' conclusions were that these subjects were more anxious and had higher systemic pain sensitivity.

The study of Bendaña et al. (2009) used a treatment sample of 52 women having problems with urinary frequency and urgency, interstitial cystitis, CPP, dysuria, and evidence of pelvic floor muscle (PFM) spasm. Initial determination of the levator ani muscle complex condition was done by manual vaginal examination. Subject criteria for selection were bladder dysfunction, including pelvic pain, and evidence of PFM tension. The therapeutic goal was to detect and reduce muscle tension and spasms in the PFMs using transvaginal SEMG and electrical stimulation. During six individual sessions the subjects observed computerized visual feedback which reflected their internal muscle tension from moment to moment. First isolating sensations of the relevant muscles from surrounding pelvic, abdominal and back muscles, they learned to increase control of the pertinent muscles in both tensing and relaxing directions.

Outcomes were good: reports of symptom improvement and reduced effect on daily life were in the range of 65–75% at 6-week and 3-month follow-up. The study's authors concluded: 'Patients gain a sense of which muscles in the pelvis they can control by manipulating feedback pathways and relaxing overall pelvic floor tone and afferent cross-stimulation, leading to symptomatic improvement'.

PFM biofeedback (neuromuscular re-education) has been found useful for men with pelvic floor dysfunction and prostatitis associated with pain.

The study of Heah et al. (1997) of men with levator ani syndrome (LAS) used manometric rectal balloon biofeedback. Average pain report after completion of biofeedback dropped to around 25% of that before biofeedback, with use of analgesics also significantly reduced.

Grimaud et al. (1991) also used a manometric technique to investigate patients with chronic idiopathic anal pain. In the 12 cases studied, the pressure in the anal canal was significantly higher than in a normal comparison group. After an average of eight biofeedback training sessions, in which patients learned voluntary control of the external sphincter, the pain disappeared, and the anal canal pressure dropped to normal or near-normal.

Cornel et al. (2005) reported treatment of 31 men with chronic prostatitis and CPP. They learned to control and relax PFM tension via biofeedback provided by a rectal SEMG sensor. Average muscle tension before treatment was 4.9 μv, and dropped to 1.7 μv afterward. Corresponding drops in symptom scores (NIH Chronic Prostatitis Symptom Index) went from 23.6 to 11.4.

Chiarioni et al. (2009) reports administering nine sessions of counselling plus electrogalvanic stimulation (EGS), massage or biofeedback randomized to 157 patients suffering from LAS. Outcomes were reassessed at 1, 3, 6 and 12 months. Among patients with LAS, adequate relief was reported by 87% for biofeedback, 45% for EGS, and 22% for massage. Pain days per month decreased from 14.7 at baseline to 3.3 after biofeedback, 8.9 after EGS, and 13.3 after massage. Pain intensity decreased from 6.8 (0–10 scale) at baseline to 1.8 after biofeedback, 4.7 after EGS, and 6.0 after massage. Improvements were maintained for 12 months. The authors conclude that biofeedback is the most effective of these treatments, and EGS is somewhat effective.

Jantos (2008) assessed vulvar pelvic muscle tension in 529 cases of vulvodynia, combined with psychological testing, to examine psychophysiological factors. The study also provided biofeedback-based intervention in the form of daily pelvic muscle exercises based on findings of SEMG using the 'Glazer Protocol' (Glazer et al. 1995) This involves use of progressively larger dilators to stretch and relax the vulvar and vaginal muscles, intravaginal EMG biofeedback, and brief psychotherapy aimed at improved psychological (anxiety, depression, fear of sexual activity) and sexual functioning. State and trait anxiety differentiated normals from vulvodynia patients, who also had lower sensory thresholds, more autonomic disturbances, and greater emotional responses. General outcomes after treatment included normalizing of muscle characteristics, capacity to accept larger dilators, and greater likelihood of resuming normal sexual activity. PFM improved in several ways, correlating with degree of improvement in the group as a whole, though not individually. Resting baseline and instability declined by more than 50%; maximum phasic and tonic contractions increased.

A unique finding in the Jantos study was the relationship between duration of symptoms and resting PFM EMG (subject characteristics at the onset of the study): severity of symptoms did not decline with time, but muscle tension did. The authors speculated that this could indicate development of contractures, which resemble muscle spasms upon palpation but are produced locally rather than by corticospinal input. As a result they are electrically silent and would not contribute to pelvic EMG. Such contractures could create pain by producing myofascial trigger points (Bornstein & Simon 2002). Trigger points produce a high local EMG signal that does not generalize to the whole muscle. These structures are sensitive to sympathetic nervous system activity (McNulty et al. 1994, Chen et al. 1998), and therefore can be aggravated by anxiety, apprehension and negative psychological states.

The psychophysiological perspective here gives a more complete understanding of how trigger points respond to physiological and emotional arousal by producing more pain (see also Chapter 4). For this reason, any arousal-reduction technique, including general relaxation methods, should be helpful for pain intensity that arises from trigger points.

Intrapelvic SEMG in the treatment of functional chronic urogenital, gastrointestinal and sexual pain and dysfunction

Biofeedback meets evidence-based medicine: The Glazer Protocol

This section of the chapter focuses on a specific methodology and protocol, the Glazer Protocol, for the diagnosis and treatment of essential CPP and dysfunction. The methodology involves the use of non-invasive intrapelvic (intravaginal or intra-anal) SEMG. The first factor differentiating this approach from the self-regulation biofeedback approach, discussed earlier, is the emphasis on the electrophysiology of the SEMG signal, rather than the psychophysiogy of self-regulation. This protocol relies more on the bioelectric information derived from the SEMG signal analysis, rather than the traditional biofeedback use of the SEMG signal to teach the patient voluntary self-regulation through enhanced interoceptive awareness. Unlike traditional biofeedback, this protocol is highly operationally defined, including diagnostic criteria (ICD), medical, psychological and sexual history, patient positioning and muscle use training, muscle activation and deactivation sequence, SEMG signal processing, recording and formatting, to create a standardized SEMG report and database. This approach facilitates the development of multicentre, multidiagnosis, multitreatment databases for statistical analysis. This operationally defined procedural and biometric/psychometric approach creates the foundation for evidence-based research and represents a substantial departure from past work in the field of clinical biofeedback (Glazer & Laine 2007).

Evidence-based medicine applies evidence from scientific methodology to health care practice. It assesses the quality of evidence relating to risks and benefits of treatments. The power of clinical evidence lies in its freedom from bias. The most powerful evidence for therapeutic efficacy comes from randomized, double-blind, placebo-controlled trials with operationally defined patient populations, diagnoses and treatment protocols. Patient testimonials, case studies, clinical experience and expert opinion have little value as scientific evidence. This in no way takes away from the importance of traditional clinical practice experience and thinking. Often clinical practice serves as an 'incubator' leading to ideas which are then transformed into more evidence-based hypotheses and subject to evidence-based medicine research. The completion of the cycle is the evidence-based research findings returning to clinical practice where their implementation can benefit clinical thinking and patient care (see Chapter 9).

The application of these scientific standards to biofeedback presents significant challenges because very little of the published literature in biofeedback reaches the higher levels of scientific evidence. The majority of biofeedback research is case histories, clinical experience and expert opinion, all subject to bias. This is largely due to the lack of standardization of technology and techniques, and failure to employ operationalized protocols, procedures and definitions.

A recent review article (Glazer & Laine 2007), summarizing the peer-reviewed literature in the use of PFM biofeedback for the treatment of functional urinary incontinence, exemplifies this. This review reports a total of 326 studies found in Medline between 1975 and 2005. Only 8.6% of these studies operationally defined independent and dependent variables, utilized prospective randomized trials with parametric statistical analyses, and used patient selection criteria to rule out organic causes of urinary incontinence. Among these 27 studies are six different operational definitions for the diagnosis, eight operational definitions for treatments, 12 operational definitions for biofeedback protocols, and six operational definitions for treatment outcome. In 30 years of peer-reviewed literature only seven studies reported a comparison of biofeedback to a matched, no treatment, control group. For these seven studies, differences in signal processing, biofeedback instrumentation, assessment and treatment protocols, biofeedback modalities, and multiple uncontrolled variables make each of these groups so different that there is no standardized definition of biofeedback. The same is true within each study, since the biofeedback groups are not comparable to their respective control groups due to non-randomized, uncontrolled variables between groups. This pervasive lack of standardization has hampered the scientific assessment of biofeedback by effectively precluding the application of evidence-based medicine standards to the field.

The hallmark of the Glazer Protocol is standardization in all aspects of clinical biofeedback research and practice. This includes the use of operational definitions for diagnoses (ICD, SEMG, history, medical exam, laboratory tests, etc.), biofeedback treatment (CPT, modality, instrumentation, signal processing, evaluation and treatment protocols, patient muscle identification training, positioning, etc.) and therapeutic efficacy (psychometrics, structural and functional organic changes, experiential self-report, lab reports, etc.). In addition, the protocol standardizes data measurement, collection, transmission and storage across multiple domestic and international site locations, languages, areas of study, etc. to produce large sample size, multinational, multi-disorder databases. These databases serve as a standard to assist in diagnosis and treatment and can be statistically queried regarding the effects of variables on therapeutic outcomes. These intrapelvic SEMG readings help identify the variables which correlate with symptoms, and eventually may help to shed some light upon the pathophysiology involved in response to biofeedback and non-biofeedback interventions such as pharmacology, acupuncture, or surgery.

Applications

The Glazer Protocol is used in the diagnosis and treatment of a wide range of PFM-related disorder specialties as shown in Table 10.1.

Patient selection

Biofeedback is used in the treatment of functional or essential disorders. These are disorders which are diagnosed by first ruling out established anatomic and physiological pathology causing the reported symptoms. Therefore it is essential that all prospective biofeedback patients have medical assessment to identify and treat or rule out well-known medical conditions as the cause of the symptoms. In addition, the patient must have intact sensory and motor pathways. Finally, a major requirement for biofeedback candidates in general, and the Glazer Protocol in particular, is sufficient motivation and discipline to conduct daily biofeedback-assisted exercise sessions for a period ranging from 4 to 8 weeks up to a period ranging from 6 to 12 months. Non-compliance and drop out rates are high; clinicians should be cautious in prescribing biofeedback for patients expressing a preference for treatments involving less commitment of time and discipline. In the experience of the author, those patients being assessed for biofeedback who request a pharmacological or surgical approach

Table 10.1 Disorders, categorized by medical specialty and ICD codes, treated with pelvic floor muscle SEMG biofeedback

Medical specialty	Diagnostic ICD-9/-10 code
Gynaecology/Dermatology/Psychiatry	
1. Vulvar vestibulitis syndrome	625.71, 625.0
2. Dysaesthetic vulvodynia	625.70, 625.9
3. Vaginismus	F94.2, 625.1
4. Dyspareunia (introital N94.1, deep 302.76)	N94.1, 302.76
Female Urology/Neurourology	
5. Dysuria	306.53, 788.1
6. Urinary stress incontinence	625.6
7. Urinary urge incontinence	N39.41
8. Urinary incontinence mixed	788.34
9a. Detrusor hyperactivity	N32.8
9b. Neurogenic bladder	N31.9
10. Urinary retention	N39.8
11. Interstitial cystitis	N30.1
Gastroenterology/Colorectal Surgery	
12. Functional fecal incontinence	787.6 R15
13. Functional constipation	K59.00
14. Anismus (anorectal pain syndrome, levator ani proctalgia fugax)	K59.4
15. Irritable bowel syndrome	564.1
Male Urology/Neurourology	
16. Mixed urinary incontinence	788.34
17. Prostatodynia	N42.81
18. Prostate cancer/prostatectomy	C61
19. Benign prostatic hypertrophy	600.0
20. Chronic pelvic or perineal pain	625.9 R10.2
Asymptomatic	
21. Healthy male (controls)	
Multiple codes limited to absence of specific organic pathology	
22. Healthy female (controls)	

to their problem are less likely to comply with home training prescriptions, and are therefore less likely to benefit from biofeedback as a primary treatment modality.

Assessment with the Glazer Protocol

The Glazer Protocol operationally defines both the intrapelvic SEMG assessment and rehabilitation of PFM. The assessment protocol starts by educating the patient on the structure and function of the PFM as they relate to their individual symptom presentation. This is accomplished with a scripted presentation, with responses to any questions the patient presents. The presentation includes instructions on private self-insertion of the intrapelvic sensor, body positioning as a critical factor in SEMG measurement, and teaching the patient the correct method for contracting and relaxing the PFM. This instruction focuses on creating the intravaginal lifting sensation associated with the correct use of PFM while permitting limited co-contractions, or overflow (Glazer & McConkay 1996) to offset fatigue during the initial stages of exercise.

The intrapelvic SEMG assessment consists of a fixed series of PFM contractions and relaxations, directed via an on-screen written script and simultaneous voice presentation. This assessment is a computer-controlled continuous process in which software (Biograph Infiniti with Glazer Protocol) directs both the instructions to the patient and the SEMG biofeedback signal processing device (Myotrac Infiniti), which continuously records raw SEMG data (2048 samples/s) and displays the integrated SEMG signal (20 samples/s) throughout the assessment. The SEMG screen presents a graphic and numeric presentation of the integrated SEMG signal as well as signal variability measures and a three-dimensional fast Fourier transformation power density spectral frequency display of the signal. This allows the clinician to view real-time changes in the spectral frequency distribution of the signal power throughout the conduct of the evaluation (Figure 10.1).

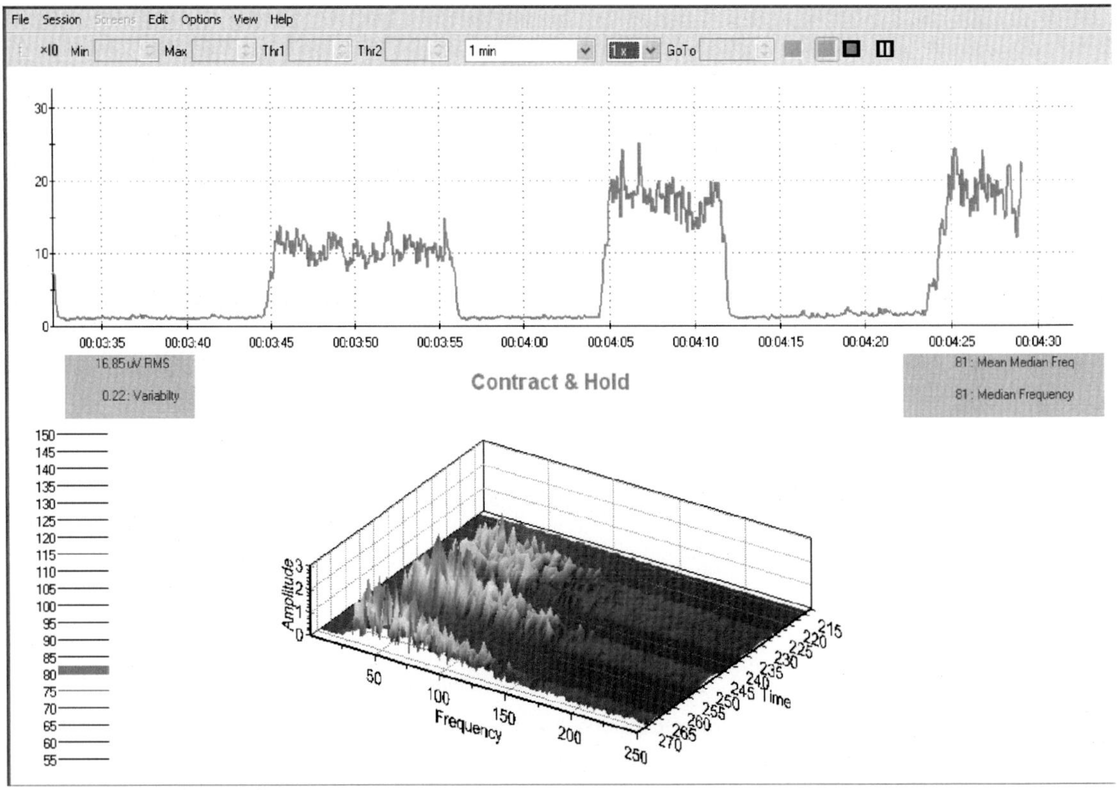

Figure 10.1 • A screenshot from the Glazer Protocol as seen by the clinician and patient in real time showing the intrapelvic SEMG tracings and numerical values for signal amplitude, muscle activation onset and release times, variability, and power density spectral frequency

The engineering of the signal processor hardware and software is a critical element in the Protocol. Only by understanding the engineering details of the instrument (Differential Amplification, Common Mode Rejection Sensitivity, Impedance, Rectification, Bandpass and Notch Filtration, Analogue to Digital Conversion, Power Density Spectral Frequency Analysis via Fast Fourier Transformation, signal re-integration methods, etc.) can the clinician understand both the utility and the limits of the SEMG data which they are observing and interpreting.

The fixed sequence of muscle activity utilized during the protocol includes pre-baseline rest, phasic contractions, tonic contractions, endurance contraction, and post-baseline rest. This traditional series of PFM assessment contractions were originally intended to reflect sexual, sphincteric and support functions of the pubococcygeus muscle (Kegel 1948, 1952). In the Glazer Protocol, SEMG measures taken continuously throughout the protocol include average SEMG amplitude, muscle recruitment and recovery latencies, median power density spectral frequency, and two measures of SEMG variability: raw (standard deviation) and amplitude corrected (coefficient of variability). Upon completion of the protocol the data are stored in raw SEMG form (2048 samples/s).

The report is maintained in the patient's electronic record and copies of the report are provided to the patient and to the referring and ongoing treating clinicians. The data derived from the raw SEMG are also exported into an SEMG database with each record categorized by diagnosis, patient demographic variables and therapeutic response variables. The database also includes data from asymptomatic volunteers to provide a matched or randomized control group for between-group statistical comparisons.

Comparing groups measured under standardized conditions is the first step in identifying SEMG characteristics associated with specific symptom patterns and diagnostic categories. This approach yields helpful data to confirm a diagnosis as well as develop hypotheses about the pathophysiology of symptoms and disorders. In addition, comparisons of SEMG measures within groups over assessment sessions can identify critical SEMG changes predictive of symptomatic and functional improvement. Once these findings have been replicated they can then form the basis of training protocols aimed at producing the SEMG changes known to be predictive of symptom reduction. Early published research findings will be reviewed later in this chapter along with a presentation of current, ongoing research and new advancements in which patients can be completely evaluated and treated via telemedicine technology over the internet.

SEMG is not a stand-alone diagnostic or therapeutic programme, no matter how well operationalized and defined its components may be. It is part of a comprehensive assessment process which often involves multiple specialists and diagnostic procedures. In CPP it is not at all unusual for patients to initially present with a history of many years of pain and visits to many physicians and non-physician healthcare practitioners (neurologists, anaesthesiologists, urologists, gynaecologists, urogynaecologists, gastroenterologists, mental health practitioners, holistic practitioners, psychopharmacologists, physiatrists, osteopaths, acupuncturists, nutritionists, physiotherapists, and many more). Satisfactory diagnosis and treatment of chronic pain is now well recognized by most practitioners as requiring an integrated biopsychosocial approach addressing organic, psychological, interpersonal and functional causes and consequences of complex pain syndromes. Biofeedback, like any procedure addressing chronic disorders, must incorporate a detailed review of medical history, systems review, medications and non-prescription agents, social and psychological status, diet, exercise and sexual functioning, in order to create a complete view of the patient. Collecting patient medical records, using standardized intake forms and acquiring input from significant others in the patient's life is an integral part of the evaluation process, and ongoing communication and information exchange among multiple treatment resources is an essential part of treatment.

Levels of interpretation and applications of SEMG evaluation data include both empirical and pathophysiological perspectives

Empirical

This level of interpretation and application is purely empirical, utilizing operationally defined intrapelvic SEMG measures as independent variables and operationally defined symptom and function measures as dependent variables. Analysis at this level serves the functions listed below, without any deductions or assumptions concerning the underlying physiology reflected in these variables.

1. Descriptive statistics help develop normative SEMG database standards.
2. Identified symptom and disorder-specific SEMG patterns assist in differential diagnosis.
3. Consistent SEMG changes and associated symptom reduction and functional improvements help develop rehabilitation protocols.

Physiological

Electrophysiology data derived from SEMG is one manifestation of local and systemic integrated physiology. The functional integration of multiple physiological systems is necessary to understand disorders such as complex regional pain syndromes. It is this physiological integration which allows the use of striated muscle SEMG to better understand the multiple physiological processes contributing to dysfunction. There are several studies which have looked at the relationship between striate muscle fatigue, SEMG, blood flow, PO_2, subjective sense of fatigue, and pain (Alfonsi et al. 1999, Yoshitake et al. 2001, Hug et al. 2004, Tachi et al. 2004, Dimitrov et al. 2006). These variables show a complex, non-linear relationship to one another, but these studies basically report that subjective sense of muscle fatigue and localized nociceptive pain are correlated with the following: SEMG increased contractile amplitude, lower median power density spectral frequency, reduced microcirculation in local muscle and surrounding tissue, and hypoxia. On a neurochemical level these changes are associated with release of neurokines, cytokines, lactic acid, interleukin, and tumour necrosis factor-α, representing localized 'defensive' responses of ischaemia, inflammation and sensitization (Mense 2004). These markers are all part of an integrated response from the most molecular cellular level to the most molar level of cognition, affect and goal-oriented intentional behaviour.

In this integrated model, intrapelvic SEMG reflects not only myofascial phenomena such as chronic tension or chronic weakness, but also neurological, neurochemical, inflammatory, vascular, blood gas levels, hormonal availability, autonomic activity, and even cognition and affect. These are all components of a single integrated response. So, we no longer restrict ourselves to looking at SEMG as representing muscle tension or weakness or asymmetry. SEMG characteristics can now represent oxygen availability, blood flow, hormone levels, tissue inflammation, and even psychological processes such as thoughts and feelings. All such processes are a part of a single response, no longer seen in a sequential or causal model but as components of a single entity. For convenience of study we may divide these functions up by anatomy, physiology, function or medical specialty, but in doing so we must understand that this deconstruction process leaves us at risk for losing the 'forest for the trees'.

If we see all responses at all levels as part of an integrated process, it now makes sense to look at the relationships which may exist among any of these components. An example of this is a recently recognized intrapelvic SEMG profile which represents atrophic vaginitis. This oestrogen loss condition may manifest as chronic, fluctuating vulvar dryness, irritation, tissue integrity compromise, dyspareunia, emotional changes, bone density loss, and pelvic organ prolapse (Mehta & Bachman 2008). There is also a highly reliable intrapelvic SEMG profile which correlates with this condition. This profile includes low-amplitude (hypotonicity), low-signal-variability resting tone, slow recruitment and recovery latencies to low-amplitude phasic, tonic, and endurance contractions. These contractions show low signal standard deviations and coefficients of variability, and a high median frequency power density spectrum on sustained isometric contractions. This SEMG pattern as a potential confirmation for oestrogen loss is still undergoing data collection to produce a sample size sufficient for parametric data analysis and publication.

Developing evidence-based biofeedback applications for pelvic pain

It is clear that the development of evidence-based biofeedback applications for pelvic pain is a major undertaking, well beyond the resources of any individual or small group of interested practitioners. Developing a structure of resources to meet this need became a major focus in the development of evidence-based biofeedback protocols for the diagnosis and treatment of CPP disorders.

Unrelated events brought clinicians, researchers, educators and patients together in Europe over 12 years ago with a mission to promote research, education and clinical use of biofeedback. What emerged was the Biofeedback Foundation of Europe (BFE). To meet their goals, the BFE developed groups which came to be known as International

Research and Education Project (IREP) teams. Each team is specific to a biofeedback application, and is made up of three subgroups (research, education and training) of six members each. Peer-reviewed publishing, clinician training and patient services are the goals of today's IREP teams.

Selected ongoing international collaborative research

The BFE/IREP team projects have led to collaboration with a team of colorectal surgeons in Nanjing, China, studying the use of intra-anal biofeedback in anal pain disorders. Urologists in Sao Paulo, Brazil, are completing a research project using the intra-anal SEMG protocol. Evaluations starting 30 days prior to patients undergoing radical prostatectomy are repeated every 3 months thereafter for a total of 12 months along with a control group. This group is also working on prediction and intervention in postpartum urinary incontinence. A second Sao Paulo group has initiated a study on a paediatric population suffering from polysymptomatic enuresis, employing a version of the Glazer Protocol. This project records simultaneous multiple SEMG measures and it is hoped that it will provide insight into this disorder and its pathophysiology.

Several recent technological and methodological advancements have also emerged from the Glazer BFE/IREP teams which have led to the introduction of clinical SEMG evaluation and treatment services via telemedicine, online, both domestically and internationally.

Research summary

The synergy between the goals of the BFE, to promote biofeedback, and the goals of Glazer, to develop evidence-based biofeedback applications for pelvic pain disorders, is clear. The BFE and Glazer have been working cooperatively for several years and the following selected studies exemplify peer-reviewed published research using intrapelvic SEMG biofeedback in diagnosis and treatment of PFM-related disorders. This representative group of studies includes SEMG diagnostic database studies, SEMG treatment studies, and protocol methodology studies.

SEMG diagnostic studies refer to the use of intrapelvic SEMG data using between-group comparison studies to determine which SEMG variable or combination of variables yield statistical significance in differentiating PFM-related disorders. The first study in this series, entitled 'Establishing the diagnosis of vulvar vestibulitis', was published in 1997 (White et al. 1997). This study compared intravaginal SEMG assessment findings from essential and organic vulvar pain patients. Six individual SEMG criteria differentiated vulvar vestibulitis patients from organic vulvar pain patients, with 88% of vulvar vestibulitis patients manifesting three or more of these criteria to a significantly greater degree than the organic vulvar pain patients. The single most statistically significant variable differentiating them was the resting baseline stability as measured by the coefficient of variability of the integrated intrapelvic SEMG. Vulvar vestibulitis patients showed significantly higher resting instability than organic vulvar pain control patients.

Another study 'Electromyographic comparisons of the pelvic floor in women with dysesthetic vulvodynia and asymptomatic women' compared SEMG PFM evaluation variables in dysaesthetic vulvodynia patients to matched asymptomatic controls (Glazer et al. 1998). Findings indicated that dysaesthetic vulvodynia patients manifest significantly greater intravaginal SEMG-sustained contractile weakness, resting hypertonicity and instability.

Two related papers (Glazer et al. 1999, Romanzi et al. 1999) studied reliability and clinical predictive validity of intravaginal SEMG. These papers reported the findings of a wide range of symptomatic patients undergoing both manual (digital) and SEMG intrapelvic repeated evaluations. At each administration, the order of procedure and clinician was randomized between a urogynaecologist and a gynaecologist conducting the digital exams and Glazer conducting intrapelvic SEMG evaluations. Reliability within and between evaluators and procedures was statistically significant but digital exam results could not significantly predict any clinical status. Intravaginal SEMG significantly predicts stress and urge incontinence, menstrual status and parity.

Hetrick et al. (2006) studied differences in intra-anal PFM SEMG readings between men suffering from chronic pelvic pain syndrome (CPPS) compared with a matched control group of pain-free men. CPPS patients were found to manifest overall greater PFM electrophysiological instability. This measure as well as chronic prebaseline resting hypertonicity and endurance contraction weakness were statistically significant in differentiating CPPS patients from their asymptomatic matched controls. It is interesting to note the similarity in these pelvic floor SEMG findings to those previously found in women suffering from essential vulvovaginal pain disorders (Glazer et al. 1995, 1998, White et al. 1997).

Intrapelvic SEMG treatment studies use intrapelvic SEMG data to develop PFM biofeedback treatment protocols. The earliest of these studies 'Treatment of vulvar vestibulitis syndrome with electromyographic biofeedback of pelvic floor musculature' (Glazer et al. 1995) was the first peer-review published study in the field. It reported a 50% rate of asymptomatic outcome on 6-month follow-up with overall self-reported improvement averaging 83%. Only the standard deviation of tonic resting periods showed significant predictive validity for pain reduction and improvement in sexual desire, arousal and orgasm. This study concluded that PFM electrophysiological stabilization through intrapelvic SEMG biofeedback-assisted exercise produces pain relief and improved sexual functioning for vulvovaginal pain patients.

Another study 'Dysesthetic vulvodynia, long term follow-up after treatment with surface electromyography-assisted PFM rehabilitation' (Glazer, 2000) reported on the 3–5-year follow-up status of 43 patients who were asymptomatic at the completion of their PFM rehabilitation treatment for vulvodynia. All 43 patients remained pain-free; recovery of sexual desire, pleasure and frequency, however, progressively improved but remained well below levels experienced prior to the onset of vulvar pain.

A doctoral dissertation from McGill University (Bergeron et al. 2001) described a prospective, randomized treatment design comparing vestibulectomy (surgical removal of a portion of the superficial tissue making up the vestibule of the vagina), Glazer Protocol biofeedback, and group cognitive behaviour therapy in the treatment of vulvar vestibulitis. Surgical outcomes were found superior to both the intrapelvic Glazer SEMG treatment protocol and the couples group cognitive behaviour therapy. When examining patient self-report measures, all three groups did equally well with a small, statistically non-significant, preference for surgery. Before biofeedback and cognitive behavioural therapy were included in the treatment of vulvar pain disorders, surgery was considered the primary treatment and 'gold standard' for many years, in spite of the significant adverse consequences as well as absence of patient satisfaction or long-term follow up.

In a study entitled 'Treating vulvar vestibulitis with electromyographic biofeedback of pelvic floor musculature' patients with moderate to severe vulvar vestibulitis syndrome underwent the Glazer intrapelvic biofeedback protocol (McKay et al. 2001). Patients received monthly in-office evaluation and daily home-trainer-assisted PFM rehabilitation. Eighty-three percent of patients demonstrated significant reduction in introital tenderness, with 69% resuming sexual intercourse and 48% reporting no discomfort during sexual intercourse.

Glazer & MacConkey (1996) published the first methodological paper 'Functional rehabilitation of pelvic floor muscles: a challenge to tradition'. Traditional PFM biofeedback-assisted rehabilitation strongly emphasized the exclusive use of the pubococcygeus without the use of supportive or accessory muscles such as gluteal, quadriceps, adductor longus and particularly abdominal muscles. This study demonstrates that the traditional practice of excluding accessory muscles in PFM re-education is not always warranted. Subjects were trained and then tested either with or without abdominal augmented PFM contractions in a 2 × 2 experimental design. Results clearly demonstrated significantly greater contractile amplitude and reduced variability (strength and coordination) in subjects tested with exclusive pubococcygeus contraction after training with abdominals, compared to subjects both trained and tested without training abdominal muscles. Clearly, where up-training and coordination are the training goals, the co-contraction of abdominals during training of the pelvic floor should not be excluded.

Glazer et al. (2002) published the first methodological paper introducing the technology of telemedicine via videoconference over the internet. This paper reported a case history demonstrating the use of a newly developed telemedicine system permitting the remote, real-time use of SEMG of pelvic floor musculature. This browser-based version of the Glazer Protocol offers a reliable and convenient diagnostic and treatment tool that overcomes the barriers of distance and time. As this technology has become more readily available, it has greatly facilitated international education and research collaboration with the standardized procedures critical to research reaching the requirements of evidence-based medicine. It also permits direct patient assessment and treatment by those with most experience in fields just beginning to utilize SEMG intrapelvic biofeedback.

Brown et al. (2003, 2004, 2005, 2006) published a series of papers reporting on the use of botulinum toxin A injected into the pelvic floor musculature as a possible treatment for vulvar vestibulitis syndrome. These studies employed intravaginal SEMG to determine if any clinical findings correlate with this measure. Data suggested that only those patients with elevated resting tone, variability and spectral frequency benefited from the injection. This is consistent with the fact that botulinum toxin A is known to selectively block type II glycolytic fibre. This finding suggests that intravaginal SEMG would serve as a valuable tool in selecting patients who would benefit from this procedure.

Summary of Medline 'biofeedback' 'pelvic pain' literature search

A peer-reviewed literature search was conducted with the use of Medline, searching all languages, all ages, and both genders, from 1975 to the present and entering the search terms 'biofeedback' and 'pelvic pain'. The search returned a total of 87 citations. Considered for inclusion in this review were only those citations reporting primary research in which at least one treatment condition was biofeedback alone, and at least one of the disorders treated had a component of chronic pelvic pain. Removed from consideration in this review were:

1. Review articles or meta-analyses without original primary research reported;
2. Studies in which biofeedback was only one component of a protocol employing multiple treatment components (e.g. biofeedback+estim, biofeedback+neuromodulation, biofeedback+trigger point release, etc.). No subjects received a biofeedback alone treatment;
3. Studies in which there are no biofeedback treatments included (e.g. pelvic floor exercises without biofeedback);
4. Studies in which there are no pelvic pain disorders treated (e.g. disorders treated are urinary or bowel symptoms without a pain component or no pain components were measured or recorded).

Applying these criteria for inclusion/exclusion results in the inclusion of 13 and the exclusion of 74 studies. The 13 studies meeting inclusion criteria break down as follows.

Design:
6 Single-group biofeedback only
1 Within-group multiple treatments randomized
3 Randomized between group no control (two or more treatment groups)
3 Randomized between group with control (two or more treatment and control groups)

Sample size: range 5–100, mean 32

Age range: range 7–74, mean 41

Gender: 4 males only, 6 females only, 3 males and females

Disorder:
1 Pelvic floor myalgia
1 Prostatitis
3 Dysmenorrhoea
2 Vulvodynia
3 Anal pain/levator ani
3 Male chronic pelvic pain syndrome

Type of biofeedback:
2 Ultrasound
4 Manometry
6 Surface electromyography
1 Thermal

Outcome:
6 Biofeedback effective (single group)
1 Biofeedback superior (within group, multiple treatment)
2 Biofeedback superior (between treatment groups)
1 Biofeedback equal (between treatment groups)
3 Biofeedback superior (treatment vs control groups)

Case study 10.1

J.A. is 44-year-old female, married, Caucasian, MBA, Corporate Executive, residing in northeastern USA with her husband of 17 years and their two teenage children. She is approximately 5'4" in height, 115 pounds and presented as neat, well-groomed, attractive, cooperative and well-spoken. Her husband, a neuroradiologist, was in attendance throughout the initial evaluation. Initial evaluation session is approximately 2 hours. She reports as follows on her initial intake form.

Health concerns

1. Vulvovaginal pain
2. Proctalgia fugax
3. Post-traumatic stress disorder – childhood abuse
4. Alcohol/drug abuse – in remission

Hospital/surgery/major illness

1. 1984 Cheekbone reconstruction from skiing trauma
2. 2006 Alcohol rehab
3. 2009 Double hernia repair

Medications currently taking

1. Gabapentin
2. Tramadol
3. Valium
4. Ambien
5. Atarax
6. Torodol

Supplements

1. Limcomin
2. Paramin
3. Calcium citrate
4. N-Acetylglucosamine
5. Psyllium
6. Fish oil
7. Dandelion root

Allergies

1. Benadryl – elevated heart rate
2. Elavil – elevated heart rate
3. Trazodone – clitoral priapism

Family history

1. Maternal cancer
2. Paternal alcohol/substance addiction
3. Paternal grandparent – seizure, alcohol/substance addiction

Systems review

1. Eyes: farsighted
2. General: worry/nervousness
3. Ears: N/A
4. Chest: N/A
5. Skin and hair: stretch marks, easy bruising, warts, split nails
6. ENT: N/A
7. Gastrointestinal: loss of appetite, nausea/vomiting, bloating, constipation
8. Cardiovascular: palpitations, low blood pressure
9. Bowel: greasy stool, rectal pain
10. Bladder: urine retention, incomplete urination, urinary tract infection (UTI), kidney stones, stress urinary incontinence (SUI)
11. Gynaecology: dysmennorrhoea, irregular menses, vaginal discharge, dryness vaginal pain, pelvic pain, dyspareunia, clitoral pain, Bartholin cysts ×3 (self-resolved)
12. Neurological: N/A
13. Musculoskeletal: back pain
14. Psychological: anxiety, substance abuse
15. Sexual: lack of arousal, pain in genitals, Bartholin cysts ×3

Psychometrics: MMPI-2

1. Valid
2. Clinical scale profile: HY, SI profile frequency 10.4%, profile stability high, supplementary scale profile: MAC-R
3. Content scale profile ANX HEA
4. Additional scales: physical, somatic, negative emotionality, generalized fearfulness, gastrointestinal symptoms, general health concerns
5. Critical items: acute anxiety states, somatic symptoms

Findings consistent with axis I chronic anxiety and somatic concerns and axis II predisposition to substance dependency.

Medical examination

Most recent gynaecological examination within the past 4 weeks indicates vaginal swab, microscopy/lab culture and bloodwork negative, visual inspection without colposcopy reports bilateral posterior vestibular inflammation and erythema with point tenderness localized 4 and 8 o'clock on cotton swab test. No cystocele, rectocele, or enterocele noted.

Patient narrative

I have been experiencing genital pain for 17 months starting 10 days after taking Cipro for a bladder infection. Symptoms improved but then I was told I had a yeast infection, although all cultures were negative, and I was given diflucan. I am negative for all STDs and ureaplasma, normal on pelvic CT scan, ultrasound and MRI to rule out pelvic congestion. My symptoms include swelling, pain with contact at vaginal opening and outside at 4 and 8 o'clock. Spontaneous raw burning getting worse over the day. Pain with sitting, tight clothes, and after urinating. Constant feeling of pressure or pushing out from lower half of vaginal opening to the anus. Severe anal pain about once a month lasting 30–60 minutes sometimes associated with sexual arousal. Intercourse abstinent for 11 months. I experience sexual arousal much less frequently and sometimes it makes pain and pressure worse. I have tried acupuncture, homeopathy, hypnosis, and meditation, which help with coping but have no effect on pain. I have tried physical therapy but after 3 months the therapist didn't think she was helping and called it off.

This condition has been very frustrating, and affects my career, my sex life, my marriage and relationships with my children, friends and colleagues. It has made my recovery from alcohol and drug addiction much more of a struggle as the pain is a trigger that makes me think about using and threatens my recovery.

Sexual evaluation

1. Menarche age 12, 28-day cycle, heavy flow, little dysmenorrhoea.
2. No history vaginal yeast, bacteria, viral or STD.
3. Intercourse initiates at age 18.
4. Reports history of variable, moderate to high, levels of desire and arousal daily with masturbation to orgasm thoughout teens.
5. G2P2 vaginal w/episiotomies. Both with large fetus and prolonged second stage labour. Patient reports postnatal recovery of desire/arousal/orgasm after breast feeding.
6. Orgasmic on clitoral stimulation manual/oral, self or partner, rarely with thrusting intercourse during which she conducts clitoral self-stimulation.
7. Since pain onset, patient reports dyspareunia, significantly reduced desire and arousal which is not discussed or 'managed' with her husband. She denies experiencing desire, arousal or orgasm since pain onset, but does engage in oral and manual stimulation of husband who also acknowledges frequent masturbation. Patient feels marriage is at risk due to her sexual abstinence.

Intrapelvic SEMG evaluation

1. Glazer Protocol administered with an intravaginal sensor after patient views information/educational and instructional video on correct use of equipment and proper position and action for PFM contractions while limiting co-contractions of leg adductors, lower abdominals and gluteal muscle groups.
2. Protocol consists of signal verification, pre-baseline rest (60 seconds), phasic (flick) contractions, tonic (10 second) contractions, endurance (60 second) contraction, and post-baseline rest (60 seconds). During the protocol pubococcygeal SEMG is taken continuously including amplitude, standard deviations, coefficients of variability, fast Fourier transformation power density spectral frequency, and recruitment/recovery latencies for all contractions and releases. At the completion of the protocol the data from the evaluation are printed out for the patient and stored in the database fore later analysis and comparison.
3. Intrapelvic SEMG findings:
   a. Mildly elevated amplitude (3.8 uv) moderately unstable (0.84 uv SD, 0.22 uv CV) pre-baseline rest.
   b. Slow recruitment (1.76 s) and recovery (2.34 s) latencies.
   c. Low flick peak average (14.62 uv).
   d. Low amplitude (12.48 uv) stable (1.62 SD, 0.13 uv CV), high FFT median spectral frequency (128.79 Hz) tonic contractions.
   e. Low amplitude (13.98 uv) stable (2.00 SD, 0.14 CV) high FFT median spectral frequency (124.76 Hz) endurance contraction.
   f. Low amplitude (2.07 uv) stable (0.31 uv SD, 0.15 uv CV) post-baseline rest.

History and data review and integration with treatment(s) prescribed

Summary of findings

Generally healthy 44-year-old female reporting 17-month history of acute onset, post Cipro for UTI, vulvar pain with both spontaneous nonlocalized chronic burning (dysaesthetic vulvodynia) and 5 and 7 pm localized provoked sharp pain on contact with introital dyspareunia (vulvar vestibulitis syndrome). Notable history includes child abuse with PTSD, alcohol and substance abuse in remission. Allergies to Benadryl, elavil and trazadone, presently taking multiple prescribed pain medications and multiple non-prescription supplements. She reports a family history of cancer and substance abuse. Systems review reveals:

1. Easy bruising, splitting nails and warts.
2. Loss of appetite, nausea/vomiting/bloating and constipation with pain on bowel movements and greasy stool.
3. Urine retention, incomplete voids, kidney stones, vaginal/rectal sensation 'like a ball pushing out from inside' and SUI.
4. Dysmenorrhoea, irregular menses, vaginal discharge, dryness, dyspareunia, vulvar, vaginal and clitoral pain spontaneous unprovoked chronic and localized provoked.
5. Reduced sexual desire arousal and orgasms with 17 months abstinence and concerned over marital relations.
6. Psychological evaluation reveals generalized anxiety and a focus on somatic concerns and a predisposition to substance abuse.
7. Gynaecological exam and labs, including complete blood count, are normal. Well-established organic causes of vulvar pain (infections, dermatoses, neuropathies, anatomic changes, pelvic inflammatory disorder, pelvic congestion, etc.) have been ruled out on multiple gynaecological and imaging procedure evaluations.
8. Intrapelvic SEMG evaluation shows mildly elevated and unstable initial rest, slow recruit/recover latencies and low peak amplitudes on phasic contractions, low amplitude, stable, high median frequency for both tonic and endurance contractions, and low-amplitude, stable post baseline.

Interpretation of findings

- Well-established organic causes of vulvar pain have been ruled out.
- Symptoms meet criteria for diagnosis of both DV and VVS, commonly overlapping conditions.
- The role of multiple prescription pain medications and non-prescription supplements to both symptom relief and/or symptom contribution must be reviewed.
- Concurrent systems disturbances include lower gastrointestinal and urogenital symptoms, commonly co-occurring with essential vulvar pain disorders which may suggest a common pathophysiology.
- Psychological factors are consistent with secondary role rather than primary aetiology. Psychological, interpersonal and sexual consequences are significant factors leading to symptomatic maintenance and resistance to functional change.
- Intrapelvic SEMG shows a pattern of pelvic floor dysfunction consistent with menstrual changes (recent onset of irregular menses), voiding disorders (retention, SUI) and essential vulvar pain disorders (DV, VVS).

Treatment

Specialty pain neurology consultation results in titration to termination of all pain, anxiolytic and soporific medications originally reported, and initiating Cymbalta 60 mg along with maintenance of hydroxazine and a lowered dose of trazadone, all taken an hour before bed. Supplements are continued as originally reported.

The patient was also referred to an endocrinologist specializing in female hormone problems including menopause transitions with sexual dysfunction. She was prescribed both topical (estrace ×2 daily) and intravaginal (vagifem daily) hormone replacement therapy (HRT).

Urological and gastrointestinal evaluations were deferred for possible later use if the initial treatment regimen did not bring about therapeutic changes in urinary and bowel symptoms.

Initiation of manualized 10-session programme of couples group sexual therapy for women suffering from vulvar pain, and their partners. This is an informational, educational, support group conducted by a psychologist using cognitive behavioural techniques and specific home assignments (Bergeron et al. 2001). For those sufferers with more profound sexual disturbances of desire, arousal and orgasm (FSFI) which offer direct interference with compliance to sexual prescriptices, brief individual therapy may also be employed, which is the case with this patient who underwent a course of brief, 10-session, weekly eclectic prescriptive therapy with a focus on addressing her general anxiety (breathing retraining), PTSD

(EMDR) from childhood abuse, somatic overconcern (systematic desensitization) and sexual avoidance (dilators, sensate focus, orgasmic restoration, etc.). Both the manualized group couples therapy and the individual therapy were conducted by the first author, who also conducted the intravaginal SEMG biofeedback.

As the patient is feeling vulnerable to relapse regarding alcohol and substance use she is encouraged to return to regular 12-step programme attendance upon completion of the manualized 10-session programme of group sexual therapy for couples in which women suffer from essential vulvar pain disorders.

The intrapelvic SEMG pattern most closely matches that pattern shown by perimenopausal women (Glazer et al. 1999, Romanzi et al. 1999). The age of the patient, recent onset of irregular menses, bowel and bladder changes, vulvar dryness, sensations associated with pelvic floor relaxation, and the findings of the endocrinologist all suggest atrophic changes may be contributory to her vulvar pain. The SEMG pattern is also consistent with the symptoms of urinary retention (elevated unstable baseline) and recent onset of SUI (slow and weak urethral closure) as well as functional faecal constipation. Intrapelvic SEMG biofeedback combined with topical and intravaginal HRT has, in my clinical practice, shown positive results with this symptom pattern.

Maintenance of collaboration with all treating resources and, as needed, availability to the patient for information and support is a key part of the ongoing treatment. The average treatment duration to maximize symptom relief and re-establish related functions is 6–12 months during which time the patient returns for office visits every 1–2 months for review of progress and modifications to treatments. The coordinating therapist is informed by the patient of upcoming appointment dates with collaborating physicians who are then asked to provide a summary of their office visit with the patient. These integrated records are, in turn, available to all members of the team, and the patient, who is encouraged to maintain a full set of her own records.

Outcomes

Medical

After 6 months of treatment the medical records report improved integrity of the vulvar vestibule tissue with greater thickness and elasticity, no erythema, reduced variable spontaneous unprovoked burning with up to 2 weeks of no discomfort, intermittent episodes of intercourse with no dyspareunia, and improved lubrication. Q-tip test shows 85% reduction in localized provoked vestibular pain. Urinary and bowel symptoms normalized with bladder intervoid interval of 2–3 hours without postvoid residual, and bowel movements average daily with well-formed stool and comfortable defecation.

Psychological, psychosexual

Patient reports reduction of generalized anxiety, somatic concerns and negative emotionality. Patient and spouse report progression from total sexual abstinence to non-sexual mutual massage, then non-genital mutual massage, then non-penetrative mutual stimulation and finally intercourse. The patient has increasingly built confidence by use of the vaginal dilator and vibrator to achieve rapid, non-irritating, pleasure and often multiple orgasms. Intercourse has resumed an average of once a week. Some attempts at intercourse must still be aborted due to dyspareunia.

Social, marital, occupational

Communication with her husband has improved, she has been much better able to perform her job tasks, spend leisure time with the family and friends and re-engage in her daily exercise routine.

Substance use

Her sense of vulnerability to relapse regarding substance use remains well controlled and she continues 3×/week attendance at 12-step meetings and remains abstinent of all substance and alcohol use throughout the treatment period.

Treatment compliance

She has maintained a high level of compliance with prescribed 20 min ×2/day pelvic floor SEMG biofeedback and has normalized her intravaginal SEMG. The patient still reports that episodic stress from environmental demands can still lead to setbacks with recurrence of vulvar vestibular burning and localized hypersensitivity to contact. The patient will continue her full compliment of treatments for the following 6 months and there are no contraindications to expectations of full recovery (Glazer 2000). However, as with all essential chronic pain disorders in which the pathophysiology is not understood, the patient must be taught a subconscious, habitual, but constant awareness of the presence of risk factors, in order to achieve a balance between prophylaxis while maintaining the highest levels of engagement possible with the least restrictions on the conduct of daily life activities. Keeping this balance between awareness of chronic predisposition (ledger, genetics) and maximization of functional engagement is the key to a healthy and satisfying life for those who suffer from any essential chronic pain disorders.

References

Alfonsi, E., Pavesi, R., Merio, I.M., et al., 1999. Hemoglobin near-infrared spectroscopy and surface EMG study in muscle ischemia and fatiguing isometric contraction. J. Sports Med. Phys. Fitness 39 (2), 83–92.

Arena, J.G., 2002. Chronic pain: psychological approaches for the front-line clinician. J. Clin. Psychol. 58 (11), 1385–1396.

Basmajian, J.V. (Ed.), 1989. Biofeedback: Principles and practice for clinicians. third ed. Williams & Wilkins, Baltimore, MD.

Bendaña, E.E., Belarmino, J.M., Dinh, J.H., Cook, C.L., Murray, B.P., Feustel, P.J., et al., 2009. Efficacy of transvaginal biofeedback and electrical stimulation in women with urinary urgency and frequency and associated pelvic floor muscle spasm. Urol. Nurs. 29 (3), 171–176. PMID: 19579410.

Bergeron, S., Binik, Y.M., Khalife, S., et al., 2001. A randomized controlled comparison of group cognitive-behavioral therapy, surface electromyographic biofeedback and vestibulectomy in the treatment of dyspareunia resulting from vulvar vestibulitis. Pain 91, 297–306.

Boersma, K., Linton, S.J., 2006a. Psychological processes underlying the development of a chronic pain problem: a prospective study of the relationship between profiles of psychological variables in the fear-avoidance model and disability. Clin. J. Pain 22 (2), 160–166.

Boersma, K., Linton, S.J., 2006b. Expectancy, fear and pain in the prediction of chronic pain and disability: a prospective analysis. Eur. J. Pain 10 (6), 551–557.

Bornstein, J., Simons, D.G., 2002. Focused review: myofascial pain. Arch. Phys. Med. Rehabil. 83 (3 Suppl. 1), S40–S47, S48–S49.

Brown, C., Vogt, V., Menkes, D., Ling, F., Glazer, H., Curnow, J., 2003. An open label trial of botulinum toxin type A in treating women with vulvar vestibulitis syndrome. Poster presentation. The International Society for the Study of Women's Sexual Health (ISSWSH), Amsterdam, Netherlands.

Brown, C., Glazer, H., Vogt, V., Menkes, D., 2005. Effect of botulinum toxin type A on sexual function in vestibulodynia. Abstract 179. Sexual Medicine Society of North America, New York, NY.

Brown, C.S., Vogt, V., Menkes, D., Bachmann, G., Glazer, H., 2004. Subjective and objective outcomes of Botulinum Toxin Type A in Vulvar Vestibulitis Syndrome, Vulvodynia and Sexual Pain Disorders in Women Conference, Atlanta, GA.

Brown, C.S., Glazer, H.I., Vogt, V., Menkes, D., Bachmann, G., 2006. Subjective and objective outcomes of botulinum toxin type A treatment in vestibulodynia: pilot data. J. Reprod. Med. 51 (8), 635–641.

Chen, J.T., Chen, S.M., Kuan, T.S., Chung, K.C., Hong, C.Z., 1998. Phentolamine effect on the spontaneous electrical activity of active loci in a myofascial trigger spot of rabbit skeletal muscle. Arch. Phys. Med. Rehabil. 79 (7), 790–794.

Chiarioni, G., Nardo, A., Vantini, I., Romito, A., Whitehead, W.E., 2009. Biofeedback is superior to electrogalvanic stimulation and massage for treatment of levator ani syndrome. Gastroenterology

Cornel, E.B., van Haarst, E.P., Schaarsberg, R.W., Geels, J., 2005. The effect of biofeedback physical therapy in men with chronic pelvic pain syndrome type III. Eur. Urol. 47 (5), 607–611.

deCharms, R.C., Maeda, F., Glover, G.H., et al., 2005. Control over brain activation and pain learned by using real-time functional MR. Proc. Natl. Acad. Sci. U. S. A. 102 (51), 18626–18631.

Dimitrov, G.V., Arabadzhiev, T.I., Mileva, K.N., Bowtell, J.L., Crichton, N., Dimitrova, N.A., 2006. Muscle fatigue during dynamic contractions assessed by new spectral indices. Med. Sci. Sports Exerc. 38 (11), 1971–1979.

Flor, H., 2002. The modification of cortical reorganization and chronic pain by sensory feedback. Appl. Psychophysiol. Biofeedback 27 (3), 215–227.

Flor, H., Fydrich, T., Turk, D.C., 1992. Efficacy of multidisciplinary pain treatment centers: a meta-analytic review. Pain 49 (2), 221–230.

Gatchel, R.J., Pent, Y.B., Peters, M.L., Fuchs, P.N., Turk, D.C., 2007. The biopsychosocial approach to chronic pain: scientific advances and future directions. Psych. Bull. 133 (4), 581–624.

Glazer, H.I., 2000. Dysesthetic vulvodynia. Long term follow-up after treatment with surface electromyography-assisted pelvic floor muscle rehabilitation. J. Reprod. Med. 45, 798–802.

Glazer, H.I., Laine, C.D., 2007. Pelvic floor muscle biofeedback in the treatment of urinary incontinence: a literature review. Appl. Psychophysiol. Biofeedback 31 (3), 187–201.

Glazer, H.I., MacConkey, D., 1996. Functional rehabilitation of pelvic floor muscles: a challenge to tradition. Urol. Nurs. 16 (2), 68–69.

Glazer, H.I., Rodke, G., Swencionis, C., Hertz, R., Young, A.W., 1995. Treatment of vulvar vestibulitis syndrome with electromyographic biofeedback of pelvic floor musculature. J. Reprod. Med. 40 (4), 283–290.

Glazer, H.I., Jantos, M., Hartmann, E., Swencionis, C., 1998. Electromyographic comparisons of the pelvic floor in asymptomatic and vulvodynia females. J. Reprod. Med. 43, 959–962.

Glazer, H.I., Romanzi, L., Polaneczky, M., 1999. Pelvic floor muscle surface electromyography; reliability and clinical predictive validity. J. Reprod. Med. 44, 779–782.

Glazer, H.I., Marinoff, S.M., Sleight, I.J., 2002. The web-enabled Glazer surface electromyographic protocol for the remote, real-time assessment and rehabilitation of pelvic floor dysfunction in vulvovaginal pain disorders. J. Reprod. Med. 47 (9), 728–730.

Granot, M., Friedman, M., Yamitsky, D., Zimmer, E.Z., 2002. Enhancement of the perception of systemic pain in women with vulvar vestibulitis. BJOG 109 (8), 863–866.

Grimaud, J.C., Bouvier, M., Naudy, B., Guien, C., Salducci, J., 1991. Manometric and radiologic investigations and biofeedback treatment of chronic idiopathic anal pain. Dis. Colon Rectum 34 (8), 690–695.

Hart, A.D., Mathisen, K.S., Prater, J.S., 1981. A comparison of skin temperature and EMG training for primary dysmenorrhea. Biofeedback Self Regul. 6 (3), 367–373.

Heah, S.M., Ho, Y.H., Tan, M., Leong, A.F., 1997. Biofeedback is effective treatment for levator ani syndrome. Dis. Colon Rectum 40 (2), 187–189.

Hetrick, D.C., Glazer, H., Liu, Y.W., Turner, J.A., Frest, M., Berger, R.E., 2006. Pelvic floor electromyography in men with chronic pelvic pain syndrome: a case-controlled study. Neurourol. Urodyn. 25 (1), 46–49.

Hug, F., Faucher, M., Marqueste, T., et al., 2004. Electromyographic signs of neuromuscular fatigue are comcomitant with further increase in ventilation during static handgrip. Clin. Physiol. Funct. Imaging 24 (1), 25–32.

Jantos, M., 2008. Vulvodynia:a psychophysiological profile based on electromyographic assessment. Appl. Psychophysiol. Biofeedback 33 (1), 29–38.

Kegel, A.H., 1948. Progressive resistance exercise in the functional restoration of the perineal muscles. Am. J. Obstet. Gynecol. 56 (2), 238–248.

Kegel, A.H., 1952. Stress incontinence and genital relaxation: a nonsurgical method of increasing the tone of sphincters and their supporting structures. Ciba Clin. Symp. 4 (2), 35–51.

McKay, E., Kaufman, R., Doctor, U., et al., 2001. Treatment of vulvar vestibulitis with electromyographic biofeedback of pelvic floor musculature. J. Reprod. Med. 46 (4), 337–347.

McNulty, W.H., Gevirtz, R.N., Hubbard, D.R., Berkoff, G.M., 1994. Needle electromyographic evaluation of trigger point response to a psychological stressor. Psychophysiology 31 (3), 313–316.

Mehta, A., Bachman, G., 2008. Vulvovaginal complaints. Clin. Obstet. Gynecol. 51 (3), 549–555.

Mense, S., 2000. Neurobiological concepts of fibromyalgia: the possible role of descending spinal tracts. Scand. J. Rheumatol. Suppl. 113, 24–29.

Mense, S., 2004. Functional neuroanatomy for pain stimuli, reception, transmission and processing. Schmerz 18 (3), 225–237 (German).

Romanzi, L., Polaneczky, M., Glazer, H.I., 1999. A simple test of pelvic muscle during pelvic examination: correlation to surface electromyography. J. Neurourol. Urodyn. 18, 603–612.

Schwartz, M., Andrasik, F. (Eds.), 2003. Biofeedback: A practitioner's guide. third ed. Guilford Press, New York.

Tachi, M., Kouzaki, M., Kanejosa, J., Fukunaga, T., 2004. The influence of circulatory difference on muscle oxygenation and fatigue during intermittent static dorsiflexion. Eur. J. Appl. Physiol. 91 (5–6), 682–688.

Turk, D.C., Dworkin, R.H., McDermott, M.P., et al., 2008. Analyzing multiple endpoints in clinical trials of pain treatments: IMMPACT recommendations Initiative on Methods, Measurement and Pain Assessment in Clinical Trials. Pain 139 (3), 485–493.

Wager, T.D., Lindquist, M., Kaplan, L., 2007. Meta-analysis of functional neuroimaging data: current and future directions. Soc. Cogn. Affect Neurosci. 2 (2), 150–158.

White, G., Jantos, M., Glazer, H.I., 1997. Establishing the diagnosis of vulvar vestibulitis. J. Reprod. Med. 42, 157–161.

Yoshino, A., Okamoto, Y., Onada, K., et al., 2009. Sadness enhances the experience of pain via neural activation in the anterior ingulate cortex and amygdale: An fMRI study. Neuroimage

Yoshitake, Y., Ue, H., Miyazaki, M., Moritani, T., 2001. Assessment of lower-back muscle fatigue using electromyography, mechanomyography and near-infrared spectroscopy. Eur. J. Appl. Physiol. 84 (3), 174–179.

Zubieta, J.K., Stohler, C.S., 2009. Neurobiological mechanisms of placebo responses. Ann. N. Y. Acad. Sci. 1156, 198–210.

Websites

http://www.ncbi.nlm.nih.gov/pubmed/7623358?itool=EntrezSystem2.PEntrez.Pubmed.Pubmed_ResultsPanel.Pubmed_RVDocSum&ordinalpos=71.

http://www.ncbi.nlm.nih.gov/pubmed/1855425?itool=EntrezSystem2.PEntrez.Pubmed.Pubmed_ResultsPanel.Pubmed_RVDocSum&ordinalpos=77.

Soft tissue manipulation approaches to chronic pelvic pain (external)

11.1

César Fernández de las Peñas Andrzej Pilat

CHAPTER CONTENTS

Introduction

There is increasing evidence demonstrating the importance of treating muscle and connective tissue in patients with chronic pelvic pain (CPP). Eighty-five percent of patients with CPP present with dysfunction or impairments in the musculoskeletal system, including poor posture and pelvic floor muscle (PFM) imbalances (Baker 1993, Hetrick et al. 2003, Prendergast & Weiss 2003, Tu et al. 2006). Shoskes et al. (2008) found that 51% of men with chronic CPP reported tenderness to palpation of the PFM, and Tu et al. (2008) demonstrated that women with CPP had a greater prevalence of musculoskeletal disorders compared with women without CPP. Furthermore, tenderness to palpation of the PFM was related to a decreased ability to relax these muscles (Tu et al. 2008).

It is apparent that proper functioning of the pelvic region is directly related to appropriate integration of the connective tissue and muscles of the lower quadrant. The presence of musculoskeletal dysfunctions may contribute to improper functioning of the pelvic region from both a biomechanical and neurophysiological perspective; for example, increasing tension and/or shortening of the PFM (Haugstad et al. 2006), and initiation or maintenance of a neurogenic inflammation

(Wesselmann 2001). In the animal model, Miranda et al. (2004) found that irritation of pelvic musculoskeletal structures promoted antidromic transmission of nociceptive inputs to bladder sensory neurons, promoting a state of neurogenic inflammation.

The diversity of clinical symptoms and physical findings found in patients with CPP emphasizes the necessity of multimodal approaches for the management of this patient population (FitzGerald & Kotarinos 2003a, Fox 2009), as outlined Chapters 8.1 and 8.2. Additionally, there is clinical and scientific evidence for suggesting that CPP can become a chronic syndrome (Bajaj et al. 2003), and hence treatment should be directed at both biomechanical and neurophysiological issues (Samraj et al. 2005). This multimodal approach is also based on the clinical relationship between CPP and pelvic girdle pain (PGP), as many patients diagnosed with PGP also suffer from CPP (Vleeming et al. 2008).

The current chapter covers external manual interventions directed at the muscles and loose connective tissues of the pelvic area that can be involved in the development or maintenance of CPP, including PGP. We discuss the neurophysiological rationale for different techniques from local muscle dysfunction (trigger points) to connective tissue entrapments (fascial tissue restrictions).

Local muscle dysfunction: Muscle trigger points

Trigger points and chronic pelvic pain

The association between CPP and myofascial pain syndrome was identified several years ago (Slocumb 1984, 1990, Schmidt 1991). Myofascial pain is also related to urogenital pain (Doggweiler-Wiygul 2004). Jarrell (2004) found that abdominal trigger points (TrPs) predicted evidence of visceral disease in 90% of a sample of 55 patients with CPP. Montenegro et al. (2009) recently proposed that abdominal myofascial syndrome should be considered in the differential diagnosis of CPP. In 2009 the European Association of Urology published guidelines suggesting that TrPs should be considered in the diagnosis of CPP (Fall et al. 2010). In fact, Anderson et al. (2009) found that TrPs in the abdominal muscles were the most prevalent in male with CPP.

Myofascial pain syndrome can be associated with both TrPs and restrictions of the fascial tissue. The most commonly accepted definition for TrP is: 'a hyperirritable spot in a taut band of a skeletal muscle that is painful on compression, stretch, overload or contraction which responds with a referred pain that is perceived distant from the spot' (Simons et al. 1999). From a clinical viewpoint, we distinguish active and latent TrPs. Active TrPs are those in which local and referred pain reproduce symptoms reported by the patient, with the pain being recognized by the patient as a 'familiar' pain (Simons et al. 1999). For instance, in patients with CPP, active TrPs will reproduce perineal or pelvic pain. Latent TrPs are those where local and referred pain do not reproduce pain symptoms, or where elicited pain is not familiar to the patient (Simons et al. 1999). For instance, in a patient with neuropathic pelvic pain, referred pain can be elicited but does not reproduce the patient's symptoms. Furthermore, a relevant feature of both active and latent TrPs is that each can induce muscle imbalances or altered motor recruitment (Lucas et al. 2004).

There are several studies demonstrating a relationship between CPP and muscle TrPs. Weiss (2001) reported the successful amelioration of symptoms in patients with interstitial cystitis using myofascial TrP release. Doggweiler-Wiygul & Wiygul (2002) found that inactivation of TrPs in PFM, gluteus and piriformis muscles improved or resolved the pain in four patients with severe CPP, interstitial cystitis and irritative voiding symptoms. Anderson et al. (2005) showed that incorporation of TrP inactivation into a multimodal approach for CPP in men resulted in an effective therapeutic approach, by providing a reduction in pain and urinary symptoms superior to that of traditional therapy. This study included voluntary isometric contractions and relaxation, to induce post-isometric relaxation and reciprocal inhibition, together with deep soft tissue mobilization (stripping, strumming, skin rolling and effleurage) as interventions directed at TrPs (Anderson et al. 2005). Anderson et al. (2006, 2009) also found that TrP inactivation was associated with significant improvement in urinary symptoms, libido, ejaculatory and erectile pain, and ejaculatory dysfunction in men with CPP. See Chapter 12 for more detail of Anderson's studies. Langford et al. (2007) demonstrated the effectiveness of TrPs inactivation of the levator ani muscle for the management of some patients with CPP. In this study 13 of 18 women improved with the first TrP injection resulting in a success rate of 72%, whereas 6 of 18 (33%) were completely pain-free.

FitzGerald et al. (2009) demonstrated a better response rate (57%) in CPP patients treated with TrP therapy as compared to the response rate (21%) in those patients receiving global therapeutic massage. In a review of prostatitis and CPP, Anderson (2002) described palpation and treatment protocols for locating muscle TrPs associated with prostatitis symptoms. In a subsequent later study, Anderson et al. (2009) confirmed a relationship between muscle TrPs and CPP in men, identifying the most common location of TrPs: pubococcygeus or puborectalis (90%), external oblique (80%), rectus abdominis (75%), adductors (19%) and gluteus medius (18%) muscles. Other relevant muscles in which TrPs also contribute to CPP are levator ani, iliopsoas, quadratus lumborum, gluteus maximus and the thoracolumbar extensor muscles (Simons et al. 1999, Carter 2000, Liebenson 2000, FitzGerald & Kotarinos 2003a, Chaitow 2007a, Montenegro et al. 2008, Anderson et al. 2009).

Why is inactivation of trigger points in chronic pelvic pain important?

The role of neurogenic inflammation has been emphasized as contributing to the pathophysiology of CPP (Wesselmann 2001). It is well accepted that noxious (nociceptive) stimuli can increase the production of pain-promoting substances at the nerve-free endings of the primary afferent nociceptors. When a sensitive nerve fibre is stimulated the impulse runs towards the spinal cord (orthodromic flow) and towards the periphery (antidromic). When the antidromic stimulus reaches the periphery, there is a release of several neuropeptides (e.g. nitric oxide, substance P, calcitonin gene-related protein) promoting neurogenic inflammation, characterized by vasodilatation, oedema and hyperalgesia (Wesselmann 2001). Clinicians should be aware of the neurophysiological theories for inactivating muscle TrPs in CPP.

1. *Trigger points are a focus of peripheral nociception.* Muscle pain is associated with the activation of nociceptors by a variety of endogenous substances, e.g. bradykinin or serotonin (Babenko et al. 1999a), substance P (Babenko et al. 1999b) and glutamate (Svensson et al. 2003). Microdialysis studies have found that concentrations of bradykinin, calcitonin gene-related peptide, substance P, tumour necrosis factor-α, interleukin-1β, serotonin or norepinephrine were significantly higher in active TrPs as compared to latent TrP or non-TrP tissues (Shah et al. 2005, 2008). Another study has demonstrated the existence of nociceptive hypersensitivity (hyperalgesia) and non-nociceptive hypersensitivity (allodynia) at the sites of muscle TrPs (Li et al. 2009). These studies support the proposal that TrPs constitute a focus of sensitization of both nociceptive and non-nociceptive nerve endings.
2. *Trigger point nociception induces central sensitization.* When muscle tissue is sensitized, nociceptors are more readily activated and respond inappropriately to normal innocuous or weak stimuli, e.g. light pressure or movement. The presence of multiple TrPs in different muscles (spatial summation), or the presence of TrPs for prolonged periods of time (temporal summation), can sensitize the spinal cord and supraspinal structures by means of a continued nociceptive afferent barrage into the central nervous system (Mense 1994). Kuan et al. (2007) demonstrated that spinal cord connections of muscle TrPs were effective in inducing neuroplastic changes in the dorsal horn neurons. Niddam et al. (2007) demonstrated that pain associated with TrPs is at least partially processed at supraspinal levels, particularly the peri-aqueductal grey matter. Readers are referred to Chapter 3 for a review of neurophysiology.
3. *Trigger points and the sympathetic nervous system.* There is evidence of an association between TrPs and the sympathetic nervous system (McNulty et al. 1994, Chen et al. 1998, Chung et al. 2004). Ge et al. (2006) found increased referred pain intensity and tenderness with sympathetic hyperactivity at muscle TrPs, suggesting a sympathetic contribution to the mechanisms responsible for the generation of referred pain. A study by Zhang et al. (2009) demonstrated an attenuated skin blood flow response after painful stimulation of latent TrPs, as compared with control non-TrPs, suggesting increased sympathetic vasoconstriction activity at latent TrPs.

Best evidence of soft tissue interventions for muscle trigger points

In this section we review the evidence for soft tissue interventions targeted at inactivating muscle TrPs. However, clinicians should consider that current evidence is based on the application of single treatments applied to TrPs, when multimodal approaches are usually practised by clinicians. Further, it is clear that management of myofascial dysfunction in patients with CPP requires a multidisciplinary approach (Srinivasan et al. 2007; see also Chapters 8.1 and 8.2). The inclusion of these techniques into a multimodal approach for patients with CPP has been found to be effective (Weiss 2001, Doggweiler-Wiygul & Wiygul 2002, Anderson et al. 2005, 2006).

Among the different interventions directed at inactivating TrPs, manual therapy is the first treatment option (Dommerholt et al. 2006). Different soft tissue interventions have been suggested, including: static compression (Hong et al. 1993, Simons et al. 1999, Fryer & Hodgson 2005, Fernández-de-las-Peñas et al. 2006, Gemmell et al. 2008, Dommerholt & McEvoy 2010), massage (Simons et al. 1999), stretching (Hong et al. 1993, Simons et al. 1999, Hanten et al. 2000), muscle energy techniques (Lewit 1999, Chaitow 2006, Rodríguez-Blanco et al. 2006), strain–counterstrain (Ibáñez-Garcia et al. 2009, Lewit 1999), neuromuscular techniques (Chaitow & Delany 2008, Ibáñez-García et al. 2009, Palomeque-del-Cerro & Fernández-de-las-Peñas 2009), positional release techniques (Chaitow 2007b) and manipulative interventions (Ruiz-Sáez et al. 2007, Fernández-de-las-Peñas 2009).

Systematic reviews have investigated the effectiveness of soft tissue manual intervention for inactivating TrPs (Fernández-de-las-Peñas et al. 2005, Rickards 2006, Vernon & Schneider 2009). These reviews found moderate to strong evidence supporting the use of static compression for immediate pain relief of muscle TrPs but limited evidence for long-term pain relief. Additionally, there is preliminary evidence demonstrating changes in muscle sensitivity after spinal manipulations (Ruíz-Sáez et al. 2006, Fernández-de-las-Peñas 2009), although further studies are required.

Application of soft tissue interventions for trigger points

In this section soft tissue interventions applied to TrPs in those muscles in which referred pain can contribute to CPP are described. Clinicians are encouraged to develop their own techniques based on a clinical reasoning process (see Chapter 7). Selection of any technique should include consideration of TrP irritability and the degree of sensitization of the central nervous system of the patient with CPP.

Compression interventions

Different compression techniques, depending on the amount of pressure applied, presence/absence of pain (Lewit 1999, Simons et al. 1999), duration of application (Hou et al. 2002), or position of the tissue (shortened or lengthened), have been described. In our clinical practice, the pressure level, duration of application, and position of the muscle, depend on sensitization mechanisms of the patient, and degree of irritability of the TrP. Table 11.1.1 summarizes clinical application of four different forms of compression: ischaemic compression (Travell & Simons 1983), TrP pressure release (Lewit 1999, Simons et al. 1999), strain/counter-strain (Jones 1981) or positional release therapies (Chaitow 2007b), and intermittent compression (Chaitow 1994).

Simons (2002) proposed that compressing the sarcomeres by direct pressure in a vertical and perpendicular manner may equalize the length of the muscle sarcomeres in the involved TrP and decrease pain. Hou et al. (2002) suggested that pain relief may result from reactive hyperaemia within the TrP or a spinal reflex mechanism for the relief of muscle tension.

Under the next heading, we describe different forms of compression interventions applied to pelvic muscle TrPs. Clinicians can apply ischaemic compression (Travell & Simons 1983), pressure release (Lewit 1999, Simons et al. 1999) or positional release therapy (Chaitow 2007b) principles depending on the patient's characteristics.

Static compression of piriformis/external obturator muscle trigger points

Typical piriformis TrP referred pain is shown in Figure 11.1.1 (Simons et al. 1999). TrPs in this muscle may contribute to pain in the lower back, buttock, hip, posterior thigh and leg, but also to pain into the groin, perineum and sometimes in the rectum during defecation. For this technique, the patient is prone with the therapist standing to the side. The therapist localizes the TrP (it can be located just lateral to the sacrum or the muscle belly), and applies a static compression directly over it. Clinicians are encouraged to use both hands during the technique (Figure 11.1.2). A similar technique may be applied over the external obturator muscle belly which has a similar pattern of referral to that of the piriformis (Cox & Bakkum 2005).

Table 11.1.1 Different compression interventions that can be applied to myofascial trigger points

	Muscle position	Degree of compression	Time of pressure	Duration of the technique
Ischaemic compression (Travell & Simons 1983)	Fully lengthened	Sufficient to maintain pain at level of between 5 and 7 – where 10 is maximum that can be tolerated (NPRS)	Until pain eases by around 50–75%	Up to 90 seconds
TrP pressure release (Simons et al. 1999)	Partially lengthened	Painless (first perception of tissue barrier)	Until the therapist perceives taut band release	Up to 90 seconds
Strain/counter-strain (Jones 1981)	Neurologically silent (shortened)	Reduction of pain by around 70%	Constant throughout	90 seconds
Pulsed ischaemic compression (Chaitow 1994)	At 'first sign of resistance' barrier – i.e. no lengthening	5-second compression to induce pain at level 7 (NPRS) – followed by 2 seconds no pressure – repeated until local or referred change reported or palpated	5 seconds pressure, 2 seconds no pressure, repeated	Up to 90 seconds – or until change in pain reported, or taut band release perceived

NPRS: Numerical Pain Rate Scale (0–10).

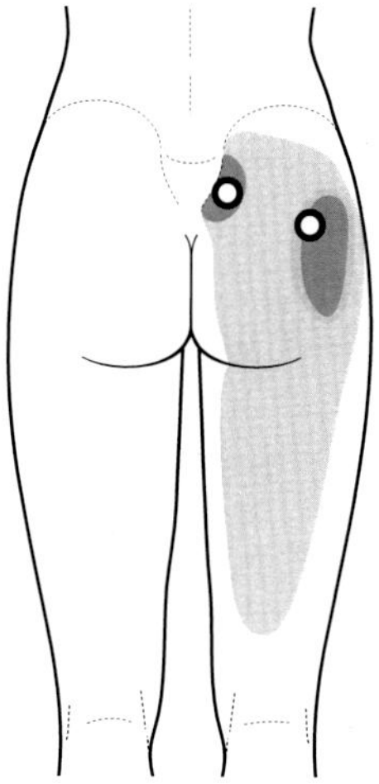

Figure 11.1.1 • Referred pain elicited by piriformis muscle TrPs

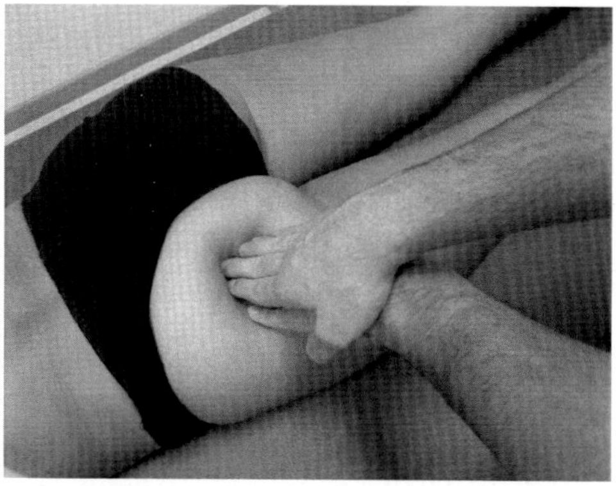

Figure 11.1.2 • Static compression of piriformis muscle TrPs

Static compression of pectineus muscle trigger points

The pectineus muscle is an important adductor muscle in relation to CPP since TrP referred pain is commonly perceived as a deep dull pain in the lateral groin area (Figure 11.1.3A). For the technique, the patient lies supine with the therapist standing to the side. The therapist localizes the TrP which is usually located in the muscle belly (just lateral to the tendon of the adductor longus muscle at the pubic bone), and applies a static compression directly over it. Clinicians are encouraged to use both hands during the compression, although the thumb is also frequently employed (Figure 11.1.4).

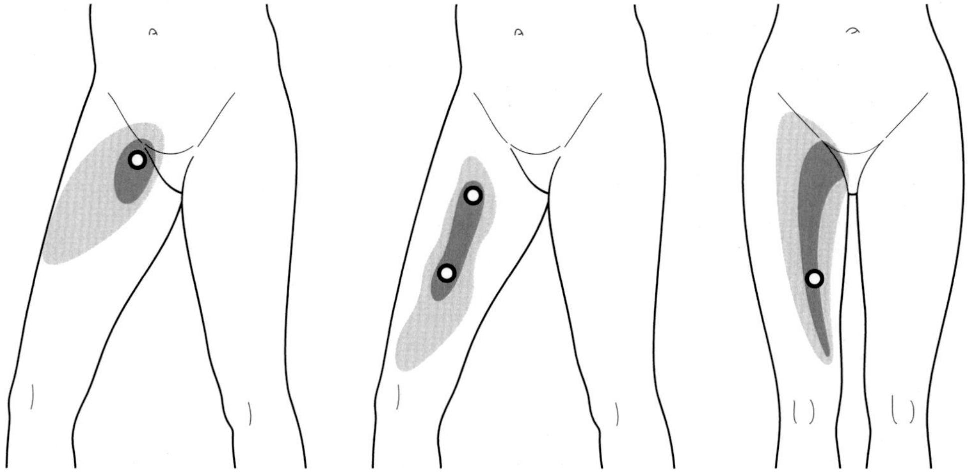

Figure 11.1.3 • Referred pain elicited by pectineus (A), adductor longus (B) and adductor magnus (C) muscle TrPs

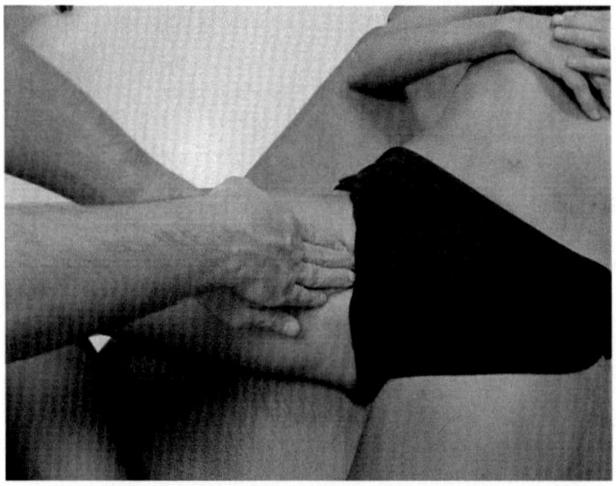

Figure 11.1.4 • Static compression of pectineus muscle TrPs

Intermittent compression of pelvic floor muscle trigger points

PFM TrPs can mimic symptoms of painful coccydynia or levator ani syndrome (Simons et al. 1999, Chaitow 2007a). In general, pelvic floor muscle TrPs refer pain toward the perineum, vagina, penile base, and give a sensation of fullness into the rectum and an urgency to urinate (Figure 11.1.5A–C). Nevertheless, it seems that TrPs in some PFM are more prevalent in CPP (Anderson et al. 2009). For instance, referred pain from pubococcygeus and puborectalis muscles spreads to the perineum and adjacent urogenital structures. Lewit & Horacek (2004) demonstrated that inactivation of pubococcygeus muscle TrPs induced secondary inactivation of erector spine TrPs. Levator ani and coccygeus TrPs refer pain to the sacrococcygeal region and also to the vagina or penis. TrPs in the internal obturator refer pain to the anococcygeal region and to the vagina. It has also been observed clinically that in some patients with CPP, pelvic floor muscle TrPs can refer pain to the sacrum.

In our clinical experience, PFM respond very well to TrP pressure release. For this technique the patient lies supine or side-lying. The therapist localizes the TrP which is usually located in a specific PFM (particularly located in the ischiorectal fossa) and applies an intermittent digital (finger or thumb) compression to it (Figure 11.1.6). Further details regarding PFM trigger point techniques can be found in Chapter 13.

Compression and contraction of gluteus maximus muscle trigger points

TrP-referred pain from gluteus maximus muscle is perceived as deep and burning pain located in the sacroiliac, coccyx and buttock areas (Figure 11.1.7). This technique consists of applying a TrP compression combined with an isometric contraction of the compressed muscle (Gröbli & Dejung 2003). For that purpose, the patient is side-lying with the therapist behind. TrPs within the gluteus maximus muscle

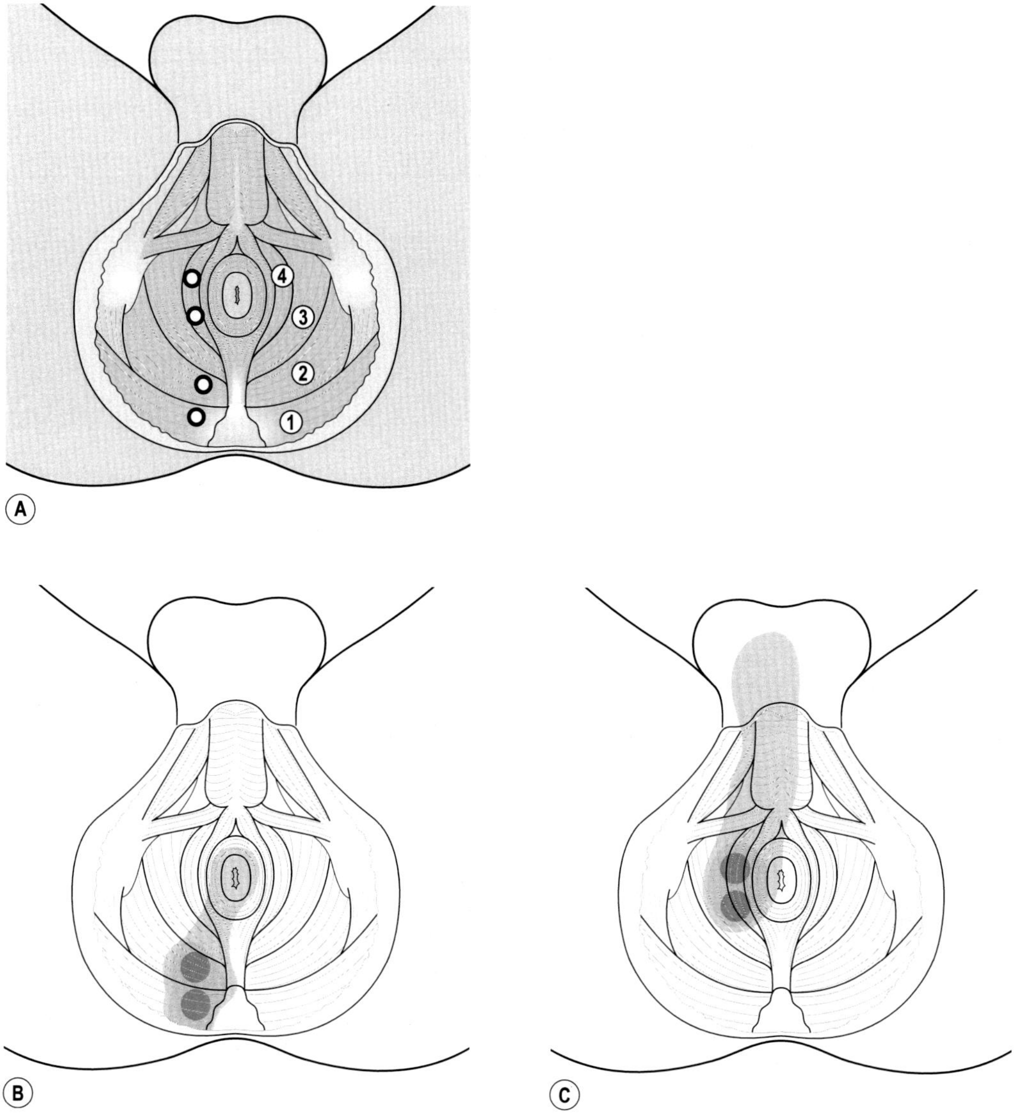

Figure 11.1.5 • (A) Scheme of pelvic floor muscles: 1. Coccygeus. 2. Iliococcygeus. 3. Pubococcygeus. 4. Levator ani. (B) Referred pain from coccygeus or iliococcygeus muscle TrPs. (C) Referred pain from pubococcygeus or levator ani muscle TrPs

are best palpated and compressed by pincer palpation. Once the therapist locates a TrP (it can placed in any part of the muscle belly) a pincer compression is applied using one or both hands (as illustrated in Figure 11.1.8). When the therapist perceives a slight relaxation of the TrP, the patient is asked to contract the muscle by squeezing both buttocks for 5 seconds. The therapist should maintain the compression during the contraction. If two hands are employed, stretching of the tissues housing the trigger point should follow the contraction, as illustrated. In the authors' clinical experience, a total of ten repetitions is usually sufficient to achieve inactivation of gluteal muscle TrPs.

Stretching compression of iliopsoas muscle trigger points

TrPs in the iliopsoas muscle refer pain to the groin area, superior part of the thigh and to the back (Figure 11.1.9). This is an important muscle since

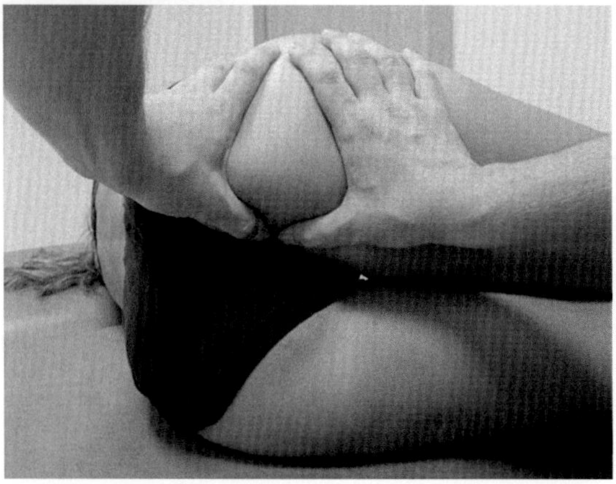

Figure 11.1.6 • Intermittent compression of pelvic floor muscle TrPs

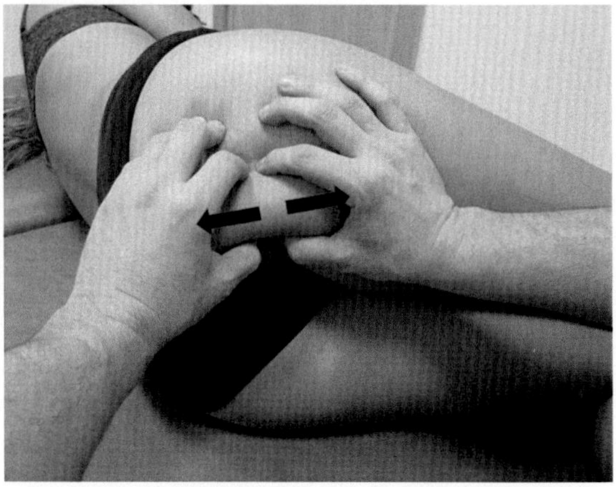

Figure 11.1.8 • Compression and contraction of gluteus maximus muscle TrPs (with accompanying stretch following contraction)

it is anatomically related to several urogenital structures and the lumbar plexus (Stepnik et al. 2006).

A stretching compression technique combines a compression intervention with passive or active stretching of the TrP taut band. For this purpose the patient is supine with the knee and hip flexed, and the foot on the table. The therapist compresses the TrP (usually located within the muscle belly reached through overlying abdominal muscles) with the tips of the fingers of one or both hands. At the time that the therapist perceives a slightly relaxation of the TrP taut band, the patient is asked to straighten the knee and the hip, either passively or actively, to increase the tension in the taut band (Figure 11.1.10). The aim of this technique is for the patient to achieve pain-free extension of the hip and knee, at the same time that the therapist maintains the compression.

Massage

Massage has multiple clinical applications with positive effects, but often lacks scientific evidence. This may be related to the fact that there are so many different forms of massage that still remain under-researched. The application of massage for inactivating muscle TrPs was discussed by Simons (2002) and Hong et al. (1993), who proposed that massage may exert a lengthening effect, similar to compression interventions. Massage can be performed along the TrP taut band (stretching longitudinal massage) or across the taut band (transverse massage). Hence, transverse massage offers transverse mobilization to the TrP taut band, whereas a longitudinal massage offers longitudinal mobilization to the taut band. In

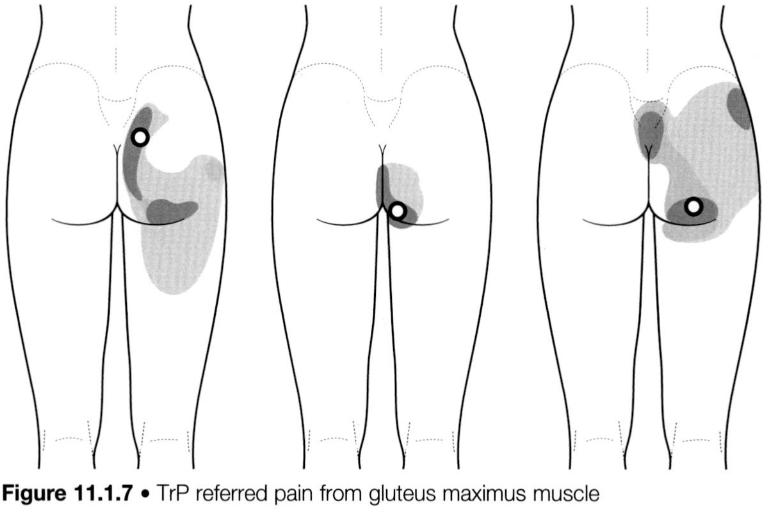

Figure 11.1.7 • TrP referred pain from gluteus maximus muscle

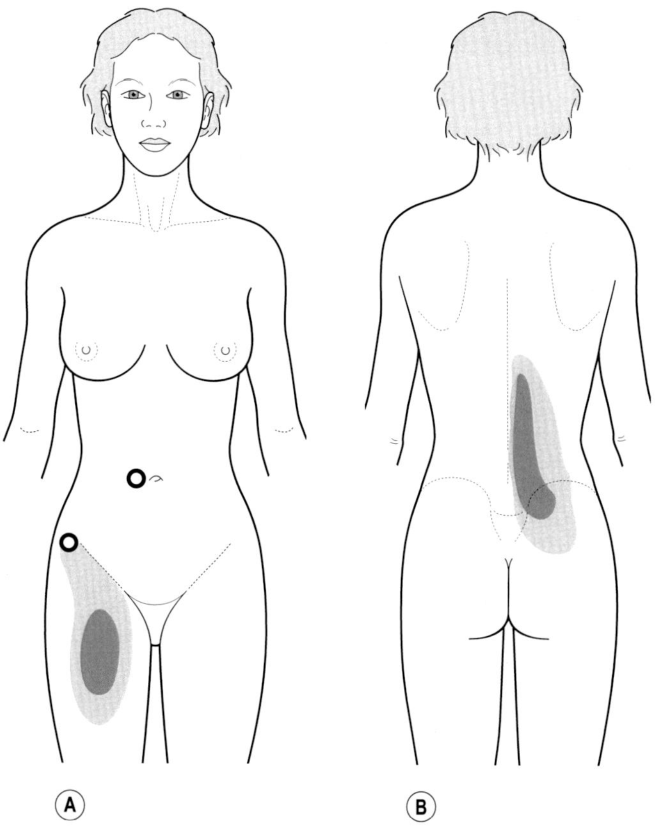

Figure 11.1.9 • Referred pain from TrPs in the iliopsoas muscle

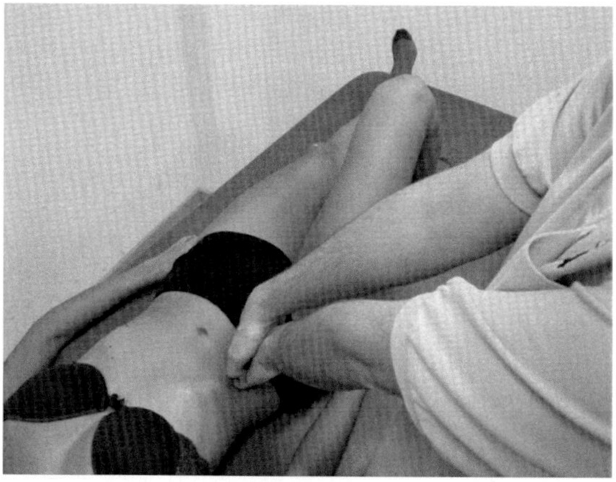

Figure 11.1.10 • Stretching compression of iliopsoas muscle TrPs

those muscles where clinicians can use pincer palpation, fingers can grasp the taut band from both sides of the TrP. Strokes centrifugally away from the TrP can lengthen the tissues (Simons 2002).

Transverse massage of quadratus lumborum muscle trigger points

Referred pain from quadratus lumborum TrPs spreads along the crest of the iliac bone, to the outer upper aspect of the groin, the greater trochanter, the sacroiliac joint and the lower buttock (Figure 11.1.11). In some patients, additional referred pain to the anterior thigh, testicle and scrotum has been described (Simons et al. 1999).

For this technique the patient is side-lying with the therapist standing in front of the patient. The ulnar aspect of the therapist's forearm should be placed over the muscle belly of the quadratus lumborum (where TrPs are usually located). The technique consists of applying a smooth and slow transverse massage over the TrP taut band (Figure 11.1.12). It is important to note that there is no established guideline (number of repetitions, time of application, or amount of pressure) for this technique. In the authors' experience, the transverse massage should be painless, and applied until the therapist feels the tissues relax.

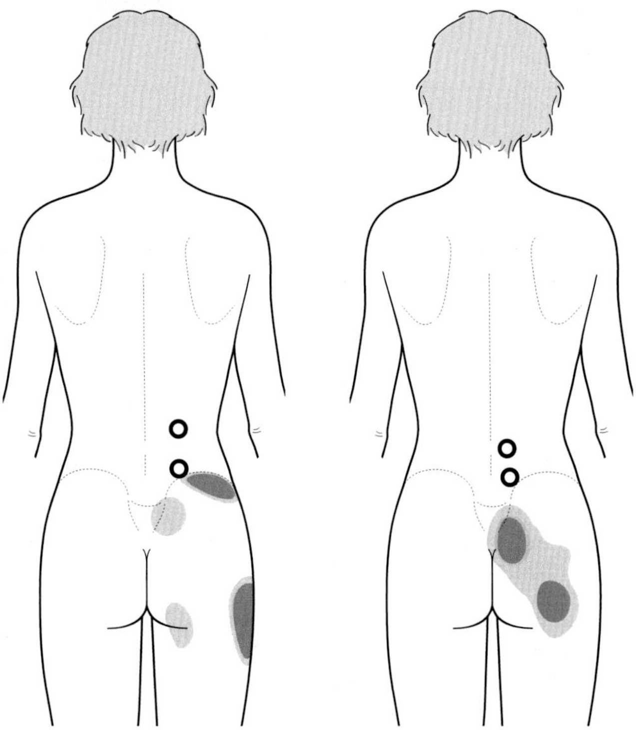

Figure 11.1.11 • TrP referred pain from quadratus lumborum muscle

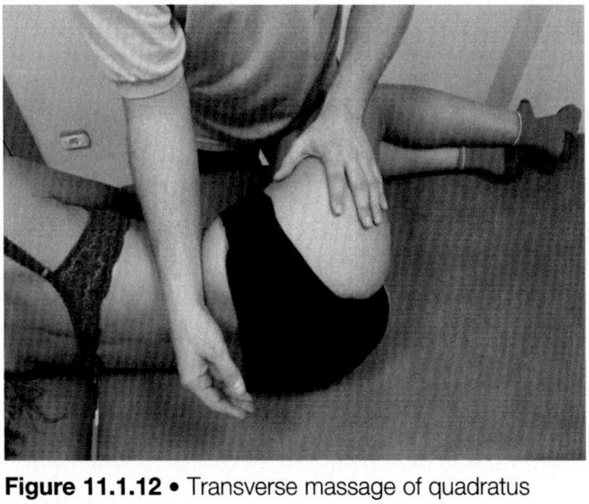

Figure 11.1.12 • Transverse massage of quadratus lumborum muscle TrPs

Stretching longitudinal massage of adductor muscle trigger points

TrPs within the adductor (brevis, longus and magnus) muscles refer pain to the medial aspect of the thigh and to the groin area (Figure 11.1.3B,C). In some patients, the adductor magnus TrPs also elicit an intrapelvic referred pain (Simons et al, 1999). For this technique the patient is supine or side-lying. Once the therapist locates a TrP (it can located in any of the adductor muscles), a pincer palpation of the TrP taut band is applied. The fingers of the therapist grasp the taut band from both sides, and stroke centrifugally away from the TrP (Figure 11.1.13).

Muscle energy interventions

There are several stretching applications targeted at inactivating TrPs: passive stretching (where the therapist passively stretches the muscle without participation of the patient), active stretching (where the patient actively stretches the muscle without participation of the therapist), spray and stretch involving a vapo-coolant spray applied during stretch (Hong et al. 1993, Simons et al. 1999), or muscle energy techniques (Fryer & Fossum 2009).

Muscle energy techniques comprise a system of manual procedures that utilize isometric and isotonic muscle contraction efforts from the patient, usually against a controlled matching counterforce from the therapist. Although there are different approaches

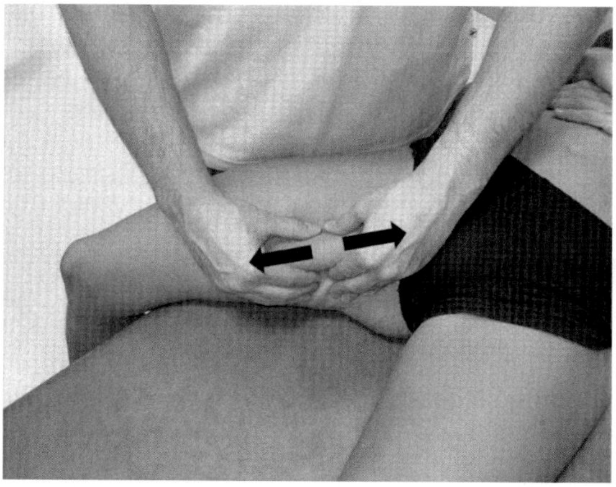

Figure 11.1.13 • Stretching longitudinal massage of adductor muscle TrPs

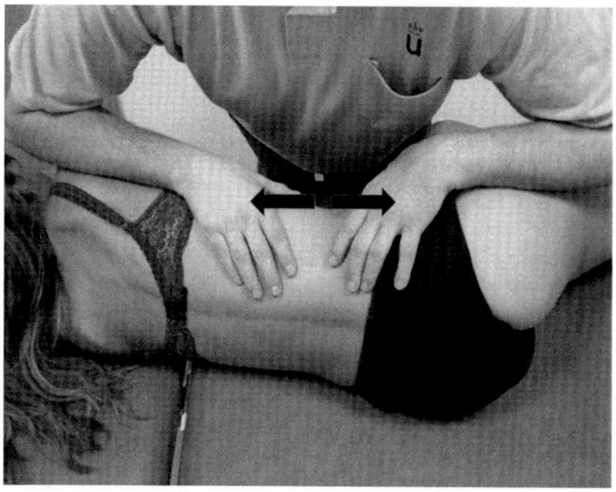

Figure 11.1.14 • Post-isometric relaxation of quadratus lumborum muscle TrPs

for application of muscle energy techniques, the 'contract–relax–release', is the most commonly utilized technique. This involves the accurate localization of an isometric contraction (3–7 seconds) at a barrier defined as 'the first sign of resistance'. An unyielding counterforce is supplied by the therapist. After the patient releases the contraction effort a new barrier is engaged, or stretching is introduced, past the previous barrier, actively or passively. The force and duration of isometric contraction can be varied, depending on the objective of the technique and the tissues involved. In fact, different durations of contraction have been proposed: 2–3 seconds (Mitchell & Mitchell 1995), 3–5 seconds (Greenman 2003), or 5–7 seconds (Chaitow 2006).

Several studies have demonstrated that muscle energy techniques increase muscle extensibility (Feland et al. 2001, Ferber et al. 2002, Ballantyne et al. 2003) and range of motion (Fryer & Ruszkowski 2004, Burns & Wells 2006) in healthy subjects. For a review of scientific evidence of muscle energy techniques, readers are referred to another text (Fryer 2006). The physiological therapeutic mechanisms by which muscle energy techniques exert their effect are speculative and controversial. Of the three most studied mechanisms that have been proposed, i.e. reflex relaxation, viscoelastic or muscle property changes (Fryer 2000), and increased tolerance to stretch, it is the latter that is most supported by the scientific literature (Fryer 2006).

Increased stretch tolerance may result from a decrease in pain perception (hypoalgesia) through the activation of muscle and joint mechanoreceptors, peripheral and central (activation of descending inhibitory pain systems) mechanisms (Fryer & Fossum 2009), and/or reduced concentrations of pro-inflammatory cytokines, and reduced sensitivity of peripheral nociceptors. Enhanced release of endocannabinoids may be one of the mechanisms of osteopathic manipulative treatment (McPartland et al. 2005), parallel to the effects of manipulative treatment upon serum endorphin levels (Vernon et al. 1986).

Muscle energy technique of quadratus lumborum muscle trigger points

The patient is side-lying with the superior leg in front of the other leg. A pillow can be placed under the waist to increase the lateral convexity of the lumbar spine. The therapist's caudal hand stabilizes the iliac bone and the cranial hand, the rib cage. The rib cage is stretched away from the iliac bone until tension is perceived (Figure 11.1.14). In that position, the patient contracts the muscle, by lifting the leg for 4–8 seconds, and then releases. When the therapist feels that the muscle is relaxed, an increase in muscle tension to the point of stretch is introduced. The patient can be asked to be actively involved by gently lengthening the leg at the start of the stretch.

Neuromuscular technique connective tissue approaches for chronic pelvic pain

TrPs represent a local muscle dysfunction; however, clinicians should consider that dysfunctional connective soft tissue is also involved in CPP. In fact, Han

(2009) has hypothesized that the afferent signals from loose connective tissue may be capable of transmitting noxious stimuli from superficial (skin) to deep (muscle) tissue (see Chapter 3 for further information on this topic). According to this theory, muscle TrP-referred pain would also be related to soft tissue dysfunction. However, this theory requires further investigation.

Neuromuscular connective tissue approaches aim to release stressful tension in fascial connective tissue (Chaitow & Delany 2008). It has been suggested that the application of a mechanical stimulus to soft connective tissue induces a piezoelectric effect, which modifies the 'gel' state of tissues to a more solute state (Barnes 1997). This effect can also be obtained with myofascial induction (release) approaches described in the following section.

Among different manual techniques, the most important manoeuvre within the neuromuscular approach is the gliding (sliding) technique. Gliding strokes are usually targeted at lengthening shortened (rigid) connective soft tissue. Longitudinal strokes are generally applied with one or both thumbs, but sometimes the elbow or the knuckles can be also used. The degree of pressure and the speed of application depend on the irritability, and tone, of the tissue. Initial pressure – which is largely diagnostic – attempts to meet-and-match tissue tension, with progressively deeper degrees of pressure being used when therapeutic objectives start. Finally, clinical experience suggests that the best result usually comes from repetitive strokes over the tissue (6–10 times).

Longitudinal stroke of abdominal wall muscle trigger points

TrPs in rectus abdominis or external oblique muscles may confuse the diagnosis by mimicking visceral pathology (Simons et al. 1999, Maloney & Newman 2005). The referred pain elicited by the external oblique muscle TrPs is perceived as burning pain over the anterior chest wall, spreading to the lower quadrant abdominal and groin area (Figure 11.1.15) The rectus abdominis muscle TrP (Figure 11.1.16A) refers pain to the lower quadrant abdominal simulating nausea and vomiting symptoms (Figure 11.1.16B, C) and also producing pain bilaterally across the upper and lower back (Figure 11.1.16D). One common mechanism of TrP activation is soft tissue scars after surgery (Simons et al. 1999). Readers are referred to treatment of scars after surgery to the connective tissue manipulation section of this chapter.

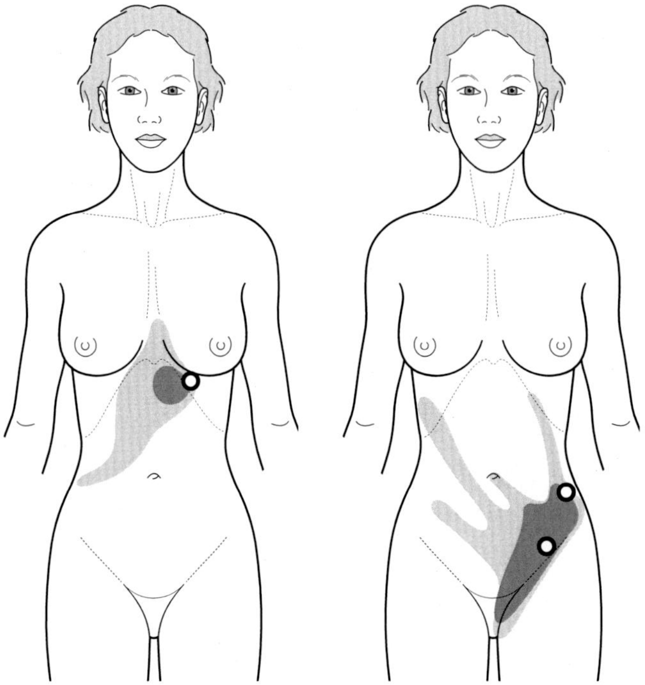

Figure 11.1.15 • TrP referred pain from external oblique muscle

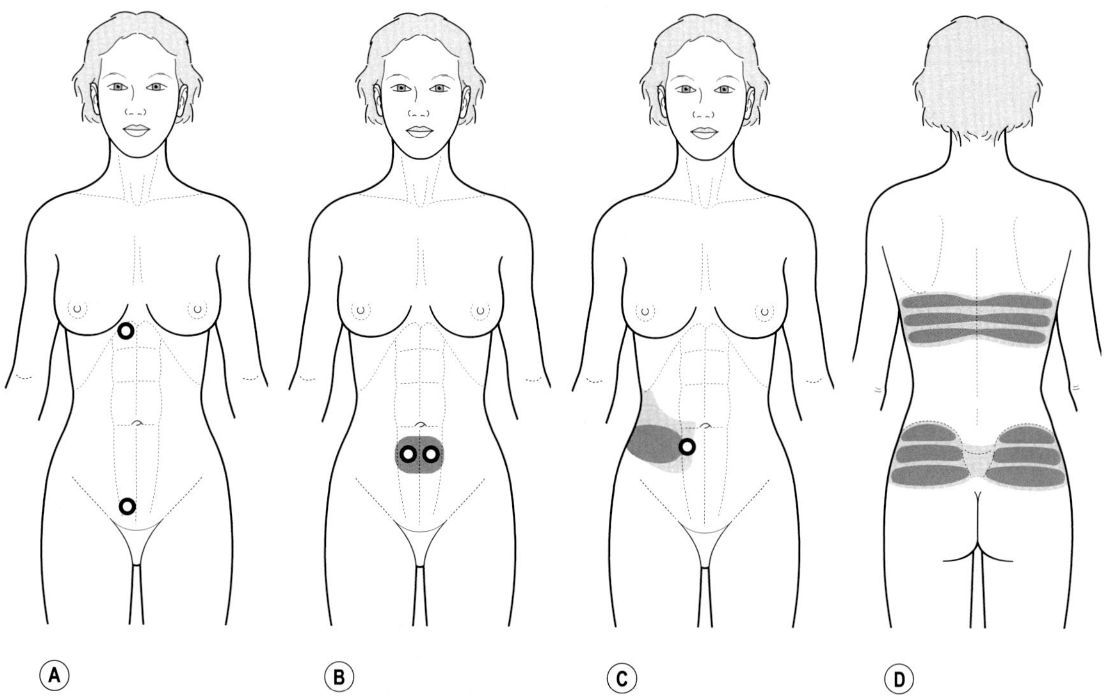

Figure 11.1.16 • Rectus abdominis muscle TrP referred pain patterns

Longitudinal strokes can be performed with the thumb over rectus abdominis muscle TrPs, from a cranial to caudal direction, with the patient supine (Figure 11.1.17). The degree of pressure applied is determined by the feedback reported by the patient or the tension felt within the patient's tissue. For external oblique muscle TrPs, the patient is side-lying, with the trunk in contralateral rotation. The strokes can be performed with the thumb or with pincer palpation (Figure 11.1.18).

Stretching stroke of gluteus medius muscle trigger points

The referred pain from gluteus medius muscle TrPs is perceived as deep pain into the lower pelvic quadrant and sacroiliac joint area (Figure 11.1.19). A stretching stroke consists of a longitudinal stroke applied over a muscle placed in a stretched position. With the patient side-lying, gluteus medius can be

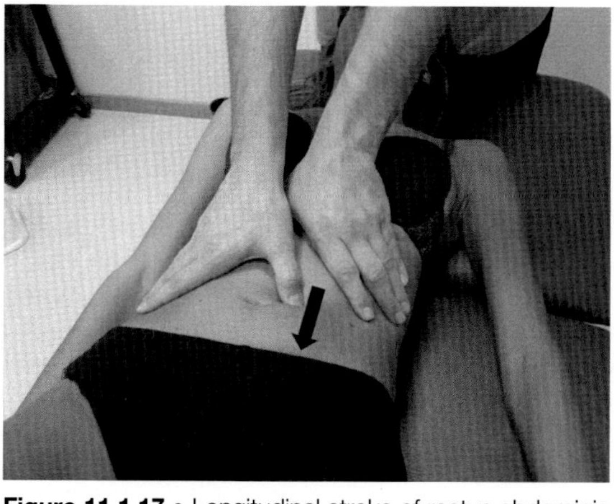

Figure 11.1.17 • Longitudinal stroke of rectus abdominis muscle taut bands

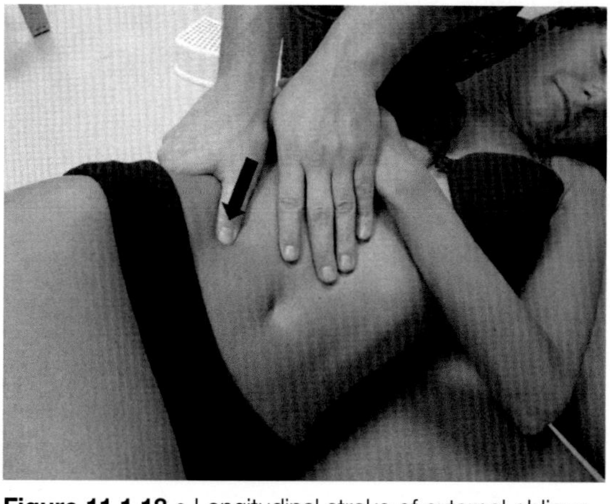

Figure 11.1.18 • Longitudinal stroke of external oblique muscle taut bands

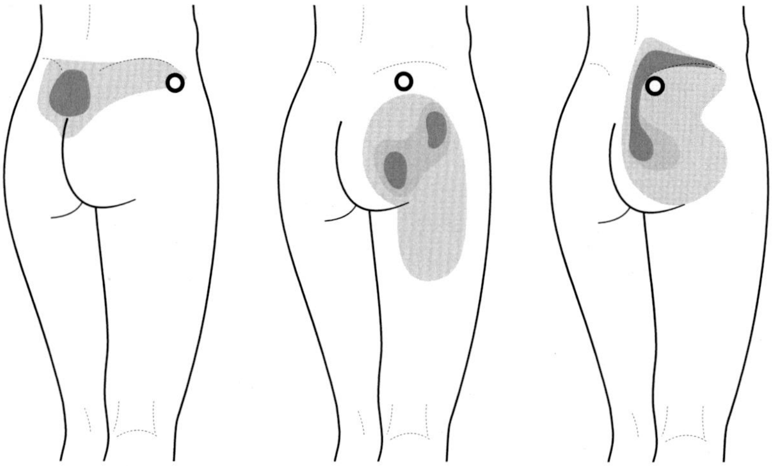

Figure 11.1.19 • Referred pain from gluteus medius muscle TrPs

stretched by adducting the leg with the knee flexed. In this stretched position, longitudinal strokes can be performed with the ulnar aspect of the therapist's forearm, from a posterior to anterior direction (Figure 11.1.20).

Dynamic longitudinal stroke of thoracolumbar extensor muscle trigger points

Thoracolumbar extensor muscle (iliocostalis lumborum and longissimus muscle) TrPs refer pain to the lower pelvic quadrant and to the buttock area (Figure 11.1.21). The proposed treatment technique combines longitudinal strokes while the patient moves the trunk into flexion (Gröbli & Dejung 2003). The patient is seated with the therapist standing behind the patient. The therapist applies longitudinal strokes over TrP taut bands with the knuckles from a cranial (neck) to caudal (lumbar spine) direction, at the time that the patient flexes the trunk (Figure 11.1.22). It is suggested that, for optimal results, the stroke should be synchronized with the motion of the patient's trunk into flexion.

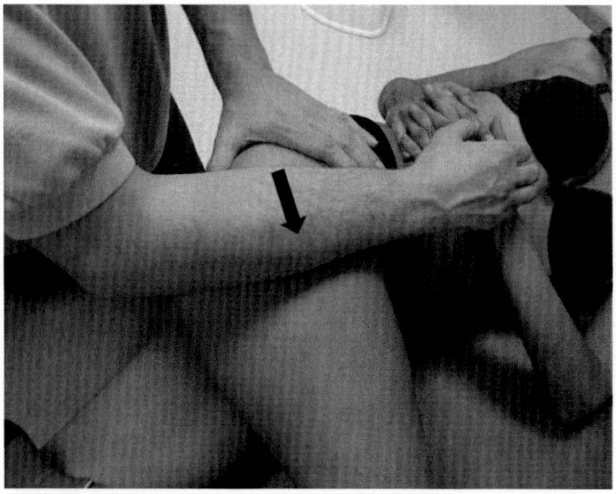

Figure 11.1.20 • Stretching stroke of gluteus medius muscle TrPs

Myofascial induction interventions

Introduction to fascial tissue

The fascia is a connective tissue that forms a continual network between the different components of the body (Pilat 2003, Langevin 2006, Vanacore et al. 2009). Its fibrous construction allows the fascial tissue to accommodate to intrinsic and extrinsic compressive and tensional body requirements (Pilat 2009). The different characteristic of fascial structures (e.g. density, distribution) allows these to act as a synergistic functional structure which absorbs and distributes local tensional and compressive forces throughout the body. This inherent synergy of the fascia may play a relevant role in functional tasks, e.g. maintenance of body posture against gravity (Langevin 2006).

Further, it is hypothesized that fascia could also integrate sensory stimuli (i.e. mechanical, thermal

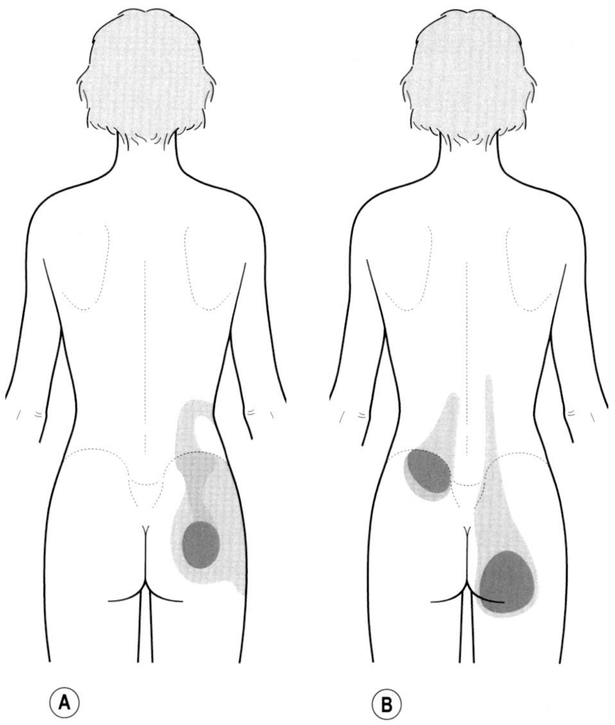

Figure 11.1.21 • Thoracolumbar extensor muscle (iliocostalis lumborum or longissimus muscle) TrPs referred pain

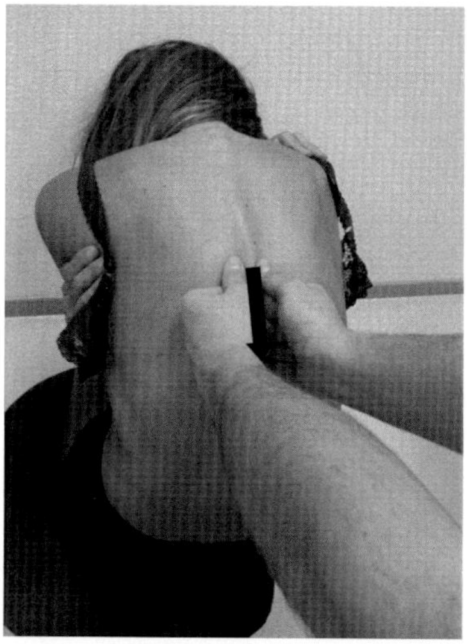

Figure 11.1.22 • Dynamic longitudinal stroke of thoracolumbar extensor muscle TrPs

or chemical) from the central nervous system (Pilat & Testa 2009, Pilat 2009). Sensory information integrated into the fascia may interact with inputs originating in the central nervous system at three different levels:

1. *Physical (mechanical–anatomical) links.* Observations on fresh cadavers show a mechanical continuity of fascial tissues where muscles that attach to the fascia act synergistically creating myofascial kinetic links which act at both macroscopic (Stecco et al. 2006, Pilat 2009) and microscopic levels. These are associated with the contraction of myofibroblasts, which are the contractile fascia cells (Maniotis et al. 1997, Vleeming et al. 1997, Hu et al. 2003, Myers 2003, Ingber 2006, Gabbiani 2007, Stecco et al. 2006, Wang et al. 2009).
2. *Functional link.* Fascial tissue is considered a mechano-sensitive structure that constitutes a particular network of mechanoreceptors, mostly interstitial ones. The mechanical modifications are created primarily in the extracellular matrix that is characterized by piezoelectric and semiconducting properties (Langevin 2006, Vaticón 2009).
3. *Chemical link.* Ingber (2006) identified the mediating structures for the mechanochemical integration process in the fascial tissue based on mechanotransduction activities. Vanacore et al. (2009) have identified networks that provide

structural integrity to the tissues. These serve as ligands for integrin cell-surface receptors related to collagen IV, the major structural component of glomerular basement membranes. It is suggested that these networks can mediate cell adhesion, migration, growth and differentiation (Wang 2009).

Some theories have suggested that the three-dimensional fascial tissue may be involved in pain transmission processes (Liptan 2010). For instance, pain experienced in the pelvic area is usually a referred pain, i.e. perceived in remote areas of the site of noxious stimulation, which does not usually follow neuropathic patterns (Travell & Bigelow 1946). The central hyperexcitability theory explains the mechanisms of pain from deep structures (Mense 1994) but does not clarify the presence of non-segmental patterns of the superficial musculature. Han (2009) has proposed an hypothesis (a *connective tissue theory*) that the signalling present in the loose connective tissue may be capable of transmitting noxious stimuli from the surface to muscles or other deep structures through the cells of the vascular and neural systems. According to this theory, some peripheral pain may have a direct origin in the connective tissue.

Fascial continuity model

The continuity of the fascial system and its links to the pelvic bones facilitate the interaction with the aponeurosis of the PFM and associated neurovascular structures. For instance, the hypogastric plexus is overlaid by the endopelvic fascia forming the complex fascial skeleton which controls the uterine, vaginal, bladder and urethral vessels. Thus, the myofascial tissue joins the viscerofascial system creating a more complex functional unit (Santos et al. 2009). Therefore, the altered load transfer through the pelvis may affect musculoskeletal dynamics, and may be associated with multiple impairments such as low back/pelvic girdle pain, pelvic adhesions, intestinal and urologic disorders, endometriosis, prolapses, orgasm difficulties, dyspareunia or nerve injuries (Delancey 1993, Snijders et al. 1993a, 1993b, Hodges & Richardson 1996, Vleeming et al. 1996, Lee & Vleeming 1998, Mens et al. 1999, Occelli 2001, Hungerford et al. 2003, Lee & Lee 2004a, Lee & Vleeming 2004, Peters & Carrico 2006, Wurn et al. 2004). Pool-Goudzwaard et al. (2003) reported that 52% of patients studied developed a combination of PGP and pelvic floor disorders during pregnancy, including voiding difficulties, urinary incontinence, sexual dysfunction and/or constipation. Of these patients, 82% stated that their symptoms began with either low or pelvic girdle pain (Pool-Goudzwaard 2003). This interaction in the manifestations of pain and/or dysfunction in the pelvic girdle make diagnosis and clinical decision-making difficult (see Chapter 9).

Which functional model may link all these requirements?

Ingber proposed the intercommunication system theory based on tensegrity principles (Ingber 1998, Pilat & Testa 2009). The tensegrity theory describes a system of shared tensions in the distribution of the mechanical forces at multiple body levels. This model attempts to explain global fascial responses to mechanical stimuli (Chicurel et al. 1998, Khalsa et al. 2000). Different studies have shown that the cell dynamics and active responses of the cytoskeleton induce a tissue remodelling at cellular and subcellular levels when the tissue absorbs mechanical forces from the extracellular matrix (Ingber 1998, 2003, 2006, Parker & Ingber et al. 2007, Stamenovic et al. 2007, Wang et al. 2009). Considering that the construction of the body follows the principles of hierarchical assembly (demonstrated at cellular and subcellular levels) this process is not limited to cells, but also involves tissues, organs and the whole body (Huang & Ingber 1999, 2000).

Jarrell (2004) reported an increasing interest in therapeutic measures that incorporate the principles of myofascial dysfunction in CPP syndromes. Lukban et al. (2001) reported a 94% improvement associated with urination in patients with chronic interstitial cystitis after the application of myofascial release interventions, muscle energy and stretching exercises. Santos et al. (2009) established the 'tensegrity connection' between the changes in pelvic girdle myofascial function and the endopelvic fascia. They described the Santos sign, which allows diagnosis of damage to pelvic ligamentous support by simple compression with the clinician's finger (Figure 11.1.23). This fascial dysfunction may be associated with urinary incontinence, coital dysfunction, orgasm dysfunctions, low back pain, and impairments in postural alignment, e.g. hyperlordosis (Santos et al. 2009).

Observations of fresh cadaver dissections confirm the hypothesis of anatomical fascial continuity

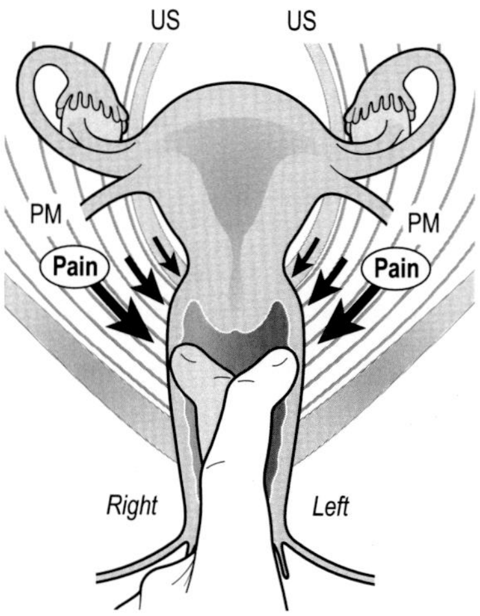

Figure 11.1.23 • The Santos sign: the viscerofascial pelvic girdle tensegrity system sign. PM, Mackenrodt ligament parameter; US, uterosacral ligaments. The vaginal exploration may be done UP with the finger compressing fascial insertions on US (cardinal of 3D endopelvic fascia) or DOWN with the finger of the clinician compressing pubo-urethral fascial ligaments. The pressure is painful in women with pelvic pain allowing an early diagnosis of uterine prolapse equivalent to dyspaurenia symptom. The pressure on the urethrovaginal insertion of the pubourethral ligament is equivalent to urinary urgency and/or incontinence

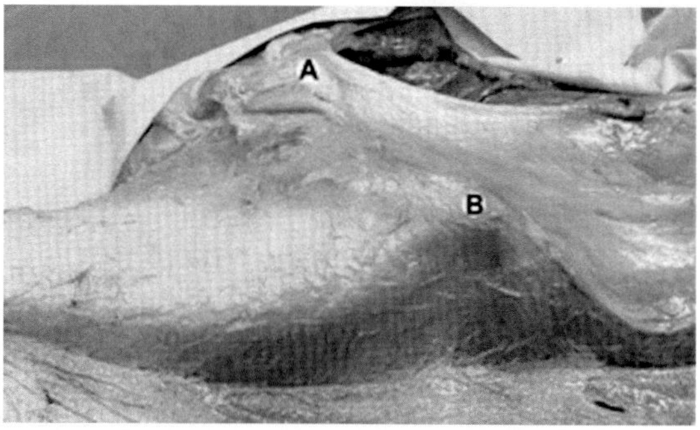

Figure 11.1.25 • Fascial continuity of the thigh and abdominal region from a fresh cadaver dissection. Note a thickening and accumulation of fat in the pubic region. A. Pubis; B. anterior superior iliac spine

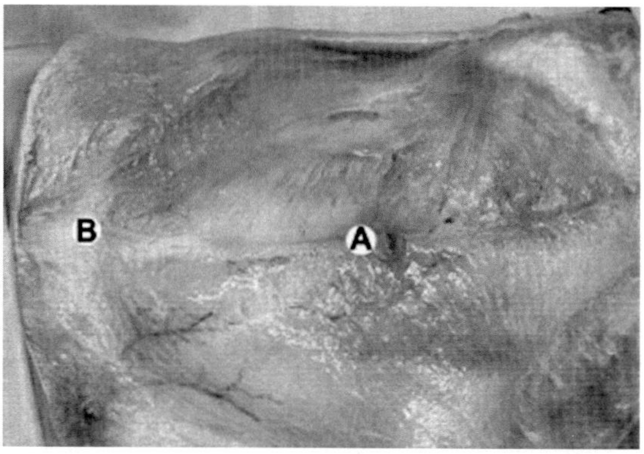

Figure 11.1.26 • Morphological differences between the superficial fascia (the lower part) and deep fascia (the upper part) in the abdominal region from a fresh cadaver dissection. Note a clear fibrous appearance of the deep fascia and the presence of veins inside the superficial fascial structure. A. Navel; B. Pubis

(Pilat 2009). At the superficial level, just beneath the skin, superficial fascia that contains a considerable amount of fat is located, which differs depending on the anatomical area (Figures 11.1.24–11.1.28). Superficial fascia is characterized by great elasticity, while deep fascia is continuous and represents a more fibrous and dense structure (Figures 11.1.26–11.1.31). At the intermuscular level fascial envelopment (Figure 11.1.32) and tendon–ligament–fascial connections can be observed (Figures 11.1.33, 11.1.34).

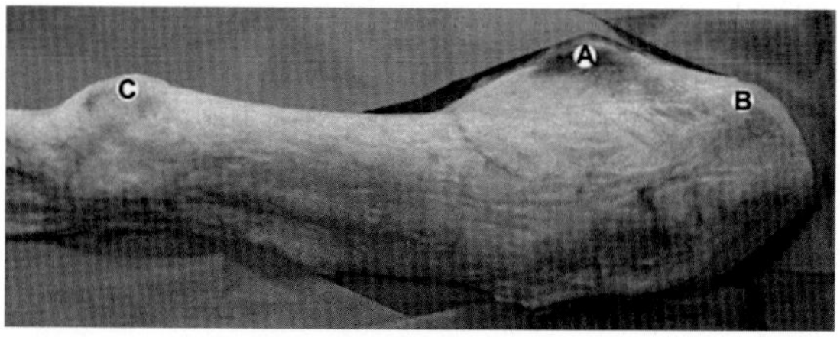

Figure 11.1.24 • Superficial fascia of the thigh from fresh cadaver dissection. Only the skin was dissected. Note the continuity of the structure. A. Pubis; B. Anterior superior iliac spine; C. Patella

Theoretical aspects for the treatment of myofascial dysfunction syndrome

Mechanics of the myofascial dysfunction syndrome

Appropriate dynamics of the fascial tissue is necessary for an optimal functioning of the body. For instance, a reduction in the mobility of the fascial

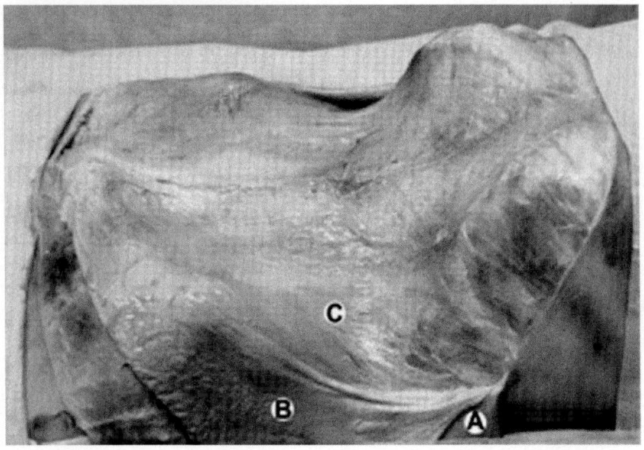

Figure 11.1.27 • Continuity of the deep fascia in the lower pectoral, abdominal and pelvic regions. Note changes in the orientation of the fibres of the deep fascia, related to the different lines of tension according to the needs in motion activity. A. Skin; B. Superficial fascia; C. Deep fascia

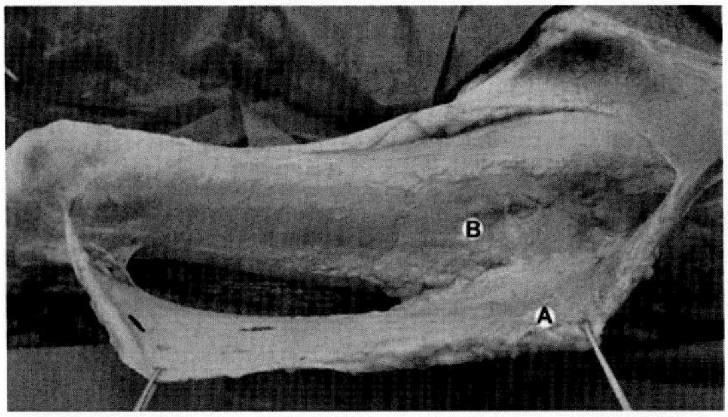

Figure 11.1.28 • Interrelationships between superficial and deep fascia of the thigh and lower abdominal region from a fresh cadaver dissection. Note the presence of fatty nodules in the intermediate plane, as well as the fibrous connections between the two fascial levels. A. Superficial fascia; B. Deep fascia

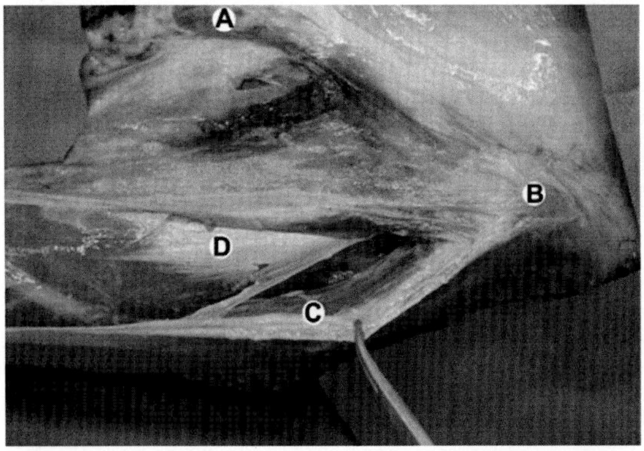

Figure 11.1.29 • Incision of the deep fascia of the thigh from a fresh cadaver dissection. Note the aponeurotic expansion of the quadriceps muscle. A. Pubis; B. Anterior superior iliac spine; C. Deep fascia; D. Quadriceps muscle

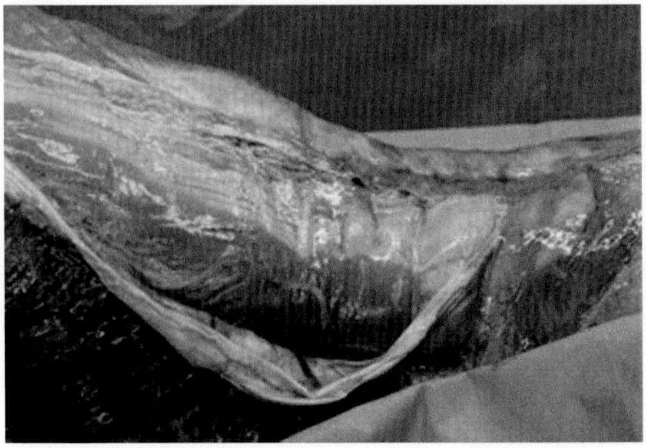

Figure 11.1.30 • Deep fascia in the superficial layer of the paraspinal muscles from a fresh cadaver dissection

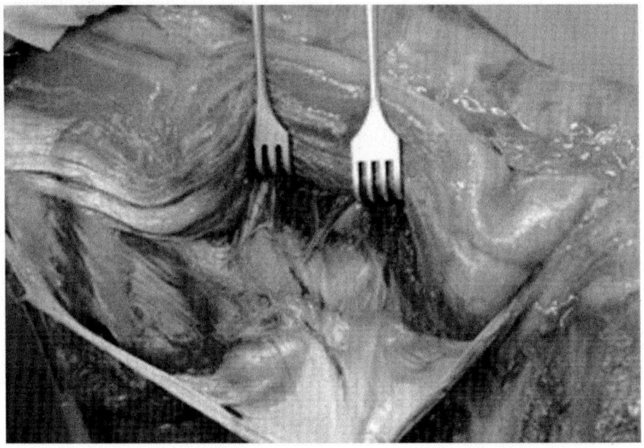

Figure 11.1.31 • Deep fascia in the deep layer of the paraspinal muscles from a fresh cadaver dissection

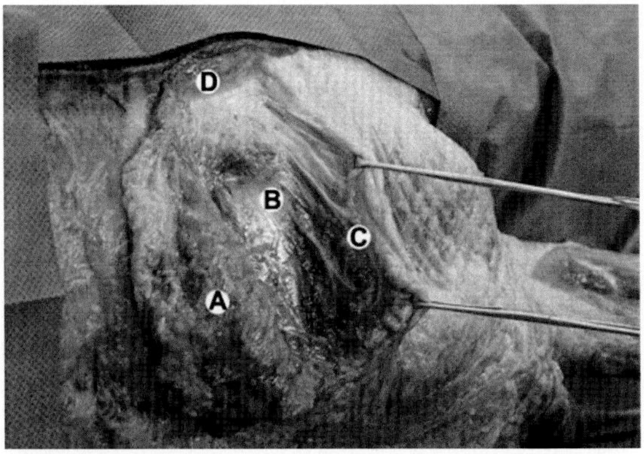

Figure 11.1.32 • Cross-section of the gluteus maximus muscle from a fresh cadaver dissection. *Note the fibrous fascial connections.* A. Cranial end of the gluteus maximus muscle; B. Deep layer of the gluteus gluteal fascia; C. Caudal end of the gluteus maximus muscle. D. Sacrum

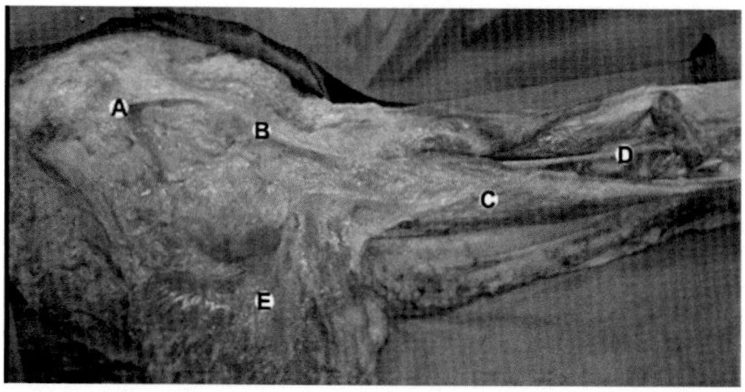

Figure 11.1.33 • Deep structures of the gluteal region and posterior thigh from a fresh cadaver dissection. The gluteus maximus muscle was removed to the side. A. Sacrotuberous ligament; B. Tendon of the large portion of biceps femoris muscle; C. Biceps femoris muscle; D. Sciatic nerve; E. Inner surface of the gluteus maximus previously sectioned

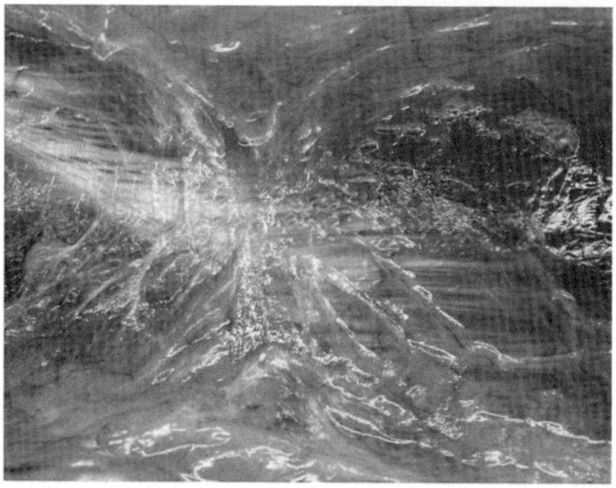

Figure 11.1.35 • Fascial entrapment

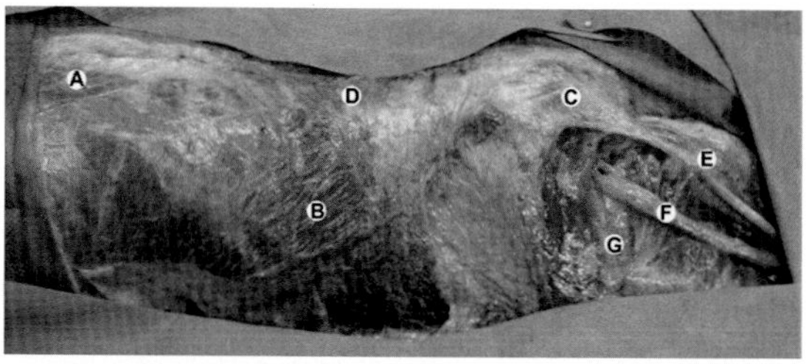

Figure 11.1.34 • Side view of the lumbopelvic region from a fresh cadaver dissection. A. Trapezius muscle; B. Latissimus dorsi muscle; C. Sacrotuberous ligament; D. Thoracolumbar fascia; E. Tendon of the biceps femoris muscle; F. Sciatic nerve; G. Piriformis muscle

tissue may alter circulation (Bhattacharya 2005, Kubo et al. 2009a, 2009b), contributing to the development of ischaemia. An excessive stimulation of collagen production can alter the quality of movement, potentially encouraging facilitating reduced physiological motion (Pilat 2009).

Fascial restrictions (Figure 11.1.35) can promote the formation of compensatory movement patterns that may lead to musculoskeletal dysfunction. These changes impact the loose connective tissue structure resulting in remodelling of the specialized structures (dense regular and irregular connective tissue) leading to fibre reorientation. Short-term tissue changes will affect local function, but long-term changes could create global dysfunctional patterns (Pilat 2003). Further research is needed to support these hypotheses.

Neurophysiological mechanisms for releasing the restrictions of the fascial tissue

The manual application of myofascial induction/release interventions creates a mechanical stimulus in the loose connective fascial tissue. The results of this mechanical stimulus occur at micro- or macroscopic levels. The theoretical mechanisms explaining the effects of myofascial induction approaches include the following.

1. *Piezoelectricity*. Since collagen tissue (a basic connective tissue component) is considered a semiconductor structure (O'Connell & Judith 2003), this tissue may be capable of forming an integrated information network enabling the interconnection of fascial components (Szent-Gyorgi 1994, Cope 1975, Bouligard 1978, Oschman 2003).
2. *Dynamics of the myofibroblasts*. The muscle is a contractile tissue that enables the body to move. Fascial tissue should be considered as an intramuscular connective tissue that forms a functional unit with muscle fibres. The fascial system is highly innervated by mechanoreceptors (Schleip et al. 2005, Langevin 2006, Stecco et al. 2008). Mechanical input (pressure or traction) received by the mechanoreceptors can create a broad range of responses in the fascial system that may result in changes at both macro- and microscopic levels related to the function of the myofibroblasts (Staubesand & Li 1997, Schleip et al. 2005, 2007). Various studies that have

focused on the Dupuytren contracture, plantar fasciitis, frozen shoulder and fibromyalgia syndrome support this reasoning (Fidzianska & Jablonska 2000, Gabbiani 2003, 2007, Satish et al. 2008). Chaudhry et al. (2008) using a 3D mathematical model for deformation of human fascia suggested that mechanical forces applied during manual therapy can create mechanical changes in the loose connective tissue (i.e. superficial nasal fascia). Schleip et al. (2007) suggested that the possible changes in resting tone of skeletal muscle fibres can transmit their tension force to the respective fascial tissues.

3. *Viscoelasticity*. These are the phenomena related to the remodeling process of the extracellular matrix hydration according to the long-term behaviour of the material. The viscoelastic properties of fascia have been observed in numerous studies which have analysed different structures: thoracolumbar fascia (Yahia et al. 1993), fascia lata (Wright & Rennels 1964), subcutaneous fascia of rats (Iatridies et al. 2003), plantar and nasal fascia (Chaudhry 2007). The clinical utilization of the viscoelastic properties of fascia has been described by various authors: Rolf (1977), Barnes (1990), Threlkeld (1992), Cantu & Grodin (2001), Barnes (1997), Pilat (2003), Schleip et al. (2005), Pilat (2009). Recent theories hypothesized that different chemical mediators may be involved in this process (Vaticón 2009), although further research is clearly needed.

Therapeutic strategies applied to the myofascial induction process

General observations related to the therapeutic process

There are different clinical approaches that target the management of dysfunctional fascial structures (Barnes 1990, Rolf 1977, Manheim 1998, Paoletti 1998, Cantu & Grodin 2001, Chaitow & Delany 2002, Pilat 2003). There is, however, a need for unification and validation of the clinical procedures through research (Remving 2007).

The applications suggested in the current chapter are based on clinical experiences of the authors (Pilat 2003) and are based on the theoretical framework previously described. It is important to note that the myofascial induction process may be applied as an exclusive treatment procedure or combined with other manual therapy strategies.

Definition of myofascial induction process

Myofascial induction (myofascial release) is a simultaneous evaluation and treatment process using 3D movements of sustained pressures, applied to the myofascial system in order to release facial restrictions. The term 'induction' is related to the fact that clinicians do not passively stretch the system but only apply an initial tension or compression force and follow the facilitating movement. The aim of the process is the recovery of motion amplitude, force and coordination (Pilat 2010).

Bases for clinical applications

General observations *(Pilat 2003, 2010)*

- The evaluation of fascial dysfunction should be included in clinical reasoning processes. We suggest that clinicians follow the common physical explorations for movement dysfunctions of each region.
- Biomechanically, the myofascial system responds to compression and traction forces. These two mechanical strategies can be used when applying myofascial induction techniques.
- Restrictions may occur in various directions and planes. They may even occur in different directions in the same plane, in the same direction in various planes, or in different planes in various directions.
- The direction of the releasing movement is towards facilitation. The therapist should refrain from performing movements in arbitrary directions.
- There is no need for active muscle contraction performed by the patient. The patient may be asked to maintain a state of active passiveness.

Clinical procedure principles *(Pilat 2003, 2007a, 2009, 2010)*

- The therapist should apply a 3D compression or traction causing the tissue to become tense. This is referred to as the first restriction barrier.
- The applied pressure is constant during the first 60–90 seconds, which is the time required for releasing the first restriction barrier (Pilat 2003, Chaudhry et al. 2007).
- During the first phase of the technique, the therapist barely causes the tissue to move.

- Upon overcoming the first restriction barrier, the therapist accompanies the movement in the direction of the facilitation pausing at each next barrier.
- In each technique, the therapist is advised to overcome three to six consecutive barriers and a minimum time of application is usually 3–5 minutes.
- The tension applied to the tissue should be constant, but the pressure applied by the therapist may be modified after overcoming the first barrier. Pressure should be reduced if there is an increase in pain and/or abundant movement activity.

Examples of clinical applications

The following techniques are examples of the therapeutic strategies used to treat myofascial restrictions related to CPP syndromes.

Transverse plane induction of the pelvic region (Figure 11.1.36)

This is a common myofascial induction procedure for the pelvic region (Barnes 1990, Upledger 1997, Pilat, 2003). The patient is supine and the therapist is seated on a chair. The therapist places the non-dominant hand under the patient's back and the dominant one over the abdominal wall, just below the navel. Both hands are placed transversely in relation to the spine. The therapist applies 3D pressure (i.e. each hand engages restriction barriers in the contacted tissues, on all planes: medial-lateral, inferior-superior, clockwise-anticlockwise rotation) and the principles of myofascial induction are followed.

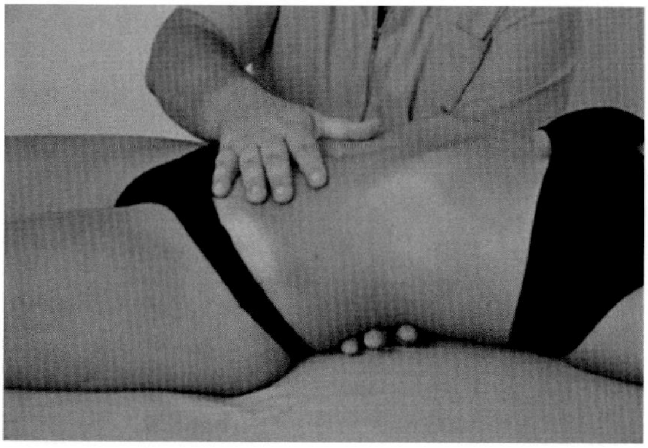

Figure 11.1.36 • Transverse plane induction of the pelvic region

Lumbosacral induction (Figure 11.1.37)

The patient is supine and the therapist is seated. The therapist places the non-dominant hand at the L5 lumbar vertebra level. The fist of the hand is closed in order to get the L5 spinous process to sit snugly in the channel formed by the fingers. The dominant hand of the therapist is placed beneath the sacrum of the patient. With the dominant hand the therapist applies a very gentle caudal traction over the sacrum. The principles of induction are followed (Barnes 1990, Upledger 1997, Pilat, 2003).

Induction of the pubic region (Figures 11.1.38, 11.1.39)

This technique consists of two phases (Pilat 2003). For phase 1, the patient is supine and the therapist is standing at the level of the patient's hip. The therapist flexes

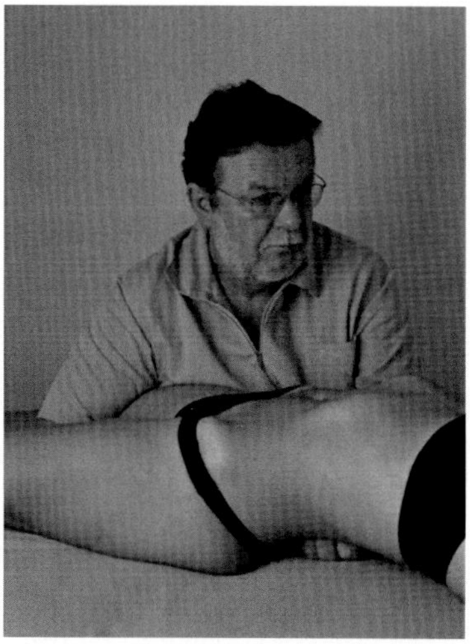

Figure 11.1.37 • Lumbosacral induction

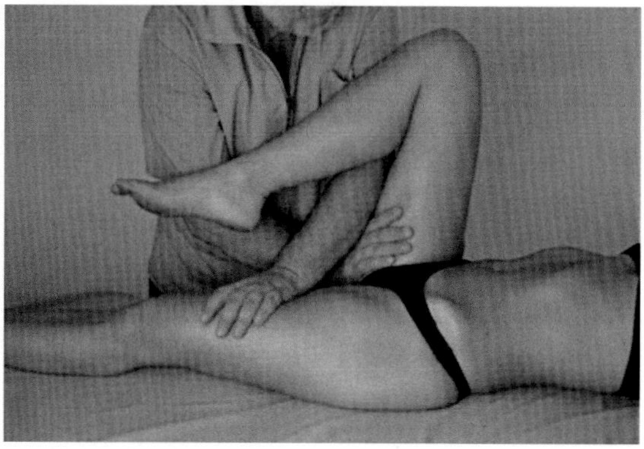

Figure 11.1.38 • Induction of the pubic region phase 1

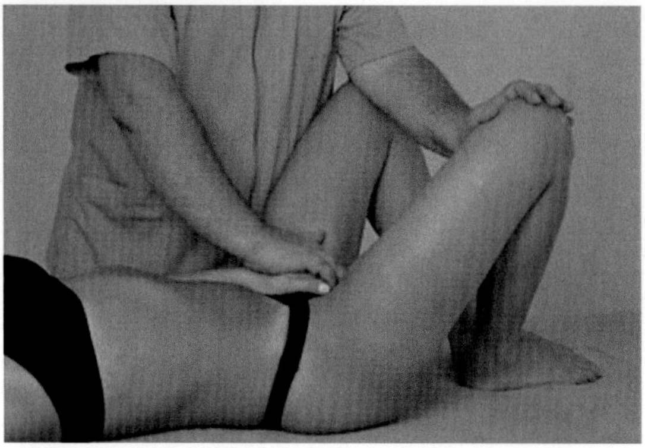

Figure 11.1.39 • Induction of the pubic region phase 2

the patient's ipsilateral hip to 90–100° leaving the contralateral leg flat on the table. Using a cross-handed contact, the therapist then places one hand on the back of the flexed (ipsilateral) thigh, and the other hand on the front of the unflexed contralateral thigh. The process involves the therapist simultaneously applying pressure in a cranial direction with the ipsilateral hand and caudad with the other contralateral hand. The therapist should avoid increasing the flexion of the thigh. The force lines should cross over the pubis, and the principles of induction should then be followed. The technique is applied bilaterally (Figure 11.1.38). For the second phase the patient lies supine with both knees flexed. The therapist stands at the level of the patient's pelvis. The therapist's caudal forearm is placed between the inner faces of both patient knees. The patient places one hand on the pubis and the therapist places the cranial hand over the patient's hand. The patient exerts a slight pressure with the knees 'squeezing' the therapist's forearm, while the therapist exerts a slight pressure on the pubis in an external direction following the movement of facilitation (Figure 11.1.39).

Cross-hand induction of the lumbar spine (Figure 11.1.40)

With the patient prone, the therapist is standing at the level of the patient's back. The therapist places the crossed hands on the patient's back and applies a slight pressure force towards the table in a craniocaudal direction (Pilat 2003). The principles of induction are then followed.

Cross-hand induction of the abdominal fascia (Figure 11.1.41)

With the patient supine, the therapist is standing at the level of the patient's waist. The therapist places the crossed hands over the abdominal fascia. The

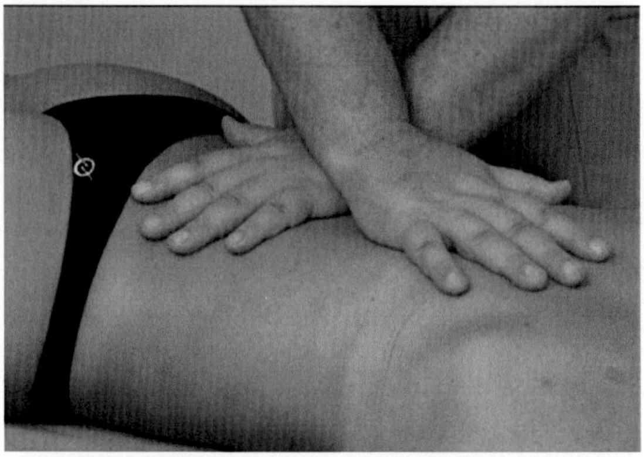

Figure 11.1.40 • Cross-hand induction of the lumbar spine

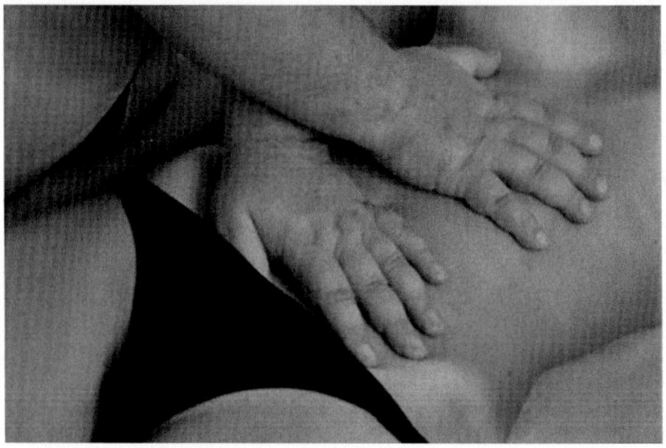

Figure 11.1.41 • Cross-hand induction of the abdominal fascia

cranial hand is placed at the level of the xiphoid process of the sternum and the caudal hand is placed at the level of the pubis (Pilat 2003). The principles of induction are then followed.

Lower induction of the thoracolumbar fascia (Figure 11.1.42)

With the patient prone, the therapist is standing at the level of the patient's pelvis. The therapist places the cranial hand on the patient's lumbar region, pressing toward the table. With the caudal hand, the therapist contacts the contralateral side at the anterior-superior iliac spine level applying traction in the direction to the ceiling. The principles of induction are then followed (Pilat 2003).

Cross-hand induction of the thoracolumbar and gluteal fascia (Figure 11.1.43)

The patient is prone and the therapist is standing at the level of the patient's pelvis. The therapist places the cranial hand at the lumbar region of the

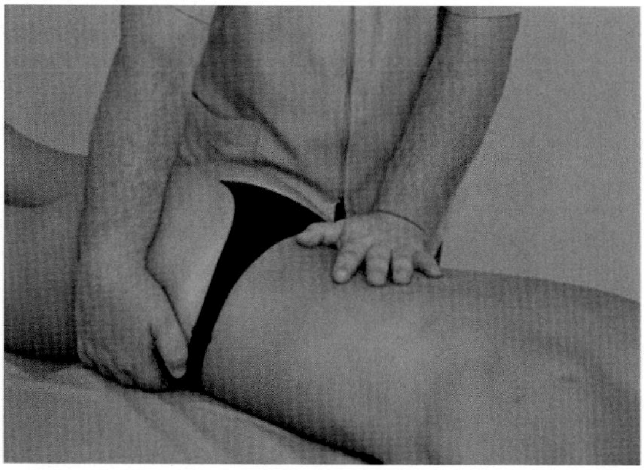

Figure 11.1.42 • Lower induction of the thoracolumbar fascia

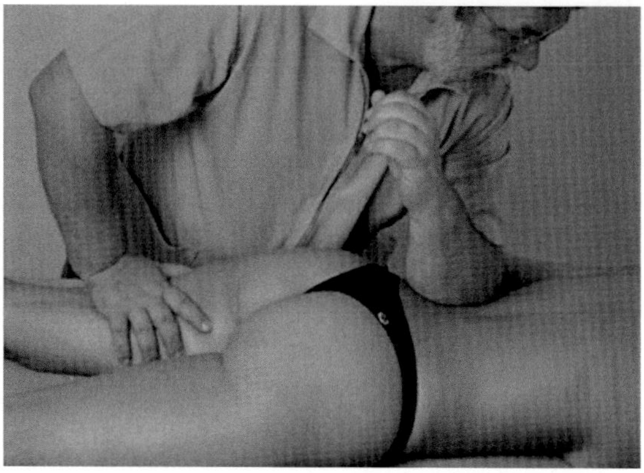

Figure 11.1.44 • Quadratus lumborum fascia induction

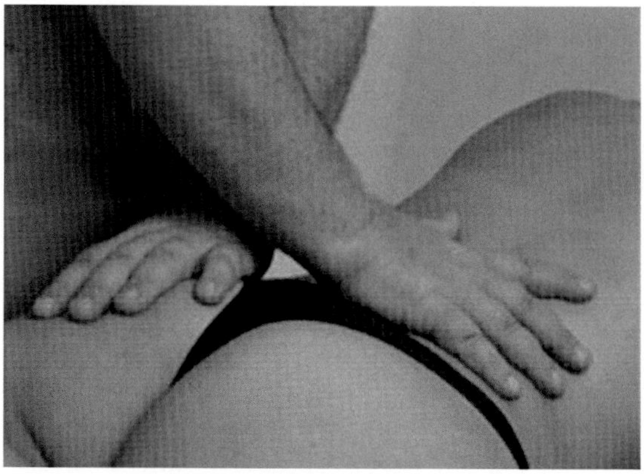

Figure 11.1.43 • Cross-hand induction of the thoraco-lumbar and gluteal fascia

contralateral patient's side and the caudal hand over the ipsilateral gluteal fascia. The principles of induction are then followed (Pilat 2003).

Quadratus lumborum fascia induction (Figure 11.1.44)

With the patient prone, the therapist is standing at the level of the pelvis facing the patient's head. The therapist places an elbow over the ipsilateral lumbar region between the last rib, the iliac crest, and laterally to the paravertebral muscles. In this position, the therapist presses with the elbow towards the table. The other hand should be placed over the patient's thigh. With this hand, the therapist pushes in a cranial direction. This manoeuvre shortens the quadratus lumborum muscle and allows easier access to its fascia. The therapist should use body weight. This position is held for approximately 3–5 minutes and the principles of induction are followed (Pilat 2003).

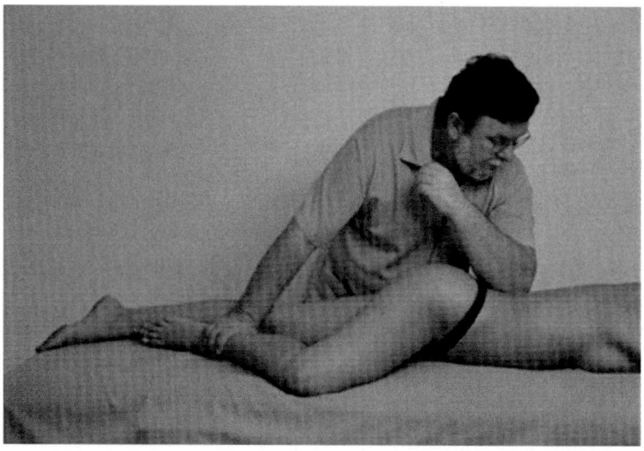

Figure 11.1.45 • Paravertebral muscles fascia induction

Paravertebral muscles fascia induction (Figure 11.1.45)

The patient is lying on his side, with the upper thorax in the prone position. The therapist leans over the patient in order to place the elbow over the lumbar paraspinal mass. Subsequently, the therapist strokes longitudinally with this elbow from L4 to T10 level. Simultaneously, the patient attempts to flex both the hip and knee while the therapist partially resists this effort. The rate of flexion of the hip and knee should take place at the same speed as the elbow movement. The active contraction of the patient's hip muscles inhibits defensive paraspinal muscle tension and thus enables deeper myofascial induction (Pilat 2003).

References

Anderson, R., 2002. Management of chronic prostatitis: chronic pelvic pain syndrome. Urol. Clin. North Am. 29 (1), 235–239.

Anderson, R.U., Wise, D., Sawyer, T., Chan, C., 2005. Integration of myofascial trigger point release and paradoxical relaxation training treatment of chronic pelvic pain in men. J. Urol. 174 (1), 155–160.

Anderson, R.U., Wise, D., Sawyer, T., Chan, C., 2006. Sexual dysfunction in men with chronic protatitis/ chronic pelvic pain syndrome: Improvement after trigger point release and paradoxical relaxation training. J. Urol. 176 (4), 1534–1539.

Anderson, R.U., Sawyer, T., Wise, D., Morey, A., Nathanson, B., 2009. Painful myofascial trigger points and pain sites in men with chronic prostatitis/chronic pelvic pain syndrome. J. Urol. 182 (12), 2753–2758.

Babenko, V., Graven-Nielsen, T., Svensson, P., et al., 1999a. Experimental human muscle pain and muscular hyperalgesia induced by combinations of serotonin and bradykinin. Pain 82 (1), 1–8.

Babenko, V., Graven-Nielsen, T., Svensson, P., et al., 1999b. Experimental human muscle pain induced by intra-muscular injections of bradykinin, serotonin, and substance P. Eur. J. Pain 3 (2), 93–102.

Bajaj, P., Madsen, H., Arendt-Nielsen, L., 2003. Endometriosis is associated with central sensitization: a psychophysical controlled study. J. Pain 4 (7), 372–380.

Baker, P.K., 1993. Musculoskeletal origins of chronic pelvic pain: Diagnosis and treatment. Obstet. Gynecol. Clin. North Am. 20 (4), 719–742.

Ballantyne, F., Fryer, G., McLaughlin, P., 2003. The effect of muscle energy technique on hamstring extensibility: the mechanism of altered flexibility. J. Osteopath. Med. 6 (1), 59–63.

Barnes, J., 1990. Myofascial Release. MFR Seminars, Paoli.

Barnes, M., 1997. The basic science of myofascial release. J. Bodyw. Mov. Ther. 1 (4), 231–238.

Bhattacharya, V., 2005. Live Demonstration of microcirculation in the deep fascia and its implication. Plast. Reconstr. Surg. 115 (2): 458–463.

Bouligard, Y., 1978. Liquid crystals and their analogs in biological systems. Solid State Phys. 14, 259–294.

Burns, D.K., Wells, M.R., 2006. Gross range of motion in the cervical spine: the effects of osteopathic muscle energy technique in asymptomatic subjects. J. Am. Osteopath. Assoc. 106 (3), 137–142.

Cantu, T.I., Grodin, A.J., 2001. Myofascial manipulation: Theory and clinical application. Aspen Publishers, Maryland.

Carter, J.E., 2000. Abdominal wall and pelvic myofascial trigger points. In: Howard, F.M. (Ed.), Pelvic Pain. Lippincott, Williams & Wilkins, Philadelphia, pp. 314–358.

Chaitow, L., 1994. Integrated neuromuscular inhibition technique. British Journal of Osteopathy 13 (1), 17–20.

Chaitow, L., 2006. Muscle Energy Technique, third ed. Churchill Livingstone, Edinburgh.

Chaitow, L., 2007a. Chronic pelvic pain: Pelvic floor problems, sacroiliac dysfunction and the trigger point connections. J. Bodyw. Mov. Ther. 11 (4), 327–339.

Chaitow, L., 2007b. Positional release techniques. Churchill Livingstone, Edinburgh.

Chaitow, L., Delany, J., 2002. Clinical application of neuromuscular techniques. vol. 2: The Lower Body. Churchill Livingstone, Edinburgh.

Chaitow, L., Delany, J., 2008. Clinical application of neuromuscular techniques. vol. 1: The upper body. Edinburgh, Churchill Livingstone.

Chaudhry, H., 2007. Viscoelastic behavior of human fasciae under extension in manual therapy. Journal of Bodywork and Movement Therapies 11 (3), 159–167.

Chaudhry, H., Schleip, R., Zhiming, J.I., et al., 2008. Three-dimensional mathematical model for deformation of human fasciae in manual therapy. J. Am. Osteopath. Assoc. 108 (8), 379–390.

Chen, J.T., Chen, S.M., Kuan, T.S., et al., 1998. Phentolamine effect on the spontaneous electrical activity of active loci in a myofascial trigger spot of rabbit skeletal muscle. Arch. Phys. Med. Rehabil. 79 (7), 790–794.

Chicurel, M., Chen, C., Ingber, D., 1998. Cellular control lies in the balance of forces. Curr. Opin. Cell Biol. 10 (2), 232–239.

Chung, J.W., Ohrbach, R., McCall Jr., W.D., 2004. Effect of increased sympathetic activity on electrical activity from myofascial painful areas. Am. J. Phys. Med. Rehabil. 83 (11), 842–850.

Cope, F.W., 1975. A review of the applications of solid state physics concepts to biological systems. J. Biol. Phys. 3 (1), 1–41.

Cox, J.M., Bakkum, B.W., 2005. Possible generator of retrotrochanteric gluteal and thigh pain: The gemelli-obturator internus complex. J. Manipulative Physiol. Ther. 28 (7), 534–538.

Delancey, J., 1993. Anatomy and biomechanics of genital prolapse. Clin. Obstet. Gynecol. 36 (4), 897–909.

Doggweiler-Wiygul, R., 2004. Urologic myofascial pain syndromes. Curr. Pain Headache Rep. 8 (6), 445–451.

Doggweiler-Wiygul, R., Wiygul, J.P., 2002. Interstitial cystitis, pelvic pain, and the relationship to myofascial pain and dysfunction: a report on four patients. World J. Urol. 20 (5), 310–314.

Dommerholt, J., McEvoy, J., 2010. Myofascial trigger point release approach. In: Wise, C.H. (Ed.), Orthopaedic manual physical therapy: from art to evidence. FA Davis, Philadelphia.

Dommerholt, J., Bron, C., Franssen, J.L.M., 2006. Myofascial trigger points: an evidence informed review. J. Man. Manip. Ther. 14 (4), 203–221.

Fall, M., Baranowski, A., Elneil, S., et al., 2010. EAU guidelines on chronic pelvic pain. Eur. Urol. 57 (1), 35–48.

Feland, J.B., Myrer, J.W., Schulthies, S.S., Fellingham, G.W., Measom, G.W., 2001. The effect of duration of stretching of the hamstring muscle group for increasing range of motion in people aged 65 years or older. Phys. Ther. 81 (5), 1100–1117.

Ferber, R., Osternig, L.R., Gravelle, D.C., 2002. Effect of PNF stretch techniques on knee flexor muscle EMG activity in older adults. J. Electromyogr. Kinesiol. 12 (5), 391–397.

Fernández-de-las-Peñas, C., 2009. Interaction between trigger points and joint hypo-mobility: A clinical perspective. J. Man. Manip. Ther. 17 (2), 74–77.

Fernández-de-las-Peñas, C., Sohrbeck-Campo, M., Fernández, J., Miangolarra- Page, J.C., 2005. Manual therapies in the myofascial trigger point treatment: a systematic review. J. Bodyw. Mov. Ther. 9 (1), 27–34.

Fernández-de-las-Peñas, C., Alonso-Blanco, C., Fernández, J., Miangolarra-Page, J.C., 2006. The immediate effect of ischemic compression technique and transverse friction massage on tenderness of active and latent myofascial triggers points: a pilot study. J. Bodyw. Mov. Ther. 10 (1), 3–9.

Fidzianska, A., Jablonska, S., 2000. Congenital fascial dystrophy: abnormal composition of the fascia. J. Am. Acad. Dermatol. 43 (Pt 1), 797–802.

FitzGerald, M.P., Kotarinos, R., 2003a. Rehabilitation of the short pelvic floor. I: Background and patients evaluation. Int. Urogynecol. J. Pelvic Floor Dysfunct. 14 (4), 261–268.

FitzGerald, M.P., Anderson, R.U., Potts, J., et al., 2009. Randomized multicenter feasibility trial of myofascial physical therapy for the treatment of urological chronic pelvic pain syndromes. J. Urol. 82 (2), 570–580.

Fox, W.B., 2009. Physical therapy for pelvis floor dysfunction. Medical Health 92 (1), 10–11.

Fryer, G., 2000. Muscle energy concepts: a need for change. J. Osteopath. Med. 3 (1), 54–59.

Fryer, G., 2006. Muscle energy technique: Efficacy and research. In: Chaitow, L. (Ed.), Muscle Energy Technique. third ed. Churchill Livingstone, Edinburgh.

Fryer, G., Fossum, C., 2009. Muscle energy techniques. In: Fernández-de-las-Peñas, C., Arendt-Nielsen, L., Gerwin, R.D. (Eds.), Tension-type and cervicogenic headache: Pathophysiology, diagnosis, and management. Jones & Bartlett Publishers, Boston.

Fryer, G., Hodgson, L., 2005. The effect of manual pressure release on myofascial trigger points in the upper trapezius muscle. J. Bodyw. Mov. Ther. 9 (4), 248–255.

Fryer, G., Ruszkowski, W., 2004. The influence of contraction duration in muscle energy technique applied to the atlanto-axial joint. J. Osteopath. Med. 7 (1), 79–84.

Gabbiani, G., 2003. The myofibroblast in wound healing and fibrocontractive diseases. J. Pathol. 200 (4), 500–503.

Gabbiani, G., 2007. Evolution and clinical implications of the myofibroblast concept. In: Findley, T.W., Schleip, R. (Eds.), Fascia Research. Basic Science and Implications for Conventional and Complementary Health Care. Urban and Fischer, Munich.

Ge, H.Y., Fernández-de-las-Penas, C., Arendt-Nielsen, L., 2006. Sympathetic facilitation of hyperalgesia evoked from myofascial tender and trigger points in patients with unilateral shoulder pain. Clin. Neurophysiol. 117 (7), 1545–1550.

Gemmell, H., Miller, P., Nordstrom, H., 2008. Immediate effect of ischaemic compression and trigger point pressure release on neck pain and upper trapezius trigger points: A randomized controlled trial. Clinical Chiropractics 11 (1), 30–36.

Greenman, P.E., 2003. Principles of Manual Medicine, third ed. Lippincott William & Wilkins, Philadelphia.

Gröbli, C., Dejung, B., 2003. Nichtmedikamentöse Therapie myofaszialer Schmerze. Schmerz 17, 475–480.

Han, D.G., 2009. The other mechanism of muscular referred pain: The "connective tissue" theory. Med. Hypotheses 73 (3), 292–295.

Hanten, W.P., Olson, S.L., Butts, N.L., Nowicki, A.L., 2000. Effectiveness of a home program of ischemic pressure followed by sustained stretch for treatment of myofascial trigger points. Phys. Ther. 80 (10), 997–1003.

Haugstad, G.K., Haugstad, T.S., Kirste, U.M., et al., 2006. Posture, movement patterns, and body awareness in women with chronic pelvic pain. J. Psychosom. Res. 61 (5), 637–644.

Hetrick, D.C., Ciol, M.A., Rothman, I., et al., 2003. Musculoskeletal dysfunction in men with chronic pelvic pain syndrome type III: a case-control study. J. Urol. 170 (3), 828–831.

Hodges, P.W., Richardson, C.A., 1996. Inefficient muscular stabilization of the lumbar spine associated with low back pain: a motor control evaluation of transversus abdominis. Spine 21 (22), 2640–2650.

Hong, C.Z., Chen, Y.C., Pon, C.H., Yu, J., 1993. Immediate effects of various physical medicine modalities on pain threshold of an active myofascial trigger point. J. Musculoskel. Pain 1 (1), 37–53.

Hou, C.R., Tsai, L.C., Cheng, K.F., et al., 2002. Immediate effects of various physical therapeutic modalities on cervical myofascial pain and trigger-point sensitivity. Arch. Phys. Med. Rehabil. 83 (10), 1406–1414.

Huang, S., Ingber, D., 1999. The structural and mechanical complexity of cell growth control. Nat. Cell Biol. 1 (5), E131–E138.

Huang, S., Ingber, D., 2000. Shape-dependent control of cell growth, differentiation, and apoptosis: switching between attractors in cell regulatory networks. Exp. Cell Res. 261 (1), 91–103.

Hungerford, B., Gilleard, W., Hodges, P., 2003. Evidence of altered lumbo-pelvic muscle recruitment in the presence of sacroiliac joint pain. Spine 28 (14), 1593–1600.

Hu, S., Chen, J., Fabry, B., et al., 2003. Intracellular stress tomography reveals stress focusing and structural anisotropy in cytoskeleton of living cells. Am. J. Cell Physiol. 285 (5), C1082–C1090.

Iatridies, J., Wu, J., Yandow, J., Langevin, H., 2003. Subcutaneous tissue mechanical behavior is linear and viscoelastic under uni-axial tension. Connect. Tissue Res. 44 (5), 208–217.

Ibáñez-García, J., Alburquerque-Sendín, F., Rodríguez-Blanco, C., et al., 2009. Changes in masseter muscle trigger points following strain-counter/ strain or neuro-muscular technique. J. Bodyw. Mov. Ther. 13 (1), 2–10.

Ingber, D., 2003. Tensegrity I. Cell structure and hierarchical systems biology. J. Cell Sci. 116 (10), 1157–1173.

Ingber, D.E., 2006. Cellular mechano-transduction: putting all the pieces together again. FASEB J. 20 (7), 811–827.

Ingber, D., 1998. The architecture of life. Sci. Am. 278 (1), 48–57.

Jarrell, J., 2004. Myofascial dysfunction in the pelvis. Curr. Pain Headache Rep. 8 (6), 452–456.

Jones, L.N., 1981. Strain and counter-strain. American Academy of Osteopathy, Newark, OH.

Khalsa, P., Zhang, C., Sommerfeldt, D., 2000. Expression of integrin alpha2beta1 in axons and receptive endings of neurons in rat, hairy skin. Neurosci. Lett. 293 (1), 13–16.

Kuan, T.S., Hong, C.Z., Chen, J.T., et al., 2007. The spinal cord connections of the myofascial trigger spots. Eur. J. Pain 11 (6), 624–634.

Kubo, K., Ikebukuro, T., Yaeshima, K., Kanehisa, H., Yata, H., Tsunoda, H., 2009a. Effects of static and dynamic training on the stiffness and blood volume of tendon in vivo. Eur. J. Appl. Physiol. 106 (2), 412–417.

Kubo, K., Ikebukuro, T., Yaeshima, K., Kanehisa, H., 2009b. Effects of different duration contractions on elasticity, blood volume, and oxygen saturation of human tendon in vivo. Eur. J. Appl. Physiol. 106 (3), 445–455.

Langevin, H.M., 2006. Connective tissue: a body-wide signaling network? Med. Hypotheses 66 (6), 1074–1077.

Langford, C.F., Udvari Nagy, S., Ghoniem, G.M., 2007. Levator ani trigger point injections: An underutilized treatment for chronic pelvic pain. Neurourol. Urodyn. 26 (1), 59–62.

Lee, D., Lee, L.J., 2004a. Stress urinary incontinence: A consequence of failed load transfer through the pelvis? In: Proceedings from the 5th interdisciplinary world congress on low back and pelvic pain. Melbourne, Australia.

Lee, D.G., Vleeming, A., 1998. Impaired load transfer through the pelvic girdle – a new model of altered neutral zone function. In: Proceedings from the 3rd interdisciplinary world congress on low back and pelvic pain. Vienna, Austria.

Lee, D.G., Vleeming, A., 2004. The management of pelvic joint pain and dysfunction. In: Boyling, J., Jull, G. (Eds.), Grieve's modern manual therapy of the vertebral column. third ed. Elsevier.

Lewit, K., 1999. Manipulative therapy in rehabilitation of the locomotor system, third ed. Butterworth Heinemann, Oxford.

Lewit, K., Horacek, O., 2004. A case of selective paresis of the deep stabilization system due to borreliosis. Man. Ther. 9 (3), 173–175.

Liebenson, C., 2000. The pelvic floor muscles and the silverstolpe phenomena. J. Bodyw. Mov. Ther. 4 (3), 195.

Li, L.T., Ge, H.Y., Yue, S.W., Arendt-Nielsen, L., 2009. Nociceptive and non-nociceptive hypersensitivity at latent myofascial trigger points. Clin. J. Pain 25 (2), 132–137.

Liptan, L., 2010. Fascia: A missing link in our understanding of the pathology of fibromialgia. J. Bodyw. Mov. Ther. 14 (1), 3–12.

Lucas, K.R., Polus, B.I., Rich, P.A., 2004. Latent myofascial trigger points: their effects on muscle activation and movement efficiency. J. Bodyw. Mov. Ther. 8 (2), 160–166.

Lukban, J., Whitmore, K., Kellog-Spadt, S., et al., 2001. The effect of manual physical therapy in patients diagnosed with interstitial cystitis, high-tone pelvic floor dysfunction, and sacroiliac dysfunction. Urology 57 (6, Suppl. 1), 121–122.

Maloney, M.L., Newman, J.M., 2005. Abdominal pain of myofascial origin. In: Ferguson, L., Gerwin, R. (Eds.), Clinical mastery in the treatment of myofascial pain. Lippincott Williams & Wilkins, Philadelphia, pp. 303–326.

Manheim, C., 1998. The Myofascial Release Manual. Slack Inc., US.

Maniotis, A., Chen, C., Ingber, D., 1997. Demonstration of mechanical connections between integrins, cytoskeletal filaments, and nucleoplasm that stabilize nuclear structure. Proc. Natl. Acad. Sci. U. S. A. 94 (3), 849–854.

McNulty, W.H., Gevirtz, R., Hubbard, D., Berkoff, G., 1994. Needle electromyographic evaluation of trigger point response to a psychological stressor. Psychophysiology 31 (3), 313–316.

McPartland, J.M., Giuffrida, A., King, J., Skinner, E., Scotter, J., Musty, R.E., 2005. Cannabimimetic effects of osteopathic manipulative treatment. J. Am. Osteopath. Assoc. 105 (4), 283–291.

Mense, S., 1994. Referral of muscle pain. Am. Pain Soc. J 3 (1), 1–9.

Mens, J.M., Vleeming, A., Snijders, C.J., Stam, H.J., Ginai, A.Z., 1999. The active straight leg raising test and mobility of the pelvic joints. Eur. Spine J. 8 (6), 468–473.

Myers, T., 2003. Anatomy Trains. Elsevier, London.

Miranda, A., Peles, S., Rudolph, C., et al., 2004. Altered visceral sensation in response to somatic pain in the rat. Gastroenterology 126 (4), 1082–1089.

Mitchell, F.L., Mitchell, P.K.G., 1995. The Muscle Energy Manual. vol. 1. MET Press, Michigan.

Montenegro, M.L.L.S., Mateus-Vasconcelos, Candido-dos-Reis, F.J., Nogueira, A.A., Poli-Nieto, O.B., 2008. Physical therapy in the management of women with chronic pelvis pain. Int. J. Clin. Pract. 62 (2), 263–269.

Montenegro, M.L.L.S., Gomide, L.B., Mateus-Vasconcelos, E.L.M., et al., 2009. Abdominal myofascial pain syndrome must be considered in the differential diagnosis of chronic pelvic pain. Eur. J. Obstet. Gynecol. Reprod. Biol. 147 (1), 21–24.

Niddam, D.M., Chan, R.C., Lee, S.H., et al., 2007. Central modulation of pain evoked from myofascial trigger point. Clin. J. Pain 23 (5), 440–448.

Occelli, B., 2001. Anatomic study of arcus tendineus fasciae pelvis. Eur. J. Obstet. Gynecol. Reprod. Biol. 97 (2), 213–219.

O'Connell, J.A., Judith, A., 2003. Bioelectric responsiveness of fascia. Tech. Orthopaed. 18 (1), 67–73.

Oschman, J., 2003. Energy medicine in therapeutics and human performance. Nature's own research Association Dover, New Hampshire.

Palomeque-del-Cerro, L., Fernández-de-las-Peñas, C., 2009. Neuromuscular approaches. In: Fernández-de-las-Peñas, C., Arendt-Nielsen, L., Gerwin, R. (Eds.), Tension Type and Cervicogenic Headache: pathophysiology, diagnosis and treatment. Jones & Bartlett Publishers, Boston, pp. 327–338.

Paoletti, S., 1998. Les fascias: role des tissus dans la mécanique humaine. Sully.

Parker, K.K., Ingber, D.E., 2007. Extracellular matrix, mechanotransduction and structural hierarchies in heart tissue engineering. Philos Trans R Soc Lond B Biol Sci 362 (1484), 1267–1279.

Peters, K., Carrico, D., 2006. Frequency, urgency, and pelvic pain: Treating the pelvic floor versus the epithelium. Curr. Urol. Rep. 7 (6), 450–455.

Pilat, A., 2003. Inducción Miofascial. McGraw-Hill, Madrid.

Pilat, A., 2007a. El lenguaje del dolor (el proceso de interpretación del dolor en fisioterapia), Libro de Ponencias XV Jornadas de Fisioterapia. EUF ONCE, Madrid.

Pilat, A., 2009. Myofascial induction approaches for headache. In: Fernández-de-las- Peñas, C., Arendt-Nielsen, L., Gerwin, R.D. (Eds.), Tension Type and Cervicogenic Headache: pathophysiology, diagnosis and treatment. Jones & Bartlett Publishers, Boston.

Pilat, A., Testa, M., 2009. Tensegridad: El Sistema Craneosacro como la unidad biodinámica, Libro de Ponencias XIX Jornadas de Fisioterapia. EUF ONCE, Madrid, pp. 95–111.

Pool-Goudzwaard, A., Hoek Van Dijke, G., Mulder, P., et al., 2003. The iliolumbar ligament: its influence on stability of the sacroiliac joint. Clinical Biomechnics 18 (2), 99–105.

Prendergast, S.A., Weiss, J.M., 2003. Screening for musculoskeletal causes of pelvic pain. Clin. Obstet. Gynecol. 46 (4), 773–782.

Remving, L., 2007. Fascia Research. Myofascial release: 5.4.5–140: An evidence based treatment concept. Elsevier Urban & Fischer.

Rickards, L.D., 2006. The effectiveness of non-invasive treatments for active myofascial trigger point pain: A systematic review of the literature. Int. J. Osteopath. Med. 9 (2), 120–136.

Rodríguez-Blanco, C., Fernández-de-las-Peñas, C., Hernández-Xumet, J.E., et al., 2006. Changes in active mouth opening following a single treatment of latent myofascial trigger points in the masseter muscle involving post-isometric relaxation or strain/counter-strain. J. Bodyw. Mov. Ther. 10 (3), 197–205.

Rolf, I., 1977. La integración de las estructuras del cuerpo humano. Ediciones Urano, Barcelona.

Ruiz-Sáez, M., Fernández-de-las-Peñas, C., Rodríguez-Blanco, C., et al., 2007. Changes in pressure pain sensitivity in latent myofascial trigger points in the upper trapezius muscle following a cervical spine manipulation in pain-free subjects. J. Manipulative Physiol. Ther. 30 (8), 578–583.

Samraj, G.P., Kuritzky, L., Curry, R.W., 2005. Chronic pelvic pain in women: Evaluation and management in primary care. Complementary Therapy 31 (1), 28–39.

Santos, G., Gonzalez, L., Hernandez, B., Lorenzo, J., 2009. Avances diagnósticos en uroginecología. Maniobra de Santos en incontinencia urinaria y prolapso. Poster No. 26 XVIII Congreso Latinoamericano de Cirugía F.E.L.A.C. Caracas Venezuela.

Satish, L., Laframboise, W.A., O'Gorman, D.B., et al., 2008. Identification of differentially expressed genes in fibroblasts derived from patients with Dupuytren's contracture. Biomedicine Central Medical Genomics 1 (1), 1–10.

Schleip, R., Klingler, W., Lehmann-Horn, F., 2005. Active fascial contractility: fascia may be able to contract in a smooth muscle-like manner and thereby influence musculoskeletal dynamics. Med. Hypotheses 65 (2), 273–277.

Schleip, R., Kingler, W., Lehmann-Horn, F., 2007. Fascia is able to contract in a smooth muscle-like manner and thereby influence musculoskeletal mechanics. In: Findley, T.W., Schleip, R. (Eds.), Fascia Research. Basic Science and Implications for Conventional and Complementary Health Care. Urban and Fischer, Munich, pp. 76–77.

Schmidt, R., 1991. Pelvic floor behaviour and interstitial cystitis. Semin. Urol. 9 (2), 154–159.

Shah, J.P., Phillips, T.M., Danoff, J.V., Gerber, L.H., 2005. An in vitro microanalytical technique for measuring the local biochemical milieu of human skeletal muscle. J. Appl. Physiol. 99 (5), 1977–1984.

Shah, J.P., Danoff, J.V., Desai, M.J., et al., 2008. Biochemicals associated with pain and inflammation are elevated in sites near to and remote from active myofascial trigger points. Arch. Phys. Med. Rehabil. 89 (1), 16–23.

Shoskes, D.A., Berger, R., Elmi, A., et al., 2008. Muscle tenderness in men with chronic prostatitis/chronic pelvic pain syndrome: The chronic prostatitis cohort study. J. Urol. 179 (2), 556–560.

Simons, D.G., 2002. Understanding effective treatments of myofascial trigger points. J. Bodyw. Mov. Ther. 6 (1), 81–88.

Simons, D.G., Travell, J.G., Simons, L.S., 1999. Travell & Simons' myofascial pain and dysfunction: the trigger point manual. In: second ed. vol. 1. Lippincott William & Wilkins, Baltimore, pp. 278–307.

Slocumb, J.C., 1984. Neurological factors in chronic pelvic pain: trigger points and the abdominal pelvic pain syndrome. Am. J. Obstet. Gynecol. 149 (5), 536–543.

Slocumb, J.C., 1990. Chronic somatic, myofascial, and neurogenic abdominal pelvic pain. Clin. Obstet. Gynecol. 33 (1), 145–153.

Snijders, C.J., Vleeming, A., Stoeckart, R., 1993a. Transfer of lumbo-sacral load to iliac bones and legs. 1: Biomechanics of self-bracing of the sacroiliac joints and its significance for treatment and exercise. Clin. Biomech. 8 (6), 285–294.

Snijders, C.J., Vleeming, A., Stoeckart, R., 1993b. Transfer of lumbo-sacral load to iliac bones and legs. 2: Loading of the sacroiliac joints when lifting in a stooped posture. Clin. Biomech. 8 (6), 295–301.

Srinivasan, A.K., Kaye, J.D., Moldwin, R., 2007. Myofascial dysfunction associated with chronic pelvic floor pain: management strategies. Curr. Pain Headache Rep. 11 (5), 359–364.

Stamenovic, D., Rosenblatt, N., Montoya-Zavala, M., et al., 2007. Rheological behavior of living cells is timescale dependent. J. Biophys. 93 (1), 39–41.

Staubesand, J., Li, Y., 1997. Begriff und Substrat der Faziensklerose bei chronisch-venöser Insuffizienz. Phlebologie 26 (1), 72–77.

Stecco, C., Porzionato, A., Macchi, V., et al., 2006. A histological study of the deep fascia of the upper limb. Ital J Anat Embryol 111 (2), 105–110.

Stecco, C., Porzionato, A., Macchi, V., et al., 2008. The expansions of the pectoral girdle muscles onto the brachial fascia: morphological aspects and spatial disposition. Cells Tissues Organs 188 (3), 320–329.

Stepnik, M.W., Olby, N., Thompson, R.R., Marcellin-Little, D.J., 2006. Femoral neuropathy in a dog with iliopsoas muscle injury. Vet. Surg. 35 (2), 186–190.

Svensson, P., Cairns, B.E., Wang, K., Arendt-Nielsen, L., 2003. Glutamate-evoked pain and mechanical allodynia in the human masseter muscle. Pain 101 (3), 221–227.

Szent-Gyorgyi, A., 1994. The study of energy-levels in biochemistry. Nature 148 (6469), 157–159.

Threlkeld, A.J., 1992. The effects of manual therapy on connective tissues. Phys. Ther. 72 (12), 893–902.

Travell, J., Bigelow, N.H., 1946. Referred somatic pain does not follow a simple "segmental" pattern. Fed. Proc. 5, 106.

Travell, J.G., Simons, D.G., 1983. Myofascial Pain and Dysfunction: The Trigger Point Manual. vol. 1. Williams & Wilkins, Baltimore.

Tu, F.F., As-Sanie, S., Steege, J.F., 2006. Prevalence of pelvic musculoskeletal disorders in a female chronic pelvic pain clinic. J. Reprod. Med. 51 (3): 185–189.

Tu, F.F., Holt, J., Gonzales, J., Fitzgerald, C.M., 2008. Physical therapy evaluation of patients with chronic pelvic pain: a controlled study. Am. J. Obstet. Gynecol. 198 (3), 272.e1–272.e7.

Upledger, J., 1997. Craniosacral therapy I: Study guide. UI Publishing.

Vanacore, R., Ham, A., Voehler, M., et al., 2009. Sulfilimine bond identified in collagen IV. Science 325 (5945), 1230–1234.

Vernon, H., Schneider, M., 2009. Chiropractic management of myofascial trigger points and myofascial pain syndrome: A systematic review of the literature. J. Manipulative Physiol. Ther. 32 (1), 14–24.

Vernon, H.T., Dhami, M.S., Howley, T.P., Annett, R., 1986. Spinal manipulation and beta-endorphin: A controlled study of the effect of a spinal manipulation on plasma beta-endorphin levels in normal males. J. Manipulative Physiol. Ther. 9 (2): 115–123.

Vleeming, A., Pool-Goudzwaard, A.L., Hammudoghlu, D., Stoeckart, R., Snijders, C.J., Mens, J.M.A., 1996. The function of the long dorsal sacroiliac ligament: its implication for understanding low back pain. Spine 21 (5), 556–562.

Vleeming, A., Albert, H.G., Ostgaard, H.C., Sturesson, B., Stuge, B., 2008. European guidelines for the diagnosis and treatment of pelvic girdle pain. Eur. Spine J. 17 (6), 794–819.

Wang, N., Tytell, J., Ingber, D., 2009. Mechano-transduction at a distance: mechanically coupling the extracellular matrix with the nucleus. Science 10 (1), 75–81.

Weiss, J.M., 2001. Pelvic floor myofascial trigger points: manual therapy for interstitial cystitis and the urgency-frequency syndrome. J. Urol. 166 (6), 2226–2231.

Wesselmann, 2001. Neurogenic inflammation and chronic pelvic pain. World J. Urol. 19 (3). 180–185.

Wright, D.G., Rennels, D.C., 1964. A study of the elastic properties of plantar fascia. J. Bone Joint Surg. Am. 46, 482–492.

Wurn, L., Wurn, B., King, C.R., et al., 2004. Increasing orgasm and decreasing dyspareunia by a manual physical therapy technique. MedGenMed. 6 (4), 47.

Yahia, L.H., Pigeon, P., DesRosiers, E.A., 1993. Viscoelastic properties of the human lumbo-dorsal fascia. J. Biomed. Eng. 15 (5), 425–429.

Zhang, Y., Ge, H.Y., Yue, S.W., et al., 2009. Attenuated skin blood flow response to nociceptive stimulation of latent myofascial trigger points. Arch. Phys. Med. Rehabil. 90 (2), 325–332.

Connective tissue and the pudendal nerve in chronic pelvic pain

11.2

Stephanie Prendergast Elizabeth H. Rummer

CHAPTER CONTENTS

Connective tissue dysfunction in chronic pelvic pain

Several different terms have been used to describe connective tissue restrictions and/or dysfunction. According to orthopaedic physician Robert Maigne, cellulagia is 'defined as neurotrophic manifestations that include subcutaneous tenderness and thickening'. It can be detected by using the 'pinch-roll' test, in which a fold of skin is rolled between the fingers causing pain, with the clinician noting thickening (Maigne 1995) (Figure 11.2.1).

Physical therapist Maria Ebner (1985) used the term trophic oedema to describe thickened hypersensitive loose connective tissue. Other literature sources have referred to dermographia, which is defined as a condition in which pressure or friction of the skin gives rise to a transient reddish mark so that a line on the skin becomes visible (Merck Manual 2008). Finally, the terms panniculosis and fibrositis have also been used to describe dysfunctional connective tissue (Travell & Simons 1993), defined as inflammatory hyperplasia of the white fibrous tissue. This text will use the term subcutaneous panniculosis to describe thickened connective tissue that is tender upon pinch rolling (i.e. dysfunctional connective tissue).

In addition to presenting as thickened or dense upon skin rolling, areas of subcutaneous panniculosis may

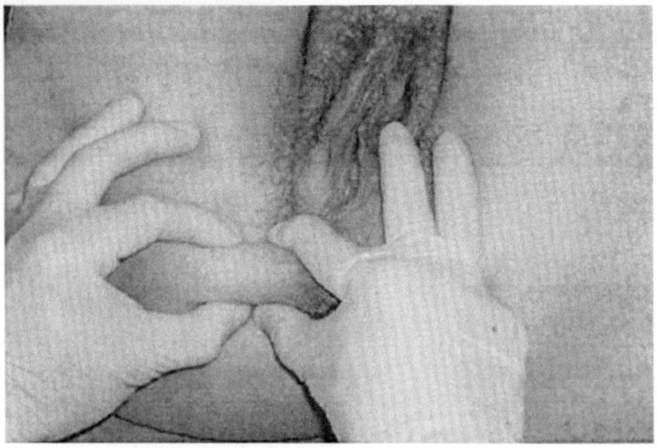

Figure 11.2.1 • Skin rolling test: the skin of the perineum is pinched just below the level of the anus and rolled to the front searching for a sharp pain at one level (Beco 2004)

show vasomotor, pilomotor and sudomotor reactions, increased subcutaneous fluid and atrophy or hypertrophy of the underlying muscles (Chaitow 2010). Underlying muscle atrophy is the resultant effect of the thickened tissue interfering with proper functioning of sodium–potassium pumping mechanisms in muscles (Ebner 1975). Panniculosis can cause local nociceptive pain via the peripheral nervous system, and it is hypothesized to cause referred pain in distant locations including the viscera through the central nervous system (Bischof & Elmiger 1963).

Mechanisms of development of subcutaneous panniculosis

When connective tissue becomes dysfunctional the problems that arise are in proportion to the support the tissues provide when they are healthy. Several mechanisms have been identified to explain how dysfunction develops in the subcutaneous tissue. These are as the result of visceral referred pain, in tissue superficial to myofascial trigger points, in the cutaneous distribution of inflamed peripheral nerves, and superficial to or referred from areas of joint dysfunction (Ebner 1975, Travell & Simons 1993, Beco 2004, Maigne 1996).

Viscerosomatic reflex

The viscerosomatic reflex is a reflex in which somatic manifestations occur in response to visceral disturbances. More specifically, the visceral-cutaneous reflex is a phenomenon where disturbances or disease in visceral organs refer pain along the distribution of somatic nerves which share the same spinal segment as the sensory sympathetic fibres to the organ affected (Head 1893). The visceral-cutaneous reflexes have been studied by many and are commonly referred to as Head's zones, Chapman's reflexes, or Mackenzie's zones (Beal 1985) (see Figures 11.2.2, 11.2.3). The reflex is initiated by afferent impulses from visceral receptors, impulses travel to the dorsal horn of the spinal cord, synapse with interconnecting neurons, connect with sympathetic and peripheral motor efferents resulting in sensory changes in the blood vessels and skin (and also muscle and viscera) (Bischof & Elminger 1963). If the pathological visceral afferent stimulation becomes chronic, neurogenic plasma extravasation will occur in the skin, thereby causing vasoconstriction in the periphery, hyperaesthesia and thixotropic changes. In more recent literature, three plausible neural mechanisms have been identified in animal models to explain visceral-cutaneous reflexes.

In 1996 Takahashi & Nakajima published that plasma extravasation occurred as a result of antidromic stimulation of C-fibres in spinal nerves. It is noted that with unilateral stimulation changes in the skin can occur unilaterally or bilaterally (Takahashi & Nakajima 1996).

Studies suggest that the actual mechanism may be a combination of the three described processes, as noted by Ursula Wesslemann et al. in 1997. One potential mechanism is described because dichotomizing sensory neurons have a branch to both the uterus and to the skin. Uterine inflammation could cause excitation of the visceral branch of the afferent neuron, leading to antidromic activation of the somatic branch causing neurogenic plasma extravasation. Wesselmann also hypothesized that visceral afferent neurons may excite cutaneous afferent neurons. The result of this spinal mechanism is antidromic activation of cutaneous afferent fibres, again resulting in plasma extravasation. Finally, the paper discussed the possibility that sympathetic post-ganglionic nerve terminals must be intact. This was demonstrated by a decrease in plasma extravasation when the anterior spinal root was not intact (Wesslemann & Lai 1993).

Similarly, basic science studies (Beal 1985, Craggs 2005) have shown that somatic disturbances cause visceral changes, otherwise known as the somatovisceral reflex.

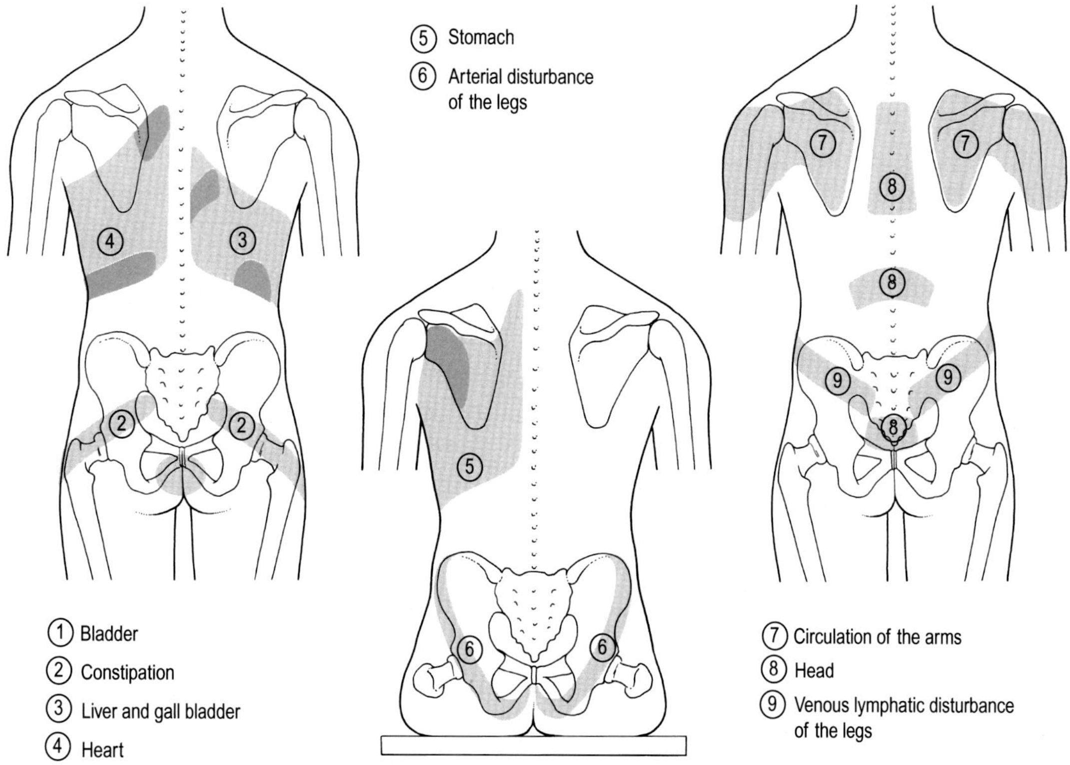

Figure 11.2.2 • Head's zones. Adapted from Chaitow (2003) Modern Neuromuscular Techniques, second ed, Elsevier.

Superficial to muscles with myofascial trigger points

Travell & Simons (1993) have reported a strong association between active myofascial trigger points and subcutaneous connective tissue restrictions. Dermographia/fibrositis commonly occurs most often over muscles of the back of the neck, shoulders and torso, and less frequently over limb muscles. In panniculosis, the subcutaneous tissue exhibits increased viscosity suggestive of thixotropy. It is proposed by Travell and Simons that the connective tissue restrictions may be related to sympathetic nervous system activity involving mechanisms operating in the underlying myofascial trigger points. Treating the panniculosis can relieve myofascial trigger point activity and/or make the underlying myofascial trigger point more responsive to treatment. Travell and Simons identify the need for a well-designed study to critically evaluate the relationship between myofascial trigger point activity and the presence of overlying panniculosis.

Dermatomes of inflamed neural structures

The 'pinch-roll' test (of the subcutaneous tissue in the territory of a peripheral nerve) is commonly accepted as a clinical indicator of inflamed neural tissue. Referred pain is accompanied by hyperalgesia of the skin and subcutaneous tissues in the involved dermatomes. This hyperalgesia or hypersensitivity can be revealed by gently grasping a fold of skin between the thumbs and forefingers, lifting it away from the trunk and rolling the subcutaneous surfaces against one another in a pinch and roll fashion. The entire dermatome may be affected or only partial tissue changes may be seen (Maigne 1996, Beco 2004).

Superficial to areas of joint dysfunction

Robert Maigne (1995, 1996) coined the term 'cellulagia' when reporting that intervertebral joint dysfunction causes neurotrophic reflexes. This cellulagia can

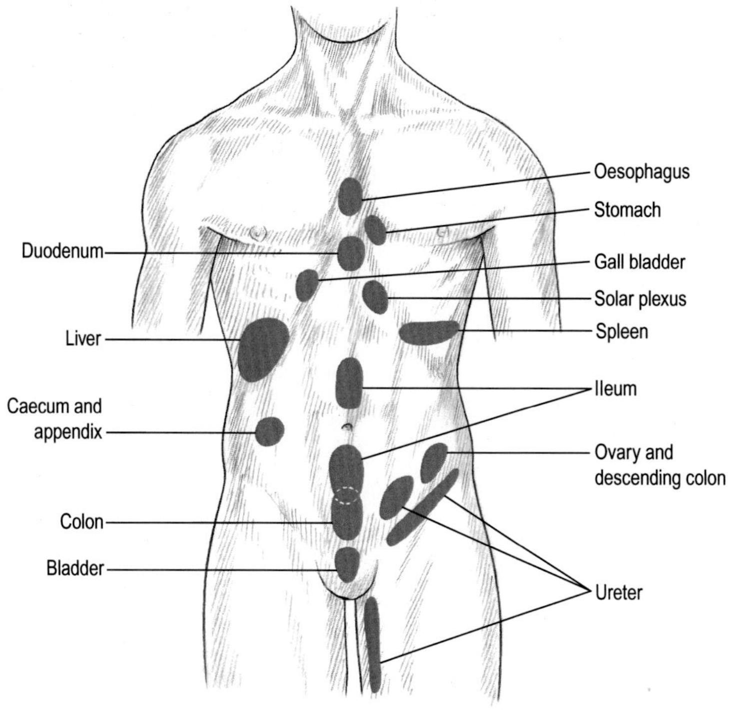

Figure 11.2.3 • McKenzie's zones. Adapted from Chaitow (2003) Modern Neuromuscular Techniques, second ed, Elsevier.

occur in the skin innervated by the corresponding nerve roots and in tissue superficial to areas of vertebral dysfunction.

The dysfunctional tissue itself and the sequellae associated with subcutaneous panniculosis can perpetuate chronic pelvic pain (CPP) and dysfunction. Subcutaneous panniculosis can cause local nociceptive pain, hypothesized visceral referred pain through the central nervous system, underlying muscle dysfunction and altered neurodynamics. The thickening of the skin causes ischaemia and therefore nociceptive pain via the peripheral nervous system (Holey 1995). In addition to local pain, the presence of increased subcutaneous fluid will cause an alteration in the osmotic pressure in cells. There is retention of sodium and associated excretion of potassium, resulting in water retention that interferes with the neuromuscular conducting mechanism (Ebner 1975). The physiological consequence of this is underlying muscle atrophy, which may then lead to the development of myofascial trigger points, a further source of pain and dysfunction. Multiple literature sources describe the mechanisms of which subcutaneous panniculosis can perpetuate visceral disturbance and that the association between cutaneous dysfunction and visceral disturbance is so high that examination of the skin can be used as a predictor of potentially undiagnosed visceral disease (Korr 1949, Wilson 1956, Grainger 1958, Beal 1985, Tillman & Cummings 1992).

Connective tissue restrictions and altered neural dynamics

As discussed below, a peripheral nerve is vulnerable to neural dynamics if its blood supply and/or normal neurobiomechanics are compromised along its path. Ischaemia or thickness associated with subcutaneous panniculosis can compromise neural gliding mechanisms, particularly when the peripheral nerves innervate or transect the dysfunctional tissue region (Butler 2004).

Any muscle and/or tissue and/or structure innervated by an affected nerve may begin to generate pain (Butler 2004). For example, a patient with connective tissue restrictions in the territory of the pudendal nerve may experience sharp, stabbing vaginal or urethral pain with increasing degrees of hip flexion. This is because the nerve must lengthen when the hip flexes; if the tissue is restricted the nerve will not be able to lengthen and the adverse tension results in neuralgic pain in the territory of the nerve. Consequently, because the and/or perineal portions of the pudendal nerve innervate the distal third of the urethra a patient may subsequently feel urethral burning. In terms of bowel function, it is not uncommon for patients with CPP to experience constipation. Connective tissue restrictions affecting the pudendal nerve can also cause neuralgia symptoms, as the restrictions will restrict the neural mobility required for lengthening when a person strains. As a result, a patient may feel neuralgic symptoms in the territory of the nerve, either immediately or with a delayed onset (Holey 1995).

The matrix of areolar connective tissue also serves to deposit collagen for the formation of scar tissue. Commonly, women with CPP have undergone laparoscopic investigation as an attempt to identify pain generators. The trochar (a surgical instrument) may have been used through the umbilicus, in the suprapubic region, or other lower abdominal sites. Formation of scar tissue here can directly create restriction of the ilioinguinal, iliohypogastric and genitofemoral nerves (Howard 2000). Peri-umbilical and suprapubic subcutaneous panniculosis secondary to incisions have been associated with urinary urgency, frequency and dysuria (Fitzgerald & Kotarinos 2003).

Efficacy of connective tissue mobilization

Over the last 20 years basic science research has confirmed the interaction between muscle, skin, viscera and central and peripheral nervous systems supporting the importance of addressing connective tissue as part of any pain-related treatment programme. Recent clinical research shows the physiological and clinical benefits of CTM (Kaada & Torsteinbo 1989, Brattbert 1999, Maddali-Bongi et al. 2009, Fitzgerald et al. 2009).

The Urological Pelvic Pain Collaborative Research Network and the National Institutes of Health examined the feasibility of conducting a randomized clinical trial to compare two methods of manual therapy, external and internal myofascial physical therapy (MPT), compared to traditional external global therapeutic massage (GTM) among patients with urologic CPP syndromes (Fitzgerald et al. 2009). Connective tissue manipulation was the primary external myofascial technique in the MPT group. They were able to standardize both treatment approaches. They found the MPT group had a response rate of 57% which was significantly higher than the rate of 21% in the GTM treatment group ($P = 0.03$). The overall response rate of 57% in the MPT group suggests that MPT represents a clinically meaningful treatment option. We can infer from these results that there is clear evidence of benefit of connective tissue manipulation in patients with myofascial pelvic pain and dysfunction.

One recent study evaluated the efficacy of a rehabilitation programme based on the combination of connective tissue massage and McMennell joint manipulation specifically for the hands of patients suffering from systemic sclerosis (Maddali-Bongi et al. 2009). In the 40 patients enrolled, 20 (interventional group) were treated for a 9-week period with a combination of connective tissue massage, McMennell joint manipulation and a home exercise programme, and 20 (controlled) were assigned only to a home exercise programme. The interventional group improved in multiple functional and quality of life tests at the end of the treatment ($P < 0.0001$) versus the control group. Therefore, they concluded that the combined treatment may lead to an improvement in hand function and quality of life.

In 1999 Brattberg investigated the effect of connective tissue massage in the treatment of patients with fibromyalgia. He randomized 48 individuals diagnosed with fibromyalgia, 23 in the treatment group and 25 in the reference group. After a series of 15 treatments of CTM he found that the treatment group reported a pain-relieving effect of 37%, reduced depression and the use of analgesics, and positive effects in their quality of life (Brattbert 1999).

In 1989, another study examined the concentration of plasma beta-endorphins in 12 volunteers before and 5, 30 and 90 minutes after a 30-minute session of CTM. They found a moderate mean increase of 16% in beta-endorphin levels from 20.0 to 23.2 pg/0.1 ml ($P = 0.025$) lasting for approximately 1 hour with a maximum in the test 5 minutes after termination of the massage. They concluded that the release of beta-endorphins is linked with the pain relief and feeling of warmth and well-being associated with the treatment (Kaada & Torsteinbo 1989).

Connective tissue manipulation

The original technique described by Dicke (1953) and more recently by Ebner (1975) and Holey (1995) involves particular strokes in very specific directions and patterns throughout the entire body depending on the pathology. The authors' use of CTM is based upon Dicke's technique in theory and practice, but the technique has been modified for the CPP population specifically. In this text, CTM will be described as the authors utilize it in practice, which has not been described previously.

Evaluation

Considerations:

- Severity of connective tissue (CT) restrictions correlate to severity of symptoms;
- Mild tissue restrictions will cause slight tissue irritation when compressed for long periods;
- Moderate restrictions may cause a hypersensitivity to touch;
- Severely restricted tissue can cause pain without touch, stretch or compression and/or skin fissures.

Prior to CT assessment:

- Skin inspection;
- Colour;
- Integrity;
- Hypertrophy or atrophy;
- Musculoskeletal evaluation;
- Areas of musculoskeletal impairments guide CT assessment.

CT assessment:

- Supine or prone position;
- Small amount of massage cream;
- Tissue assessed by rolling tissue between tips of thumbs and fingers;
- Thumbs slide underneath CT while fingers grasp tissue and pull towards thumb;
- Tips of fingers used, not pads, therefore short fingernails are required;
- Grasp is firm and fairly superficial;
- Pressure to skin is minimal;
- Direction of force is parallel to tissue, not perpendicular;

Less restricted tissue is easier to mobilize, more restricted tissue is more difficult:

- Initial strokes palpate tissue for:
- Contour;
- Temperature;
- Sensitivity;
- Elasticity;
- Turgor;
- Bulk.

Restricted tissue will be:

- Colder;
- Hypersensitive;
- Less elastic;
- Thickened;
- Bulkier.
- Begins distally at knee and progresses proximally to torso until entire area from knees to ribs is assessed.

Areas of particular interest:

- Pubic symphysis/suprapubic tissue;
- Medial to the ischial tuberosities;
- Along the pubic rami;
- Vulvar tissue;
- Peri-anal tissue;
- Tissue lateral to coccyx.

Treatment

- Treatment identical to assessment in technique;
- Tissue mobilized until:
  - Improvement in mobility;
  - Decrease in sensitivity;
  - Increase in warmth is detected.
- Short- or long-term treatment depending on severity of CT restrictions;
- Series of treatments typically required, effects are cumulative;
- Treatment sessions 30 minutes to 2 hours.

Patient response

- Report of cutting or scratching sensation or feeling of dull pressure;
- Severely restricted tissue is very painful;
- Severity of tension correlates to severity of response;
- As tissue mobility improves treatment becomes less painful;
- Patient may report dizziness, nausea, increased sweating, or, in a minority of patients, even fainting (Bischof & Elmiger 1963, Ebner 1975, Frazer 1978);
- Often patients will report an immediate relief in visceral or myofascial pain or dysfunction (Ebner 1975, Gifford & Gifford 1988).

Tissue response

- 'Triple response', in this order: appearance of a red line, red flush in tissue if stroke is repeated, slight swelling called a wheal (Lewis 1927);
- First reaction always occurs if there is tension in CT, last two reactions occur depending on strength of stimulus and number of repetitions on area;
- Skin response will lessen as tension in CT decreases;
- Bruising somewhat common in first 2–4 treatments;
- Tissue will be sore for 2–3 days following treatment;
- Tissue soreness diminishes after a series of treatments.

Special considerations

- Overweight patients will have more tension;
- Older patients will have looser CT;
- Certain anatomic sites will have more or less tension;
- Imperative to educate patient about what to expect during and after treatment.

Goals

- Improve circulation;
- Improve tissue integrity;
- Decrease ischaemia;
- Reduce nocigenic chemicals in restricted CT;
- Decrease or eliminate visceral pain or dysfunction;
- Decrease adverse neural tension on peripheral nerve branches.

Contraindications (Goats & Keir 1991)

- CT over malignancy;
- Acute inflammation or closed abscesses;
- Women in third trimester of pregnancy.

The pudendal nerve in chronic pelvic pain

As discussed in Chapter 2, the pudendal nerve supplies the majority of the pelvic floor musculature, the skin of the genitals and peri-anus, and a portion

Box 11.2.1

Physiological characteristics of connective tissue and subcutaneous panniculosis

Important physiological functions of areolar, or loose connective tissue

- Binds structures and holds them in their anatomical space
- Stores fat and helps conserve body heat
- Aids in tissue repair and forms scar tissue
- Involved in nutrient and metabolite exchange between vessels and individual cells
- Fibroblasts and mast cells inversely related to suprarenal hormones (water retention)

Symptoms of subcutaneous panniculosis (Dicke 1953, Ebner 1975)

- Hypersensitivity to touch (i.e. vestibulitis)
- Intolerance to tight-fit clothing such as underwear
- Pain during tissue compression (i.e. pain with sitting)
- Pain upon stretch (i.e. posterior thigh pain during a hamstring stretch)
- Cutaneous pain without provocation (i.e. unprovoked vulvodynia)
- Itching (i.e. vulvar itching in the absence of infection)
- Poor tissue integrity (i.e. skin tearing during intercourse)

Physiological effects of connective tissue manipulation

- Mechanical effects (Ebner 1975)
- Vasodilation
- Improved tissue mobility
- Decreased nocigenic chemicals
- Autonomic reactions
- Decreased hyperalgesia
- Improved tissue integrity
- Hypothesized reflexive effects (Ebner 1975)
- Decreased adverse visceral reactions on organs sharing the same or neighbouring spinal cord segments

Unresolved connective tissue restrictions can cause

- Visceral disturbance
- Muscle dysfunction
- Adverse neural tension
- Further connective tissue restrictions
- Urinary, bowel and sexual dysfunction
- Perseverance of myofascial impairments and pelvic pain

(Ebner 1975, Travell & Simons 1993, Butler 2004, Kotarinos 2008)

of the rectum, vagina and urethra (for a comprehensive review see Hibner et al. 2010). It is a mixed nerve, featuring both autonomic and somatic components; therefore, it carries motor, sensory and autonomic fibres affecting both the afferent and efferent pathways (Gray & Williams 1995). Due to its autonomic fibres, a patient with pudendal neuralgia could experience sympathetic symptoms such as an increase in heart rate, decreased mobility of the large intestine, constricted blood vessels, dilated pupils, piloerection, perspiration, or an increase in blood pressure (Reitz et al. 2003).

The pudendal nerve arises from the sacral nerve roots 2, 3 and 4 and has three branches: the perineal nerve, the inferior rectal nerve and the dorsal nerve to the clitoris or penis (Robert et al. 1998, Benson & Griffis 2005) (Figure 11.2.4). It runs through three main regions: the gluteal region, the pudendal canal and the perineal region (Thoumas et al. 1999).

The perineal nerve supplies both somatic and visceral structures, innervating the inferior third of the vagina and urethra, the skin of the labia/scrotum, the transverse perineum, bulbospongiosus, ischiocavernosus, urethral sphincter, and the anterior portion of the external anal sphincter.

The inferior rectal nerve innervates the anal canal, the caudal third of the rectum, the peri-anal skin, and the posterior portion of the external anal sphincter.

The dorsal nerve to the clitoris or penis innervates the skin of the penis or clitoris.

Yet, there is no general consensus regarding the precise anatomy of the nerve, although it is widely agreed that it enters the gluteal region through the greater sciatic foramen, hooks around the sacrospinous ligament near its attachment to the ischial spine, enters the perineum through the lesser sciatic foramen and passes through the ischioanal fossa to Alcock's canal (Figures 11.2.4, 11.2.5, 11.2.6). Anatomical studies have indicated that the pudendal nerve either gives rise to the inferior rectal branch before or after Alcock's canal (Robert et al. 1998). This anatomical variation is critical when considering decompression surgery of the pudendal nerve. After Alcock's canal the pudendal nerve further divides into two terminal branches: the perineal nerve and the dorsal nerve to the clitoris or penis (Figure 11.2.4, 11.2.5, 11.2.6) (Robert et al. 1998).

Pudendal neuralgia

Pudendal neuralgia can be described as a severe, throbbing or stabbing pain distributed along the defined course of the nerve. As discussed comprehensively in this text, the pudendal nerve is just one of many possible contributors to CPP.

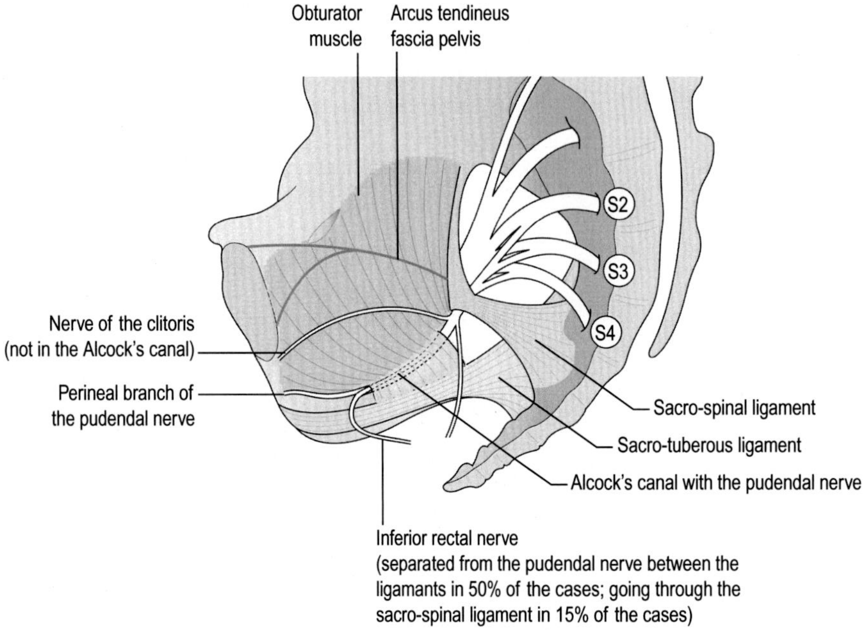

Figure 11.2.4 • S2, S3 and S4: sacral roots forming the pudendal nerve. Adapted from Beco (2004) Pudendal nerve decompression in perineology: a case series. BMC Surg. 4, 1–17

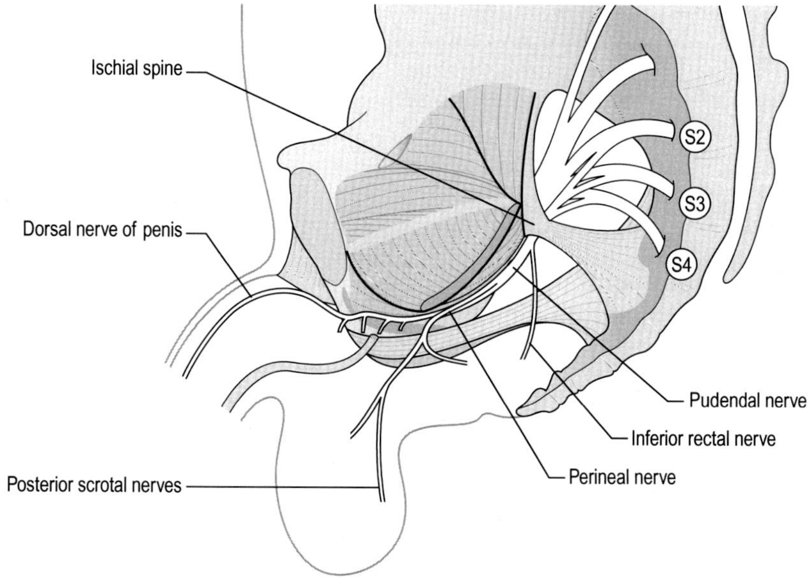

Figure 11.2.5 • Pudendal nerve anatomy

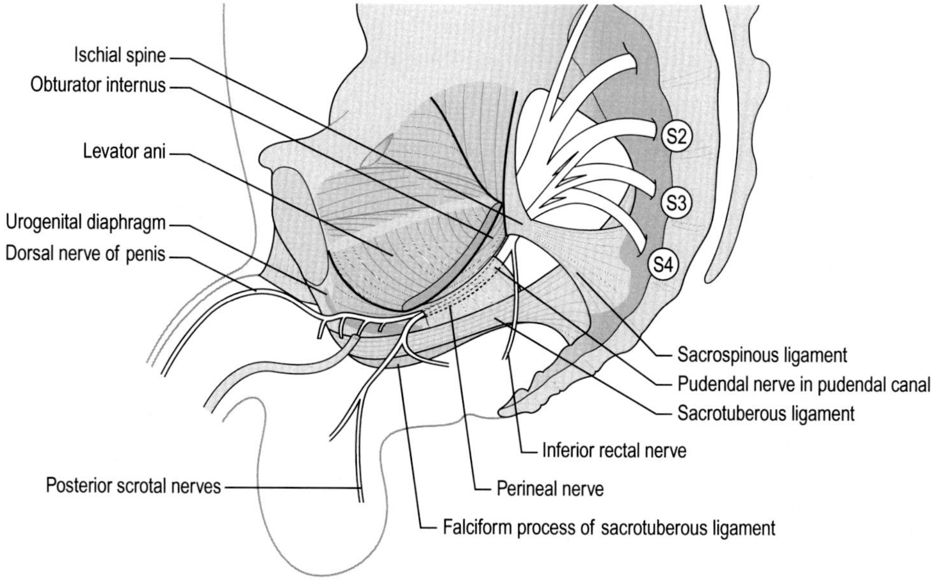

Figure 11.2.6 • Schematic diagram showing the relationship between the pudendal nerve and muscles and ligaments of the pelvis

Differentially diagnosing pudendal neuralgia relies on a few basic subjective complaints and objective findings. The patient must report pain that is severe, throbbing, stabbing or burning in the territory of the nerve. Pain that is described as 'achey' or 'tender like a bruise' is likely not neuropathic pain.

Additionally, upon palpation of the pudendal nerve per vagina and/or anus, the patient should report tenderness and/or pain in the distribution of the nerve (positive Tinel's sign) (Tinel 1978, Hibner et al. 2010) (Figure 11.2.5).

There are four primary mechanisms from which pudendal neuralgia can develop.

The first is via a tension injury. This occurs when the pudendal nerve is overstretched or repetitively stretched to the point of injury. Common examples include constipation, strenuous squatting exercises (see Chapter 6) and childbirth (Kiff et al. 1984, Snooks et al. 1990).

The second mechanism is through compression. Horseback riding, or prolonged sitting compress the pudendal nerve creating an ischaemic environment which eventually leads to a loss of conduction (see discussion of cycling in Chapter 6). If the nerve is chronically compressed, it results in venous stasis, increased vascular permeability, oedema and scar formation (Benson & Griffis 2005).

The third mechanism of injury is surgical insult or acute injury. Occasionally the pudendal nerve can incur injury during surgical procedures such as pelvic reconstruction procedures or hysterectomies. In rare cases, the pudendal nerve can be injured after a fall (Benson & McClellan 1993).

Lastly, pudendal neuralgia can develop due to the visceral–somatic interaction. Through this reflex, visceral disturbances, such as chronic bladder infections and chronic yeast infections, can contribute to pudendal neuralgia (Head 1893, Bischof & Elminger 1963, Beal 1985, Giamberardino et al. 2005, Giamberardino 2008).

Pudendal nerve entrapment

The aetiology of pudendal nerve entrapment (PNE) is unclear and two scoring systems have been described to positively diagnose the condition (Table 11.2.1). Bautrant et al. (2003a) suggested that a positive diagnosis of PNE must include one major and two minor criteria or two major criteria and lack of other painful cause such as (endometriosis, cyst, etc.).

Labat et al. (2008) emphasize that the diagnosis of pudendal neuralgia by PNE is essentially clinical. They state that only the operative finding of nerve entrapment and post-operative pain relief can formally confirm PNE as the cause of the neuralgia.

Table 11.2.1 Scoring systems described to positively diagnose pudendal nerve entrapment

Major criteria	Minor criteria
Pain in the territory of the nerve	Neuropathic pain
Positive Tinel's sign	Pain aggravated by sitting
Positive anaesthetic block	Existence of an aetiological factor or trigger

Labat et al. (2008) go on to describe the five Nantes criteria suggestive of a diagnosis of pudendal neuralgia by PNE:

- Pain in the anatomic territory of the pudendal nerve;
- Worsened by sitting;
- The patient is not woken at night by the pain;
- No objective sensory loss on clinical examination;
- Positive anesthetic pudendal nerve block.

The aetiology is unclear, but PNE may occur secondary to an elongated ischial spine which rotates the sacrospinous ligament. Robert et al. (1998) and Antolak et al. (2002) hypothesize that hypertrophy of the pelvic floor causes the ischial spine to elongate; see Chapter 6. Two areas of potential nerve entrapment have been described in the literature (Robert et al. 1998, Antolak et al. 2002, Bautrant et al. 2003b). The most common site of entrapment is between the sacrospinous and sacrotuberous ligaments: the 'clamp' (Bautrant et al. 2003b). The second position of entrapment is in Alcock's canal, compressed by the falciform process (the medial portion of the sacrotuberous ligament) or by the thickened obturator internus fascia (Robert et al. 1998) (Figure 11.2.6).

Possible consequences of pudendal neuralgia

Pudendal neuralgia is associated with an array of impairments due to the nerve's vast presence throughout the pelvic floor (Robert et al. 1998, Benson & Griffis 2005). Pudendal neuralgia and/or entrapment can cause pelvic floor muscle dysfunction, connective tissue restrictions and neural mechanosensitivity (Beco 2004, Maigne 1996). Neurodynamics refers to integrated biomechanical, physiological and morphological functions of the nervous system (Shacklock 1995a, Butler 2000, Shacklock 2005). A well-functioning nervous system must be able to undergo particular mechanical events such as elongation, sliding, cross-sectional change, angulation and compression. If the nervous system is unable to tolerate these mechanical events, it is vulnerable to neural oedema, ischaemia, fibrosis and hypoxia which can alter neurodynamics (Shacklock 1995, Butler 2000).

The blood supply of the pudendal nerve can be compromised by surrounding connective tissue restrictions or muscles such as the obturator internus, piriformis, gluteals or pelvic floor muscles (Butler 1991). The nerve's neurobiomechanics can become compromised through structural or soft tissue changes, involving the ischial spine, the obturator fascia or the sacrospinous ligament, causing stretch, compression, or fixation along mechanical interfaces (Butler 1991, Shacklock 1995, Shafik 2002). Pudendal neuralgia can contribute to pelvic floor muscle hypertonus which can cause structural and biomechanical abnormalities to develop (Baker 1993). Due to the range of symptoms associated with pudendal neuralgia or entrapment and the impact of the symptoms on a patient's life, coupled with the challenges of a successful treatment programme, patients who suffer from pudendal neuralgia often also suffer from depression and/or anxiety (Mauillon et al. 1999). Lastly, as discussed in depth in Chapter 3, central sensitization is another impairment that often co-occurs with a neuropathic pain syndrome such as pudendal neuralgia.

Symptoms

Common symptoms of pudendal nerve dysfunction include pain with sitting, urinary dysfunction, bowel dysfunction, sexual dysfunction, burning, shooting, stabbing genital and/or anal pain, feeling of fullness in the rectum or vagina, and decreased pain while sitting on a toilet (Robert et al. 1998). The pain during sitting is secondary to the irritated or inflamed pudendal nerve being compressed; hence, when sitting on a toilet, the pain is decreased because the same area is not being compressed. Urinary dysfunction can include hesitancy, urgency, frequency, dysuria and nocturia (Fitzgerald & Kotarinos 2003). Bowel dysfunction can include dyschezia and constipation. Sexual dysfunction for women can include dyspareunia, dysorgasmia and aorgasmia (Basson et al. 2010); for men, post-ejaculatory pain or erectile dysfunction. The feeling of fullness in the vagina or rectum is a result of pelvic floor muscle hypertonus. When irritated, the pudendal nerve causes hypertonus of the muscles it innervates.

The array of symptoms caused by pudendal neuralgia can result in many functional limitations. These limitations include decreased sitting tolerance, urinary dysfunction, bowel dysfunction, difficulty completing activities of daily living, decreased tolerance to exercise and sexual dysfunction. These functional limitations lead to disabilities. Common disabilities of this patient population include the inability to work, attend school, maintain relationships, care for self, care for dependants, meet financial responsibilities and engage in sexual intercourse.

Evaluation

Pudendal neuralgia can be a source of pelvic pain. Similar to the diagnosis of pudendal nerve entrapment, there are no valid diagnostic tests confirming pudendal neuralgia and the diagnosis is essentially clinical. It is accepted to use a diagnosis of pudendal neuralgia when a patient describes burning, stabbing pain in the territory of the nerve.

As described in Chapter 8, many pelvic pain diagnoses do not dictate a standard treatment protocol. Instead, an appropriate treatment plan comes after a thorough physical examination to identify impairments that may be causal of pelvic pain, and in this case, pudendal neuralgia.

Differentially diagnosing a patient with CPP to determine if he/she has pudendal neuralgia requires a comprehensive examination of the following potential impairments:

- Subcutaneous panniculosis;
- Myofascial trigger points;
- Pelvic floor dysfunction;
- Biomechanical and/or structural abnormalities;
- Neural mechanosensitivity.

In addition to these five components, a clinician must also palpate the pudendal nerve for tenderness and/or a positive Tinel's sign (Figure 11.2.5). Palpation of the pudendal nerve is done digitally per vagina and/or anus. The nerve is most commonly palpated at the ischial spine and within Alcock's canal, but can also be palpated at the dorsal clitoral/penile branch and the inferior rectal branch:

- Pudendal nerve palpation (see Chapter 13 for further detail regarding practical anatomy palpation);
- Ischial spine: palpate bony prominence of ischial spine in lower lateral section of vagina/rectum;
- Alcock's canal: find obturator internus by resisting hip external rotation, rotate finger medially;

- Dorsal clitoral/penile branch: follow inferior pubic rami to portion of ramus that is level with the clitoris/base of penis, flex distal interphalangeal joint and palpate;
- Inferior rectal branch: palpate lateral to coccyx.

The nerve has a positive Tinel's sign if the patient reports sharp pain upon palpation of the nerve as well as radiating pain in the distribution of the nerve. With regards to the pudendal nerve, the patient would report sharp pain radiating to the vagina, scrotum, perineum, urethra, rectum, clitoris/penis, anus and/or peri-anal tissue. Tenderness upon palpation of the nerve only is not a positive Tinel's sign.

Treatment

To effectively treat pudendal neuralgia the clinician must address all of the potential impairments outlined above. However, there are specific treatment techniques that focus on the pudendal nerve itself. The following neural mobilization techniques aim to improve the neurodynamics of the pudendal nerve and its terminal branches, thereby decreasing neural mechanosensitivity. The frequency and duration of the treatment are dependent upon the patient response.

Neural mobilization

- Supine with hip flexion (Figure 11.2.7);
- Place tip of thumb medial to ischial tuberosity;
- With increasing degrees of hip flexion move thumb posteriorly and caudally.

Bridging (Figure 11.2.8)

- Place tip of thumb medial to ischial tuberosity;
- When patient initiates bridging move thumb posteriorly and caudally.

Prone with hip internal rotation (Figure 11.2.9)

- Therapist on contralateral side;
- Place thumb medial to ischial spine;
- Shear tissue with thumb cephalad and medial, towards rectum.

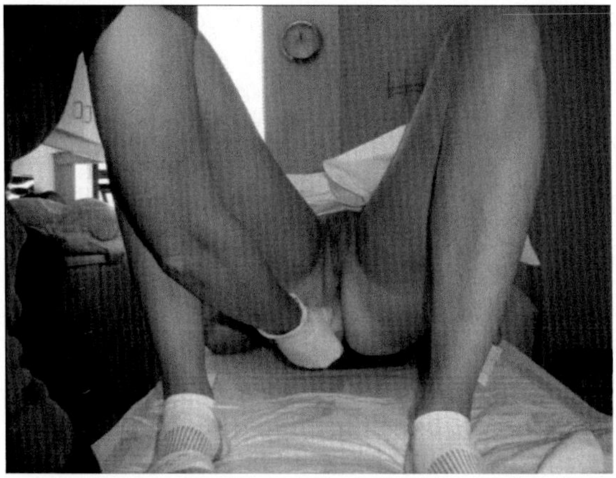

Figure 11.2.8 • The therapist places the tip of the thumb medial to the ischial tuberosity of the patient lying supine, knees flexed and abducted, feet on the table. When the patient initiates bridging, the thumb is moved posteriorly and caudally

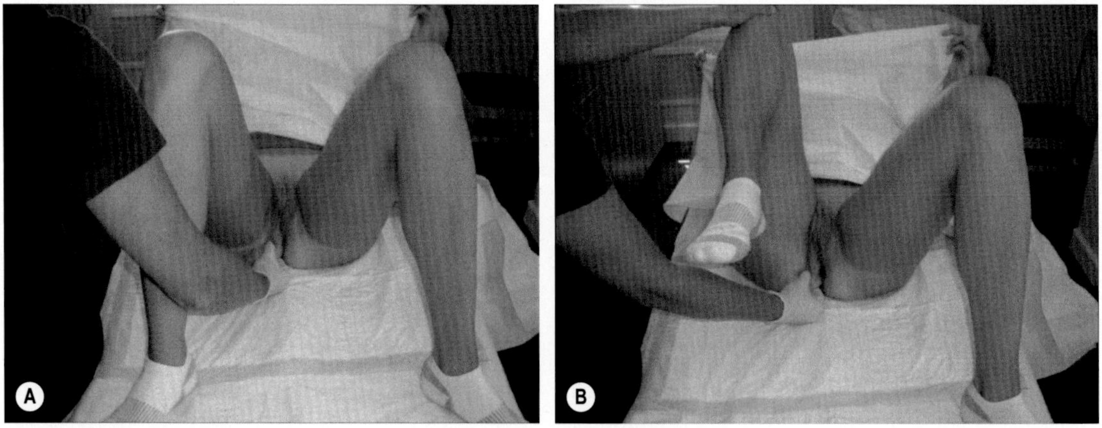

Figure 11.2.7 • The therapist places the tip of thumb medial to ischial tuberosity, and with increasing degrees of hip flexion moves the thumb posteriorly and caudally

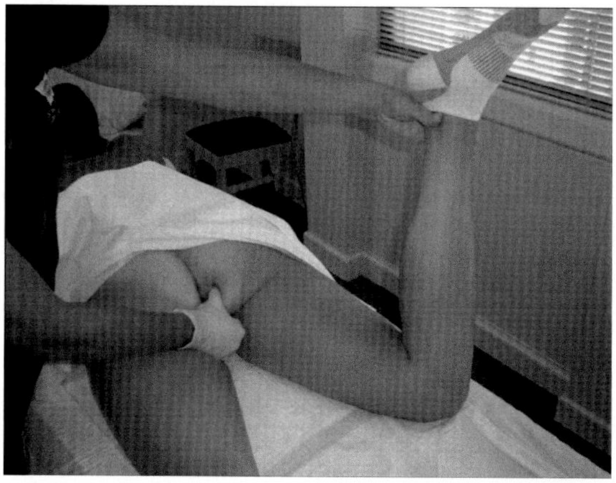

Figure 11.2.9 • The therapist places the thumb medial to ischial spine and shears the tissue with thumb cephalad and medial, towards the rectum

Clinical response

- Limited range of motion initially that improves upon consecutive repetitions.

Patient response

- Sharp pain that may radiate in the distribution of the pudendal nerve with the initial 1–3 repetitions;
- Pain should progressively decrease upon consecutive repetitions.

Home exercise programme

A patient is able to self-mobilize the pudendal nerve best by assuming a deep squat position then progressively leaning away from the side being mobilized. This exercise is only appropriate for patients who are virtually symptom-free towards the end of their treatment programme.

Special considerations

These treatment techniques can provoke increased pain if initiated too early in the treatment plan or performed incorrectly. Specialized training is required for the clinician to perform the techniques effectively. If the patient reports continued or increased pain after approximately three repetitions the clinician should discontinue the treatment technique at that time. It is appropriate to re-initiate the treatment technique 2–3 weeks later to reassess the patient's response. Because neural mobilizations can provoke an increase in symptoms and/or pain, self-mobilization of the pudendal nerve as part of a home exercise programme should be used cautiously.

Case study 11.2.1

- Lise: 27-year-old female
- Diagnosis: vaginismus
- Duration of symptoms: 10+ years
- Initial symptoms
  - Inability to insert tampon as teenager
  - Unable to engage in intercourse due to severe vaginal tightness and pain
- Current symptoms
  - Vaginal burning, increased with sitting and exercise
  - Pain with sexual arousal
  - Severe clitoral hypersensitivity
- Evaluation
  - Visual inspection: vulvar tissues very darkened (Figure 11.2.10A), white clitoral hood
  - Severe CT restrictions along bony pelvis and moderate restrictions in thighs and gluteals
  - Q-tip test: severe hypersensitivity to all points
  - Hypertonic pelvic floor musculature, adverse neural tension on dorsal clitoral branches bilaterally
- Treatment
  - CTM, myofascial release to pelvic floor musculature, neural mobilization
  - After 3 months
    - Decrease in pelvic floor muscle hypertonus, increase in CT mobility in thighs and gluteals, improved vulval colour.
    - Patient noted considerable decrease in unprovoked vaginal pain, decrease in pain with sitting, slight decrease in vestibule and clitoral hypersensitivity
  - After 6 months
    - Pelvic floor muscles starting to normalize, but unstable, CT mobility continues to improve, colour of vulvar tissues and clitoris improving (Figure 11.2.10B) vestibule had

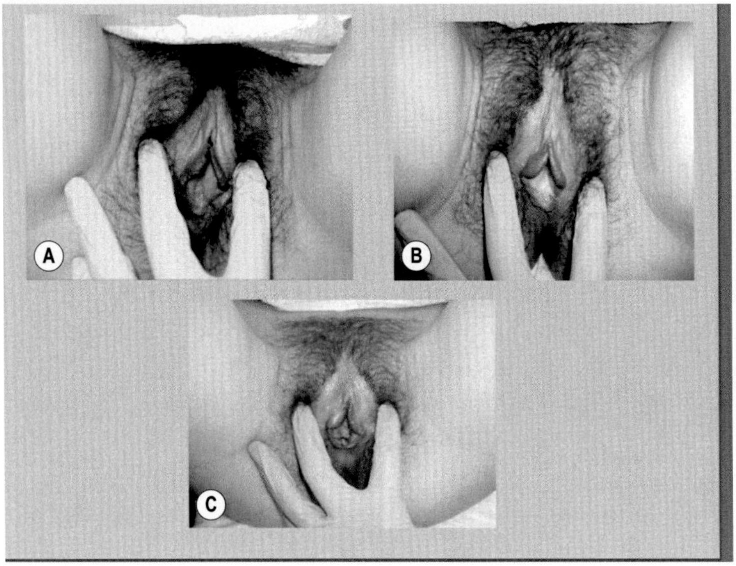

Figure 11.2.10 • The changes in the colour of the vulvar tissue after CTM and neural mobilization at (A) assessment, (B) 9 months of treatment, (C) 11 months of treatment

less hypersensitivity with Q-tip testing, dorsal clitoral branch mobility improving
- Patient tolerance to sitting and walking improving, vaginal pain minimal, vulvar and clitoral hypersensitivity decreasing

- After 9 months
  - Colour of vulvar tissues and clitoris improved, minimal vestibule sensitivity, pelvic floor muscles within normal limits
  - Patient reported mild hypersensitivity of vulva and clitoris, mild sitting discomfort, mild to moderate discomfort with arousal and walking
- After 11 months
  - Colour of vulvar tissue improved dramatically (Figure 11.2.10C), minimal to zero sensitivity in vestibule
  - Patient able to insert medium dilator without pain, minimal to zero vulvar and clitoral hypersensitivity with provocation, mild itching with arousal and mild discomfort with long term sitting and moderate walking.

This chapter has illustrated the interconnectedness of subcutaneous panniculosis, ANT, and underlying muscle dysfunction. Thorough musculoskeletal investigation can identify these impairments, allowing the provider to assess and treat the patient with CPP.

References

Antolak, S., et al., 2002. Anatomical basis of chronic pelvic pain syndrome: the ischial spine and pudendal nerve entrapment. Med. Hypothesis 59 (3), 349–353.

Baker, P.K., 1993. Musculoskeletal origins of chronic pelvic pain. Obstet. Gynecol. Clin. North Am. 20 (4), 719–742.

Basson, R., et al., 2010. Summary of the recommendations on sexual dysfunctions in women. J. Sex. Med. 7 (1 Pt. 2), 314–326.

Bautrant, E., et al., 2003a. New Method for the treatment of pudendal neuralgia. J. Gynecol. Obstet. Biol. Reprod. 32, 705–712.

Bautrant, E., DeBisshop, E., Vaini-es, V., 2003b. Modern algorithm for treating pudendal neuralgia: 212 cases and 104 decompressions. J. Gynecol. Obstet. Biol. Reprod. 32, 705–712.

Beal, M.C., 1985. Viscerosomatic reflexes: a review. J. Am. Osteopath. Assoc. 85 (12), 786–801.

Beco, J., 2004. Pudendal nerve decompression in perineology: a case series. BMC Surg. (4), 1–17.

Benson, J.T., Griffis, K., 2005. Pudenal neuralgia, a severe pain syndrome. Obstet. Gynecol. 192, 1663–1668.

Benson, J.T., McClellan, E., 1993. The effect of vaginal dissection on the pudendal nerve. Obstet. Gynecol. 82, 387–389.

Bischof, I., Elmiger, G., 1963. Connective tissue massage. In: Licht, S. (Ed.), Massage, Manipulation and Traction. Krieger, Huntingdon, New York.

Brattbert, G., 1999. Connective tissue massage in the treatment of fibromyalgia. Eur. J. Pain 3 (3), 235–244.

Butler, D.S., 1991. Mobilisation of the Nervous System. Churchill Livingstone, Edinburgh.

Butler, D., 2004. Mobilization of the nervous system. Churchill Livingstone, Edinburgh.

Butler, D.S., 2000. The Sensitive Nervous System. Noigroup Publications, Adelaide, Australia.

Chaitow, L. (Ed.), 2003. Modern Neuromuscular Techniques, second ed. Elsevier.

Chaitow, L., 2010. Modern Neuromuscular Techniques, third ed. Elsevier, Edinburgh.

Craggs, M., 2005. Pelvic somato-visceral reflexes after spinal cord injury: Measures of functional loss and partial preservation. Prog. Brain Res. (152), 205–219.

Dicke, E., 1953. Meine Bindegeweb-massage. Marquardt, Stuttgart.

Ebner, M., 1975. Connective Tissue Massage: Theory and Therapeutic Application. Churchill Livingstone, Edinburgh.

Fitzgerald, M.P., Kotarinos, 2003. Rehabilitation of the short pelvic floor part 1 and 2. Int. J. Urogyn. 14 (4), 269–275.

Fitzgerald, M.P., Anderson, R., Potts, J., et al., 2009. Randomized multicenter feasibility trial of myofascial physical therapy for the treatment of urological chronic pelvic pain syndromes. J. Urol. 182 (2), 570–580.

Frazer, F.W., 1978. Persistent post-sympathetic pain treated by connective tissue massage. Physiotherapy 64 (7), 211–212.

Giamberardino, M.A., 2008. Women and visceral pain: are the reproductive organs the main protagonists? Mini-review at the occasion of the "European Week Against Pain in Women 2007. Eur. J. Pain 12 (3), 257–260.

Giamberardino, M.A., et al., 2005. Relationship between pain symptoms and referred sensory and trophic changes in patients with gallbladder pathology. Pain 114 (1–2), 239–249.

Gifford, J., Gifford, L., 1988. Connective tissue massage. In: Wells, P.E., Framptom, V., Bowsher, D. (Eds.), Pain: Management and Control in Physiotherapy. Chapter 14. Heinemann Medical, London.

Goats, G.C., Keir, K.A., Connective tissue massage. Br. J. Sports Med. 25 (3), 131–133.

Grainger, H.G., 1958. The somatic component in visceral disease. In: Academy of Applied Osteopathy 1958 Yearbook, Newark, Ohio.

Gray, H., William, P.L., Bannister, L.H., 1995. Gray's anatomy: the anatomical basis of medicine and surgery. thirty-eighth ed. Churchill Livingstone, New York.

Head, H., 1893. On disturbances of sensation with especial reference to the pain of visceral disease. Brain (16), 1–130.

Hibner, M., et al., 2010. Pudendal neuralgia. J. Minim. Invasive Gynecol. 17, 148–153.

Holey, L.A., 1995. Connective tissue manipulation: towards a scientific rationale. Physiotherapy (80), 730–739.

Howard, F., 2000. Diagnosis and management of pelvic pain. Lippincott, Williams &Wilkins, Philapdelphia.

Kaada, B., Torsteinbo, O., 1989. Increase of plasma beta endorphins in connective tissue massage. Gen. Pharmacol. 20 (4), 487–489.

Kiff, E.S., Barnes, P.R., Swash, M., 1984. Evidence of pudendal neuropathy in patients with perineal descent and chronic straining stool. Gut 25, 1279–1282.

Korr, I.M., 1949. Skin resistance patterns associated with visceral disease. Fed. Proc. 8, 87.

Labat, J.J., Riant, T., Robert, R., et al., 2008. Diagnostic criteria for pudendal neuralgia by pudendal nerve entrapment (Nantes criteria). Neurourol. Urodyn. 27 (4), 306–310.

Lewis, T., 1927. The blood vessels of the human skin and their responses. Shah, London.

Maddali-Bongi, S., Del Rosso, A., Galluccio, F., 2009. Efficacy of connective tissue massage and McMennell joint manipulation in the rehabilitative treatment of the hands in systemic sclerosis. Clin. Rheumatol. 28 (10), 1167–1173.

Maigne, R., 1995. Thoraco-lumbar junction syndrome: a source of diagnostic error. J. Ortho. Med. (17), 84–89.

Maigne, R., 1996. Diagnosis and Treatment of pain of vertebral origin. Williams and Wilkins, Baltimore.

Mauillon, J., et al., 1999. Results of pudendal nerve neurolysis-transposition in twelve patients suffering from pudendal neuralgia. Dis. Colon Rectum 42 (2), 186–192.

Merck Manual Online, 2008.

Reitz, A., et al., 2003. Autonomic dysreflexia in response to pudendal nerve stimulation. Spinal Cord 41, 539–542.

Robert, R., et al., 1998. Anatomic basis of chronic perineal pain: role of the pudendal nerve. Surg. Radiol. Anat. 20, 93–98.

Shacklock, M.O., 1995a. Clinical applications of neurodynamics. In: Shacklock, M.O. (Ed.), Moving in on Pain. Butterworth-Heinemann, Chatswood, UK, pp. 123–131.

Shacklock, M.O., 2005. Clinical Neurodynamics: A New System of Neuromusculoskeletal Treatment. Butterworth-Heinemann, Oxford, UK.

Shafik, A., 2002. Pudendal canal syndrome: a cause of chronic pelvic pain. Urology 60 (1), 199.

Snooks, S.J., Swash, M., Mathers, S.E., Henry, M.M., 1990. Effect of vaginal delivery on the pelvic floor: a 5-year follow-up. Br. J. Surg. 77, 1358–1360.

Takahashi, Y., Nakajima, Y., 1996. Dermatomes in the rat limbs as determined by antidromic stimulation of the C-fibers in spinal nerves. Pain (67), 197–202.

Thoumas, D., et al., 1999. Pudendal neuralgia: CT-guided pudendal nerve block technique. Abdom. Imaging 24, 309–312.

Tillman, L.J., Cummings, G.S., 1992. Biologic mechanisms of connective tissue mutability. In: Dynamics of Human Biologic Tissue. FA Davies, Philadelphia.

Tinel, J., 1978. The 'tingling sign' in peripheral nerve lesions (translated by E.B. Kaplan). In: Spinner, M. (Ed.), Injuries to the major branches of peripheral nerves of the forearm. second ed. WB Saunders, Phildelphia, pp. 8–13.

Travell, J., Simons, D., 1993. Myofascial pain and dysfunction, the trigger point manual. vol. 1 and 2. Lippincott Williams & Wilkins, Philadelphia.

Wesslemann, U., Lai, J., 1997. Mechanisms of referred visceral pain: uterine inflammation in the adult virgin rat results in neurogenic plasma extravasation in the skin. Pain (73), 309–317.

Wilson, P.T., 1956. Osteopathic cardiology. Academy of Applied Osteopathy 1956 Yearbook. Newark, Ohio.

Evaluation and pelvic floor management of urologic chronic pelvic pain syndromes

12

Rodney U. Anderson

CHAPTER CONTENTS

Introduction

Urologic disorders and pelvic pain present an obvious relationship. A large proportion of the human population has endured pain or discomfort of a simple urinary tract infection. And one of the earliest adventures in human surgical intervention arose in the centuries BC as the Greeks 'cut for stone' to relieve the obstruction and pain of urinary bladder calculi. However, now that most of the urogynaecologic organ maladies of infection, neoplasia and obstruction are understood, we are still left with a noisome bag of discomforts lacking any clear pathogenesis. These are the urologic chronic pelvic pain syndromes (UCPPS). The majority of these conditions arise from either a possible urinary bladder source known as bladder pain syndrome/interstitial cystitis (BPS/IC) or prostate source known as prostate pain syndrome (PPS), named chronic prostatitis/chronic pelvic pain syndrome (CP/CPPS) in the United States. The European Association of Urology attempted to update and provide a classification of pelvic pain disorders to suggest avenues for further management (Fall et al. 2010). Their pelvic pain descriptions fit into neat little boxes of urological, gynaecological, anorectal, neuromuscular and 'other' categories. These non-malignant pain conditions or syndromes perceived in structures related to the pelvis of both males and females do not deserve more specific diagnoses because the aetiology and pathogenesis remains a mystery – 'a riddle wrapped in a mystery inside an enigma' – and we depend on a complex symptomatic analysis to help guide us in evaluation and therapy. Regrettably the final common pathway often defaults as a referral to a pain management team. While awaiting elucidation of the cellular and molecular pathogenic mechanisms of UCPPS, we should rely on a diagnostic and therapeutic algorithm to direct logical evaluation and multimodal management. We must develop alternative ways of thinking about managing these urologic pain conditions. UCPPS needs to be viewed as much more than an organ-specific disease, but rather as a biopsychosocial disorder. The central problem is pain. Traditional biomedical treatment for UCPPS has failed (Anderson 2006). Antibiotics, α-blocking agents and anti-inflammatory agents as well as virtually all other pharmaceuticals have shown unimpressive outcomes in ameliorating the effects of these disorders. The biopsychosocial model of this condition rather than the biomedical model holds the key to understanding the pathogenesis and possible future treatments. Phenotyping is one current trend and we recommend it for approaching patients with these disorders allowing specific guideline development for multimodal therapy (Baranowski et al. 2008, Nickel et al. 2009, Shoskes et al. 2009). Some of the recent developments and approaches arose from clinical investigation and treatment protocols supported by the National Institutes of Health (NIH) in the United States over the past 10 years. A descriptive phenotyping classification allows understanding of epidemiology, aetiology and potential design of randomized clinical trials. Clinically identifiable domains suggested include: urinary, psychosocial, organ specific, infection, neurological/systemic and muscle tenderness (Nickel & Shoskes 2009, Shoskes et al. 2009) (Table 12.1).

The early chapters of this book present a diverse range of symptoms and describe multiple aetiological possibilities for chronic pelvic pain (CPP). The aim of this chapter is to review evidence regarding urologic conditions associated with pelvic pain, provide a description of good urologic evaluation, and focus on one specific management approach involving manipulation of the pelvic floor neuromuscular tissue using both physiotherapeutic and psychological maneuvers (the Wise-Anderson Stanford Protocol).

Table 12.1 Percentage of patients with specific myofascial trigger point tenderness

Muscle groups	% Patients with trigger point tenderness, N = 72
Internal muscles	
Puborectalis/pubococcygeus	90.3
Coccygeus	34.7
Sphincter ani	16.6
External muscles	
Rectus abdominis	55.6
External oblique	52.8
Adductors	19.4
Gluteus medius	18.1
Gluteus maximus	6.9
Bulbospongiosus	12.5
Transverse perineal	11.1

Urologic diagnostic evaluation

Prostate pain syndrome

Chronic prostatitis is an incorrect label; we are dealing with a variable set of pain conditions with no objective markers and multivariate symptoms. The disorder is not prostatocentric symptomatology and pain sites exist between the umbilicus to above the mid thigh. The European Community has promoted the term prostate pain syndrome (PPS) as a more generic term over the NIH category III chronic prostatitis/chronic pelvic pain syndrome (CP/CPPS). Still, it smacks of a prostatocentric approach, which is probably to be avoided for lack of evidence, and it encourages the use of antibiotics as standard therapy that clearly lacks efficacy. By definition, PPS is persistent discomfort or pain in the pelvic region with sterile specimen cultures and either significant or insignificant white blood cell counts in prostate specimens: semen, expressed prostatic secretion or urine collected after prostate massage. There does not appear to be any diagnostic or therapeutic advantage to differentiating between those patients with significant or insignificant leucocytes from the prostate (Schaeffer et al. 2002); however, in the author's experience, men with no prostate inflammation appear to suffer greater degrees and longer duration of pelvic pain on average.

Medical history

The typical patient is a young to middle-age man with variable symptoms of chronic, irritative and obstructive voiding accompanied by moderate to severe pain in the pelvis, low back, perineum and genitalia. To qualify as CPP the condition should occur for longer than 6 months and, for research purposes, continuous within the previous 3 months. The healthcare burden of PPS is exemplified by approximately two million physician office visits per year in the United States. It is one of the most common genitourinary diagnoses in men under the age of 50 years. The urologist's first order of business when referred such a patient is to accept the challenge seriously and treat the man suffering with this condition with respect, interest and compassion. The patient is understandably tense, wary and defensive, having encountered frustration and rejection previously. The physician should listen to the patient's complaints and accurately document the circumstances surrounding the onset of the disorder – sensory descriptions, various treatment modalities and outcomes, noting particularly the time course of events and associated triggers that may have caused a flare in his symptoms. The US national cohort study by the NIH reported a typical duration of patient complaints averaging 4 years.

The urologist evaluating pelvic pain in a male must rule out associated urinary bladder or prostate diseases. Errors in diagnosis and inappropriate therapeutic pathways may ensue if less than a systematic evaluation is undertaken. Both prostate and bladder cancer as well as urinary calculus disease have been missed because of an inappropriate diagnosis of 'chronic prostatitis'. It is crucial to have empathy for the suffering patient, documenting his description of the physical characteristics of the pain complex: what makes it worse, what helps, where is the pain referred, and what associations exist with sexual function? The psychosexual behaviour and influence of sexual partner relationships play a significant role. How has the chronic pain affected libido, the ability to attain adequate penile erections, accomplish intercourse, reach orgasm and have pleasurable ejaculation? Associated alimentary tract complaints such as irritable bowel disorder, constipation, dietary exacerbations and bowel function may point to further clarifying aspects of the disorder. Further, the psychosocial medical history should probe for genetic or acquired personality types: tense, anxious, chronic tension-holding patterns, possible childhood issues of sexual or physical abuse, traumatic toilet training, abnormal bowel patterns, teen sexual problems, excessive masturbation, suppressed homosexuality, excessive weight lifting, gymnastic manoeuvres and activities such as dance training. Identifying such issues helps to create a specific phenotype of the pain condition and may ultimately suggest appropriate multimodal therapy.

We utilize symptom questionnaires and validated instruments to detail patient psychological issues. These tools help quantify the baseline, eventual progress and outcome of our management techniques. The most widely used research tool is the National Institutes of Health Chronic Prostatitis Symptom Index (NIH-CPSI). An alternative type of CPPS symptom questionnaire – the Pelvic Pain Symptom Score (PPSS) – has also been useful in our hands. The PPSS expands the description of named painful anatomical locations and grades the severity of pain (0 to 4+); it includes urinary symptoms that mimic the International Prostate Symptom Score (IPSS), and scores sexual dysfunction aspects of the patient condition as a separate domain. Our group utilized this questionnaire in the treatment outcome analyses of pelvic floor therapy (Anderson et al. 2005, 2006). We have also used other psychosocial instruments including Brief Symptom Inventory, Beck Anxiety, and Perceived Stress Scale to study neuroendocrine psychiatric influences associated with CPPS (Anderson et al. 2008).

Physical examination

After carefully documenting a thorough medical history of the pelvic pain, it is time to examine the patient. He should be informed that the examination is discovery in nature and will be gentle and avoids any exacerbation of the existing discomfort. The patient removes all clothing from the waist down and assumes a dorsal lithotomy position with the legs spread and heels in the stirrups (as in a female examination). The abdominal exam is easily accomplished under these circumstances. Prior to a prostate examination and massage we palpate the pelvic muscles seeking actual trigger points (TrPs) or specific discomfort zones, particularly the endopelvic muscles and tissue surrounding the prostate. Examination in this position allows palpation of the suprapubic region over the sigmoid bowel, bladder and rectus abdominis and oblique muscles. With the physician sitting at the foot of the examining table the genitalia, spermatic cord and anal areas are inspected. The pull-out extension of the examining table allows the examiner to have elbow leverage for internal pelvic muscle palpation and direct visualization of the penis and the urethral opening to collect prostatic fluid. We find it convenient and efficient to collect the fluid with a sterile glass pipette, the prostatic secretion drops accumulating with capillary action as they appear at the penile meatus; very important when only one or two precious drops are visible to examine and culture. We typically ask the patient not to urinate prior to the examination. This allows palpation of the partially full bladder and tenderness may be found. Furthermore, the patient should void a small amount of urine after a prostate massage to collect prostatic fluid by centrifugation if none is expressed and to provide a culture and sensitivity specimen.

In our evaluation at Stanford, as do most urologists, we examine the prostate for gland consistency, whether it is soft or 'boggy', whether there are areas of induration or hardness – this may represent fibrosis or scarring from previous inflammation – but we must remain ever vigilant for adenocarcinoma. It would not be appropriate to massage a prostate gland containing cancer. After checking muscles and tender points, we methodically massage the prostate gland, beginning at the base and milking it toward the centre on each side to express prostatic fluid into the urethra. The prostate is composed of 20–30 small microscopic tunnels (acini) emanating from the periphery of the prostate. Each glandular unit is connected to the outside world by a tiny duct that opens into the urethra on each side of the primary seminal vesicles' ejaculatory duct in the centre of the prostate – the verumontanum. These tiny prostate ducts expel the enzyme-rich prostatic secretion with smooth muscle prostate contractions at the time of sexual ejaculation. Once the prostatic fluid has been collected, the patient then voids a small volume to provide a washout of prostatic fluid that can be separated, analysed and submitted for bacterial culture. We advise patients to refrain from any sexual ejaculation for 7 days prior to coming in for the examination to afford a better opportunity to maximize collection of prostatic fluid. Older men typically have more prostatic fluid because the gland is larger, having increased in size with age. Younger men find it a challenge to refrain from sexual ejaculation for a week.

We examine the prostatic fluid microscopically in our office laboratory after staining with safranin red and crystal violet; this staining helps identify white cells and improves the microscopic review. We quantify the number of white cells in the prostatic fluid using a haemacytometer and record the result as number of leucocytes per microlitre. This allows us to compare with counts from normal, asymptomatic men and to track changes as a treatment programme is instituted. We conduct this careful analysis of the prostatic fluid partly for academic reasons of clinical research. However, quantifying the degree of inflammation from massaged ducts has failed to yield any correlation with patient pain symptoms. This relationship between pain and prostate gland inflammation is poorly understood.

Prostatic massage has been utilized as treatment for CP by several generations of urologists, particularly prior to the advent of antibiotics. In a report from a popular Philippine study, repeated prostatic massages reveal occult micro-organisms. Therapeutic benefit from massage derives from expression of poorly emptying ductal acini and may diminish smooth muscle prostatic pressure. Some have proposed massage plus antibiotic treatment (Shoskes & Zeitlin 1999). In their study, prostate massage plus antibiotics for 2–8 weeks produced 40% resolution of symptoms, 20% significant improvements; however, 40% had no improvement. There was no correlation between inflammatory content and bacterial cultures. Our opinion favours repetitive massage of the prostate, not for emptying the gland, but rather to relieve pelvic tension and release myofascial TrPs. We continue to be extremely sceptical of the concept of occult bacteria that need to be 'massaged out'.

The prudent physician must rule out other diagnostic possibilities, including urethral stricture, urethritis, epididymitis, seminal vesicle cysts, cancer of the prostate, urethra, bladder or testis, tuberculosis of the urinary or genital tract, urinary calculus disease (urolithiasis) and other treatable entities. A serum PSA (prostate-specific antigen) laboratory test should be done for men over the age of 40, and men with a long smoking history or age greater than 60 years should have a urinary cytology done. Some of these other diagnostic possibilities associated with UCPPS may require ancillary examinations such as cystoscopy, transrectal ultrasound, CT scans, urodynamic studies and even magnetic resonance studies of the pelvis and lower spine. These ancillary examinations should be carefully considered and selected out of significant clinical suspicion, not as a systematic course of evaluation.

Imaging of the prostate in chronic prostatitis

We recommend transrectal ultrasound (TRUS) to image the prostate gland. It has not gained wide acceptance as a method of evaluation for PPS but may provide valuable information demonstrating inflamed tissue, the presence of stones in the ducts (representing urinary mineral deposits), swelling and thickening of seminal vesicles (semen storage organs behind the prostate) and accurate measurement of the size of the gland. Abdominal ultrasound and CT are inaccurate and magnetic resonance of the prostate is not cost-effective. Many urologists have observed intraprostatic calcifications on TRUS. Older men (55+) develop benign prostatic hyperplasia (BPH) and it commonly associates with PPS. Most workers believe the ultrasound hyperdense areas represent deposits of urinary metabolite crystals and inspissated secretions within the ducts. These concretions are commonly seen exuding from the peripheral zone of the prostate at the time of transurethral resection. It has been noted, however, that a substantial percentage of younger men with chronic prostate or pelvic pain have such calcifications (Geramoutsos et al. 2004). Shoskes et al. (2007) imaged 47 men with PPS symptoms averaging 60 months and reported 47% of them had such calcifications. There was no difference in the CPSI score between those who did or did not have the finding; however, the men with stones had less discomfort and greater leucocyte presence.

Japanese investigators utilized computerized X-ray images and angiography to evaluate CPP. They demonstrated excellent three-dimensional graphic images of veins around the prostate and found considerable congestion in these veins behind the bladder and along the sides of the prostate in patients suffering with pain. The veins on the surface of the prostate were much thicker in diameter than in subjects with no pain – essentially varicose veins of the prostate. It suggests heightened tension in the muscles of the pelvic floor and supports our view that CPP syndromes are associated with chronic pelvic muscle tension.

Cystoscopy

It is common for urologists to use cystoscopy to visualize the urethra, prostate and bladder in patients suffering from CPP. This consists of passing a pencil-sized flexible probe with magnifying optical lenses, high-intensity fibreoptic light and associated video camera up the penile urethra. However, cystoscopy may be the least productive investigative procedure. Some urologists say to the patient, 'Oh, yes, I see some inflammation in the prostate'. This is anatomically impossible as they are only looking at the surface of the urethra and not at the prostatic tissue itself. There is rarely, if ever, any obvious inflammation on the surface of the prostatic urethra in the condition of CP/CPPS.

Urodynamics

One investigative tool to evaluate urinary and prostate function consists of neurophysiological measurements with urodynamics. This diagnostic approach evaluates sensory and physiological function of the related smooth and striated muscle in the bladder, prostate and external sphincter. This testing consists of placing a small pressure-sensing catheter into the bladder to detect changes in bladder pressure with filling, sensation of urgency, simultaneously monitoring the urethral voluntary sphincter pressure activity and associated pelvic floor function. An important component of this testing requires a pressure sensor in the rectum to monitor simultaneous abdominal pressure. We utilize electrical sensors patched to the skin around the anal verge to detect action motor potentials within the superficial pelvic floor, both with relaxation and voluntary contraction, but primarily to determine how much relaxation is achieved when attempting to urinate. Bladder pressure and flow dynamics reveal the synergy with the pelvic floor, demonstrating the effects of chronic tension or lack of efferent stimulation. At the minimum one should perform a urinary free-flow rate with voided volume, resting water cystometry, a pressure-flow study of micturition and electromyographic (EMG) studies of external sphincter. Independent anal or vaginal probe EMG studies as performed with biofeedback can also be quite revealing in these patients.

Many workers suggest relationships between chronic pain and smooth or striated muscle function of the urinary bladder, prostate or sexual organs. Small, undocumented reports of findings in PPS patients suggest possible avenues of scientific pursuit. Comparison of symptoms, morphological, microbiological and urodynamic findings in patients with PPS have existed for decades (Strohmaier & Bichler 2000, Lee 2001, Hetrick et al. 2006, Hafez 2009). A common theme emerges suggesting functional obstruction at the level of the bladder neck and external sphincter, high sensitivity during filling cystometry, and poor or interrupted urinary flow. Abnormally low urinary flow rates <15 ml/s were found in 65% of patients. Some patients respond to α-blocking agents as therapy for UCPPS while most do not.

Isolated male orchalgia (pain in the testicles)

Chronic orchalgia, or pain in the testis, vexes a lot of young men and they reluctantly bring this to the attention of their physician. Some would suggest that isolated male orchalgia does not belong with the phenotypes of PPS. However, pelvic floor dysfunction studies suggest an extremely large proportion of these patients (88%) exhibit an increased pelvic floor resting tone at a mean of 6.7 μV – values >3.0 μV are considered abnormal (Planken et al. 2010). Testicular pain occurs most commonly in young men in their 20s and 30s and requires a careful history and physical examination because this is also the age group where testicular cancer most commonly occurs.

Usually the examination is negative, with the patient complaining of pain localized to one side or the other but occasionally bilateral, and when the epididymis is squeezed during examination it reproduces the pain for the patient. Rarely does a vasectomy result in such tenderness or chronic orchalgia. The common urologic diagnosis is sterile epididymitis, but there is virtually no evidence for any inflammatory condition.

We must understand the nerve supply to the testis so that the diagnostic evaluation makes functional sense. Scrotal pain may arise from numerous factors and any organ that shares the same nerve pathway with the scrotal contents can present as referred pain in this region, such as the ureter and the hip. Sensory nerve fibres are carried in the branches of the genitofemoral and ilioinguinal nerves. Increased fluid around the testicle (hydrocele), varicocele, or epididymal cysts (spermatocele), are usually coincidental and are rarely the cause of the chronic orchalgia. This pain is almost always spermatic cord/epididymal neurological pain and not testicular organ pain.

Removal of the epididymis as an approach to treat chronic testis pain has met with variable success and positive results range from 32% (Sweeney et al. 2008) to 85% in post-vasectomy pain (Hori et al. 2009). Selective denervation is also successful using a microscopic method to remove all nerve fibres from the spermatic cord arising from the testicular tissue or the scrotal contents. We always perform at least three selective long-acting anaesthetic spermatic cord nerve blocks as a diagnostic trial, usually with a cortisone solution. Several of these nerve blocks at intervals may relieve the cyclical nature of this syndrome. Microscopic denervation after successful spermatic cord block has shown successful results with complete relief of pain in 76–97% of selected patients (Levine & Matkov 2001, Heidenreich et al. 2002). A recent report suggests that sacral nerve root electrical stimulation may be beneficial in these patients, and in some cases skin surface electrical stimulation has been helpful (McJunkin et al. 2009).

Pudendal nerve entrapment (pudendal neuralgia)

We should mention the concept of the pudendal nerves being compressed, stretched or entrapped in the pelvis as a potential cause of chronic pelvic pain. There are five essential diagnostic criteria (Stav et al. 2009):

1. Pain along the anatomical distribution of the pudendal nerve;
2. The pain aggravated by sitting;
3. The patient is not awakened at night by the pain;
4. There is no objective sensory loss on clinical examination;
5. The pain is improved by an anaesthetic pudendal nerve block.

Neurophysiology tests such as pudendal nerve motor latency test and EMG may serve as complementary diagnostic measures. Surgical procedures, which are very controversial and have little convincing evidence as to efficacy, presumably release fascia and ligaments of the pelvis and transpose nerves away from these impinging structures. Patients thought to have this syndrome typically have considerable pain while sitting and then completely relieved when standing. It is also relieved by sitting on a toilet seat, although both of these criteria exist to some degree in PPS. There are theories that athletic endeavours may have caused distortion in the nerve pathway. Similarly, chronic constipation may contribute to the presumed condition.

Bladder pain syndrome

BPS occurs most commonly as a UCPPS in the female patient with a prevalence of about 300 per 100 000 women and 10–20% of that number in men. Using a 'high-sensitivity' definition of the disease it is thought that as many as 6% of women in the US meet the BPS symptom criteria. This syndrome was previously known by the diagnosis of interstitial cystitis (IC). The IC diagnosis implies an inflammation within the wall of the urinary bladder, involving gaps or spaces in the bladder mucosa. However, not all patients have this histological picture and there is no histology pathognomonic of this syndrome that remains a broad clinical diagnosis. The term BPS focuses on the total pain symptom complex occurring for longer than 6 months rather than any specific organ disease. The primary symptom is pelvic pain, pressure or discomfort perceived to be related to the urinary bladder. There has been considerable effort devoted to define objective diagnostic criteria, but the typical clinical picture includes pain upon bladder filling and often immediately after emptying. Urinary voided volumes are typically lower than normal. Many workers feel that IC associated with inflammatory mucosal lesions, neovascularity and ulcers originally described by Hunner represent a more advanced or serious level of disease. The disorder of BPS, as in PPS, has manifestations clearly characterized as a biopsychosocial disorder and often appears simultaneously with other pain syndromes such as irritable bowel, fibromyalgia and chronic fatigue syndrome.

Medical assessment

The initial evaluation should include a urinary frequency and voided volume chart (preferably including timed fluid intake as well), focused physical examination looking for TrPs, urinalysis and urine culture. Surprisingly, about 30% of patients are found to have a bacterial infection history and these patients will often demonstrate recurrent bacteriuria when followed on a long-term basis. However, the presence of bacteria does not impact the pelvic pain symptoms and treating with antibiotics makes no difference in the symptom complex. There has been no scientific evidence that bacteriuria itself induces or plays a pathogenic role in IC.

Cytology and cystoscopy are recommended if clinically indicated. It is reasonable to consider urodynamics if there are elements of dysfunctional voiding, particularly if overactive bladder contractility is suggested. Pelvic imaging should be reserved for specific indications. Most of the time gynaecologic evaluation has been accomplished utilizing laparoscopy if there exists any suspicion of gynaecologic disorder.

If cystoscopy is indicated then it is most appropriate to perform the examination with hydrodistension of the bladder under general or spinal anaesthesia to physical capacity at 80 cm water pressure. More advanced and longer-duration bladder disease often associates with lower physical capacity at these pressures. Upon endoscopic emptying, typical petechial haemorrhages appear within the submucosal capillary vessels, with or without evidence of mucosal ulceration. This has been an accepted diagnostic and research criterion for diagnosis of IC when occurring with the clinical picture of painful bladder syndrome (PBS). The hydrodistension under anaesthesia may provide beneficial therapy in that about 30% of patients find relief from their bladder pain, often for several months. Aside from bladder stretching under anaesthesia, local therapy includes intermittent vesical instillations of agents such as heparin, cortisone, buffered lidocaine, and experimental approaches such as capsaicin solution to eliminate C-fibre activation. There are current clinical trials underway demonstrating the safety and efficacy of detrusor muscle injections of botulinum toxin A to alleviate the pain of IC. When pelvic pain involves the fascia and muscles outside of the bladder a neuromuscular approach is more effective.

Neuromuscular treatment

It is beyond the scope of this chapter to discuss the myriad therapeutic modalities that have been utilized to relieve UCPPS. We refer the reader to previous chapters and review articles with the caveat that very few level 1 or 2 evidence-based treatments have been documented and most cannot be recommended (Hanno et al. 2010). Traditional therapy includes antibiotics, α-blockers, anti-inflammatory agents, phytotherapy, minimally invasive therapies, heat therapy, neuromodulation and surgical invasion, including the extreme of radical extirpation of the urinary bladder and/or prostate. While urologists are trained surgeons, surgical procedures have failed to offer any solution to the CPPS. Urologists should carefully consider alternative and complementary methods of patient care, especially in relationship to CPP. At the same time, medical practice guidelines should be evidence-based and not advocated solely on opinions of efficacy. Well-educated patients and patient advocates seek greater control of their treatment and the planning thereof by focusing on preventative maintenance issues and partnering with physicians in managing their disorder.

Neuromuscular basis for therapy

Many investigators believe that the source of pain and dysfunction in men and women with CPP, including chronic testicular pain, relates to chronically tense myofascial tissue in and around the pelvic floor (Anderson et al. 2005, Berger et al. 2007, Planken et al. 2010). In simple and broad terms we can describe the neuromuscular disorder as pelvic myoneuropathy. Traditionally, the diagnosis of UCPPS depends upon a descriptive symptom complex. However, it is now clear that UCPPS is multifaceted and not all patients have the same constellation of symptoms, or respond in the same way to single treatment modalities. Because the pathogenic mechanisms associated with the development of pelvic genitourinary symptoms are unknown, it remains difficult to explain the role of painful myofascial tissue. One of the phenotypes proposed for UCPPS includes a domain of tenderness of skeletal muscle and this has been the focus of a growing number of clinical research trials and publications. A recent NIH-sponsored, multicentre study demonstrated the feasibility of performing clinical therapeutic trials utilizing muscle and connective tissue physiotherapy (myofascial physical therapy) to treat UCPPS (Fitzgerald et al. 2009). A comparator group of subjects was randomized to receive total-body traditional Western massage with no myofascial release or internal pelvic therapy. In the NIH trial the original physician investigators quantified the degree of tenderness in muscle groups prior to corroboration by physical therapists trained in such techniques. A clear discrepancy existed between what physicians scored for subjective pain on examination and what the physical therapists reported; physicians found 28% less tenderness on their examination ($P < 0.01$). Patients randomized to the myofascial physical therapy group underwent connective tissue manipulation to all body wall tissues of the abdominal wall, back, buttocks and thighs as well as internal pelvic muscles clinically found to contain connective tissue abnormalities and/or myofascial TrP release to painful myofascial TrPs. This was done until a texture change was noted in the treated tissue layer. Manual techniques such as TrP barrier release with or without active contraction or reciprocal inhibition, manual stretching of the TrP region and myofascial release were used on the identified TrPs. A secondary outcome of the pilot study revealed good patient response to the internal and external myofascial physical therapy as compared to generalized external Western massage only (57% versus 28%, respectively). This form of therapy was expanded to a larger trial in women suffering from IC/PBS and the results show an equally impressive response to the manual physical therapy.

We are not the first doctors to have considered the kind of treatment we are describing in this book. As early as 1934 there were a few physicians who understood that pelvic pain is related to tension or spasm of the pelvic muscles. The following sequence lists a chronological description of development.

Progress of discovery and understanding of chronic pain syndromes and myofascial trigger points

- 1838 Recaimer – First describes syndrome of tension myalgia of pelvic floor in 'Stretching massage and rhythmic percussion in the treatment of muscular contractions'.
- 1937 Thiele – Describes tonic spasms of levator ani, coccygeus and piriformis muscles and their relationship to pain.
- 1942 Travell et al. – First description of myofascial TrPs as common cause of chronic muscle pain.
- 1951 Dittrich – First recognized pelvic pain occurring as a result of referral from TrPs in subfascial fat and perifascial tissue.
- 1963 Thiele – Successful use of digital massage of spastic levator muscles subsequently described as 'Thiele massage'.
- 1977 Sinaki et al. – Consolidates various syndromes of pelvic musculature under one terminology: tension myalgia of the pelvic floor. Uses combined treatment with rectal diathermy, Thiele's massage and relaxation exercises.
- 1983 Travell and Simons – Publish the first edition of *Myofascial Pain and Dysfunction: The Trigger Point Manual* in 1983; identifying internal muscles and areas of referred pain from myofascial TrPs. Second edition published in 1992.
- 1984 Slocum – Treats TrPs related to the abdominal pelvic pain syndrome in women using locally injected anaesthetic. Indicates emotional stress frequently a potentiating factor, not a cause for CPP.
- 1994 Hong – Developed rabbit animal model to identify myofascial TrPs. With colleagues, subsequently publishes 36 animal clinical and 12 basic science articles to advance our understanding.
- 2004 Simons – Reviews the present understanding of myofascial TrPs as they relate to musculoskeletal dysfunction.

George Thiele, M.D., was a colorectal surgeon who developed a physical treatment for pelvic pain that he generally included under the name coccygynia (pain of the coccyx or tail bone). Thiele's findings were later confirmed by Shapiro in 1937, who referred to pain around the coccyx as the Thiele syndrome. In an article in 1963, Thiele reported on 324 patients who had pelvic pain in and around the rectum and anus. He, along with several other researchers, realized that removal of the coccyx failed to help anyone with pelvic pain other than those who had severe trauma to the tailbone. Furthermore, he acknowledged that there was no evidence of any disease of the coccyx or adjacent areas.

Mehrsheed Sinaki, M.D., was a physician at the Mayo Clinic in the department of physical medicine and rehabilitation throughout most of the 1970s. Doctor Sinaki reviewed the medical records of patients who had a diagnosis of pelvic pain in general, but at that time more often referred to by the terms piriformis syndrome, coccygodynia, levator ani spasm syndrome, proctalgia fugax, or simply rectal pain. Absent were reports of urinary symptoms or of diagnoses including prostatitis, IC, or some of the other conditions we include in this book. Sinaki acknowledged that the conditions he examined were obscured by many vague and chronic complaints. Furthermore, he found, as we do today, that a general medical exam and routine laboratory and X-ray exam are unremarkable. He wrote:

> The neurologist finds no neurological abnormalities and the orthopedist usually finds no bone, disk, bursa, or tendon . . .hemorrhoids or fissures may be inadequate (to diagnose the problem) because the levator ani, coccygeus and piriformis muscles and their attachments are often not carefully palpated.

Sinaki believed that the definitive test for the conditions he was reviewing was the digital–rectal examination in which the doctor inserts a gloved lubricated finger into the rectum to feel the state of the muscles. He observed, however, that the normal digital–rectal examination was inadequate to assess the tenderness of the muscles. Figures 12.1–12.5 demonstrate the internal pelvic muscle palpations and typical referral of discomfort when a TrP is involved. Figures 12.6 and 12.7 show typical pain referral patterns from external palpations.

We previously indirectly measured the internal pelvic level of muscle tension via the rectum and vagina of patients consulting us for pelvic pain and dysfunction. Men with PPS show an increased level of pelvic floor muscle tension on EMG. Many women demonstrate weakness and inability to contract pelvic muscles; however, this is only a surface recording of the anal or vaginal muscles not the entire pelvic floor or deeper pelvic muscles around the prostate. There is emerging interest in utilizing behavioural pelvic floor rehabilitation techniques in treating male CPPS. A group from Northwestern University Medical School in Chicago used biofeedback in pelvic floor re-education as well as bladder training for this disorder (Clemens et al. 2000). They recognized that pelvic floor tension myalgia contributes to the symptoms. They studied a small group of 19 men, average age of 36 years, and treated them with this non-interventional process. The men showed improvement, particularly in their urinary scores, but also had a significant decrease in their median pain scores, from 5 to 1 on a scale of 0 (no symptoms) to 10 (worse symptoms). Dr. Howard Glazer reports on his extensive experience utilizing biofeedback in a previous chapter.

The International Association for the Study of Pain defines pain using descriptions and does not address the mechanism of pain. Zermann et al. (2001) found 88% of men with PPS had tender myofascial palpation. Berger et al. (2007) also showed that pelvic tenderness is not limited to the prostate in men with PPS. They studied 62 men with PPS and 98 men without pelvic pain, examining tenderness of ten external pelvic tender points, seven internal pelvic tender points, and other tender points as described by the American College of Rheumatology for evaluation of fibromyalgia. They found 75% of men with PPS had prostate tenderness but so did 50% of normal controls. They also observed no correlation with leucocytosis in expressed prostatic fluid.

Similarly, a recent collaborative network study of 384 symptomatic men with PPS and 121 asymptomatic controls revealed that 51% of PPS patients had tenderness at 11 anatomical sites versus 7% of controls. The most common tender site in this survey was the prostate itself, but once again tenderness specifically did not correlate with any inflammation in the gland as determined by analysis of expressed prostate secretion. The prostate is anatomically intimate with the levator muscles and fascia of puborectalis and pubococcygeus and therefore these muscles would undoubtedly be stimulated during prostate manipulation.

Sites of pain have also been recently described for PBS by Warren and colleagues (2008) who hypothesized that careful, systematic analysis of pain experienced by such patients would indicate patterns that might provide clues to pathogenesis. In the 226 women surveyed, 66% reported two or more pain sites; mean of 2.1 sites per patient. Suprapubic prominence and changes in the voiding cycle are consistent with the bladder being the site of pain generation, but do not prove the point. Women with vulvodynia or urethral syndrome do not differ in these pain sites. When specific TrPs are discovered in females, it is feasible to augment myofascial release therapy with TrP injection utilizing local anaesthetic. In a limited study by Langford et al. (2007) 18 women were treated with localized

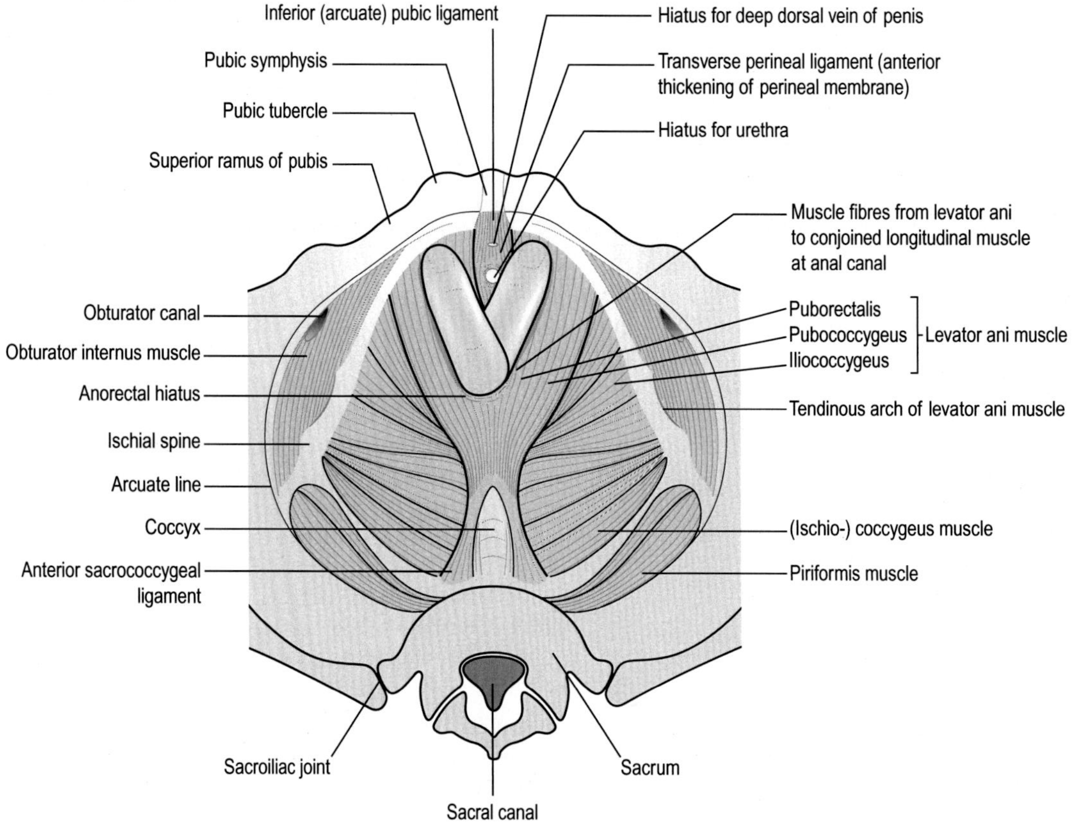

Anterior levator ani, superior portion (or puborectalis)

This is one of the most important trigger point sites in male pelvic pain, and palpating high enough up and firmly enough is critical in proper treatment. Frequently this area is the site of trigger points that are responsible for the tip-of-the-penis and shaft-of-the-penis pain. Furthermore, trigger points in this area can refer to the bladder, urethra, pressure and fullness in the prostate.

- One of the most important trigger point sites for male pelvic pain
- Can refer tip-of-the-penis, shaft-of-the-penis, bladder and urethral pain
- Can refer pressure/fullness in prostate

Figure 12.1 • Anterior levator trigger points and typical pain referral pattern

injection and 13 of the 18 women (72%) were improved at 3 months follow-up; six were completely pain-free.

Wise-Anderson Stanford Protocol

After many years of treating patients with UCPPS utilizing both manual physical therapy as well as cognitive behaviour relaxation training, we determined that intensive or immersion therapy over several days was an ideal method to break long-term pain cycles and teach patients to care for themselves. Patients are evaluated as above by a urologist and then immerse themselves into daily physical therapy and paradoxical relaxation training over a 6-day period. We have conducted over 80 monthly sessions of this type, and several months of follow-up (3–24 months) have revealed significant benefit to a large proportion of patients. There has been a significant decrease in NIH-CPSI scores ($P < 0.001$) and more than 50% of the patients have global response assessments categorized as moderately or markedly improved. In addition a large number of the patients have shown significant psychological benefit (Anderson et al. 2010).

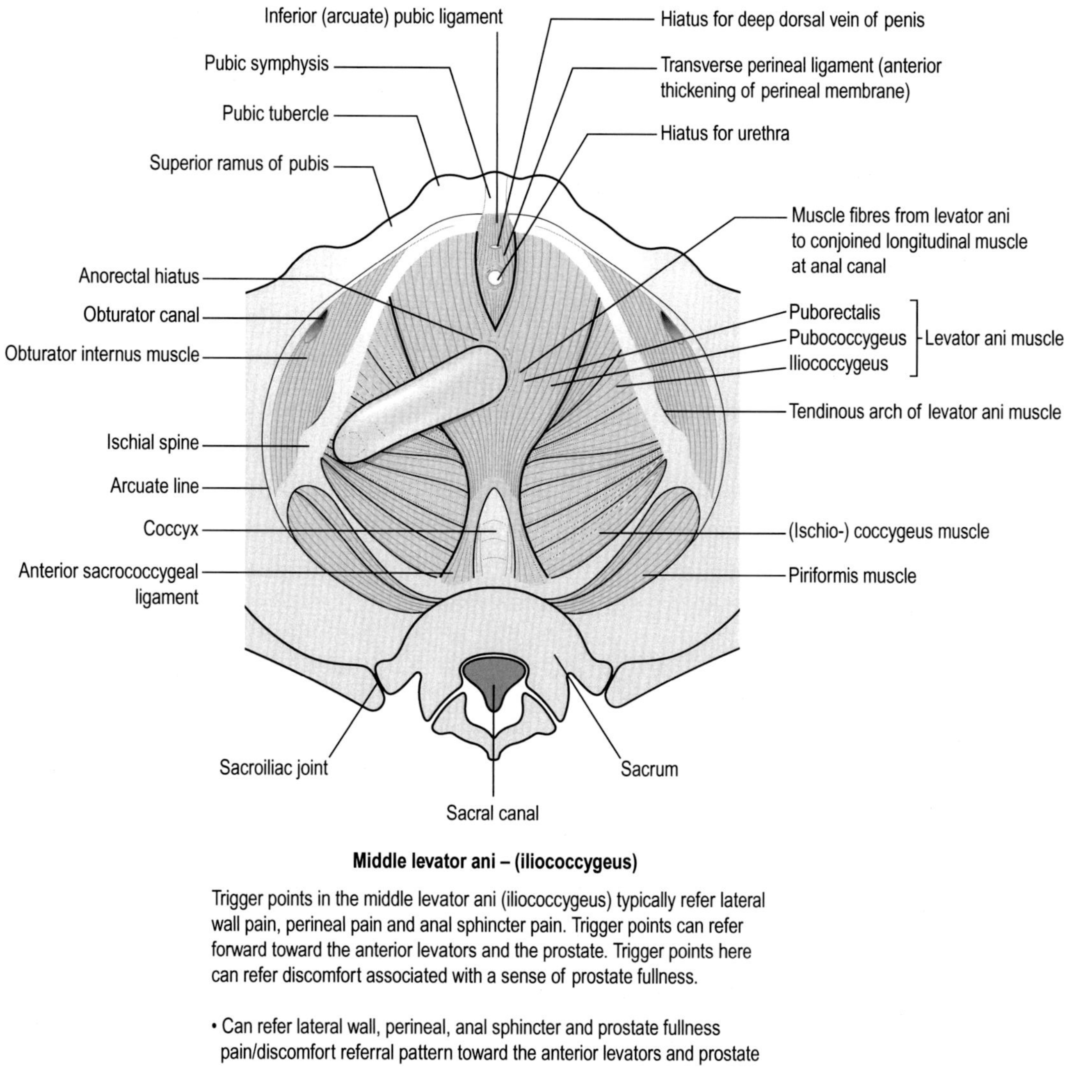

Figure 12.2 • Mid-level levator muscle trigger points and typical pain referral pattern

We reported a case series study of self-referred men with longstanding CPPS and attempted to describe the relationship between the locations of myofascial TrPs or restrictive muscular tissue, both internal and external to the pelvis, and the sites of pain initially described by the patients at the time of their evaluation (Anderson 2009). We hypothesized that palpation of certain myofascial TrPs would reproduce the pain sensations experienced by the patients.

The same physical therapist performed manual myofascial tissue palpation on all subjects. A traditional palpation force of approximately 4 kg/cm^2 for tender points (recommended for examination of fibromyalgia) was used for the assessment of pain. Pain was ranked as 0 (none) to 3+ (severe) for each area examined. Only categorical pain levels of 2+ or 3+ were counted as 'Yes – pain is present', while scores of 0 or 1+ were counted as 'No pain'. Sets of muscles that typically reproduced pain sensation in specific locations referred from TrPs were chosen for the investigation.

The median age of the 72 men with CPPS in this analysis was 40 years (range 20–72; IQR = 32, 49) with a median duration of symptoms of 44 months (range 4–408 months). The severity of symptoms at the time of the initial examination was measured by the pain VAS (visual analogue scale) score and

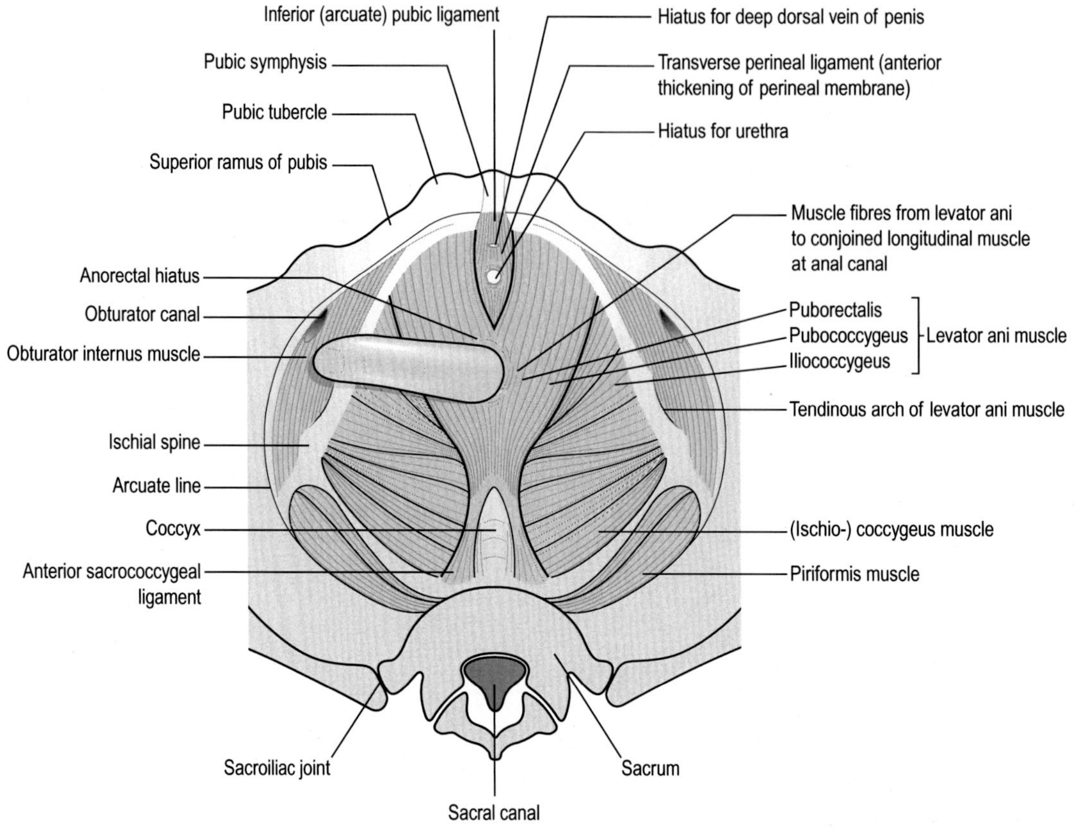

Obturator internus

Trigger points in the obturator can refer pain to the perineum, outward toward hip, to the whole pelvic floor both anteriorly and posteriorly. The obturator is intimate with the pudendal nerve and can refer a dull ache and burning in the pelvic floor on the side that it is being palpated. Trigger points in the obturator can refer the golf-ball-in-the-rectum feeling, symptoms to the coccyx, hamstrings and posterior thigh. In women, tigger pionts in the obturator can refer to the urethra, the vagina and specifically the vulva and is a very important point in the treatment of vulvar pain.

- Can refer dull ache on the side palpated, golf-ball-in-the-rectum sensation, coccyx, hamstrings, posterior thigh, urethra, vagina and vulva (important in vulvodynia)

Figure 12.3 • Obturator internus muscle trigger points and typical pain referral pattern

NIH-CPSI score with higher scores representing greater severity. The median VAS score was 5 out of 10 (range 1–9). The median NIH-CPSI overall score was 27 (43 is the maximum possible) with a median pain domain score of 13 (possible maximum = 21), urinary complaints of 5 (possible maximum = 10) and quality of life score of 10.5 (possible maximum = 12). The median total number of self-reported locations of pain was 4 (IQR = 3, 5) out of a possible 7 pre-designated sites. There was no correlation between pain VAS score and total number of painful locations (R = –0.195; P = 0.11). Furthermore, there was no statistically significant difference in pain VAS score by the presence of pain in any specific location. However, we did find that tenderness in the puborectalis and/or pubococcygeus muscles was associated with a higher pain VAS score (P = 0.013, Mann-Whitney test). Table 12.2 presents the internal and external muscles palpated and how frequently they elicited a painful response. For example, 90.3%

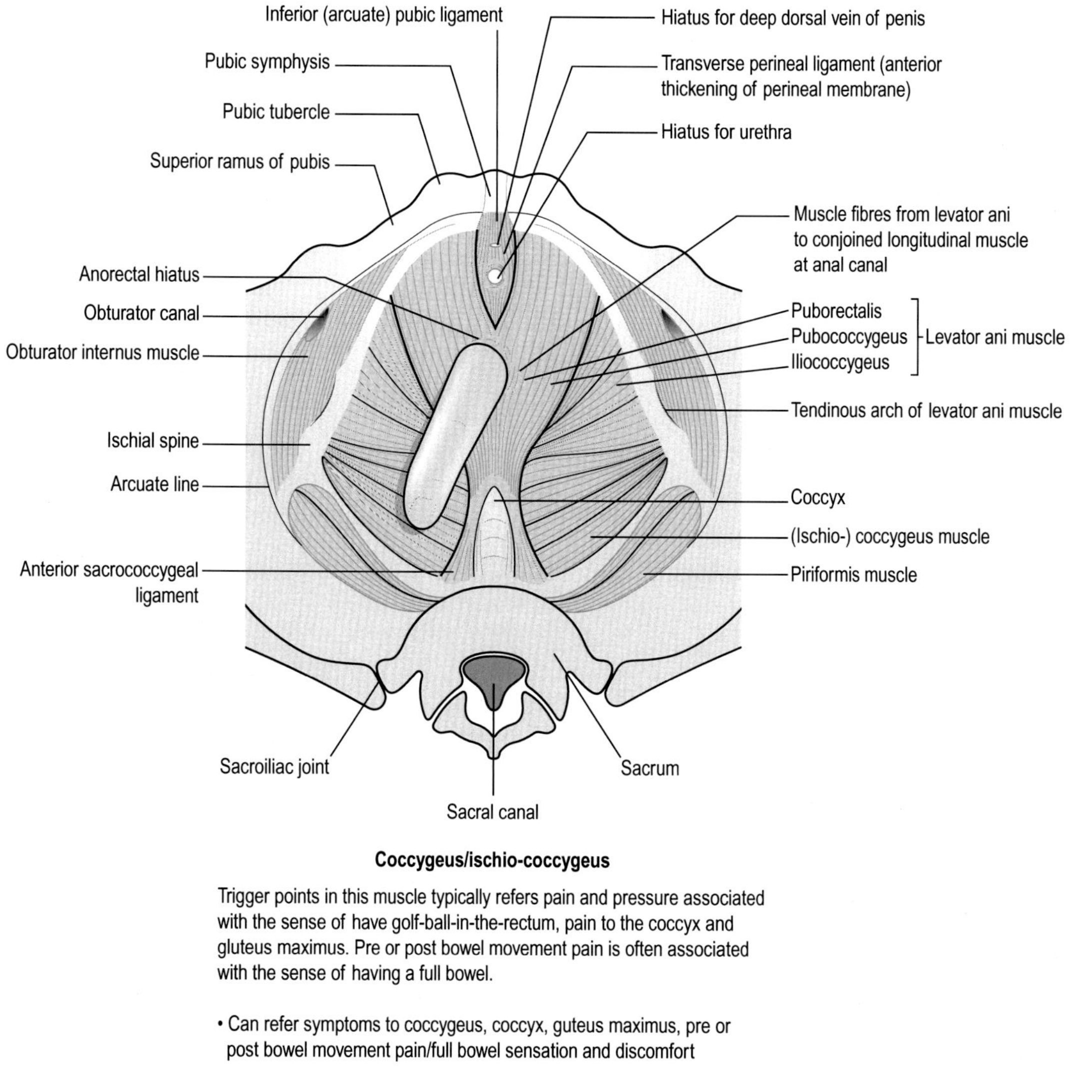

Figure 12.4 • Coccygeus muscle trigger points and typical pain referral pattern

(65/72) of men stated that they felt pain associated with palpation of the puborectalis and/or pubococcygeus muscles.

Painful TrPs, areas of restriction and associated pain location

Table 12.3 presents the muscles palpated and frequencies of referred pain to specific locations, whether or not the patient had initially complained of pain in that anatomical area. For example, palpation of the puborectalis and/or pubococcygeus muscles elicited pain in the penis in 93% (67/72) of the patients. At least two of the ten TrPs could elicit or refer pain to every one of the anatomical sites in a statistically significant proportion of patients (P values determined by the Fisher's exact test) and every TrP was able to reproduce pain in at least one site. The most reactive muscles were the rectus abdominis and external obliques; palpation of TrPs in these muscles elicited pain in four of the seven sites. Perineal pain was the most reproducible, being elicited by eight out of ten TrPs.

The frequency with which TrP palpation referred pain to a patient's self-reported chronic pain location is presented in Table 12.3. The odds ratio is shown when calculable. For example, among the 66 patients

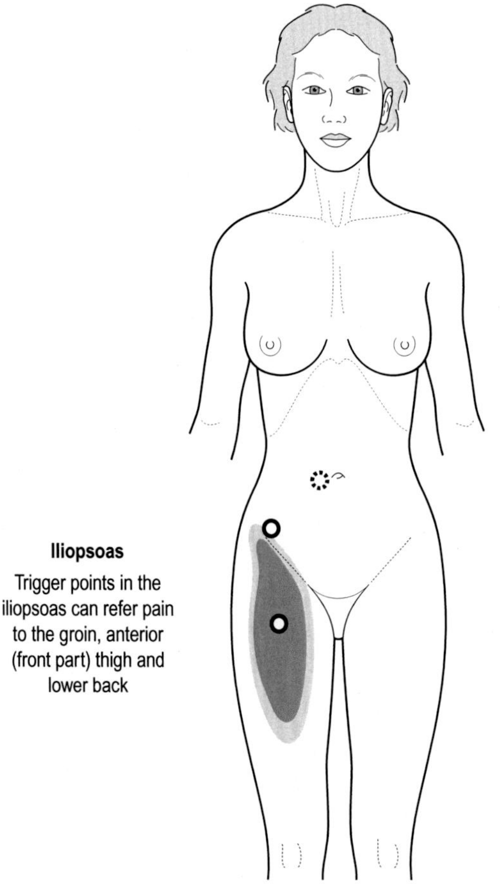

Iliopsoas
Trigger points in the iliopsoas can refer pain to the groin, anterior (front part) thigh and lower back

Figure 12.5 • Iliopsoas muscle trigger point pain referral pattern

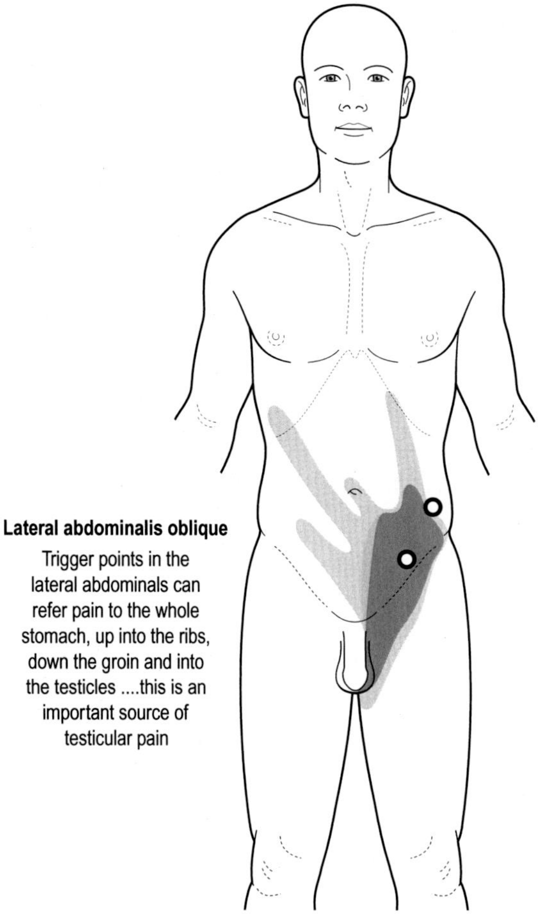

Lateral abdominalis oblique
Trigger points in the lateral abdominals can refer pain to the whole stomach, up into the ribs, down the groin and into the testicles ....this is an important source of testicular pain

Figure 12.6 • Lateral abdominal muscle trigger point pain referral pattern

with penile pain, 64 (97%) experienced this pain after palpation of TrPs in the puborectalis and/or pubococcygeus muscles. The odds ratio of 32.0; 95% CI (2.3, 461.0) implies that these patients were 32 times more likely to have penile pain reproduced with this muscle palpation than patients without penile pain. However, a more conservative interpretation lies with the lower limit of the CI. Thus with 95% certainty, patients with penile pain are at least 2.3 times more likely to have their pain reproduced with this TrP than patients who do not report penile pain. The odds ratio or P value could not be derived in some cases because of zero cell counts. For example, eight of 20 patients (40%) had coccyx or buttocks pain elicited by palpation of the gluteus maximus. None of the patients without coccyx or buttocks pain experienced pain in this location after palpation (0/52 without pain versus 8/20 with pain, $P < 0.001$, Fisher's exact test); the odds ratio was not calculable because of the zero cell count. Table 12.3 reveals that pain in each location could be reproduced by at least one TrP in a statistically significant proportion of patients with that prior pain report; rectal and coccyx/buttocks pain were each elicited by four different TrPs. Palpation of the external oblique muscles referred pain to the suprapubic area, testes and groin at least 80% of the time in patients with pain in these locations. Moreover, 80% (8/10) of the TrP palpations reproduced pain in at least one location, and palpation of the rectus abdominis elicited pain in four locations (penis, perineum, rectum and suprapubic area). Repeated palpation of a muscle group had a consistent effect in pain referral. These physical examination findings may lead to greater understanding of pathogenic mechanisms and lead to more focused therapy.

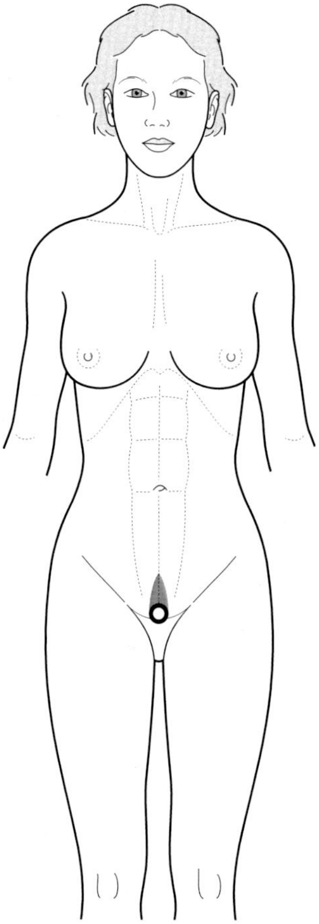

Pyramidalis
The pyramidalis is not present in some individuals but when it is present and has trigger points, they can refer pain and sensation to the bladder, pubic bone and urethra

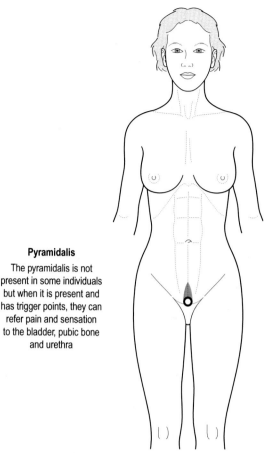

Figure 12.7 • Pyramidalis muscle trigger point and pain referral pattern

Our sample size of 72 subjects is small, although we were able to demonstrate both statistically and clinically significant associations between certain TrPs and specific pain locations. No asymptomatic men were examined as control subjects; therefore we are unable to compare how patients without CPPS would respond to these palpations. However, the purpose of this study was to examine patients with CPPS rather than compare their responses to normal subjects. Finally, it is difficult to objectively measure pain and thus we relied on patients' self-reported responses. If a painful location was not reported during the initial history, we could not account for it in our later analyses. We recognize that some individuals may be naturally more sensitive to muscle palpations and pressure that could cause pain in the pelvic region even though they do not suffer from CPPS.

The personal therapeutic wand for chronic pelvic pain

The ideal therapeutic provider combination for care of UCPPS should include a urologist evaluating the urologic signs and symptoms in a systematic fashion, a knowledgeable psychologist to provide psychosocial interpretation, psychological support and cognitive behaviour training such as progressive relaxation therapy and possible medical hypnosis, and a skilled physiotherapist who understands myofascial TrPs, how to release them and how to teach the patient self care. It is not always possible for patients to find follow-up physiotherapy from those who may be appropriately trained and skilled in the techniques required. We have introduced and taught patients self-treatment utilizing a personal therapeutic wand that can be inserted into the rectum or vagina to seek and release TrPs (Figures 12.8–12.10). Previous self-treatment devices have been inadequate to reach appropriate TrPs accurately and safely. Patients are carefully instructed regarding the location of their TrPs and then observed and guided to using the wand within specific pressure ranges to avoid any mucosal trauma or induction of internal tissue damage. These pressures have ranged between 2 and 6 pounds per square inch. Fibromyalgia TrP testing is typically performed at 4 kilograms per square centimetre. In some instances we have been able to train a spouse or significant other to assist in administering the therapeutic wand. Aside from one or two limited minor rectal bleeding episodes, no significant adverse effects have been noted. Patients are prospectively enrolled into a clinical trial under Institutional Review Board approval and followed for a period of 6 months, evaluating safety and efficacy. The intention is to enrol and evaluate 200 patient subjects.

Paradoxical relaxation

An important foundation of the Wise-Anderson Stanford Protocol was established early by Dr. David Wise in an attempt to achieve pelvic floor relaxation effortlessly (Wise 2010). He stated that 'Paradoxical Relaxation was a method that emerged in the trenches of chronic pain where I closed my own eyes, brought my attention to the inside, and dealt with the question of how I could stop the physical pain and anxiety in which I found myself.' Nothing that he proposes is theoretical, but shared outcomes from the personal laboratory of his own relaxation practice.

Table 12.2 Frequencies of specific locations of pain elicited by palpation of myofascial trigger points

Muscles palpated for trigger points	Location of reproduced pain symptom, % of 72 men with CPPS						
	Penis	Perineum	Rectum	Suprapubic	Testicles	Groin	Coccyx or buttocks
Internal muscles							
Puborectalis/ pubococcygeus	**93.1**	**19.4**	2.8	**56.9**	5.6	2.8	0
Coccygeus	1.4	**36.1**	**50.0**	1.4	0	0	**26.4**
Sphincter ani	0	**26.4**	**36.1**	0	0	0	4.2
External muscles							
Rectus abdominis	**73.6**	**65.3**	**45.8**	**38.9**	0	0	0
External oblique	**12.5**	4.2	1.4	**51.4**	**45.8**	**51.4**	0
Adductor magnus	0	**41.7**	**41.7**	0	0	**41.7**	0
Gluteus medius	0	**16.7**	6.9	0	**8.3**	1.4	**11.1**
Bulbospongiosus	**44.4**	**8.3**	0	0	1.4	0	0
Transverse perineal	2.8	**22.2**	**11.1**	0	0	0	0
Gluteus maximus	0	5.6	6.9	0	0	0	**8.3**

Frequencies that are significantly not zero, $P < 0.05$ (by Fisher's exact test) are in boldface and lightly shaded; frequencies >50% are boldface and shaded darker.

Initially we used anal and vaginal electrodes to teach reduction of the electromotive impulses. Gradually it became more useful to enlist cognitive behavioural therapy and an adoption of the Dr. Edmund Jacobson method of progressive relaxation. Dr. Wise developed and now teaches and trains patients to perform intensive paradoxical relaxation for 25–45 minutes as well as daily moment to moment relaxation. It is possible to reliably calm tension, agitation and anxiety with pharmacological agents. The silver lining of suffering anxiety is that it motivates one to learn to profoundly relax. Frequently the patients learn respiratory sinus arrhythmia breathing to assist in reaching the levels of relaxation that are beneficial. The term 'paradoxical' relaxation refers to accepting the tension or other sensation associated with the pain but letting go of the effort to try to relax. The secret is learning to focus attention and prevent the mind from wandering away from the presence of mind to quiet the nervous system and achieve profound relaxation. Relaxation occurs when attention rests in sensation and not in thought. It is not letting go of focused attention and letting your mind go anywhere it wants to. If one is able to sustain long periods of focused attention, the ability to profoundly relax the pelvic floor and lower the activity of the autonomic nervous system will have a chance of becoming reliable or deep. When attention cannot be sustained long enough to permit the patient to become aware of the unconscious holding and guarding he or she is doing, the guarding tends to remain in place. The task is to remain focused and simultaneously relinquish any unnecessary effort in doing so. One teaching pearl reminds patients to observe the sensation of sitting on a toilet to urinate or move their bowels. It is the sensation of a slight drop in the pelvic

Table 12.3 Frequencies and odds ratios of pain reproduced at specific sites after trigger point palpation among men with CPPS who pre-identified a site of chronic pain

	Typical location of pain reported by patient (total N = 72 patients)						
No. patients (% with pain present at specified location)	Penis	Perineum	Rectum	Suprapubic area	Testicles	Groin	Coccyx or buttocks
	66 (91.7)	56 (77.8)	51 (70.8)	45 (62.5)	37 (51.4)	34 (47.2)	20 (27.8)
Trigger point palpation in specific muscle	**% Patients with symptom present that was elicited with trigger point palpation (P value*) [odds ratio]**						
Puborectalis and pubococcygeus	**97.0 (0.005) [32.0]**	(0.72) [1.9]	3.9 (1.0) NA	**86.7 (<0.001) [81.5]**	10.8 (0.12) NA	(0.22) NA	0 NA
Coccygeus	1.5 (1.0) NA	**42.9 (0.04) [5.3]**	**(<0.001) NA**	(1.0) NA	0 NA	0 NA	**80.0 (<0.001) [65.3]**
Sphincter ani	0 NA	(0.53) [1.7]	**(<0.001) NA**	0 NA	0 NA	0 NA	**(0.02) NA**
Rectus abdominis	**78.8 (0.001) [18.6]**	**76.8 (<0.001) [9.9]**	**60.8 (<0.001) [14.7]**	**62.2 (<0.001) NA**	0 NA	0 NA	0 NA
External oblique	(0.44) NA	(1.0) NA	2.0 (1.0) NA	**80.0 (<0.001) [104.0]**	**89.2 (<0.001) NA**	**94.1 (<0.001) [105.6]**	0 NA
Adductor magnus	0 NA	**51.8 (0.001) [16.1]**	**56.9 (<0.001) [26.4]**	0 NA	0 NA	(0.10) NA	0 NA
Gluteus medius	0 NA	(0.06) NA	(0.3) NA	0 NA	**(0.03) NA**	(0.47) NA	**(<0.001) NA**
Bulbospongiosus	27.3 (0.50) [1.95]	7.1 (0.61) [0.5]	0 NA	0 NA	2.7 (1.0) NA	0 NA	0 NA
Transverse perineal	3.0 (1.0) NA	(0.50) [2.3]	(0.10) NA	0 NA	0 NA	0 NA	0 NA
Gluteus maximus	0 NA	(0.07) NA	(0.31) NA	0 NA	0 NA	0 NA	**(<0.001) NA**

*P value from Fisher's exact test comparing the given frequency to those who experienced referral pain but were asymptomatic. Frequencies in boldface and shaded are $P < 0.05$. Odds ratios were calculated and have 95% certainty; NA indicates odds ratio not calculable due to cell with zero count.

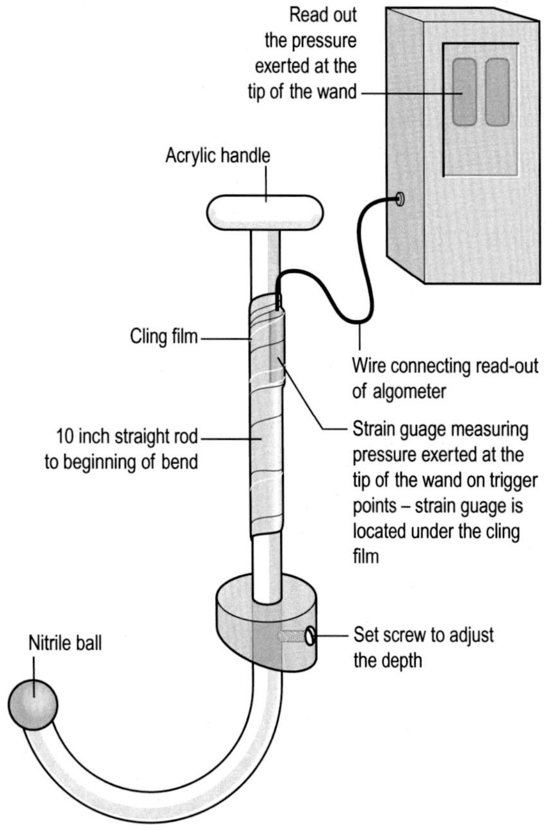

Figure 12.8 • Illustration of personal massage wand to release trigger points with safety pressure monitoring

floor through relaxation of both the sympathetic and parasympathetic nervous system simultaneously.

We have instituted recent clinical trials using medical hypnotherapy and patient self-hypnosis administered by an experienced psychologist experienced in this therapy. In addition we utilize parallel cognitive behavioural approaches. We are analysing the preliminary results of this pilot trial to consider expansion of research application. But it is apparent to virtually every clinician that therapeutic management must address the psychosocial and mental behaviour aspects of the problem.

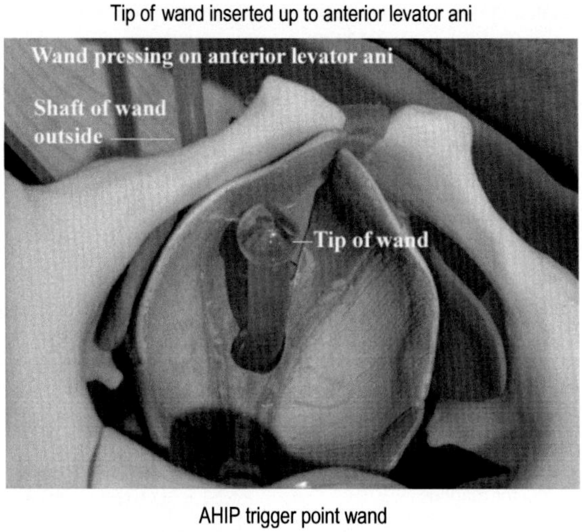

Figure 12.10 • Illustration of internal protuberance of personal massage wand

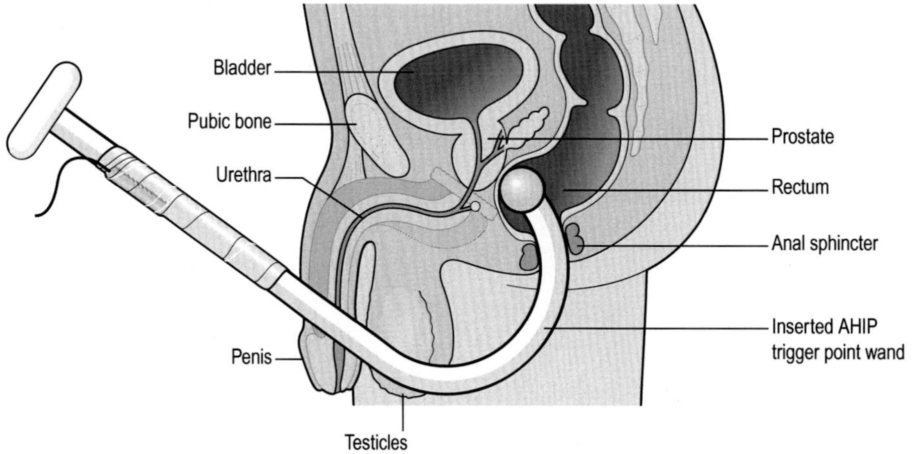

Figure 12.9 • Illustration of angulation of personal massage wand to facilitate reaching painful trigger points

References

Anderson, R.U., 2006. Traditional therapy for chronic pelvic pain does not work: what do we do now? Nat. Clin. Pract. Urol. 3, 145–156.

Anderson, R.U., Wise, D., Sawyer, T., et al., 2005. Integration of myofascial trigger point release and paradoxical relaxation training treatment of chronic pelvic pain in men. J. Urol. 174, 155–160.

Anderson, R.U., Wise, D., Sawyer, T., et al., 2006. Sexual dysfunction in men with chronic prostatitis/chronic pelvic pain syndrome: Improvement after trigger point release and paradoxical relaxation training. J. Urol. 176, 1534–1539.

Anderson, R.U., Orenberg, E.K., Chan, C.A., et al., 2008. Psychometric profiles and hypothalamic-pituitary-adrenal axis function in men with chronic prostatitis/chronic pelvic pain syndrome. J. Urol. 179, 956–960.

Anderson, R.U., Wise, D., Sawyer, T., Glowe, P., Orenberg, E., 2010. 6-day intensive treatment protocol for refractory chronic prostatitis/chronic pelvic pain syndrome using myofascial release and paradoxical relaxation training. J. Urol. 185, 1294–1299.

Baranowski, A.P., Abrams, P., Berger, R.E., et al., 2008. Urogenital pain–time to accept a new approach to phenotyping and, as a consequence, management. Eur. Urol. 53, 33–36.

Berger, R.E., Ciol, M.A., Rothman, I., et al., 2007. Pelvic tenderness is not limited to the prostate in chronic prostatitis/chronic pelvic pain syndrome (CPPS) type IIIA and IIIB: comparison of men with and without CP?/CPPS. Biomedical Center Urology 7, 17.

Clemens, J.Q., Nadler, R.B., Schaeffer, A.J., et al., 2000. Biofeedback, pelvic floor re-education, and bladder training for male chronic pelvic pain syndrome. Urology 56, 951–955.

Fall, M., Baranowski, A.P., Sohier, E., et al., 2010. EAU guidelines on chronic pelvic pain. Eur. Urol. 57, 35–48.

Fitzgerald, M.P., Anderson, R.U., Potts, J., et al., 2009. Randomized multicenter feasibility trial of myofascial physical therapy for the treatment of urological chronic pelvic pain syndromes. J. Urol. 182, 570–580.

Geramoutsos, I., Gyftopoulos, K., Perimenis, P., et al., 2004. Clinical correlation of prostatic lithiasis with chronic pelvic pain syndromes in young adults. Eur. Urol. 45, 333–337.

Hafez, H., 2009. Urodynamic evaluation of patients with chronic pelvic pain syndrome. Urotoday International Journal 2.

Hanno, P., Lin, A., Nordling, J., et al., 2010. Bladder pain syndrome international consultation on incontinence. Neurourol. Urodyn. 29, 191–198.

Heidenreich, A., Olbert, P., Engelmann, U.H., 2002. Management of chronic testalgia by microsurgical testicular denervation. Eur. Urol. 41, 392–397.

Hetrick, D.C., Glazer, H., Liu, Y.W., et al., 2006. Pelvic floor electromyography in men with chronic pelvic pain syndrome: A case-control study. Neurourol. Urodyn. 25, 46–49.

Hori, S., Sengupta, A., Shuklaw, C.J., et al., 2009. Long-term outcome of epidiymectomy for the management of chronic epididymal pain. J. Urol. 182, 1407–1412.

Langford, C.F., Nagy, S.U., Ghomeim, G.M., 2007. Levator ani trigger point injections: An underutilized treatment for chronic pelvic pain. Neurourol. Urodyn. 26, 59–62.

Lee, J.C., Yang, C.C., Kromm, B.G., et al., 2001. Neurophysiologic testing in chronic pelvic pain syndrome: A pilot study. Urology 58, 246–250.

Levine, L.A., Matkov, T.G., 2001. Microsurgical denervation of the spermatic cord as primary surgical treatment of chronic orchialgia. J. Urol. 165, 1927–1929.

McJunkin, T.L., Wuollet, A.L., Lynch, P.J., 2009. Sacral nerve stimulation as a treatment modality for intractable neuropathic testicular pain. Pain Physician 12, 991–995.

Nickel, J.C., Shoskes, D.A., Irvine-Brid, K., 2009. Clinical phenotyping of women with interstitial cystitis/painful bladder syndrome: A key to classification and potentially improved management. J. Urol. 182, 155–160.

Planken, E., Voorham van der Zaim, P.J., Lycklama Nijeholt, A.B., et al., 2010. Chronic testicular pain as a symptom of pelvic floor dysfunction. J. Urol. 183, 177–181.

Schaeffer, A.J., Knauss, J.S., Landis, J.R., et al., 2002. Leukocyte and bacterial counts do not correlate with severity of symptoms in men with chronic prostatitis: The National Institutes of Health chronic prostatitis cohort study. J. Urol. 168, 1048–1053.

Shoskes, D.A., Zeitlin, S.I., 1999. Use of prostate massage in combination with antibiotics in the treatment of chronic prostatitis. Prostate Cancer Prostatic Dis. 2, 159–162.

Shoskes, D.A., Lee, C.T., Murphy, D., et al., 2007. Incidence and significance of prostatic stones in men with chronic prostatitis/chronic pelvic pain syndrome. Urology 70, 235–238.

Shoskes, D.A., Nickel, J.C., Dolinga, R., et al., 2009. Clinical phenotyping of patients with chronic prostatitis/chronic pelvic pain syndrome and correlation with symptom severity. Urology 73, 538–542.

Stav, K., Dwyer, P.L., Roberts, L., 2009. Pudendal neuralgia fact or fiction? Obstet. Gynecol. Surv. 64, 190–199.

Strohmaier, W.L., Bichler, K.H., 2000. Comparison of symptoms, morphological, microbiological and urodynamic findings in patients with chronic prostatitis/pelvic pain syndrome. Is it possible to differentiate separate categories? Urol. Int. 65, 112–116.

Sweeney, C.A., Oades, G.M., Fraser, M., et al., 2008. Does surgery have a role in management of chronic intrascrotal pain? Urology 71, 1099–1102.

Warren, J.W., Langenberg, P., Greenberg, P., et al., 2008. Sites of pain from interstitial cystitis/painful bladder syndrome. J. Urol. 180, 1373–1377.

Wise, D., 2010. Paradoxical relaxation. In: Wise, D., Anderson, R.U. A Headache In The Pelvis: A new understanding and treatment for chronic pelvic pain syndromes. sixth ed. National Center for Pelvic Pain, Sebastapol, CA.

Zermann, D.H., Ishigooka, M., Doggweiler-Wiygul, R., et al., 2001. The male chronic pelvic pain syndrome. World J. Urol. 19, 173–179.

Practical anatomy, examination, palpation and manual therapy release techniques for the pelvic floor

13

Maeve Whelan

CHAPTER CONTENTS

Introduction

The aim of this chapter is to describe in detail the practical anatomy of the pelvic floor as the practitioner would evaluate it in the clinic, followed by specific manual therapy techniques to treat the pelvic floor tissues that may be contributing to chronic pelvic pain.

Female practical anatomy

Introduction

The organs, muscles, ligaments and fascial tissue as well as their origins, insertions and supports are explained in a way that helps direct the evaluator in the examination process. The orientation and the accessibility of the structures are described throughout as the examination starts from external proceeding to internal.

Planes of examination

'It is important to recognise that the pelvic diaphragm is not flat or bowl-shaped as is frequently depicted. At the urogenital and anal hiatus the muscles lie in a near vertical configuration and behind the anus they flatten to form a nearly horizontal diaphragm' (Brooks et al. 1998). The examination of the patient most frequently takes place in the crook lying position. As the examiner faces the patient the perineum from the pubic bone to the supporting surface is visualized on a clock; this was first described by Laycock & Jerwood (2001).

On this clock the pubic bone is at 12 o'clock and the perineal body is at 6 o'clock, palpation for example of a contraction of the levator ani would be at 4 o'clock and 8 o'clock. This is referred to here as the 'vertical clock' of examination. Examination on this plane accesses the structures on the perineum first externally then circumferentially at the introitus and at the front, back and side walls of the lower vagina in a caudal to cranial direction.

During this part of the examination palpating from the vertical clock to the horizontal clock it should be visualized that the vagina extends inward from the vestibule at a 45° angle and then turns horizontal over the levator plate (Brooks 2007). The 'horizontal clock' runs for purposes of description perpendicular to the vertical but is clearly not completely perpendicular; the coccyx here is at 12 o'clock and the perineal body again is at 6 o'clock (Figures 13.1, 13.2) (Whelan 2008). It should also be stated that the pelvic floor and the structures of the pelvis are multidimensional and it can be difficult to visualize the many different planes. This suggested method of examination is based on two planes only but the examiner will appreciate the overlap into other planes.

Practical anatomy on the vertical clock – External perineal

The examination on the vertical clock has two parts, the external first and then the internal. The external genitalia are observed for lesions, erythema and colour

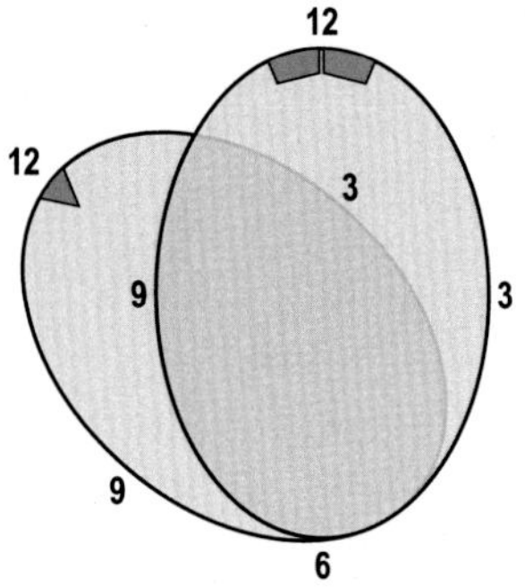

Figure 13.1 • Clocks of examination

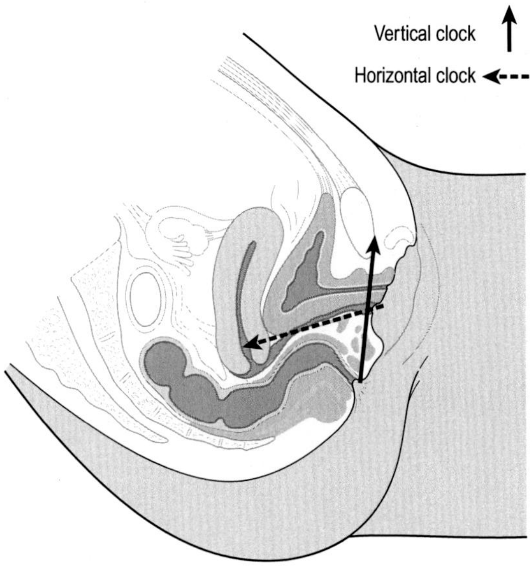

Figure 13.2 • Clocks shown on sagittal section of pelvis. Reproduced from Haslam, J., Laycock, J. (Eds.), (2007) Therapeutic Management of Incontinence and Pelvic Pain: Pelvic Organ Disorders, second revised ed.Springer-Verlag

changes before the soft tissue assessment begins. The conditions that may affect the external genitalia in chronic pelvic pain are discussed in Chapter 8; however, the therapist should be familiar with symptoms and appearance of dermatological conditions such as dermatitis, lichens planus and lichens sclerosus and be aware of the occurrence of thrush and sexually transmitted infections including genital herpes and genital warts.

As the patient lies in the crook lying position the pubic bone is observed in the 12 o'clock position on the vertical clock and the perineal body is at 6 o'clock. The mons pubis is the area of skin overlying the pubic bone. Inferior to this is the anterior commissure of the labia majora; this is where the divide of the labia majora starts. The labia majora ends at the posterior commissure of the labia majora superior to the perineal body. Inferior to the anterior commissure of the labia majora is the area of tissue superior to the glans of the clitoris called the prepuce of the clitoris. Lateral here is the pudendal cleft which is the space between the labia majora. The frenulum of the clitoris is the area just below the clitoris. The labia minora start at the clitoris and extend down to the frenulum of the labia minora superior to the perineal body. The vestibule of the vagina is the space surrounded by the labia minora. Below the frenulum of the clitoris is the external urethral orifice and below this again is the vaginal orifice. Lateral to the vaginal orifice in the 5 o'clock and

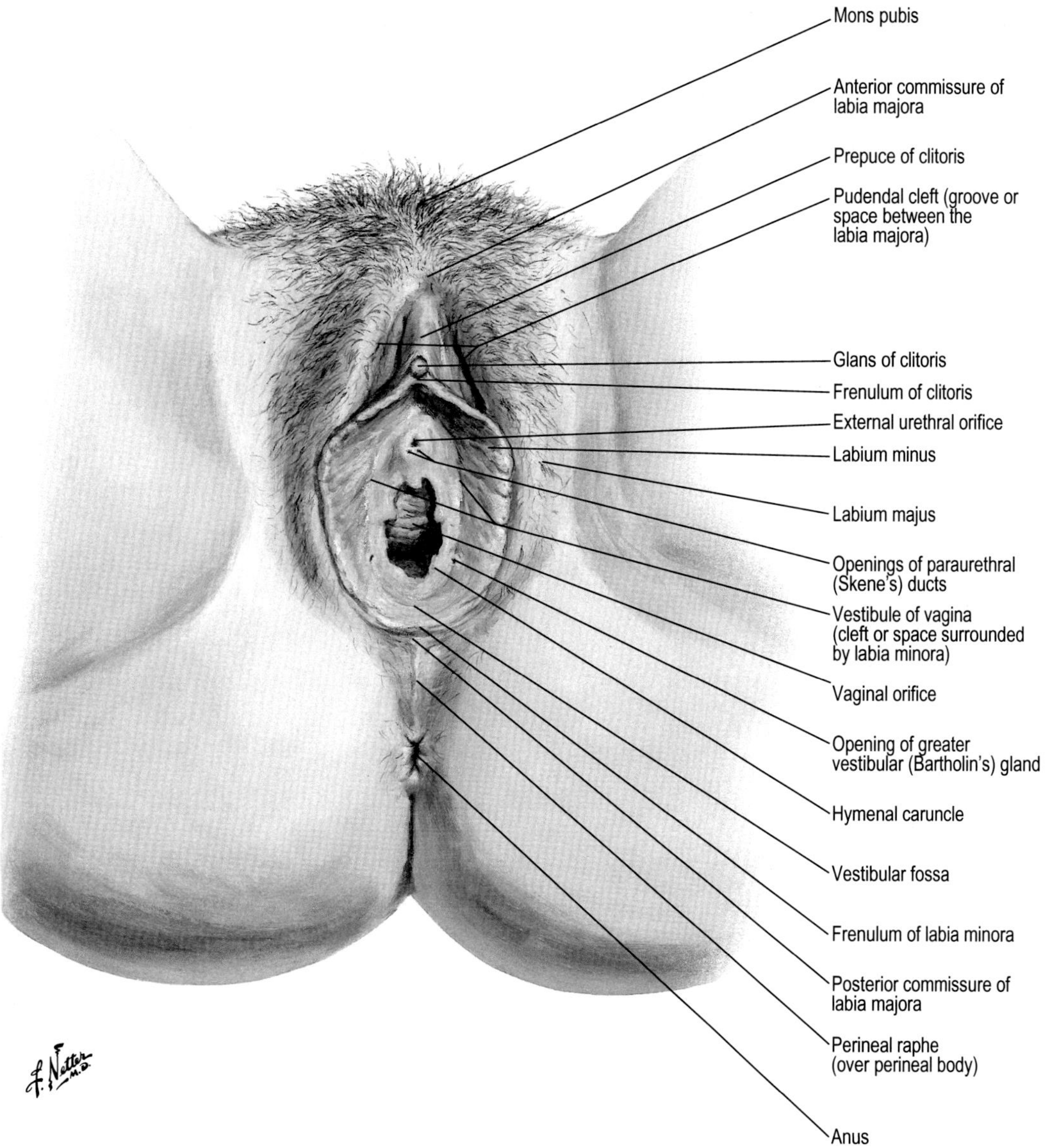

Figure 13.3 • External genitalia

7 o'clock positions are the openings of the Bartholin's glands (Figure 13.3).

The perineal body is positioned between the posterior commissure of the labia majora and the anus; it forms the centre point of the perineum and lies deep to the external genitalia. Attaching to the perineal body centrally are the superficial transverse perineii muscles and they extend bilaterally to the ischial tuberosities. The ischiocavernosus muscles arise from the ischiopubic ramus and extend upwards to the crus of the clitoris. The bulbospongiosus muscles attach to the perineal body, the fibres run on either side of the vagina covering the superficial part of the vestibular bulb and vestibular glands and insert below the clitoris (Figure 13.4). Palpation of the bulbocavernosus and the transverse perineii is best performed by pincer palpation where the pad of the palpating finger is inserted just inside the vagina and met by the opposition of the thumb on the outside. The tissue is stretched or rolled between the finger and the thumb revealing the resting tone, tension, taut bands and trigger points. The

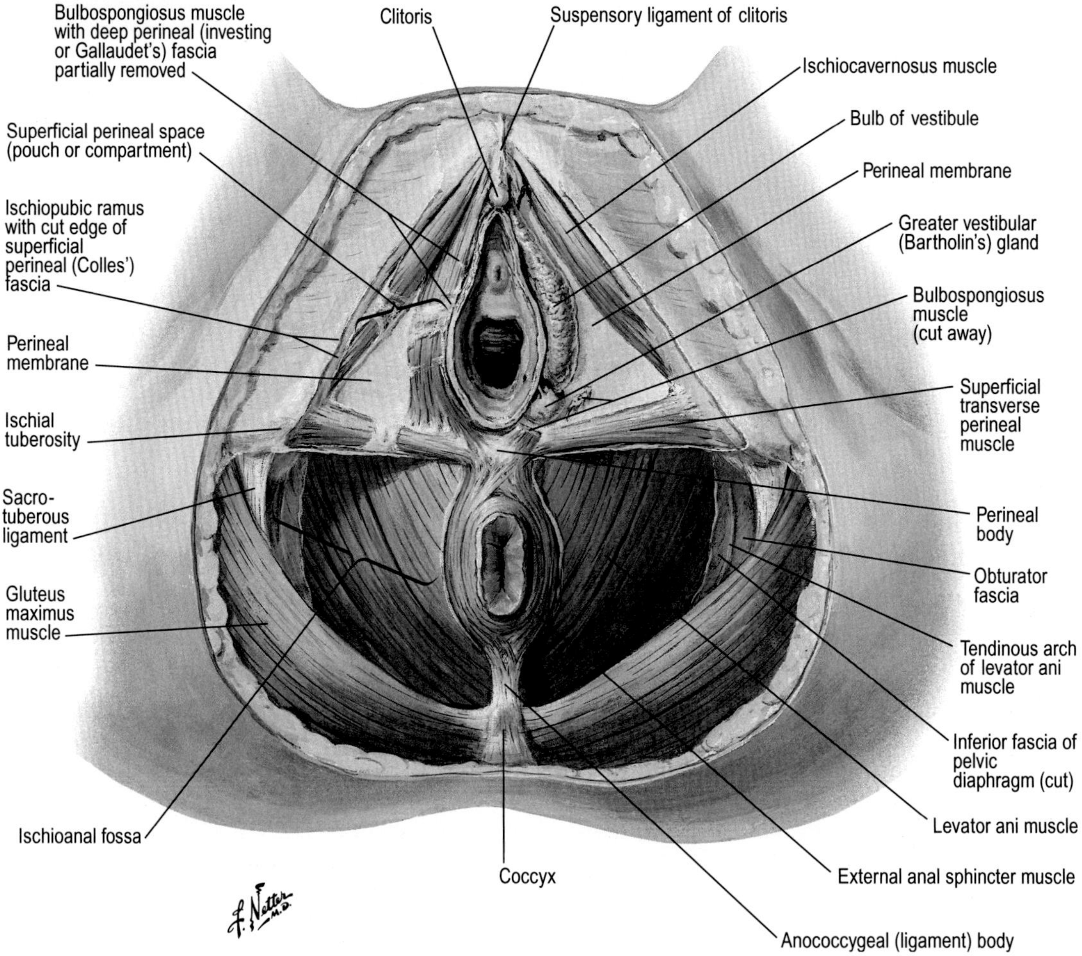

Figure 13.4 • Perineum and deep perineum

ischiocavernosus is palpated against the ischiopubic ramus behind.

The deep perineal membrane extends from the ischiopubic ramus laterally to the vagina medially overlying what were previously referred to as the deep transverse perineal muscles but are the compressor urethrae muscle and the urethrovaginal sphincter muscles (DeLancey 1990). The urethrovaginal sphincter surrounds the vaginal wall and extends along the inferior pubic rami above the perineal membrane as the compressor urethrae. Superficial to these are the ischiocavernosus, bulbocavernosus and transversus perineii and the fascia superficial again to this layer is the superficial (Colles) fascia. The bulb of the vestibule is deep to the bulbospongiosus muscle and attaches to the deep perineal membrane. The perineal membrane is also referred to as the urogenital diaphragm (Herschorn 2004).

Practical anatomy on the vertical clock – Internal vaginal

The internal examination is started at the introitus with the pad of the finger palpating the perineal body, which is the central tendon of the superficial pelvic floor; resistance and length of the pelvic floor should be appreciated here. A short pelvic floor will be palpated where the dorsum of the finger just inside the vagina is held tight up against the pubic bone (Fitzgerald & Kotarinos 2003).

The anterior attachments of the levator ani muscle group are palpated on this plane by moving the palpating finger laterally to feel for resistance and attachment to the pubic bone. The most superficial part of the levator ani group is the puboperineal portion attaching from the pubic bone to the perineal

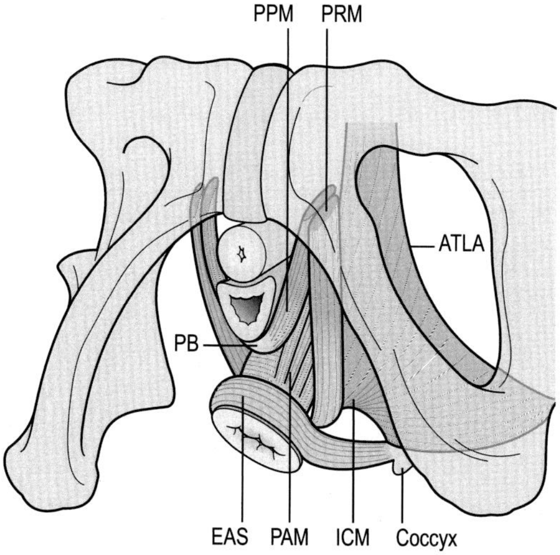

Figure 13.5 • Levator ani. ATLA, arcus tendineus levator ani; EAS, external anal sphincter; ICM, iliococcygeal muscle; PAM, puboanal muscle; PB, perineal body uniting the two ends of the puboperineal muscle (PPM); PRM, puborectal muscle. Reproduced from Kearney et al (2004) Levator ani muscle anatomy evaluated by origin-insertion pairs. Obstet. Gynecol. 104, 168–173

body; the pubovaginalis muscle attaches from the pubic bone to the posterior vaginal wall and the puboanal portion inserts into the anal canal and skin (Figure 13.5). These muscles are part of the pubovisceralis muscle group, they were previously referred to as the pubococcygeus muscle but were renamed to reflect the orientation of the different parts of the muscle in the pelvic floor (Lawson 1974, Kearney et al. 2004). Now the pubococcygeus muscle refers distinctly to the muscle attaching from the pubic bone to the coccyx only. The puborectalis is distinct from the other pubovisceralis muscles as it attaches to the pubic bone and forms a sling behind the rectum and creates an angulation of the rectum whereas the other muscles elevate the anus perineal body and vagina (DeLancey & Ashton-Miller 2007).

Loss of attachment of the puborectalis will be palpated as bony end feel laterally on the pubic bone and high tone will be noted as thickened and resistant, often with acute pain at this point in the symptomatic patient. If the finger can be moved over the inferior pubic ramus without encountering any contractile tissue for 2–3 cm then this implies an avulsion injury to the puborectalis on that side. This may be the case in 15–30% of women who have given birth normally (Dietz 2009). This is compared from side to side. The palpating finger then tracks along the posterior vaginal wall evaluating resistance and this resistance can change from the vertical to the horizontal clocks as the pubovaginalis to the puborectalis muscles are palpated. The pubovaginalis or puborectalis muscles are short if the palpating finger is held up against the pubic bone. It may be difficult to stretch or lengthen the muscle and deep palpation may reveal a specific point of tension or a taut band within the muscle. There may be increased sensitivity in this localized taut band indicating the presence of a trigger point. On moving the finger slightly more posteriorly into the vagina, the rectovaginal fascia is palpated overlying the rectum, the rectum and its contents are palpated. Just lateral to the rectum, tone of the puborectalis is palpated, high tone will flex the palpating finger and there will be strong resistance on downward pressure.

The pad of the palpating finger is turned upwards towards the urethra. The anterior wall is covered by the pubocervical fascia and the urethra is palpated through this fascia. The pubocervical fascia extends from the symphysis pubis along the anterior vaginal wall to blend with the fascia that surrounds the cervix. The urethra is followed posteriorly behind the pubic bone up to the urethrovesical junction and finally the base of the bladder is palpated. Immediately in front of the cervix the base of the bladder rests on the vaginal wall (Brooks 2007). Descent of the anterior wall either low down or up higher is felt as a soft 'bogginess'. The vesical neck should lie 2–3 cm above the insertion of the pubourethral ligaments and the inferior surface of the pubic bone (DeLancey 1990). The pubourethral ligaments form the periurethral connective tissue and attach to the white line of the arcus tendineus fascia pelvis close to its pubic end (Standring 2008).

The urethra is palpated by a longitudinal or lateral stretch of the overlying tissue, sensation, resistance and painful points are evaluated. Posterior to and arising just lateral to the pubic symphysis is the arcus tendineus fascia pelvis (ATFP). The ATFP corresponds to the lateral attachment of the anterior bladder wall to the pelvic side wall and is joined by fibres of the superficial fascia of the levator ani. Its connection to the pubis lies 1 cm above the inferior margin of the pubic symphysis and 1 cm lateral to the midline (DeLancey 1990). The anterior portion is palpable at its attachment to the pubic bone and posteriorly it becomes less well defined and more difficult to palpate as it broadens out towards its attachment to the ischial spine (Figure 13.6).

On palpation along the anterior wall of the vagina, the end point will be the anterior fornix. At this point the anterior wall is attached to the cervix of the uterus, the cervix is palpated and then the posterior fornix is palpated, depending on the position of the

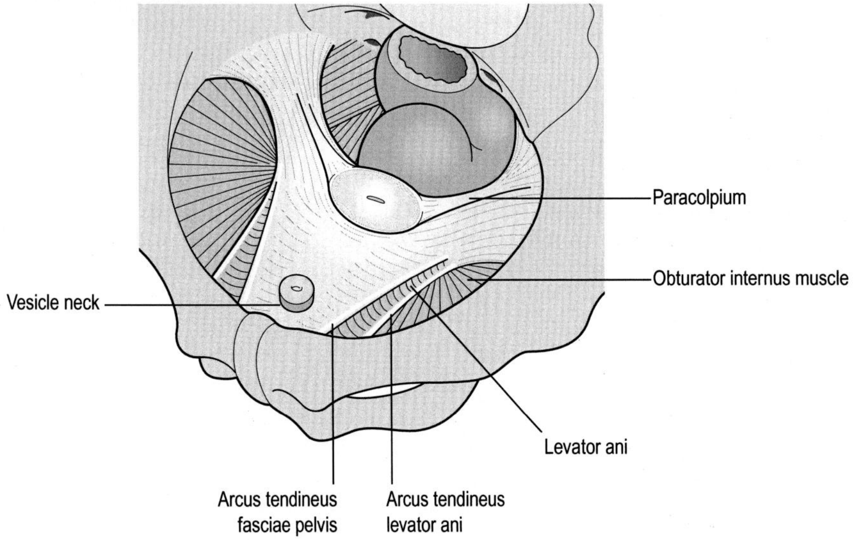

Figure 13.6 • Arcus tendineus fascia pelvis. Reproduced, with permission, from DeLancey

uterus, the posterior fornix may be difficult to palpate. The apex of the vagina is palpated and total vaginal length is noted. It is worth noting both position and the resistance of the uterus on palpation as clinical observation has shown this may change with treatment and can be retested. The paracolpium is the connective tissue surrounding the mid to upper vagina and uterus and fuses with the pelvic wall and fascia laterally. The cardinal ligaments extend from the lateral margins of the cervix and upper vagina and lateral pelvic walls, to an area expanding from the greater sciatic foramen to the piriformis and the lateral sacrum as far as the sacroiliac joints. The uterosacral ligaments are attached to the cervix and upper vagina posterolaterally and posteriorly to the fascia in front of the sacroiliac joints (Herschorn 2004). The paracolpium can be palpated but the uterosacral and cardinal ligaments are too deep to be palpated to their attachments. The apex of the vagina and uterus are held in place by the uterosacral and cardinal ligaments anchoring the pelvic viscera over the levator plate (Figure 13.7).

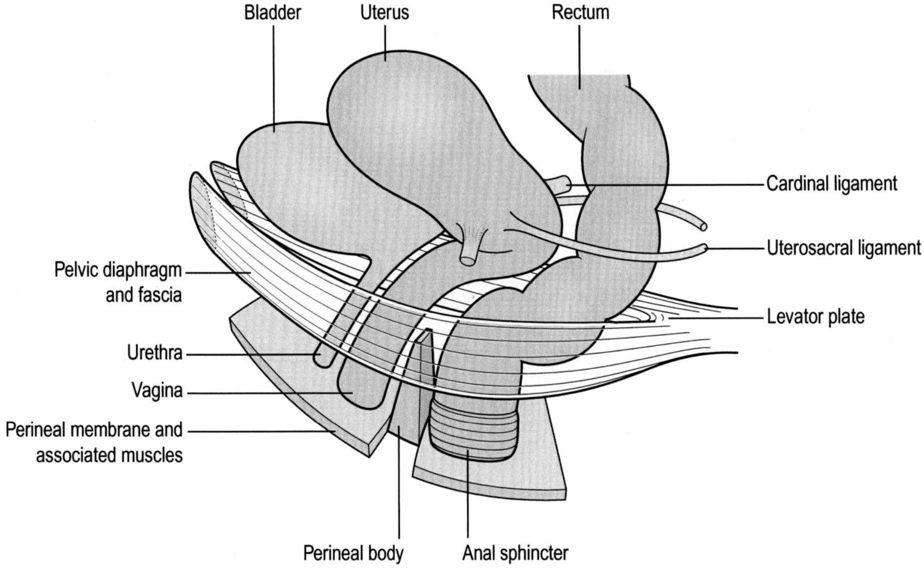

Figure 13.7 • Upper horizontal vaginal axis and upper vaginal supports. Reproduced from Herschorn, S., Carr, L.K., 2002. In: Campbell's Urology

Practical anatomy on the vertical clock – Internal anal

The external anal sphincter is depicted in many anatomy diagrams as being on the same vertical plane as the pubic bone when in fact it is slightly more posterior. It lies between the two clocks of examination as described. This will be dependent on the patient being in a neutral spine position, i.e. when there is a slight hollow in the lumbar spine. If the patient is posteriorly tilted as they often might be when anxious at the initiation of an exam it may appear to be on the same plane. The structures described below assessed vaginally on the horizontal plane can be accessed through the sphincter as well, but examination may be more restricted because of the size of the anal orifice. However the coccyx, ischiococcygeus and piriformis may be more easily accessed anally as these structures lie more posteriorly.

The examination of the anal sphincter is started by asking the patient to bear down gently as this prevents a contraction against the examiner's finger. The external anal sphincter has three parts: the subcutaneous, superficial and deep portions. It surrounds the internal anal sphincter which is the inner layer of rectal smooth muscle. The puboanal portion of the levator ani muscle inserts along the anal canal. Tone is evaluated by attempting to move the finger in the anus; if there is high tone, movement of the finger will be difficult. The length of the anus is also assessed; it should be approximately 3 cm long. Fissures or haemorrhoids should also be noted.

Once inside the rectum, examination of the anterior structures will be on the vertical clock and the rectovaginal fascia is palpated anteriorly towards the pubic bone. The presence of stool should be noted as the rectum should be empty once the bowel has been evacuated. The tip of the cervix may be palpated through this fascia depending on its position. Centrally the rectum should be open; rectal prolapse will be palpated as a fold of tissue overlying the entrance to the anus from the rectum or intussusception, where a more proximal part of the bowel descends into a more distal segment. The puborectalis sling position, resistance and contractility is also evaluated as described in the examination on the horizontal clock.

Examination can be carried out in the side lying or in the crook lying position; prone lying is also a possibility. Consideration should be given to the examiner's dexterity as palpation of the structures on the left can be difficult for the right-handed examiner, in which case examination could be carried out in left side lying, particularly where treatment of these structure may be required and therefore a prolonged examination. The examiner could also change hands, with the right hand being used to examine the patient's right and the left hand being used to examine the patient's left with the patient in supine crook lying.

Practical anatomy on the horizontal clock – Internal vaginal

The examination so far has involved evaluation of the structures palpable in a circumferential and caudal to cranial direction. Now on examination of the deep pelvic floor the orientation changes in that the palpating finger examines across the posterior, lateral and posterolateral walls (Figure 13.2).

The palpating finger faces downwards towards the base of the spine and starts with palpation of the coccyx. The most posterior of the pelvic floor muscles is the ischiococcygeus attached from the coccyx to the ischial spine. Anterior to this is the iliococcygeus part of the levator ani group, a thin fan-shaped muscle extending from the tendinous arch of the levator ani (TALA) and with some fibres extending from the anus, to the last two segments of the coccyx (Figure 13.8). The fibres from both sides fuse and will form a raphe contributing to the anococcygeal ligament; this raphe is called the levator plate and provides shelf-like support to the organs. This is important for the configuration of the upper horizontal vaginal axis and support to the rectum and upper two-thirds of the vagina (Singh et al. 2001, Herschorn 2004).

On palpation there should be some sponginess but the iliococcygeus in dysfunction is often palpated as a tense immobile structure. The belly of the iliococcygeus will be palpated at 10 o'clock on the right and 2 o'clock on the left on this horizontal clock. The TALA arises from the fascia overlying the obturator internus and the levator ani muscle and is palpated from the ischial spine forward to the pubic bone anteriorly. It can be palpated more laterally and superiorly than the ATFP posterior to the pubic bone and tracked backwards to the ischial spine.

The ischial spine is palpated as a bony point but the surrounding structures can have a taut end feel so it is not always easy to discriminate between bone and soft tissue. Anterior and inferior to the ischial spine is the pudendal nerve which can then be tracked anteriorly in Alcock's canal (see Chapters 2.3 and 11.2). The obturator internus attaches to the

TALA medially and the ilium laterally; it extends anteriorly to the pubic bone and posteriorly to the ischial spine. The belly of the obturator internus is palpated through the overlying obturator fascia; the obturator canal carrying the obturator nerve is palpated by tracking anteriorly towards the pubic bone.

To maintain contact with these structures while examining, the pad of the finger will now be facing towards the examiner from its internal position on the obturator internus. The structures are then palpated on the left side of the pelvis; for the right-handed examiner it is even more difficult to stay in contact with these deep, lateral structures. The examiner's body position needs to change into the left lateral side flexed position in order to maintain contact with the structures on the patient's left. It is therefore suggested that in order to palpate the patient's left side, the right-handed therapist changes sides and palpates with the left hand.

The attachments of the puborectalis muscle are palpated on the vertical clock at the pubic symphysis. The muscle can be tracked unilaterally backwards by the palpating finger to the rectum in the direction of the coccyx. The continuity of palpation is lost by the rectum and it is then picked up again on the opposite side and tracked forwards to the attachment to the pubic bone. The puborectalis muscle kinks the rectum and forms the anorectal junction. As a sling muscle, the puborectalis should be flexible and stretch should be possible, so tension and resistance can be evaluated by exerting pressure backwards towards a point anterior to the coccyx.

The portion of the levator ani muscle attaching to the anal canal is named the puboanal muscle (Figure 13.8). The orientation here changes and the direction of stretch to determine resistance is towards the anus. The sphincter can be palpated vaginally by opposing the pad of the palpating finger overlying the sphincter and the thumb externally. Tension points can be successfully picked up using this method. A separate anal examination should also take place where indicated (see below).

The puboperineal and pubovaginalis portions of the levator ani have been described in the section on evaluation on the vertical plane; the puborectal and puboanal portions are described above. The pubococcygeal portion arises from the pubic bone and extends to its attachment at the coccyx; the term pubococcygeus can only properly be used to describe the few fibres that join bone to bone (Strobehn et al. 1996). It is palpated laterally to the puborectalis. The pubovisceralis muscle as described by Lawson (1974) is the correct term used to describe the levator ani muscle with its attachment primarily to soft tissue as well as to bone.

Posterior to the ischiococcygeus muscle is the piriformis muscle; the lower portion is palpable vaginally but this may be difficult depending on the length of the examiner's finger. It is attached from the undersurface of the sacrum at levels S2–S4 to the hip at the greater trochanter. Internal palpation is easier rectally. This muscle is successfully accessed and treated externally.

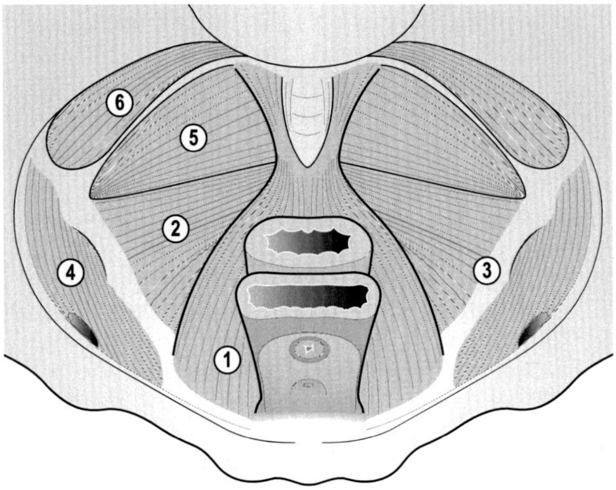

Figure 13.8 • Structures of the pelvic floor examined on the horizontal clock. 1. Pubovisceralis. 2. Iliococcygeus. 3. Tendinous arch of the levator ani. 4. Obturator internus. 5. Ischiocavernosus. 6. Piriformis

Practical anatomy of the male pelvic floor

For the purposes of this chapter, the anatomy of the male pelvic floor is described on the vertical and horizontal planes of examination, with the patient in the crook lying position in the same way as the female pelvic floor was described.

Introduction

The male perineum has been described as fitting into two triangles: an anterior or urogenital perineum, formed by a line through the perineal body extending to the ischial tuberosities on either side and upwards to the symphysis pubis, and posterior perineal triangle formed by the base line through the perineal body and ischial tuberosities where the apex of the triangle is the coccyx (Figure 13.9). On most textbook anatomical views the anus and coccyx on this posterior triangle are depicted on exactly the same plane as the urogenital triangle; however, it can be observed clinically that the anus is slightly more posterior and the coccyx is even more posterior on the supporting surface with the patient in the crook lying position. The urogenital triangle can be useful when observing the structures on the perineum for orientation.

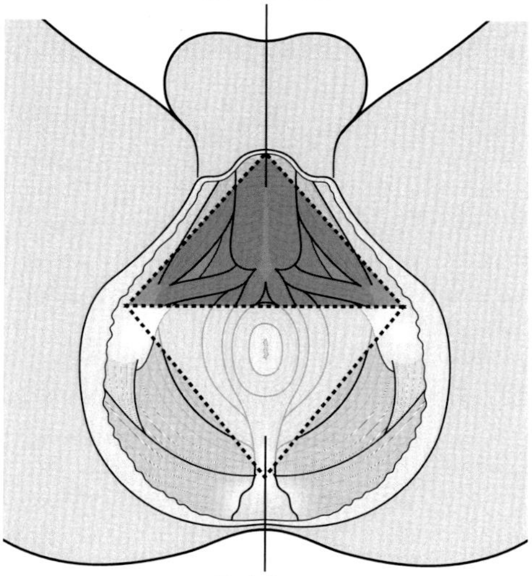

Figure 13.9 • Male perineum, urogenital triangle.
Reproduced from Anson, McVay (1984) Surgical Anatomy, sixth ed. WB Saunders

The vertical clock as described for the female pelvic floor is less practical here without the common access point anterior to the perineal body. Therefore the common base of the clock at 6 o'clock will be the anus with 12 o'clock as the pubic symphysis on the vertical clock and 12 o'clock as the coccyx on the horizontal clock, with the patient in supine crook lying position (see Figure 13.1). Structures accessed through the anus and rectum in a caudocranial direction circumferentially around the examining finger are described on the vertical clock; structures examined on the deep posterior and posterolateral wall are described on the horizontal clock.

Practical anatomy on the vertical clock – External perineal

On the urogenital triangle, the pubic symphysis is at the apex underlying the scrotum, which is lifted up for purposes of examination, and the perineal body is at the central point of the base of the triangle. Attached to the perineal body are the superficial transverse perineii muscles extending out to the ischial tuberosities laterally to the corners of the urogenital triangle. These corners are slightly below the central point of the perineal body. The bulbocavernosus attaches to the perineal body inferiorly and extends upwards inserting into the dorsum of the penis and the perineal membrane. The ischiocavernosus muscles arise from the ischiopubic rami laterally and cover the corpora cavernosa (Figure 13.10).

Deep to these superficial muscles is the perineal membrane which lies in between the triangular shape formed by the two ischiopubic rami on either side and the base formed by the superficial transverse perineal muscles. It is pierced by the urethra and the deep artery and nerve of the penis.

The crus of the penis arises laterally from the ischiopubic ramus to the pubic bone at which point it extends away from the pubic bone becoming external from the body. It becomes the corpora cavernosa of the penis as it extends distally. Medial and deep to this and arising superior to the perineal body is the bulb of the penis which extends centrally becoming the corpus spongiosum and ends in the glans of the penis.

The superficial perineal fascia (Colles' fascia) extends from the ischiopubic ramus across the perineum; the deep perineal fascia (Gallaudet's fascia)

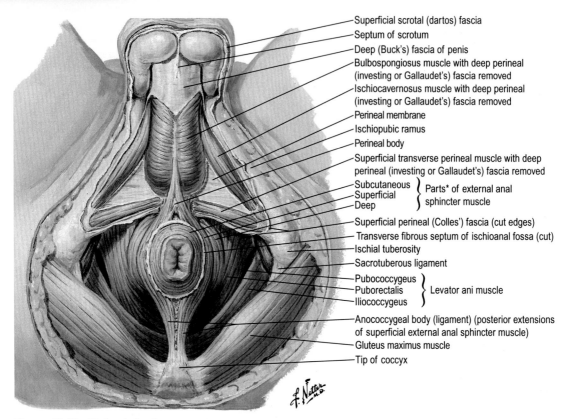

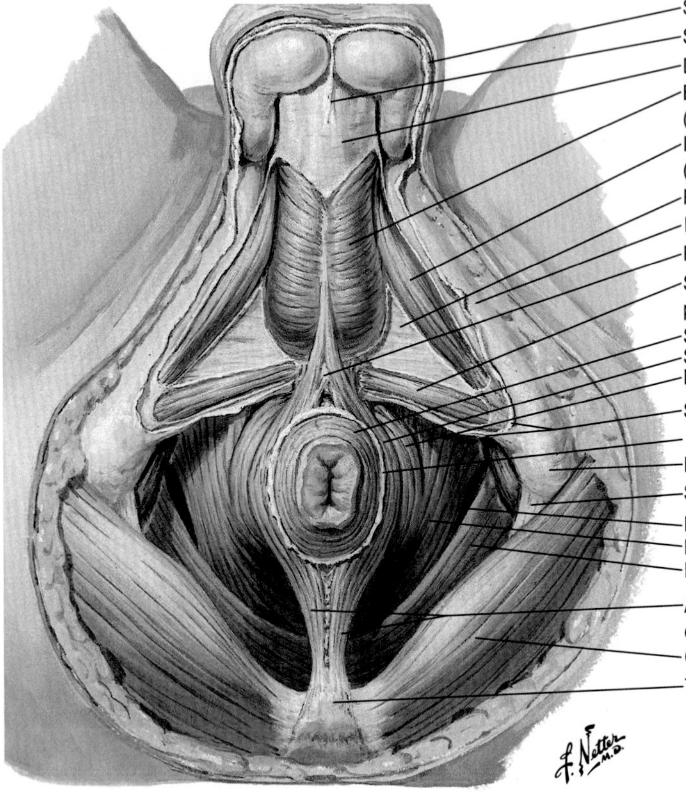

Figure 13.10 • Perineal structures

covers the superficial perineal space of the triangle formed by the bulbospongiosus, ischiocavernosus and superficial transverse perineal muscles. Another fascial layer deeper to this is the Buck's fascia of the penis; it overlies the crus and the bulb of the penis extending up to the glans of the penis.

The scrotum and scrotal tissue overlie the base of the penis. Deep to the skin is the superficial (dartos) fascia of the scrotum. The septum of the scrotum formed by the dartos fascia extends up to the deep Buck's fascia of the penis creating the sac separating right from left. Deep to the dartos fascia each side is the cremaster muscle and fascia and deeper again is the testis. Extending upwards from the testis is the spermatic tissue, arteries and veins.

Practical anatomy on the vertical clock – Internal anal

The assessment is carried out in the crook lying position for descriptive purposes although examinations clinically can take place in side lying or prone lying as well. It can help to run the palpating finger from the coccyx forward along the perineum till the sphincter is reached. Ensuring a well-gelled gloved examining finger the patient is asked to bear down gently to allow easier introduction of the finger. In the case of very overactive pelvic floor muscles this may be extremely painful and it may be necessary to spend time on release techniques before this is even attempted. The sphincter examination is described on the vertical clock although it is slightly more posterior than the other structures on the vertical clock on the perineum.

The anal sphincter has an internal and an external component. The external anal sphincter surrounds the internal anal sphincter. The internal anal sphincter is a thickening of the inner circular smooth layer of the rectum. The external anal sphincter muscle has a subcutaneous, a superficial and a deep portion which are variable and often indistinct. The subcutaneous part attaches to the perineal body. The superficial part also attaches to the perineal body and to the coccyx as the anococcygeal raphe (Figure 13.11). At the posterior inflection of the rectum the deep

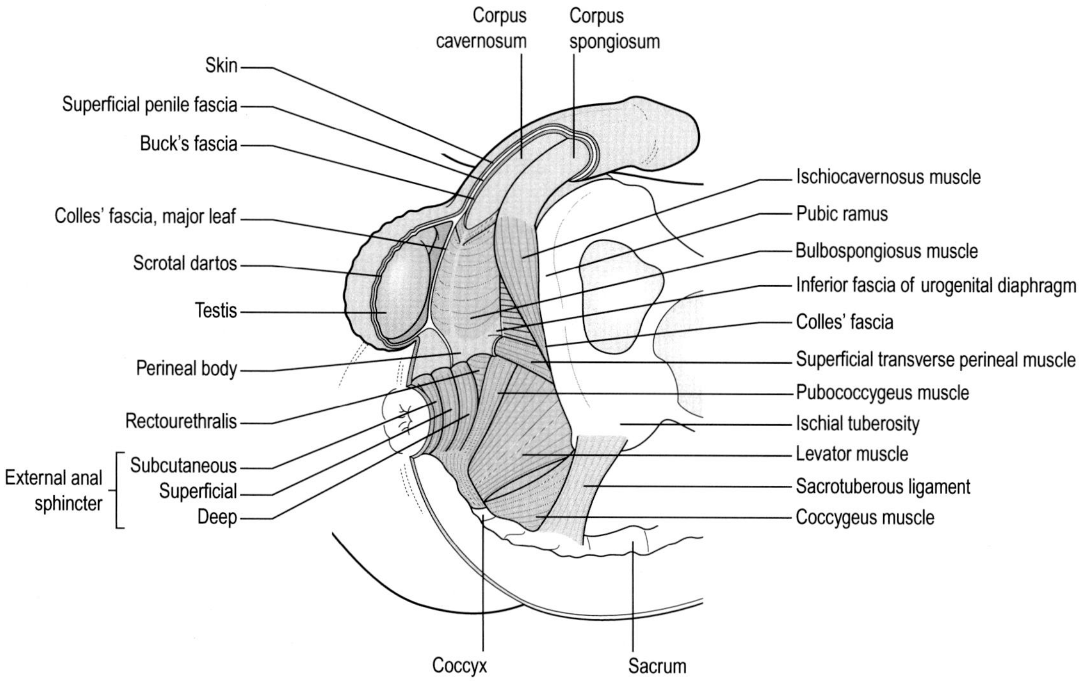

Figure 13.11 • External anal sphincter.

sphincter blends with the puborectalis sling of the levator ani. Along the anal canal, posteriorly is the attachment of the puboanal portion of the levator ani muscle and fascia of the pelvic diaphragm. The corrugator cutis ani muscle situated around the anus is a thin layer of involuntary muscle fibre radiating from the orifice and blending with the skin. It raises the skin into ridges around the margins of the anus.

The pad of the examining finger palpates the full circumference of the sphincter, palpating at first downwards towards the coccyx and then facing upwards towards the pubic bone followed by laterally either side. Movement may be difficult where the sphincter is tight. It should be possible for the patient to be able to relax with the examining finger in place. Overactivity of the sphincter is when it remains difficult to move the examining finger even with the application of release techniques (see Chapter 11).

Practical anatomy on the vertical clock – Internal rectal

Once inside the sphincter the examination on the vertical clock continues. The pad of the palpating finger is turned upwards and the prostate is palpated (Figure 13.12). The prostate has anterior, posterior and lateral surfaces, it has a narrowed apex inferiorly and a broad base superiorly. The base is contiguous with the base of the bladder. It is a glandular and fibromuscular structure, 3 cm in length, 4 cm in width and 2 cm in depth (Brooks 2007). The pubic bone can be palpated below and on either side of the prostate. Deep to and traversing the length of the prostate is the urethra; inferiorly the apex is continuous with the sphincter urethrae muscle and the deep transverse perineal muscles.

The urethra is 18–20 cm long and extends from the bladder neck through the prostate and the penile shaft to its meatus at the glans penis. It is divided into the proximal (sphincteric) portion and the distal (conduit) segment (Dorey 2002). The prostate and bladder base are palpated through the rectal fascia, the rectovesical space and rectovesical and rectoprostatic fascia. There is a further space between the bladder and the pubic bone called the retropubic (Retzius) space. From the rectum towards the prostate there are muscle fibres from the levator ani to the conjoined longitudinal muscle of the anal canal, prerectal muscle fibres from the levator ani muscle and the rectourethralis superior muscle. There are fibromuscular extensions of the levator ani muscle extending from the prostate up to the insertions of the levator ani on to the pubic bone.

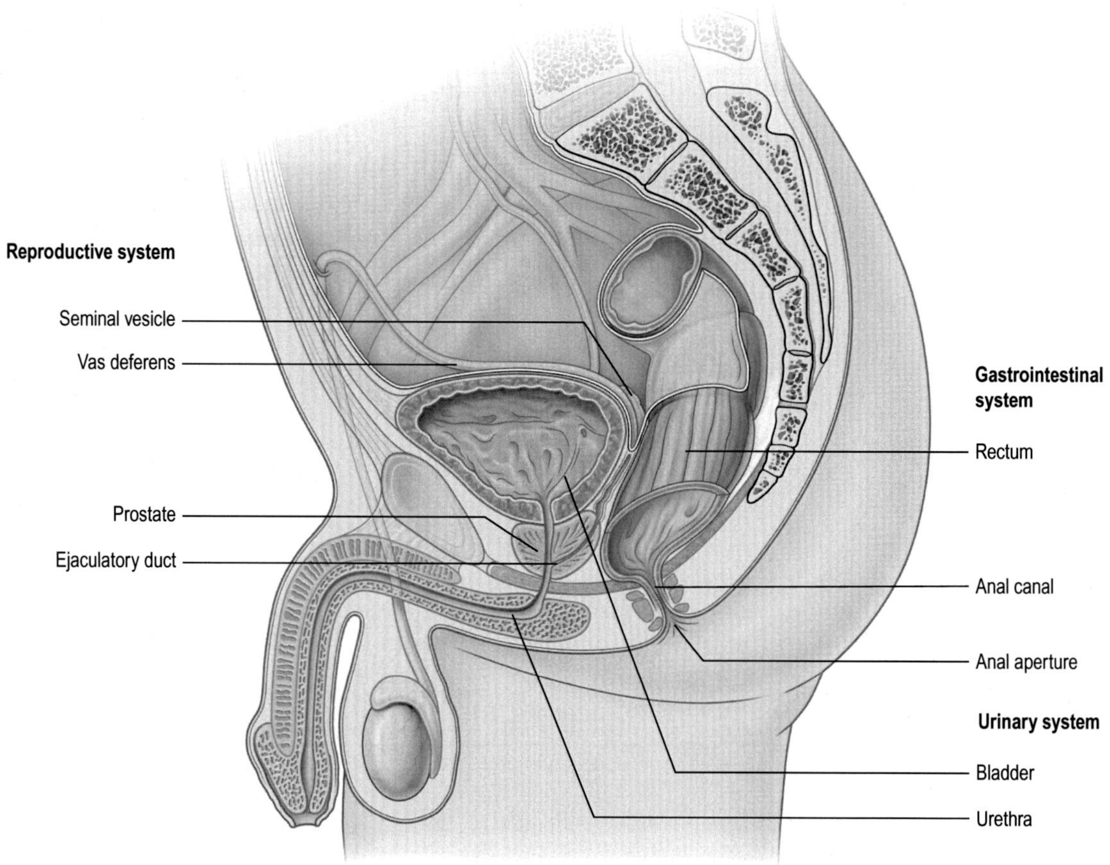

Figure 13.12 • Sagittal pelvic floor

The arcus tendineus fascia pelvis (ATFP) in the male extends from the puboprostatic fascia or the pubourethral ligament to the ischial spine. This fascia forms the junction of the endopelvic fascia and the visceral fascia. The ATFP is found at the base of a sulcus between the pelvic side wall and the prostate and bladder.

Practical anatomy on the horizontal clock – Internal rectal

It is at the apex of the prostate that the anus will open out into the rectum as it extends 90° posteriorly. It is important that there is sufficient relaxation at the sphincter to be able to carry out this examination. The pad of the palpating finger faces down reaching posteriorly towards the examining surface till it comes in contact with the coccyx. The coccyx for purposes of description is at 12 o'clock on the horizontal clock. The ischiococcygeus muscle is palpated extending laterally to the ischial spine from the coccyx. The iliococcygeus muscle arises from the ischial spine and the tendinous arch of the levator ani (TALA) which can be felt all the way to the pubic bone anteriorly (Figure 13.13). The iliococcygeus inserts into the coccyx bone joining with the iliococcygeus from the other side forming the levator plate. Posteriorly the anococcygeal body or ligament is palpable. The pudendal nerve is palpated anteromedially to the ischial spine (see Chapters 2.3 and 11.2).

The puborectalis muscle arises from the pubic bone and extends backwards around the rectum. The puboanal portion of this levator ani muscle joins with fibres of the external anal sphincter, the finger will pull back out from the rectum and pressure is now exerted posteriorly into the anus. The pubococcygeal portion of the levator ani muscle extends backwards to the levator plate and more posteriorly will become the anterior sacrococcygeal ligament on the sacral bone. The TALA arises from the fascia of

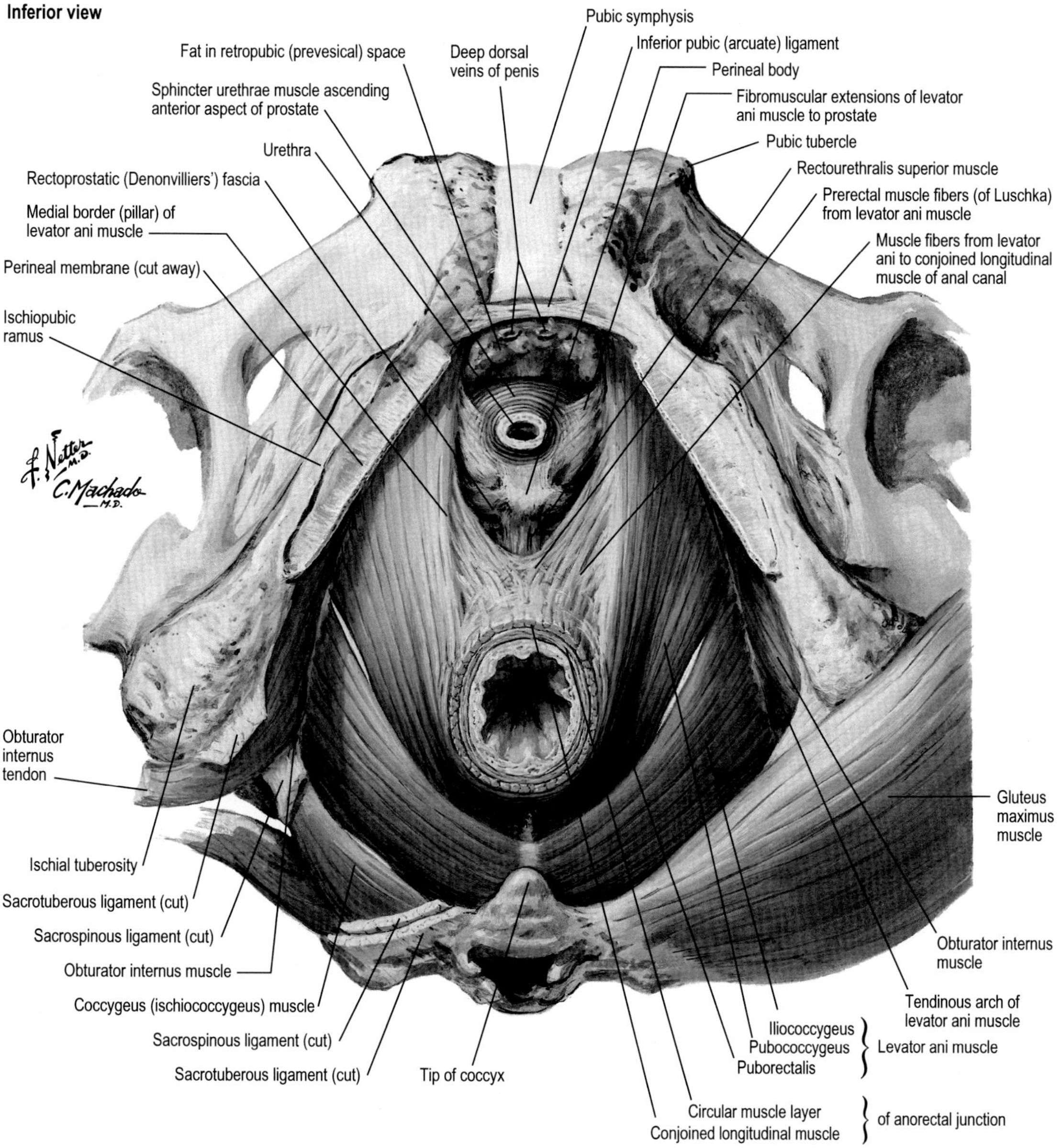

Figure 13.13 • The pelvic diaphragm

the obturator interus and levator ani muscles; it is palpated from the pubic bone laterally and then runs posteriorly to the ischial spine. Lateral to the TALA and attaching to it is the obturator muscle; it attaches in turn laterally again to the ilial bone. The obturator canal carrying the obturator nerve is palpated anteriorly closer to the muscle's attachment to the pubic bone.

The examination is systematically repeated on the other side. If the examiner is right-handed it can be more difficult to remain in contact with the structures as described; if the patient lies on his left side this will be easier, particularly if structures need to be treated and the examination is prolonged. Ideally the examiner will assess the patient's right side with his right hand and the patient's left side with his left hand. This level of dexterity should be developed on an ongoing basis as it can be difficult to change if one has developed the sensitivity in one hand only for both evaluation and treatment.

Direction-specific manual therapy of the pelvic floor

Introduction

Tension and trigger points are associated with chronic pelvic pain conditions and their treatment forms part of the multidisciplinary approach (Weiss 2001, Anderson et al. 2005, 2006, Srinivasan et al. 2007). The background and mechanism of trigger points are discussed in depth in Chapter 11. Trigger points can be treated successfully externally and internally and manual therapy is the first treatment of choice (Dommerholt et al. 2006). External treatment of the pelvic floor is described in Chapter 11. This section explores the release of trigger points and tension in the pelvic floor specifically using the concept of the direction of movement of the pelvic floor to maximize the effect.

The pelvic floor has a specific direction of activation: a contraction will squeeze the vagina, urethra and rectum closed against the pubic bone and lift the organs in a cephalic direction (Ashton-Miller & DeLancey 2007), but the direction of contraction will not always be cranioventral where dysfunction exists (Jones et al. 2006). If a pelvic floor contraction is normally cranioventral then release should normally be dorsocaudal. The levator ani will have a slightly different direction of activation depending on the part of the muscle and the fibre orientation, the puborectalis kinks the anorectal junction and will lift cranioventrally, the pubovaginalis, puboperinealis and puboanal muscles will elevate the perineal body and anus (Peschers & DeLancey 2008).

Part of the principle of treatment of a trigger point is to sufficiently elongate the muscle, producing a maximum palpable distinction between the normal tonus of the uninvolved fibres and increased tension of the taut band fibres. Optimal tension is usually about two-thirds of the muscle's normal stretch range of motion but may be only one-third or less with very active trigger points (Travell & Simons 1999).

If muscle length is affected by the existence of trigger points then it would seem logical to consider the direction of the muscle contraction in order to maximize the release. This section looks at direction-specific manual therapy of the pelvic floor, taking into account muscle function and fibre orientation. The techniques are mainly internal as they are specific to movement of the pelvic floor although the superficial muscles of the perineum are also described.

Release of muscle and fascia externally is also key in treatment of chronic pelvic pain disorders. These techniques are described separately in Chapter 11.

Techniques

The direction-specific manual therapy techniques in this section are described on the vertical and horizontal planes following a system of examination outlined above.

The exact techniques can vary according to the clinician's findings; however, the techniques used may be limited because of the reduced accessibility with single-digit palpation vaginally or rectally. Generally the palpation techniques described by Travell & Simons (1999) will cover all muscles in the pelvic floor: flat palpation, pincer palpation and deep palpation. These will generally be static compression techniques as transverse friction is not advisable in the deep pelvic floor as the tissue can be delicate and the condition is not visible.

- Flat palpation is where the finger tip slides the overlying fascia aside and palpates across the fibres to be examined.
- Pincer palpation is performed by grasping the muscle between the finger tip and thumb and pressing the fibres or rolling forwards and backwards to locate taut bands; these techniques will be for the superficial or more accessible tissue.
- Deep palpation is when intervening tissue overlies the muscle containing the trigger point and palpation through tissue is necessary. 'Sufficient pressure on a trigger point always elicits at least withdrawal, wincing or vocalization by the patient' (Travell & Simons 1999).

The amount of time spent on restricted tissue and the amount of pressure exerted will vary according to the sensitivity of the tissue. General treatment of central and attachment trigger points has been well documented by Chaitow & DeLany (2002) and the timing described by the same authors in integrated neuromuscular inhibition technique (Chaitow 1994) has been found by the author to be effective. They describe a pressure sufficient to activate the trigger point is maintained for 5–6 seconds followed by 2–3 seconds release and repeated for up to 2 minutes until the patient reports that the local or referred symptoms have reduced. Importantly the ischaemic pressure is stopped if there is an increase in pain or if the pain has ceased. This is followed in the original description by positional release techniques but can also be followed in the pelvic floor by direction-specific breathing techniques to maximize the release, and other breathing techniques as described in Chapter 7.

Transverse massage or longitudinal stretch massage can be used to lengthen the tissue (Hong et al. 1993). Massage of the pelvic floor can be performed rectally or vaginally; this was first described rectally by Thiele (1963). He recommended rubbing the fibres along their length, with a stripping motion from attachment at the pubic bone to insertion at the coccyx. Levator ani massage was also described by Grant et al. (1975) in successful treatment of patients with levator ani syndrome. Travell & Simons (1999) described stripping massage as a powerful tool in activation of accessible myofascial trigger points. Malbohan et al. (1989) described successful levator ani massage with a dorsal movement of the coccyx to stretch the levator ani in treatment of low back pain attributed to coccygeal spasm.

Treatment timing will vary according to the patient's sensitivity. Patients do however tolerate treatment well as 'the' pain has been identified. An internal vaginal treatment may be tolerated well for 15–20 minutes with good effect varying between passive treatment as described above, breathing release and patient-assisted release (see description later in this chapter). Rectal treatment may be less well tolerated due to the more restricted tissue mobility and its sensitivity.

Manual techniques on the vertical plane

Travell & Simons (1993) have stated that none of the superficial muscles are likely to be identifiable unless they have taut bands lying parallel to the direction of the muscle fibres. Furthermore they are likely to present as single muscle syndromes with pain referral locally and into the urethra, perineum and the vulva in women and the penis in men, whereas levator ani and coccygeus are more likely to exhibit multiple muscle involvement.

Superficial transverse perineii

In the female the perineal body is palpated posteriorly at the introitus of the vagina. The transverse perineii are palpated centrally from the perineal body to the ischial tuberosities laterally with flat palpation from the outside. The pad of the palpating finger is then inserted into the vagina turned to face the examiner palpating the transverse perineii from the inside and opposing the thumb on the outside. The belly of the muscle is palpated as it is pressed between the finger and the thumb moving medially to laterally; the muscle can be moved in a forward and backwards direction as it is held between the finger and the thumb to evaluate mobility and treat existing taut bands or trigger points. This manoeuvre is repeated, extending out laterally as far as the attachment point to the ischial tuberosities. In the male, flat palpation can be used as described, or pincer grip with the index finger inserted into and past the anus until the pad faces upwards and forwards towards the examiner and opposes the thumb placed along the transverse perineii muscles externally.

Bulbospongiosus

Bulbospongiosus can be pressed by finger pad pressure externally as it extends along the two sides of the entrance of the vagina from the perineal body to below the clitoris, or the pad of the finger is placed inside the vagina and the thumb opposes from the outside using the pincer palpation techniques and the muscle is palpated for taut bands. If present they are rolled between the finger and thumb until there is a change in either tension or pain referral. In the male the bulbospongiosus can be palpated from the perineal body up to the base of the penis surrounding the corpus spongiosum using flat palpation. Pincer palpation can also be applied as the pad of the palpating finger remains at the perineal body end and the thumb opposes at the corpus spongiosum end both externally. Alternatively pincer palpation is applied medial to lateral across the width of the muscle and at intervals along its length.

Ischiocavernosus

In the female the ischiocavernosus muscle can be pressed with flat palpation as it is rolled over the length of the pubic ramus by the palpating finger or fingers from outside against the bone. The upper insertion can be palpated with the bulbospongiosus changing from pincer palpation as described with bulbospongiosus to flat palpation with the thumb against the ischiocavernosus and the index finger remaining inside the vagina facing outwards to oppose. In this way the insertion can be mobilized with a forward and backwards and rolling motion. In the male, flat palpation is applied externally and the ischiocavernosus can be rolled against the underlying ischiopubic ramus; one finger can be used or the pads of three fingers simultaneously.

Anterior to posterior levator ani stretch

This anterior to posterior stretch has already been described by Weiss (2001) in the female pelvic floor (Figure 13.14). The distal phalynx of the palpating finger rests on the posterior vaginal wall from the perineal body to approximately 2 cm inside. The puboperineal muscle and the pubovaginal muscles are stretched posteriorly and taut bands or points of referral are identified and treated by ischaemic pressure until the tension eases or the referral decreases. The attachments are followed laterally up to the pubic bone and the pressure becomes more specific laterally to evaluate the insertions on either side. Attachment trigger points result from sustained increased tension of the muscle fibres to their bony insertion. This sustained tension can produce swelling and tenderness described as enthesopathy where the muscle fibres attach (Travell & Simons 1999). This is an important point for evaluation and resistance may be high at these points especially with pelvic floor overactivity.

Arcus tendineus fascia pelvis

The ATFP are tensile structures corresponding in the female to the lateral attachment of the anterior bladder wall to the pelvic side wall and the base of a sulcus between the pelvic side wall, the prostate and bladder in the male (Brooks 2007). They are palpable as well-defined fibrous bands at the origin near the pubic bone becoming less well defined as they pass posteriorly to insert into the ischial spine fusing with the endopelvic fascia and merging with the levator ani (Ashton-Miller & DeLancey 2007) (Figure 13.6).

The ATFP connection to the pubis lies 1 cm above the inferior margin of the pubic symphysis and 1 cm lateral to the midline (DeLancey 1990); it is palpated with the pad of the finger along the undersurface of the pubic bone on the anterior vaginal wall and the anterior rectal wall in the male. Contact is soon lost as the fascia extends posteriorly superiorly alongside the base of the bladder in the direction of the ischial spine. This structure is distinguished from the attachment of the tendinous arch of the levator ani described in the next section as it extends across from the vertical to the horizontal plane.

Damage to this fascia and its attachments has been implicated in cystocele, urethrocele and stress urinary incontinence in females, so its presence and presentation will be variable (Brooks 2007).

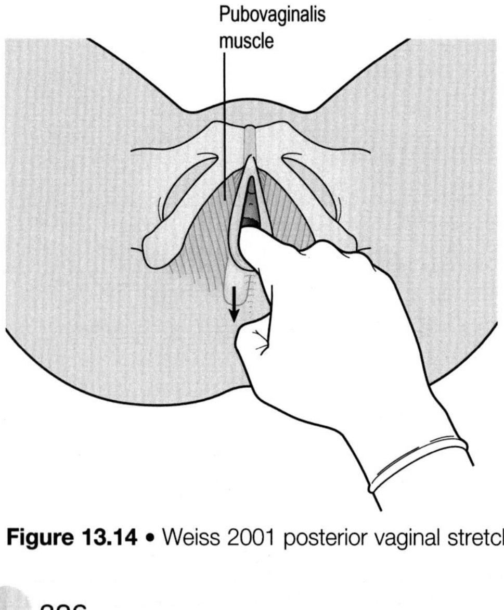

Figure 13.14 • Weiss 2001 posterior vaginal stretch

Urethra

The urethra is palpated on the vertical plane with the pad of the palpating finger facing upwards from the urethral meatus cranially to the urethrovesical junction posterior to the pubic bone and as far as the bladder base. The overlying connective tissue will be variable in sensitivity and mobility; quality of movement can be tested by gliding the pad of the finger either caudocranially along the urethra posterior to the pubic bone or transversely moving the urethra laterally. These lateral distraction techniques have been described by Weiss (2001) (Figure 13.15) and under connective tissue manipulation in Chapter 11.2.

Pain on palpation from the pubic bone as far as the urethrovesical junction on the anterior wall of the vagina is frequently secondary to other superficial and deep trigger points. This area should be tested at the start of the examination and retested following intervention.

In the male the urethra traverses the prostate centrally and is therefore only palpable through the prostate in this prostatic portion on internal examination. Prostatic massage has been described as therapeutic in the treatment of urologic chronic pelvic pain (Anderson et al. 2009).

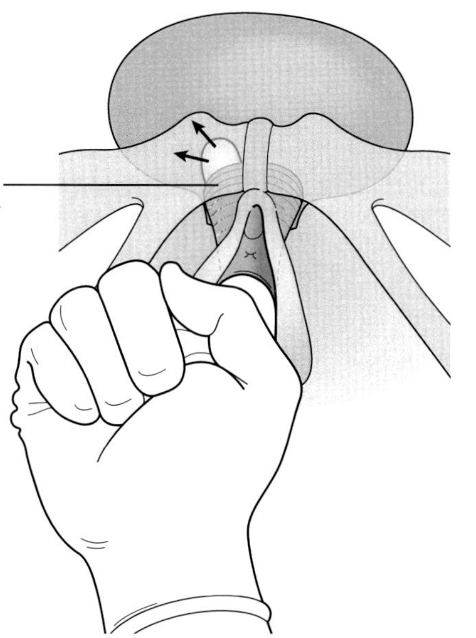

Figure 13.15 • Weiss 2001 lateral mobilization of urethral sphincter

External anal sphincter

Treatment through the external anal sphincter is commenced by asking the patient to bear down as the gelled examining finger is introduced. If the sphincter is tight, as it may be with chronic pelvic pain or defecation disorders, then extreme care should be taken and other external manual techniques may be necessary before proceeding. Treatment techniques are commenced as the pad of the finger faces the supporting surface in crook lying position, the sphincter eases out as the finger is introduced at first 1–2 cm and then further to 3–4 cm incorporating the puborectalis muscles (Dorey 2002). If sufficient range of movement is available the finger can be turned the full circumference of the sphincter turning towards the right and towards the left and feeling for resistance and differences throughout the higher portion and the lower portion of the sphincter, then pressing into areas of resistance.

Stretching of the sphincter can manually be a challenge in men who have a lot of pelvic floor tension. The tissue will usually be more mobile in women even when the sphincter is overactive. Care needs to be taken in case of fissures and haemorrhoids, although these are not contraindications to treatment.

A further technique to treat the external anal sphincter is using pincer palpation with the thumb externally over the sphincter opposing the index finger internally resting over the vaginal tissue on the sphincter. This way the entire sphincter can be palpated for any tension and mobilized accordingly. In the male this pincer palpation is also possible through the anus but only segmental mobilization is possible between finger and thumb (see Figures 13.5 and 13.11).

Manual techniques crossing over vertical to horizontal plane

Puborectalis

Puborectalis is accessed either vaginally (as a first choice) or rectally in women and rectally in men. It is stretched from the attachment at the pubic bone anteriorly to behind the rectum posteriorly and deep in the direction of a point anterior to the coccyx (Figure 13.16). Deep in the pelvic floor, the

Figure 13.16 • Anterior to posterior puborectalis stretch

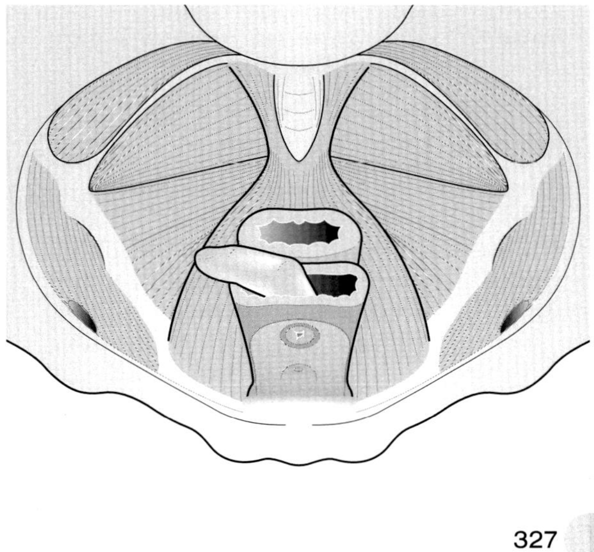

puborectalis spans from just posterior to the anus supporting the rectum, to just anterior to the coccyx. The entire muscle is evaluated for trigger points, areas of referral and taut bands. When symptomatic, the patient may report a strong feeling of faecal urge or a shooting pain up into the rectum or pain referring elsewhere inside the vagina in the female or perineum and penis in the male. The patient may also describe pain referral into the coccyx. The terms proctalgia or proctalgia fugax are often used as an umbrella term to describe the symptoms of referred pain with elicitation of a puborectalis trigger point; proctalgia by definition is a disorder of the internal anal sphincter. Right and left are evaluated and compared. The downward stretch will feel very resistant on the overactive pelvic floor and it may take a few sessions to unfold a specific referring trigger point. If there is loss of attachment, the surrounding and contralateral muscle may hypertrophied as it is overloaded (Dietz 2009). Deep palpation will be needed in the puborectalis muscle.

Puboanalis

The puboanal muscle is distinct from the puborectalis; it is further forwards and the direction of stretch changes from towards the coccyx to towards the anus. The attachment point is picked up at the pubic bone and the direction is steeper than with puborectalis to the anal canal. Pressure onto the anus often reproduces a faecal urge which is stronger the more symptomatic the patient is. The patient may also get a strong sensation that stool is present and needs to be reassured by the examiner. The stretch starts off as the posterior vaginal stretch but as the finger extends approximately 3 cm back into the vagina the palpating finger flexes to follow the muscle into the anal canal. In the male the examining finger needs to pull out so that the pad of the finger is pressing on the superficial sphincter.

Tendinous arch of levator ani

The TALA inserts anteriorly into the pubic bone and posteriorly to the ischial spine as does the ATFP but the orientation is different. The TALA is palpated more laterally and superiorly on the pubic bone than the ATFP. Contact can be maintained throughout as it is followed laterally and posteriorly to the ischial spine. Palpation is started with the finger pad facing upwards on the vertical plane and laterally along the pubic bone until the thin tendinous attachment is identified, then the finger will need to turn facing downwards, laterally towards the side wall of the pelvis and posteriorly as it follows the arch backwards to its attachment at the ischial spine (see Figure 13.8).

As the TALA is the tendon of the fascia of the levator ani, it can be tender on palpation and reproduce painful symptoms in the pelvic floor. Frequently as the levator ani muscles are released, this tenderness can change and palpation for tenderness should be repeated following intervention.

Manual techniques on the horizontal plane

In the case of an overactive pelvic floor or chronic pelvic pain it may be necessary to spend time first on manual therapy on the vertical plane and on other myofascial release techniques and learned breathing techniques before any of these muscles can be accessed on the horizontal plane. These techniques are carried out vaginally in women as a first choice, and rectally in men.

Posterior fibres of puborectalis and pubococcygeus

The posterior fibres of the puborectalis around the back of the rectum can often be involved with defecation and rectal pain disorders. The direction of release here is very specific in a downward motion towards the supporting surface anterior to the coccyx. Visualization from the patient during treatment of lengthening the arms of the U-shaped sling muscle backwards or opening the back passage backwards can assist release.

The few fibres of the levator ani that attach onto the coccyx are the pubococcygeus muscle. The coccyx is identified and palpated on its ventral surface and the muscle attachments are palpated applying pressure downward towards the supporting surface both onto the bone itself and anterior to the bone; taut bands are evaluated as the finger pressure is applied both perpendicular to and along the length of the muscle fibres.

Iliococcygeus and the levator plate

The iliococcygeus is described as the shelf support muscle of the pelvic floor; it is a thin fan-shaped muscle extending from the tendinous arch of the levator ani to the coccyx. The fibres are more horizontal centrally as they insert into the coccyx and form part of the anococcygeal raphe (Strohbehn et al. 1996). The raphe between the anus and coccyx is the levator plate; it is formed by the fusion of the iliococcygeus and the posterior fibres of the pubococcygeus (Herschorn 2004). The point of palpation to identify tension in the belly of the muscle is, on the horizontal clock, at 10 o'clock on the right and 2 o'clock on the left in a posterolateral direction towards the supporting surface (see section on anatomy). When the iliococcygeus muscle has been overloaded there is no 'give' in this direction and deep pressure reveals a taut, fibrous muscle (see Box 13.1, Figure 13.17).

Downward and lateral pressure is exerted into the belly of the muscle and the fibres are stretched towards the supporting surface. The muscle can be quite taut throughout and it can take time and significant pressure to pick out symptomatic taut bands and trigger points. The description by Wilson (1936) of the muscle fibres being 'matted together' works well here. During treatment, the patient often describes a feeling of a hard bar on the supporting surface under the pelvis. There may be pain referral to the hip area or to the coccyx and this area can also reproduce some rectal symptoms. It can be acutely painful but frees up over the course of a session of manual therapy and activation can be felt to change where the cranioventral activation of the pelvic floor improves (see Box 13.1).

Box 13.1

Note on iliococcygeus specific to female anatomy

The iliococcygeus muscle is not thought to have a role in the cranioventral activation of the pelvic floor because of the orientation of the fibres. It is injured in childbirth considerably less often than the pubovisceral portion of the levator ani (DeLancey et al. 2003). It was reported in one study that only three out of 32 birth injuries were to iliococcygeus; the rest were to the pubovisceral portion of the muscle (DeLancey et al. 2003). A contractile iliococcygeus will elevate the pad of the palpating finger uniform with the rest of the levator ani. When inhibited a levator ani contraction will flex the palpating finger and the iliococcygeus does not stay in contact with the pad of the palpating finger. It has been reported that surrounding muscles are overloaded by trigger-pointed muscles or by loss of attachment (Weiss 2001, DeLancey & Ashton-Miller 2007, Dietz 2009). It could therefore be that inhibition of the iliococcygeus indirectly affects the cranioventral activation of the other levator ani muscles because of its proximity to them and its attachments laterally and posteriorly pulling the muscles in this posterolateral direction. The significance of this is that if the shelf support role of the iliococcygeus is lost then the load of the organs on the pelvic floor will be greater, causing further stress inhibition and trigger points on the pelvic floor muscles.

Ischiococcygeus

Access to the ischiococcygeus muscle may be difficult vaginally depending on the length of the examiner's finger. The muscle is considerably narrower than the iliococcygeus. It extends from the ischial spine to the lateral border of the sacrum and coccyx. Downward pressure perpendicular to the fibre orientation is exerted towards the supporting surface and slightly cranially under the tip of the palpating finger. In cases where the coccyx is involved in a pain syndrome, this may be acutely painful. As the muscle

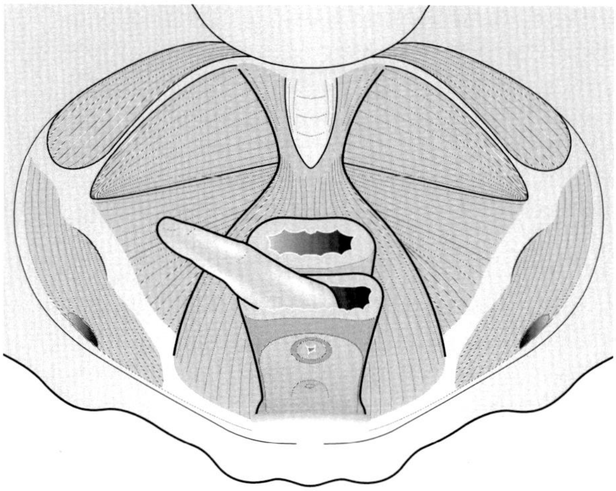

Figure 13.17 • Posterolateral stretch and facilitation

is so far posterior it is difficult to exert the pressure that may be necessary to identify and release taut bands or trigger points. Release of this muscle can be successfully performed anally and mobilization of the coccyx may be indicated as well. The palpating index finger presses into the ischiococcygeus internally and the index finger or thumb of the opposite hand opposes the finger externally. This can be repeated to the coccyx as the muscle and/or the coccyx is moved in a forward and backwards motion. The ischiococcygeus can also be massaged in the direction of the muscle fibres medially to laterally. These techniques can be repeated for iliococcygeus.

Both the iliococcygeus and the ischiococcygeus muscles can be accessed through the ischiorectal fossa, the area between the ischial spine and anus externally. Palpation internally and simultaneously externally can confirm the point to be accessed externally as an inwards pressure from the external point can be easily felt internally on the muscle. It can help the patient as they palpate the point externally at the same time as the therapist palpates internally to become familiar with the point as they self treat at home.

The use of a tennis ball can be successful for home programmes. The patient locates the point of the ilio- or ischiococcygeus muscle in the ischiorectal fossa and sits into a hard surface to release the muscle either rolling or staying in the one position for up to 20 seconds on each point until the pain, tension or pain referral eases. The patient should be warned not to press onto the coccyx itself as the skin is thin here and may break down particularly where connective tissue restrictions exist.

Obturator internus

The obturator internus extends over to the side wall of the pelvis. Palpation is still best described on the horizontal plane. The fibres are palpated using flat pad pressure as the therapist turns the palpating finger downwards and then over and slightly upwards to the side wall, the TALA is palpated and the obturator internus lies laterally. The fibres are followed all the way forwards to their attachment point on the inner surface of the pubic bone and posteriorly to the ischial spine. If the therapist is right-handed then the palpating finger will be facing around towards the therapist as the therapist stands on the patient's right when in contact with the obturator internus. Resisted hip abduction will confirm the correct location. In the symptomatic patient the obturator nerve in the obturator canal may be painful; this can be used as a retest point once some of these manual techniques have been tried. Pain referral can sometimes be into the posterior proximal region of the thigh.

When palpating the left side of the patient the therapist will be in a left laterally side bent position with the right elbow high in order to access these left lateral structures. Ideally the therapist will have developed ambidextrous skills to be able to treat the patient's left side with the therapist's left hand. Alternatively for the right-handed therapist the patient could be positioned in left side lying to access the left side. The obturator internus is successfully accessed for treatment externally (see Chapter 11.1).

Weiss (2001) described palpation of the obturator internus with simultaneous stretch of the muscle in lateral hip rotation (see Figure 13.18).

Direction-specific breathing release

The guidelines described below and illustrated in the DVD on direction-specific breathing release are designed to achieve pelvic floor relaxation. They should not be confused with the specific breathing rehabilitation exercises described in Chapter 9 and its video demonstration.

Introduction

In recent years there has been much literature describing the effects and importance of breathing on the musculoskeletal system; these are investigated

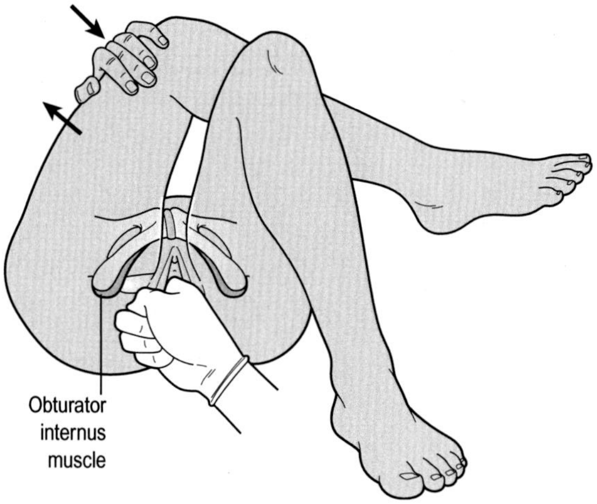

Figure 13.18 • Obturator internus treated with hip in rotation. Reproduced from Weiss (2001) Pelvic floor myofascial trigger points: manual therapy for interstitial cystitis and the urgency-frequency syndromes. J. Urol. 166, 2226–2231

in detail in Chapter 9. The involvement of the abdomen has also been well documented and is now an integral part of any physiotherapy treatment for chronic pelvic pain (Slocumb 1984, Fitzgerald et al. 2009, Kotarinos et al. 2009, Montenegro et al. 2009).

If a patient is in acute pain then internal manual techniques will be difficult to tolerate and it will be prudent to spend time learning breathing release and abdominal release techniques to counteract tension. Studies have looked at the interaction of the pelvic floor with breathing (O'Sullivan et al. 2002, O'Sullivan & Beales 2007, Pool Goodzward 2004, Hodges et al. 2007) and the descent of the pelvic floor has been described as a normal consequence of inspiration (Talasz et al, 2010). Paradoxical relaxation has been described in Chapter 12, and its success has been documented (Anderson et al. 2005, 2006). The technique described below has been developed by the author in its current form to help with direction-specific release.

The current technique involves inspiration, diaphragmatic descent and simultaneous release of the abdomen in order to produce a direction-specific release of the pelvic floor. This release is passive in the pelvic floor and should happen as a consequence of the correctly performed in-breath; however, the ability of the patient to maximally release the posterior pelvic floor helps the quality of the release. The 'cylinder' is explained and an image portrayed of a taut elastic band between the diaphragm and the pelvic floor (Figure 13.19). The taut band represents the tension within the muscles and fascia between the diaphragm and the pelvic floor. As the patient breathes in the diaphragm descends and the abdomen fills out, the elastic band is slackened allowing a release of the pelvic floor (Figure 13.20). This release is dependent on the abdomen being maximally released at the same time as it expands. Any tension at all in the abdomen will stop the release happening in the pelvic floor. The patient learns to visualize the direction of release of the pelvic floor and how to use their in-breath to control it. This is described to the patient as 'sniff, flop and drop' and is broken down for teaching purposes as follows.

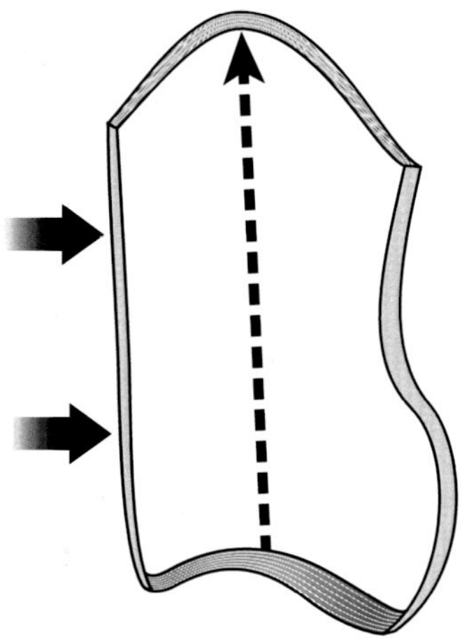

Figure 13.19 • Taut band showing tension in cylinder

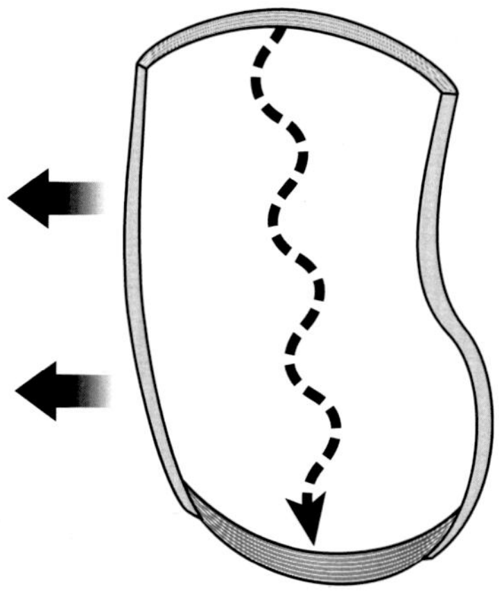

Figure 13.20 • Slackened band showing release in cylinder

Sniff, flop and drop technique

Abdominal palpation

The patient lies supine with legs out straight so that the abdominal muscles are somewhat on stretch. The patient learns to identify their points of tension through the abdomen from the ribs to the pubic bone but the upper abdomen is the key point in allowing the diaphragm to descend. The upper triangle formed by the lower ribs up to the xiphisternum is the area that should be focused on at first to allow optimal descent of the diaphragm. The patient is shown self-palpation using deep perpendicular pressure through the rectus abdominis, the oblique muscles and abdominal fascia. They may also work with a manual therapist to achieve better release. In addition the use of a therapeutic 'spikey' ball or tennis ball at home may be helpful as the patient lies on the ball starting off supported on the elbows, to identify a tension point, and then lowering gradually onto the ball and wriggling on it to identify specific areas of tension. The patient can then breathe with emphasis on breathing out, while relaxing as the pressure from the ball eases the local tension. This

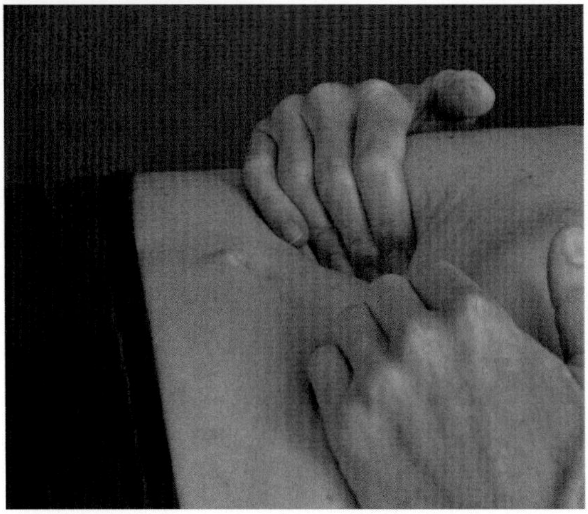

Figure 13.21 • Patient palpating upper abdomen

technique should be performed starting with any tension on the lower right abdomen and working around to the upper right, upper left and lower left to follow the direction of the colon into the bowel. The patient should not spend more than 10 seconds on each point before rolling slightly off onto another adjoining point (Figure 13.21).

Sniff

The patient learns to breathe into the abdomen rather than the chest, and learns how to expand the abdomen without raising the chest or blocking the breathing. The patient palpates the upper abdomen all the time maintaining softness. The breath in is described as a *sniff* to put emphasis on the volume of air that is needed to make the diaphragm descend. It therefore needs to be loud but not forced. Generally if the inhalation is too shallow it is hard to create sufficient diaphragmatic descent, and if it is not quick enough, the muscles will push the abdomen out rather than allowing the passive filling with breathing. The patient can be shown an example of the elbow letting go from a flexed position. If it is let go slowly the biceps will work eccentrically, but if dropped quickly there will be no muscle control, just letting go.

If the in-breath has been performed correctly, with the abdomen letting go, then the exhalation that follows will be short and soft, as if all the air had 'disappeared'. This can be compared with the short and soft out-breath, used to clean a pair of spectacles (Figures 13.22 and 13.23).

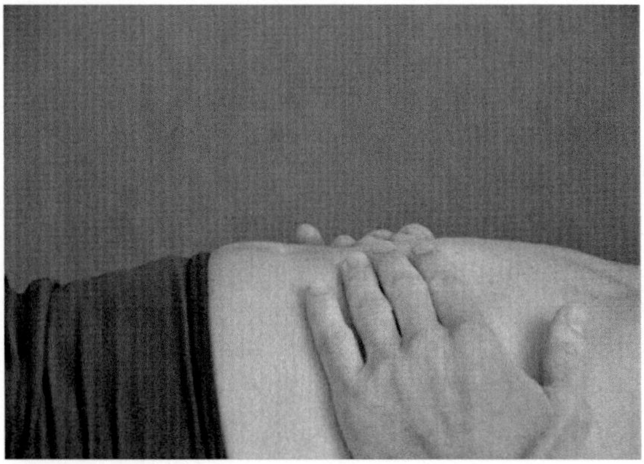

Figure 13.22 • Correct inhalation with sniff

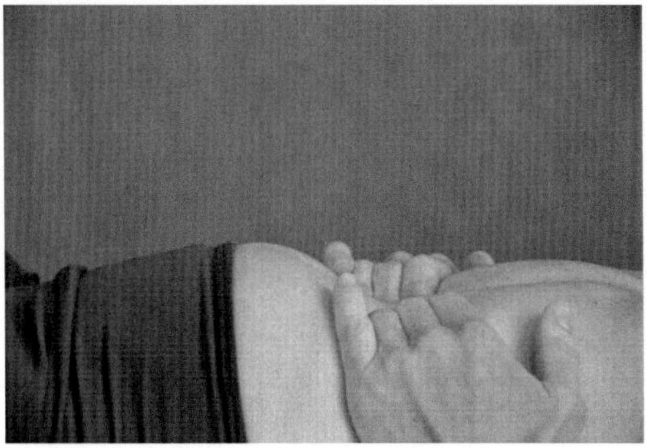

Figure 13.23 • Incorrect inhalation with sniff

Flop

The patient is taught to identify their stomach-holding pattern and to learn where their flexion/holding line may be. The patient also learns how to let go from the ribs down to the pubic bone or just *flop* the stomach out. Again this is assisted by palpation and manual therapy. The flop may be more productive in side lying as gravity assists and the patient has the image of letting go into the supporting surface. This can also be worked on in forward kneeling, e.g. resting arms on a gym ball or in four-point kneeling. It can be counterintuitive to flop up against gravity (Figures 13.24 and 13.25).

Drop

The patient learns to release the pelvic floor in an action that is called a *drop*. The patient is taught that the pelvic floor releases backwards, visualization and demonstration with diagrams helps the individual to feel a release in the direction of the coccyx. It is

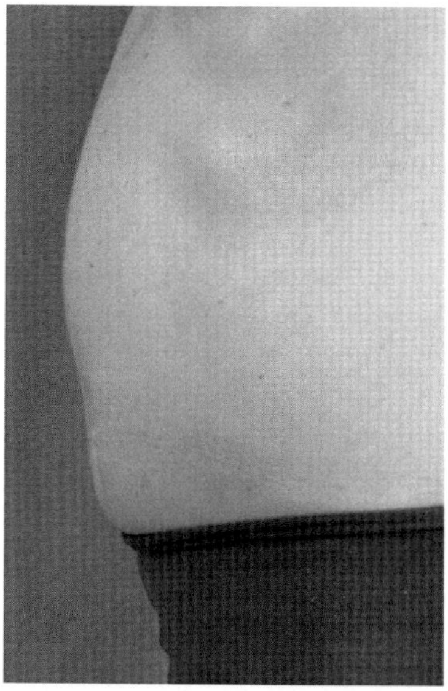

Figure 13.24 • Correct abdominal flop

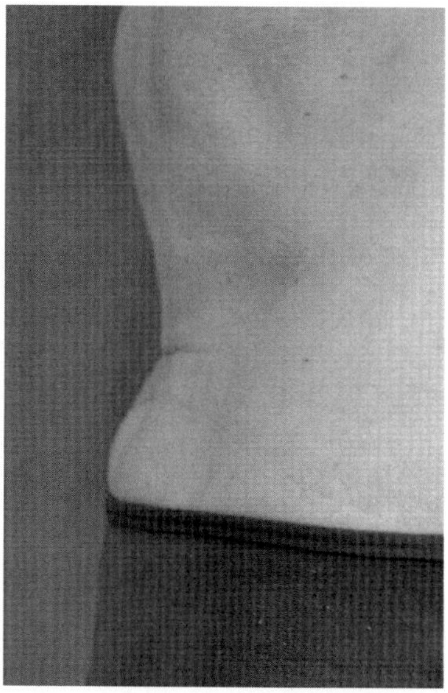

Figure 13.25 • Incorrect abdomen held

explained that the pelvic floor has some tone even at rest and it is this resting tone that is being changed with the release. The release can be described as an opening of the sphincter muscle or a lengthening of the U-shaped sling muscle backwards towards the supporting surface or coccyx. The patient can also think of opening or flaring the coccyx backwards towards the supporting surface (Figures 13.26 and 13.27).

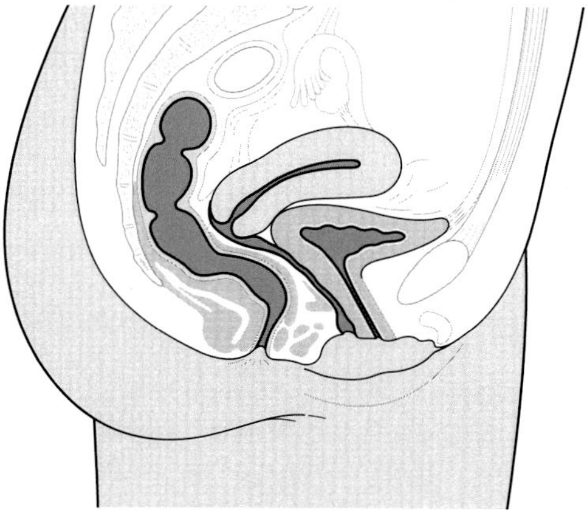

Figure 13.26 • Pelvic floor released

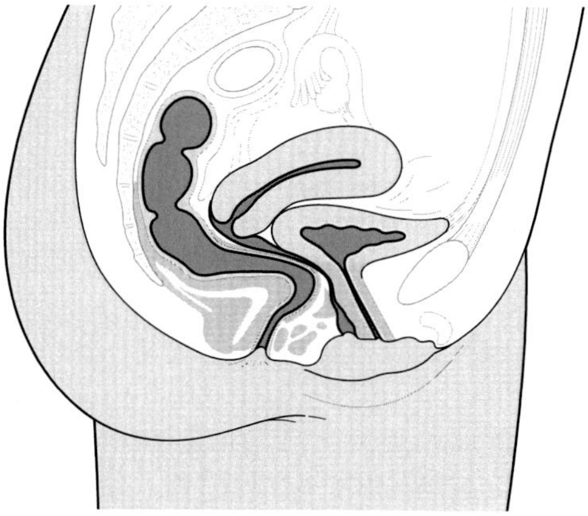

Figure 13.27 • Pelvic floor contracted

Sniff, flop and drop

When sniff and flop as well as flop and drop can be successfully coordinated, then sniff, flop and drop is practiced as one coordinated movement. The patient sniffs in as the stomach flops out, and the pelvic floor drops at the same time. This is held for approximately 3 seconds and the movement is appreciated by the patient. A better drop can be felt if the patient can actively release, and the earlier in the sniff that the drop is performed the better the quality of release. This is not easy, particularly when the pelvic floor is holding tension, but nonetheless the majority of patients will grasp the concept either on the first session or within a few sessions. The motor control required is significant and therefore a lot of concentration is required. It is important to emphasize to the patient that the less effort they use, the more successful the techniques will be.

It is important not to combine these three components until diaphragmatic breathing and abdominal release have been practised or else the tendency is to force the pelvic floor to overcome the tension. This can result in negative downwards pressure of the organs which should never happen as the release is posterior or dorsocaudal and not caudal.

Pelvic floor contraction

When the release of the pelvic floor has been practised then the patient can progress to contraction for balance and strengthening and to use the contraction for better quality of release according to the principle of post-isometric release (see below). The instruction for a pelvic floor contraction is to pull in the back passage as if to stop oneself from passing wind, and to continue lifting upwards and forwards towards the pubic bone. This instruction has been shown to be successful in producing a cranioventral contraction (Jones et al. 2006, Lovegrove-Jones 2010). Although this sounds to be specific to the back passage, it does cross the pelvic floor from back to front and this is explained to the patient as they are shown the diagrams (see Figures 13.26 and 13.27).

Pelvic floor contraction to drop or flop and drop or sniff, flop and drop

When the patient has learned to contract they must then learn to completely release after each contraction. The direction of release is explained in the 'drop' section above. The patient practises pelvic floor contraction to drop initially, then flop and drop to maximize the drop and then sniff, flop and drop when they can coordinate this movement.

Transversus abdominis and pelvic floor contraction

The pelvic floor contraction can be facilitated by transversus abdominis (TrA), as this method has been shown to facilitate a contraction of the levator ani muscles (Sapsford et al. 2001, Jones et al. 2006, Junginger et al. 2010). It may not always be a good idea to use the TrA muscle as this may encourage negative muscle activity patterns. This should be evaluated by the therapist in assessment of the pelvis and trunk. The following instruction for contraction is based on the assumption of correct activation of the TrA muscle, with no bracing of the upper abdomen, hardening of the stomach on palpation, or drawing of the ribs downwards. The patient is instructed without breathing to slowly and gently draw the lower stomach in, as if away from the zip of the trousers, or drawing the navel towards the spine (see Figures 13.28 and 13.29). The pelvic floor may start contracting on its own at this stage. The back passage is then drawn upwards and forwards towards the pubic bone.

Transversus abdominis and pelvic floor contraction to flop and drop or sniff, flop and drop or with breathing to sniff, flop and drop

The patient is instructed to draw in the TrA and pelvic floor as described, to hold it for just 5 seconds and then to release both TrA and pelvic floor maximally, i.e. flop and drop. When it is possible to do this the next challenge is to be able to breathe and hold.

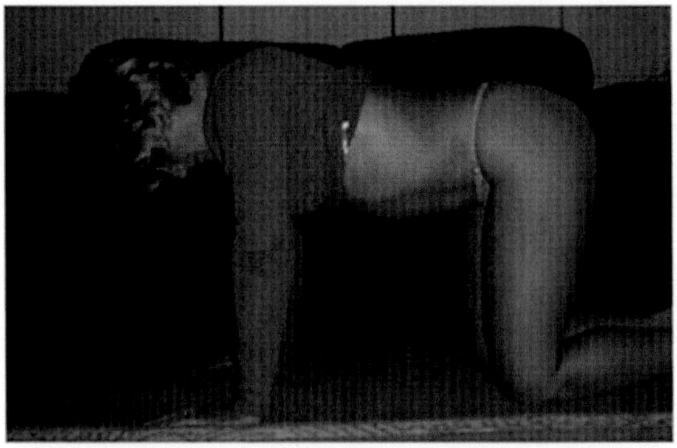

Figure 13.28 • Transversus abdominis contraction

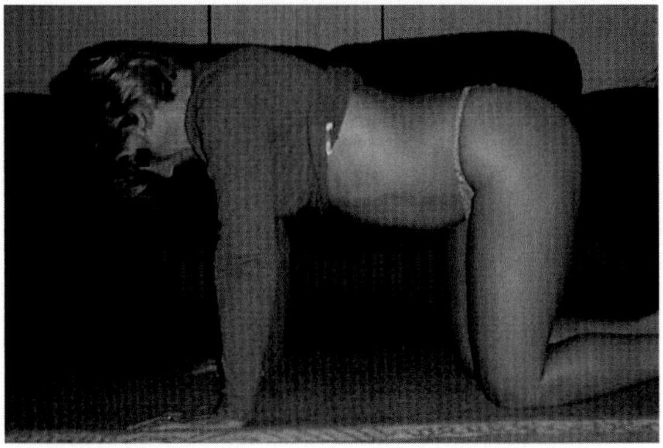

Figure 13.29 • Transversus abdominis release

The TrA is drawn in and the pelvic floor is contracted, this is held for 5 seconds. The patient must make sure that the chest has not lifted or that breath has not been drawn in while contracting. The patient ensures that the lungs are empty before releasing. The release is then the sniff, flop and drop as before.

The next step is to contract TrA and the pelvic floor and hold, take in a small breath, not filling the stomach, breathe all the way out, training the muscle by trying to hold firm or reinforcing throughout the exhalation. At the end of this out-breath the patient then releases with sniff, flop and drop. Continuing on from this TrA is contracted with the pelvic floor as above and the patient breathes normally for approximately 10 seconds. At the end of the contraction, the lungs must be emptied with an out-breath before the sniff, flop and drop to release. The patient will need to be prompted at intervals over the 10 seconds to keep the back passage engaged. The usual principles of progression of muscle strengthening in rehabilitation are applicable hereafter.

Home programme

A home programme involves the patient lying on a relatively hard surface in pelvic neutral position with knees bent. Alternatively the individual can try side lying, lying with the lower legs supported on a low stool, lying with knees bent and rolled down to one side, in forward kneeling or four-point kneeling. The choice of position has to do with the individual patient and their musculoskeletal system. It is explained that concentration is needed and that there should be no noise or family disturbances. At first it will take at least 10 minutes to find the connection with the pelvic floor through breathing and often longer but concentration will often wane putting a limit on the session. Particularly early on in their rehabilitation, patients encounter the frustration of not feeling the connection and consequently may be less compliant with their exercises. It should be explained that, with sustained practice, the time taken to find the connection becomes shorter and ultimately the patient will be in control with just a few in-breaths. However, it may take a few weeks of practice and the help of a pelvic floor manual therapist to find this connection. It should be emphasized that it is always the less effort the better and that trying harder, with more effort, does not help the connection to the pelvic floor.

The patient may ask if it is necessary to be lying down and the answer is initially 'yes' until the connection has been established. Then the exercises can be practised in sitting and standing as a progression; however, the patient should always do a release session, in lying, to achieve the maximum release eliminating gravity and the postural muscles, even during the final stages of a rehabilitation or a maintenance programme.

A suggested programme would involve 10 minutes breathing, followed by a shorter session of contract/relax, depending on the stage the patient is at. There should not be progression to the strengthening stage until the ability to sniff, flop and drop has been achieved. The author has found that a short session of 10–15 repetitions, twice per day, along with 10 minutes breathing beforehand, is effective in changing both activation and release of the pelvic floor. The patient should be warned not to carry tension from one contraction to the next when doing a contract/relax session as this can often be perceived as the muscle fatiguing when it is actually just getting shorter. It can be helpful to 'sniff, flop and drop' 2–3 times, again with the emphasis on the in-breath to achieve optimal release before progressing to the next contract/relax.

The patient can also be encouraged to stretch their pelvic floor muscles themselves at home. It is suggested that while sitting on the toilet, the right thumb or index finger could be inserted in order to stretch the left levator ani backwards towards the coccyx, or the left thumb or index finger may be inserted to stretch the right levator ani backwards. Accessible trigger points can be self-treated in this way. Some patients will take to this idea and others will not. An alternative is to use an instrument which can be introduced through the vagina or the back passage and used to maintain pressure on the trigger point. Examples of two such devices are the wand developed by Wise & Anderson (2008) (which is described and illustrated in Chapter 12) and the EZ Magic angled probe available at www.icrelief.com.

The patient must also learn to not carry tension in the affected muscles throughout the day. Techniques to address this have been described by Wise & Anderson (2008).

Further techniques to maximize release

Once direction of release has improved then it will be noticed that amplitude of contraction has improved. This can then be used to good effect by incorporating the principle of post-isometric relaxation. The patient is asked to contract the levator ani muscle group by the instruction to lift the back passage upwards and forwards against the downward pressure of the examiner's finger. Following maximal contraction the patient is then instructed to completely release the muscle in a direction downwards and backwards towards the supporting surface.

How exactly proprioceptive neuromuscular facilitation (PNF) works continues to be investigated and remains inconclusive (Chalmers 2004, Sharman et al. 2006). There are various hypotheses regarding the mechanisms of action of post-isometric relaxation; however, it is likely to involve both neurological and circulatory influences (Fryer & Fossum 2009). Clinically it can be observed that if a patient works on a maximal contraction into end of range and reinforces for example 5 times, the maximal release afterwards is even more effective.

The 'sniff, flop and drop' technique makes use of the 'quick stretch' theory described in proprioceptive neuromuscular facilitation (PNF). The stretch stimulus has been defined as 'an increased state of responsiveness to cortical stimulation that exists when a muscle is placed in an elongated position' (Saliba et al. 1993). The stretch reflex is facilitated by a rapid elongation of the muscle that stimulates the muscle spindle fibres to fire resulting in a reflex contraction. This reflex response produces a short-lived contraction, where volitional control then takes over. Earlier in this section it was suggested that a quicker inhalation with a greater volume of air is more effective in releasing the pelvic floor than a slower in-breath with a slower pelvic floor release. It may be that this technique follows the principles of PNF.

If the patient learns how to control breathing during treatment this should assist release of tension. Once the 'sniff, flop and drop' technique has been learnt, the patient can assist the therapist by releasing the pelvic floor during manual therapy as the pelvic floor is being passively stretched.

The patient's understanding of the physiology of the pelvic floor region and the concept of releasing and contracting the pelvic floor muscles through full range of motion leads to greater awareness of the pelvic floor muscles and should lead to improved motor control. In turn, improved motor control should lead to the patient being able to reach their goal sooner and maintain the changes achieved through therapy in the long term.

This chapter has described the functional anatomy of the female and male pelvic floors and described direction-specific manual therapy and breathing techniques to release the pelvic floor. It has highlighted how breathing, the abdominal muscles and the pelvic floor can be used interactively to facilitate improved function of the pelvic floor. The next chapter moves away from the pelvic floor and discusses an osteopathic perspective on evaluating and treating patients with pelvic girdle pain whilst incorporating European guidelines for physical diagnosis and treatment.

References

Anderson, R.U., Wise, D., Sawyer, T., Chan, C., 2005. Integration of myofascial trigger point release and paradoxical relaxation training in treatment of chronic pelvic pain in men. J. Urol. 174 (1), 155–160.

Anderson, R.U., Wise, D., Sawyer, T., Chan, C., 2006. Sexual dysfunction in men with chronic prostatitis/chronic pelvic pain syndrome: Improvement after trigger point release and paradoxical relaxation training. J. Urol. 176 (4), 1534–1539.

Anderson, R.U., Sawyer, T., Wise, D., et al., 2009. Painful myofascial trigger points and pain sites in men with chronic prostatitis/chronic pelvic pain syndrome. J. Urol. 182, 2753–2758.

Anson, B.J., McVay, C.B., 1984. Surgical anatomy. sixth ed. WB Saunders, Philadelphia, p. 893.

Ashton-Miller, J.A., DeLancey, J.O.L., 2007. Functional anatomy of the female pelvic floor. In: Bo, K., Berghmans, B., Morkved, S., Van Kampfen, M. (Eds.), Evidence Based Physical Therapy for the Pelvic Floor, p. 25.

Brooks, J., 2007. Anatomy of the lower urinary tract and male genetalia. In: Wein, A., Kavoussi, L., Nivick, A. et al., (Eds.), Campbell-Walsh Urology, ninth ed., pp. 61, 65.

Brooks, J.D., Chao, W.M., Kerr, J., 1998. Male pelvic anatomy reconstructed from the visible human data set. J. Urol. 159, 868–872.

Chaitow, L., 1994. Integrated neuromuscular inhibition technique. Br. J. Osteopathy 13 (1), 17–20.

Chaitow, L., DeLany, J., 2002. Summary of modalities. In: Clinical Application of Neuromuscular Techniques. Churchill Livingstone, Edinburgh, pp. 201, 208.

Chalmers, G., 2004. Re-examination of the possible role of Golgi tendon organ and muscle spindle reflexes in proprioceptive neuromuscular facilitation muscle stretching. Sports Biomech. 3 (1), 159–183.

DeLancey, J.O.L., 1990. Anatomy and physiology of urinary continence. Clin. Obstet. Gynecol. 33 (2).

DeLancey, J.O., Kearney, R., Chou, Q., et al., 2003. The appearance of levator ani muscle abnormalities in magnetic resonance images after vaginal delivery. Obstet. Gynecol. 101, 46–53.

DeLancey, J.O.L., Ashton-Miller, J.A., 2007. MRI of intact and injured female pelvic floor muscles. In: Evidence Based Physical Therapy, p. 94.

Dietz, H.P., 2009. Pelvic floor assessment. Fetal Maternal Med. Rev. 20 (1), 49–66.

Dommerholt, J., Bron, C., Franssen, J.L.M., 2006. Myofascial trigger points: an evidence informed review. J. Man. Manip. Ther. 14 (4), 2003–221.

Dorey, G., 2002. Anatomy and physiology of the male lower urinary tract. In: Conservative treatment of male urinary incontinence and erectile dysfunction, p. 8.

Fitzgerald, M.P., Kotarinos, R., 2003. Rehabilitation of the short pelvic floor.1: Background and patient evaluation. Int. Urogynecol. J. 14, 261–268.

Fitzgerald, M.P., Anderson, R.U., Potts, J., et al., 2009. Randomised multicenter feasibility trial of myofascial physical therapy for the treatment of urological chronic pelvic pain syndromes. J. Urol. 182, 570–580.

Fryer, G., Fossum, C., 2009. Muscle energy techniques. In: Fernández-de-las-Peñas, C., Arendt-Nielsen, L., Gerwin, R.D. (Eds.), Tension-type and cervicogenic headache: Pathophysiology, diagnosis, and management. Jones & Bartlett Publishers, Boston.

Grant, S.R., Salvati, E.P., Rubin, R.J., 1975. Levator syndrome: An analysis of 316 cases. Dis. Colon Rectum 18, 161–163.

Haslam, J., Laycock, J. (Eds.), 2007. Therapeutic Management of Incontinence and Pelvic Pain: Pelvic Organ Disorders, second revised ed. Springer-Verlag, London.

Herschorn, S., 2004. Female pelvic floor anatomy: The pelvic floor, supporting structures and pelvic organs. Rev. Urol. 6 (Suppl. 5), S2–S10.

Herschorn, S., Carr, L.K., 2002. In: Campbell's Urology 1092–1139.

Hodges, P.W., Sapsford, R., Pegel, L.H.M., 2007. Postural and respiratory functions of the pelvic floor muscles. Neurourol. Urodyn. 26 (3), 362–371.

Hong, C.Z., Chen, Y.C., Pon, C.H., Yu, J., 1993. Immediate effects of various physical medicine modalities on pain threshold of an active myofascial trigger point. J. Musculoskeletal Pain 1 (1), 35–53.

Jones, R.C., Peng, Q., Shishido, K., Constantinou, C.E., 2006. 2D ultrasound imaging and motion tracking of pelvic floor muscle activity during abdominal manoeuvres in stress urinary incontinent women. Neurourol. Urodyn. 25 (6), 596–597.

Kearney, R., Sawhney, R., Delancey, J.O., 2004. Levator ani muscle anatomy evaluated by origin-insertion pairs. Obstet. Gynecol. 104, 168–173.

Kotarinos, R., 2009. Physical findings in patients with urologic chronic pelvic pain findings. Neurourology and Urodynamics Proceedings of ICS 264.

Lawson, J., 1974. Pelvic anatomy. I. Pelvic floor muscles. Ann. R. Coll. Surg. Engl. 54, 244–252.

Laycock, J., Jerwood, D., 2001. Pelvic floor muscle assessment: The PERFECT scheme. Physiotherapy 87 (12), 631–642.

Lovegrove Jones, R.C., 2010. Dynamic Evaluation of Female Pelvic Floor Muscle Function Using 2D Ultrasound and Image Processing Methods. PhD thesis. University of Southampton, Faculty of Medicine, Health and Life Sciences.

Malbohan, I.M., Mojisova, L., Tichy, M., 1989. The role of coccygeal spasm in low back pain. J. Man. Med. 4, 140–141.

Montenegro, L.L.S., Gomide, L.B., Mateus-Vasconcelos, E.L., et al., 2009. Abdominal myofascial pain syndrome must be considered in the differential diagnosis of chronic pelvic pain. Eur. J. Obstet Gynecol Reprod. Biol. 147, 21–24.

O'Sullivan, P., Beales, D., 2007. Changes in pelvic floor and diaphragm kinematics and respiratory patterns in subjects with sacroiliac joint pain following a motor learning intervention: A case series. Man. Ther. 12 (3), 209–218.

O'Sullivan, P.B., Beales, D.J., Beetham, J.A., 2002. Altered motor control strategies with sacroiliac joint pain during the ASLR test. Spine 27 (1), E1–E8.

Peschers, U.M., DeLancey, J.O.L., 2008. Laycock, J., Haslam, J. (Eds.), Therapeutic management of incontinence and pelvic pain, 9–20.

Pool-Goudzwaard, A., 2004. Contribution of pelvic floor muscles to stiffness of the pelvic ring. Clin. Biomech. 19 (6), 564–571.

Saliba, V., Johnson, G.S., Wardlaw, C., 1993. Rational Manual Therapies. Ch 11 Proprioceptive Neuromuscular Facilitation. Williams & Williams, p. 249.

Sapsford, R.R., Hodges, P.W., Richardson, C.A., Cooper, D.H., Markwell, S.J., Jull, G.A., 2001. Co-activation of the abdominal and pelvic floor muscles during voluntary exercises. Neurourol. Urodyn. 20 (1), 31–42.

Sharman, M.J., Cresswell, A.G., Riek, S., 2006. Proprioceptive neuromuscular facilitation stretching: mechanisms and clinical implications. Sports Med. 36 (11), 929–939.

Singh, K., Reid, W., Berger, L., 2001. Assessment and grading of pelvic organ prolapse by use of dynamic magnetic resonance imaging. Am. J. Obstet. Gynecol. 185, 71–77.

Slocumb, J., 1984. Neurological factors in chronic pelvic pain: Trigger points and the abdominal pelvic pain syndrome. Am. J. Obstet. Gynecol. 149, 536.

Srinivasan, A.K., Kaye, J.D., Moldwin, R., 2007. Myofascial dysfunction associated with chronic pelvic floor pain: management strategies. Curr. Pain Headache Rep. 11 (5), 359–364.

Standring, S. (Ed.), 2008. The Anatomical Basis of Clinical Practice. fortieth ed. Section 8 Abdomen & Pelvis. Churchill Livingstone Elsevier.

Strohbehn, K., Ellis, J., Strohbehn, J., DeLancey, J.O., 1996. Magnetic resonance imaging of the levator ani with anatomic correlation. Obstet. Gynecol. 87, 277–285.

Talasz, H., Kofler, M., Kalchschmid Pretterklieber, M., Lechleitner, M., 2010. Breathing with the pelvic floor? Correlation of pelvic floor muscle function and expiratory flows in healthy young nulliparous women. Int. Urogynecol. J. 21 (4), 475–481.

Thiele, G.H., 1963. Coccydynia: cause and treatment. Dis. Colon Rectum 6, 422–436.

Travell, J., Simons, D., 1993. Myofascial Pain and Dysfunction: The trigger point manual, vol 2: The lower extremities, pp. 117, 119, 122, 126.

Travell, J., Simons, D., 1999. Myofascial Pain and Dysfunction: The trigger point manual, vol 1: The upper half of body, pp. 11–93.

Weiss, J., 2001. Pelvic floor myofascial trigger points: manual therapy for interstitial cystitis and the urgency-frequency syndromes. J. Urol. 166, 2226–2231.

Whelan, M., 2008. Laycock, J., Haslam, J. (Eds.), Therapeutic management of incontinence and pelvic pain, pp. 60–61.

Wilson, T.S., 1936. Manipulative treatment of subacute and chronic fibrositis. Br. Med. J. 1, 298–302.

Wise, D., Anderson, R., 2008. A Headache in the Pelvis, fifth ed. National Center for Pelvic Pain.

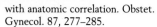

Patients with pelvic girdle pain: An osteopathic perspective

14

Michael A. Seffinger   Melicien Tettambel
Hallie Robbins

CHAPTER CONTENTS

Introduction

An osteopathic perspective on caring for patients with pelvic girdle pain (PGP) begins with an understanding of the osteopathic philosophy. The philosophy and its tenets help the clinician to organize scientific knowledge and apply a rational approach to patient care. This approach considers all aspects of health, including physical, mental, emotional and spiritual. It is a patient-centred, health-oriented approach that includes utilization of manual diagnosis and treatment. Viewpoints and attitudes arising from this approach give practitioners an important template for clinical problem solving, health restoration and maintenance, and patient education.

Based on the sciences of anatomy and physiology, the osteopathic philosophy emphasizes the following tenets:

1. The human being is a dynamic unit of function.
2. The body possesses self-regulatory mechanisms that are self-healing in nature.
3. Structure and function are interrelated at all levels.
4. Rational treatment is based on these principles.

(Ward & Sprafka 1981, Lesho 1999, Educational Council on Osteopathic Principles 2009)

Though anatomy and physiology are commonly taught in parts and systems, the first tenet recognizes that the person is a dynamic unified whole, not the mere compilation of anatomical parts or physiological systems. The pelvic girdle is anatomically linked to the entire spine and upper and lower extremities; it is an integral component to standing and sitting postures and motions (Beal 1982, Ronchetti et al. 2008). Therefore, in search of the cause of PGP and dysfunction, the clinician should examine the entire musculoskeletal system while the patient is walking, standing and sitting, as well as in the passive postures of lying supine and prone. The pelvic girdle is also intimately associated with the pelvic viscera that it protects (Beal 1985, Tettambel 2005). Additionally, the person's environment, social life, diet and nutrition, drugs used or abused, sleep patterns, emotions, beliefs and other behavioural factors play a role in the generation and recovery from PGP (O'Sullivan & Beales 2007, Vøllestad & Stuge 2009).

The second tenet stresses that the body is *capable* of self-regulation, self-healing and health maintenance.

This capability is inherent, but at times may require assistance in the form of manual therapy, surgery, exercise, nutritional advice, pharmacology or counselling (Tettambel 2007, Fall et al. 2010).

The third tenet states that structure and function are inter-related. Bodies have architectural (anatomical) form and engineering (physiological) processes that intimately influence each other. In the pelvic girdle, if there is sacroiliac dysfunction or lumbosacral torsion, a patient may have mechanical or structural back pain that might contribute to bowel dysfunction or urinary problems (Beal 1985, Browning 1990, Tettambel 2005). Conversely, if a woman has a difficult pregnancy or childbirth, she may develop pelvic pain as a result of a caesarean section or vaginally delivering a very large baby with or without instrumentation. Over time, the pain may become chronic, affecting her posture and gait (Ronchetti et al. 2008); and she may not anticipate another pregnancy with a positive attitude. Thus, the fourth osteopathic key tenet is pertinent: rational treatment is based upon the three previous principles. In this instance, to restore normal functionality, rational treatment may consist of postpartum spinal and extremity manual therapy; exercise to maintain stability and encourage flexibility of her musculoskeletal system; and perhaps family planning counselling to allow her to care for herself and her family.

Each of the above principles is important to the understanding of somatic dysfunction. Somatic dysfunction can be defined as 'impaired or altered function of related components of the somatic (body framework) system: skeletal, arthrodial and myofascial structures and their related vascular, lymphatic and neural elements' (Educational Council on Osteopathic Principles 2009). When a patient presents with PGP, the clinician should consider whether there is a somatic component to the chief complaint, injury or illness:

- Where in the soma might the problem exist?
- How does it manifest?
- Although the presenting painful condition may involve the pelvic girdle, could other bones, muscles, ligaments, nerves, vasculature, pelvic organs, fascia and/or related structures be primary features? (See Chapter 9.)

There may also be other relationships between the pelvic container and its contents, potentially affected by posture, gait and pulmonary ventilation (see Chapter 11). Somatic dysfunction could also be the result of a neurophysiological phenomenon, i.e. peripheral or central sensitization (Howell & Willard 2005) (see Chapter 3 for physiological mechanisms). Reflex loops of visceral and somatic excitation and facilitation may also be involved, introducing autonomic and referred pain to the equation (Janig 2008).

If there is a disturbance of the normal function of somatic structures, how might the problem best be addressed? Somatic dysfunction possesses characteristics identifiable by means of palpation to appreciate static or motion asymmetry of the body, as well as changes – structural and physiological – in other body tissues or systems. Osteopathic clinicians who perform osteopathic manipulative treatment (OMT) commonly use a combination of tests that evaluate the patient for signs of sensitive or tender points, tissue texture abnormalities in the soft tissues surrounding the spinal and pelvic joints, asymmetry of anatomical landmarks and alterations in quality or quantity of range of joint motion (Dinnar et al. 1982, Beal 1982, Fryer et al. 2009). A useful mnemonic, 'STAR', may be helpful to establish a palpatory structural diagnosis that may be amenable to manipulative treatment (Educational Council on Osteopathic Principles 2009) (see Box 14.1).

When the pelvic girdle is restricted, gait and posture change (van Wingerden et al. 2008). Persistent PGP can negatively affect the patient's attitude about ability to function, sometimes to a state of depression and altered sensorium due to chronicity of the problem (Gutke et al. 2007). Pelvic girdle motion may also be restricted by pelvic organ pathology (Beal 1985). A bimanual pelvic exam may detect a mass, pelvic inflammatory disease, adhesions from infection or surgery, or possibly signs of endometriosis (Tettambel 2005). In addition to restriction of motion, pain may be elicited (Boyle 2008). However, in a patient with PGP due to somatic dysfunction, the primary objective should be to treat the dysfunction underlying the pain (Damen et al. 2001).

Used alone, digital pain provocation for sensitivity of the soft or osseous tissues is the most reliable of the four types of palpatory tests in the neck and back regions (Seffinger et al. 2004, Stochkendahl et al. 2006). Lumbar percussion for pain provocation is very specific, so it can be used as a screening test; if it reproduces the patient's reported pain, then there is indeed a truly painful condition at that location (Kristiansson & Svardsudd 1996). It must be understood that reliability of pain provocation tests does not indicate that more than one examiner can reliably feel or interpret the sensitivity of the palpated tissues; rather that a patient can reliably state repetitively that a palpated site is sensitive when palpated by different practitioners (Seffinger et al. 2004,

Box 14.1

STAR mnemonic used to establish a palpatory structural diagnosis amenable to manipulative treatment

- 'S' represents sensitivity. Sensitivity may occur as the result of tissue contact or pressure that would not be sufficient to cause discomfort in 'normal' tissues.
  This may be reported as tender or painful by the patient when being palpated. To establish a diagnosis of somatic dysfunction, sensitivity may or may not be present. Sensitivity may be subjective and not always a reliable indicator of dysfunction. However, a patient may not be aware of any pain until a structure is palpated. Usually, a patient with a complaint of pain may be anxious about the performance of a palpatory exam and report increased tenderness on palpation of a structure because the structure was palpated (Fryer et al. 2004a).
- 'T' represents tissue texture abnormality that is palpable evidence of physiological dysfunction. Palpable changes found in skin, subcutaneous tissue, fascia and muscles reflect disturbances in local tissues, related organs or specific spinal segments.
  Tissue changes can be acute or chronic somatic dysfunctions. In acute dysfunction, one can palpate warmth, moisture, as well as bogginess and increased tension of tissues. Oedema may be present. Conversely, in chronic dysfunction, the tissues may feel cool, thin, dry and ropey (O'Connell 2003, Fryer et al. 2005).
- 'A' represents structural asymmetry, which may be observed or palpated. Anatomical landmarks, such as iliac crests or trochanter heights, can be visualized to compare bilateral location. These landmarks can also be palpated to assess position bilaterally (Beal 1982).
- 'R' represents range of motion. This motion may be either active or passive with quantitative and qualitative features. To evaluate joints of the pelvic girdle by palpation, one must note how much the joint moves and how well it moves. What restrictions to normal motion are present? Where are the anatomical, restrictive and pathological barriers in both active and passive motion testing? How do these barriers affect local joint motion as well as the rest of the pelvis (Beal 1982)? Ultimately how does this dysfunction affect the body as a unit of function (Tettambel 2005)?

Haneline & Young 2009). Soft tissue tests assessing for tissue texture abnormalities, altered compliance or presence of muscle tension are in general not reliable when used as the sole source of palpatory information (Seffinger et al 2004, Stochkendahl 2006, Haneline & Young 2009). Although regional range of motion tests are more reliable than segmental range of motion tests, motion tests for SIJ or lumbar mobility are not in general reliable (Hestbaek & Leboeuf-Yde 2000, van der Wurff et al. 2000a, 2000b, Seffinger et al. 2004, Stochkendahl 2006, Robinson et al. 2007). However, using a cluster of pain provocation tests combined with motion tests improves reliability (Arab et al. 2009). Likewise, combinations of pain provocation tests have demonstrated validity (Van der Wurff et al. 2006, Hancock et al. 2007, Szadek et al. 2009). Pelvic distraction, thigh thrust, compression and sacral thrust tests in combination are accurate in detecting the SIJ as a source of pain (Laslett et al. 2003, 2005). When all tests do not provoke pain, the SIJ can be ruled out as a source of the pain. One study demonstrated that the maximum interexaminer reliability occurs when only the result of the most reliable test is used to determine the side of SIJ dysfunction, sacral base position and innominate bone position (Tong et al. 2006).

The European guidelines for physical diagnosis of PGP (Vleeming et al. 2008) recommend using the following tests as they have demonstrated reliability:

- Posterior pelvic pain provocation test (P4);
- Patrick's Faber (hip flexion, abduction, external rotation);
- Palpation for sensitivity of the long dorsal SIJ ligament;
- Gaenslen's test;
- Palpation for sensitivity of the pubic symphysis;
- Modified Trendelenburg's test of the pelvic girdle;
- Active straight leg raising test.

In pregnant women, the most accurate combination of pain provocation palpatory tests to detect the location of sacroiliac or lumbosacral pain is:

- Motion tests of femoral compression, lumbar movement and supine iliac gapping (Kristiansson & Svardsudd 1996, DonTigny 2005a, 2005b);
- Digital pressure to assess the sacrospinous ligament and posterior superior iliac spine (Kristiansson & Svardsudd 1996);
- Lumbar spine percussion (Kristiansson & Svardsudd 1996).

Using a combination of reliable lumbar and pelvic motion and sensitivity assessment tests in pregnant patients with non-specific lumbopelvic pain, two examiners were able to reach substantial agreement in differentiating patients as having either lumbar pain or PGP (Gutke et al. 2009). This is useful since up to 25% of patients presenting to a spine specialist pain clinic with low back pain are likely to actually have PGP (sacroiliac and/or hip as pain generator) (Sembrano & Polly 2009). If primary care clinicians were better at screening patients with low back pain, unnecessary referrals to specialists would result, limiting unnecessary expenditures of precious personal and healthcare industry financial resources.

Evaluation of the pubic symphysis and tubercles for levelness and tenderness is used to determine imbalance of forces attached there, including the rectus abdominis muscles and sheath, thigh adductor muscles (adductor magnus, longus and brevis, the gracilis and the pectineus), inguinal ligament and pelvic floor muscles (levator ani and coccygeus) (Greenman 2003).

The information outlined above forms a foundation for understanding an osteopathic approach to assessing and treating patients with PGP (Jordan 2006). Beyond palpatory evaluation for evidence of somatic dysfunction (i.e. assessing for STAR), additional information may help to determine treatment plans. Patient gender, age, professional and social activities, attitude, as well as other factors help determine the approach to evaluation and a care plan.

- Dancers, for example, commonly complain of lumbopelvic and various musculoskeletal pain at various times in their career depending on the demands placed upon them by the choreographer, the environment, their skill, age, coping ability and experience (Demann 1997, Hincapié et al. 2008).
- Athletes of sports that entail increased mechanical load on the lumbosacral spine and pelvis are at higher risk for PGP and low back pain (Bahr et al. 2004).
- The elite athlete has special considerations as well (Bo & Backe-Hansen 2007).
- The type of employment may affect the cause and nature of PGP. For example, the main biomechanical risk factors identified for the development of low back work-related musculoskeletal disorder were heavy physical work, awkward static and dynamic working postures, and lifting; the psychosocial risk factors identified were negative affectivity, low level of job control, high psychological demands and high work dissatisfaction; individual risk factors identified were younger age and high body mass index (da Costa & Vieira 2009).
- Motor vehicle collision survivors might have injuries from steering wheel blows to the pelvis, compression of door panels into the hip, lapbelt-incurred lumbopelvic torsions, or femoropelvic compression from floorboard and pedal ground forces at time of impact; or when bracing in preparation of the impending event.
- Older adults may have developed posture or gait disorders due to trauma (falls, accidents), or disease (neurological, vascular, cataracts) that can affect pelvic girdle mechanics.
- Young females who participate in sports may have ligamentous laxity, making them more susceptible to injury (Bo & Backe-Hansen 2007). Pelvic ligamentous laxity is helpful in childbearing years, but not desirable in menopause (Gabbe 2007).
- Pregnancy and birth trauma may result in chronic PGP (Latthe 2006, van der Hulst 2006).
- Sexual trauma may also result in pelvic pain and dysfunction.
- Postmenopausal women are at risk for pelvic organ prolapse, bladder or bowel incontinence, osteoporosis and degenerative arthritis (Prather 2007). Hormonal factors also influence pelvic structures, function and pain (O'Sullivan & Beales 2007, Eberhard-Gran & Eskild 2008).
- Women who work outside the home may develop pain due to 'wardrobe malfunctions' of restrictive clothing or uncomfortable shoes (Chen et al. 2005), as well as postural challenges that accompany manual labour or repetitive actions.
- Obesity as a result of pregnancy, endocrine problems, or poor nutritional habits contributes to pelvic girdle dysfunction (Mottola 2009).

An osteopathic approach to the patient with PGP would start with collection of historical information and the performing of a comprehensive physical examination, including a palpatory structural examination. A patient-centred treatment approach would investigate what would be required to promote health in the presence of challenging situations. In osteopathic literature there are five conceptual treatment models to promote health and modify disease (pathological) processes (Educational Council on Osteopathic Principles 1987, 2009, Hruby 1991, 1992). As the body is an integrated whole, posture, neural responses, respiration/circulation, metabolic processes and behaviour are tightly woven together; dysfunction of any of these coordinated body functions will therefore compromise the entire organism. Each of these models is discussed in this chapter, with intended therapeutic benefits, within the four key principles outlined above.

Biomechanical model

The biomechanical model requires knowledge of posture and motion as they relate to PGP and dysfunction (see Box 14.2). The patient should be observed in active posture as well as in the resting supine position. Palpatory examination using the combination of elements of STAR should be employed. It is necessary to consider how motions of the pelvic container affect both motion and function of the pelvic contents. Also requiring consideration is how pelvic dysfunction relates, from cause-and-effect perspectives, to the spine, abdomen, rib cage, lower and upper extremities. The spinal curves, lateral as well as anterior-posterior, require assessment, with consideration of their effect on muscle length and tension. Posture is assessed when standing or sitting from anterior, posterior and lateral views. Notes on postural influences are to be found in Chapter 11. Orthopaedic tests help determine structural and functional involvement of particular lumbopelvic components (Liebenson 2004, 2007). When evaluating the patient, painful structures usually denote muscle spasm or hypertonicity, but may also indicate peripheral and/or central sensitization (Howell & Willard 2005) or the result of decreased muscle activity (Fryer et al. 2004b). The antagonists to hypertonic muscles may be inhibited. Short- and long-term (up to 2 years) outcomes improve with an individualized exercise programme addressing muscle imbalance to relieve such weakness or inhibition (Stuge et al. 2004a, 2004b). Presence of rectus abdominis muscle diastasis, especially in post partum women, should be assessed and treated due to the

Box 14.2

Biomechanical aetiological features

The bony pelvic girdle comprises right and left ilia (with pubes and ischia) which constitute the hemipelvis, plus the sacrum. Each hemipelvis arises embryologically from three bony islands that join flexibly in the acetabulum by the age of 8 years. Each side also has three joints – sacroiliac, hip, pubic symphysis – and so can be considered most balanced and stable when all three 'legs' of the stool are level and moving well. Because the pelvis serves for ambulation and stance, as well as for containment of truncal contents and passage of bodily functions, such a balancing act is dynamic even at rest.

- Congenital deformities such as small hemipelvis, club foot, facet asymmetry in the lumbosacral spine, partial or complete sacralization of the fifth lumbar, spondylolisthesis, spina bifida occulta, or butterfly (or bat) wing process can alter lumbopelvic biomechanics (Bailey & Beckwith 1937). Most of these conditions are discovered by X-ray, when there is an unsuccessful course of conservative care, which may have included manipulation. They may or may not be related to PGP and may or may not require surgical correction. Spine surgical consultation is indicated if symptoms do not improve or worsen with conservative measures.
- Anatomical short leg can cause sacral base unlevelling and pelvic asymmetry related to lumbopelvic pain (Juhl et al. 2004). Posture and gait can be affected with resultant musculoskeletal imbalance, scoliotic spinal curves and pain (Juhl et al. 2005). Heel lift therapy should be considered in patients with PGP and low back pain associated with unlevel sacral base due to anatomical short leg (Lipton et al. 2009).
- Injury to the coccyx due to trauma or childbirth can affect sacral motion via its ligamentous attachments (Meleger & Krivickas 2007). Ligamentous strains of the coccyx can also affect motion of the ilia and ischia, as well as cause pain in the pelvis, perineum and lower extremities. Coccygeal muscle pain can persist despite normalization of sacral dynamics due to the strong ligamentous spans retaining positional strain patterns; the authors have noted that some patients with persistent coccydynia complain of coccygeal pain with bowel movements, micturition, coitus, and upon sitting, standing or moving, likely because two-thirds of the levator ani sling muscles involve the coccyx.
- Lumbopelvic somatic dysfunction can compromise pelvic diaphragm (levator ani and coccygeus muscles) balance and functions, resulting in pelvic floor pain and bladder dysfunction (Pool-Goudzwaard et al. 2005, Arab et al. 2010). Bowel function may also be compromised (Ng 2007).
- Pelvic obliquity can arise from imbalances of the iliopsoas muscles and quadratus lumborum muscles. These form the deepest of the lumbopelvic core muscle layers.
- Difficult childbirth may induce pubic shears or avulsions. In addition to painful gait, dyspareunia with sexual dysfunction and bladder voiding dysfunction can result.
- In the Mitchell model of the 'walking cycle', the transverse axis for gait is through the pubic symphysis. Shears and compression strains would not only affect gait, but posture and pelvic bowl tilt as well (Greenman 2003). Movement at the pubic symphysis may be small, but intense pain on standing (on one leg) or walking may be reported by the patient when dysfunction exists (Greenman 2003).

effect it can have on the integrity of the abdomino-pelvic 'canister' and its functions in providing postural stability, controlled bladder function and efficient breathing mechanics (Lee et al. 2008).

Mitchell (1958) was an osteopathic pioneer in the development of a biomechanical model to explain the role of the pelvis in posture and gait. Mitchell also collaborated in the development of muscle energy technique (MET), a modality employed to treat somatic dysfunction (Goodridge 1981). This approach and his techniques have been adopted widely across professions and cultures. When joints such as SIJ are altered from their ideal positioning, or if inflammation or joint fluid pressures are elevated, inhibited motion occurs, often with resultant pain (Howell & Willard 2005). Muscle energy techniques (MET) may be used to balance muscle tone (i.e. stretch hypertonic muscles and strengthen hypotonic muscles), relieve asymmetrical forces upon spinal and peripheral joints, and enable restoration of normal joint motion (Wilson et al. 2003, Selkow et al. 2009). Benefits of MET manipulation alone, and combined with exercise, are beginning to be assessed by randomized clinical trials (Wilson et al. 2003, Selkow et al. 2009). Further studies are needed, especially in the contexts of the patient's age and other activities of daily living.

Gait (or other means of locomotion) should be assessed for its cadence, symmetry, rate and reported ease through repeated visual or kinematic observation. Specific patterns of muscle activity have been fitted into the six determinants of the gait cycle (Kerrigan et al. 2000, 2001, Esquinazi & Mukul 2008). In patients with PGP, muscle activity patterns are not only altered during gait (Wu et al. 2008), but also during the active straight leg raising (ASLR) test as compared with pain-free subjects (O'Sullivan et al. 2002, Beales et al. 2009a, 2009b). Researchers found increased minute ventilation, decreased diaphragmatic excursion (O'Sullivan et al. 2002), increased intra-abdominal pressure (Beales et al. 2009a, 2009b) and increased pelvic floor descent (O'Sullivan et al. 2002, Beales et al. 2009a, 2009b) during the ASLR test in PGP patients, indicating considerable widespread effects on the neuromuscular control of respiration and pelvic floor function. Interestingly, enhancement of pelvis stability via manual compression through the ilia reversed these differences (O'Sullivan et al. 2002, Beales et al. 2009a, 2009b). Hu et al. (2010) therefore reasoned that since manual pelvic compression restores normal abdominal and pelvic motor control in patients with PGP during the ASLR test, a pelvic compression belt worn while walking might provide similar stabilizing effects. Nulligravid women walked on a treadmill at increasing speeds while wearing or not wearing a belt. Simultaneously, there was fine-wire electromyography (fwEMG) of the psoas, iliacus and transversus abdominis muscles and surface EMG (sEMG) of other hip and trunk muscles. Wearing a pelvic belt while walking reduced core abdominal muscle activity and induced contralateral activation of biceps femoris and gluteus maximus, thus promoting anterior tilting of the pelvis and enhancing force closure effects. Thus, poor force closure of the SIJs may be a key component of the altered gait, respiration and pelvic floor mechanics observed in some patients with PGP. Pregnancy adds another mechanical challenge to the patient with form and force closure problems. Wu et al. (2004) compared gaits of healthy women who were pregnant or nulligravid and found them to be very similar except for increased antiphase pelvis–thorax coordination among pregnant subjects walking quickly; the difference is greater among women with PGP while pregnant (Wu et al. 2008).

Pelvic mechanics are also altered in men who have PGP. Hungerford et al. (2004) did kinematic assessment of pelvic bone motion in men with posterior pelvic pain (PPP) compared to men without PPP. Posterior rotation of the weight-bearing innominate was observed in controls, while anterior rotation during weight-bearing occurred in symptomatic men.

Sacral motion can occur around a variety of axes: anteroposterior, vertical, horizontal or oblique (Beal 1982). It is most likely, however, that there is no stationary sacral axis and that the axis shifts with the introduction of movement (Beal 1982). Sacral and lumbar spine motions are often impaired in patients with PGP (Beal 1982, van Wingerden et al. 2008). Sacroiliac motion can be restricted at the superior or inferior aspects of the SIJ; compression can also occur (Beal 1982, Vleeming et al. 1990a, 1990b). There are no muscle attachments directly connecting the sacrum to the pelvic girdle. The sacrum is suspended between the ilia by ligaments. Its motion is influenced by joint surface (form closure) and myofascial and ligamentous function (force closure) (Vleeming 1990a). Ligamentous strains or laxity during pregnancy can disrupt joint mechanics, cause low back and pelvic girdle pain (Damen et al. 2001), and contribute to muscle imbalances in the pelvis, lower extremities and trunk of the body. In gynaecology patients, evaluation of sacral motion and dysfunction, along with pelvic girdle motion, should be assessed. On clinical gynaecological examination, strains of the broad ligament and uterine malpositioning may be inter-related with altered bone and joint mechanics (Barney 2008, Boyle 2008). The abdominal, lumbar, pelvic and lower extremity myofascial tension affects SIJ stiffness and stability (Van Wingerden et al. 2004). Patients with PGP with or without low back pain have altered standing posture and forward-bending motions (Van Wingerden et al. 2008). Therefore, it is important to assess and treat not only contiguous bony and ligamentous structures but the back, pelvic and extremity muscles and fascia as well, in helping the patient resolve not only the PGP, but to restore and maximize gait, posture and motion.

Hip range of motion impacts lumbopelvic integrity (Liebenson 2004, 2007) and should be checked in all directions to assess its six muscle groups. Janda (1977, 1986) found that prone hip extension reveals hamstring strain substitution for gluteus maximus activation. Nadler et al. (2002) associated impaired hip extension with propensity for low back pain in women. Vleeming and colleagues (2007) have written extensively about the biomechanical integration of rectus femoris muscle and sacrotuberous ligament as a key component of form closure and force closure affecting the long dorsal sacroiliac ligament and other pelvic girdle structures. Janda (1977, 1986) and Nadler et al. (2002) also found that weak hip abductors contribute to lumbopelvic instability and motor control substitution. Hip pain is also increased with lumbar hyperflexibility more frequently than stiffness (Biering-Sorensen 1984). Hip external rotation is likely to show lumbopelvic dysfunction than internal rotation (Liebenson 2007).

There is marked similarity between osteopathic and physical therapy assessments of dysfunction present in patients with PGP as evidenced by correlating the reports from Greenman (1996) with the integrated pelvic girdle model of Vleeming et al. (2007) and Lee (2004) (see Table 14.1).

Table 14.1 Osteopathic and physical therapy assessments of dysfunction

Somatic dysfunctions (SD) in persistent low back pain (Greenman 1996)	Integrated model of pelvic girdle: form closure, force closure, motor control, emotional awareness (Lee 2004, Vleeming et al. 2007)
Non-physiological pelvic SD (pubic shears)	Core, abdomen, pelvic floor and hip adductor muscles imbalance at pubic tubercles and rami
Non-physiological pelvic SD (sacroiliac shears)	Improper load distribution of sacroiliac joint (SIJ)
Sacral nutation failure (including non-neutral and backward sacral torsion SD)	Flexion (nutation): sacrotuberous ligament-biceps femoris Extension (counternutation): long dorsal sacroiliac ligament
Pelvic tilt/'Short-leg syndrome'/unlevel sacral base	Impaired pelvic–trunk coordination
Muscle imbalance (including psoas syndrome)	Global muscle and core muscle faulty recruitment
Lumbar single level (Type II) lumbar SD	L5 associated with SIJ dysfunction

Osteopathic manipulative treatment options (see Box 14.3)

Osteopathic manipulative treatment (OMT) has been shown to be efficacious in treating chronic low back and pelvic pain (Licciardone et al. 2005), low back pain during pregnancy (Licciardone et al. 2010), pelvic pain from chronic prostatitis (Marx et al. 2009), and is advocated for women with chronic pelvic pain (Tettambel 2007) and patients with PGP (Greenman 2003). When diagnosing and treating somatic dysfunction with OMT, choosing the type of manipulative procedure appropriate for the patient requires training and experience.

In addition, knowing when and how much OMT to provide is important.

- Diagnosis of recent, acute strains or sprains from trauma requires early biomechanical intervention, but in small and frequent doses.
- Chronic conditions respond to larger doses of manipulation given at longer intervals (Kimberly 1976, Ferreira et al. 2003, Greenman 2003, Bronfort et al. 2006). Taking into consideration the age of the patient is another factor in determining the dose of OMT.
- Younger (adolescent) patients may tolerate more vigorous muscular and ligamentous treatment procedures; however, theoretically, due to the

Box 14.3

Osteopathic terminology (ECOP 2009)

- *Somatic dysfunction*. Impaired or altered function of related components of the somatic (body framework) system: skeletal, arthrodial and myofascial structures, and their related vascular, lymphatic and neural elements. Somatic dysfunction is treatable using osteopathic manipulative treatment.
- *Osteopathic manipulative treatment*. The therapeutic application of manually guided forces by an osteopathic physician (US) or practitioner to improve physiological function and/or support homeostasis, which have been altered by somatic dysfunction. OMT employs a variety of techniques, including:
  - *Articulatory treatment system (ART)*. A low-velocity/moderate- to high-amplitude technique where a joint is carried through its full motion with the therapeutic goal of increased range of movement. The activating force is either a repetitive springing motion or repetitive concentric movement of the joint through the restrictive barrier.
  - *Balanced ligamentous tension (BLT)*. 1. According to Sutherland's model, all the joints in the body are balanced ligamentous articular mechanisms. The ligaments provide proprioceptive information that guides the muscle response for positioning the joint, and the ligaments themselves guide the motion of the articular components. (Foundations) 2. First described in 'Osteopathic Technique of William G. Sutherland', that was published in the *1949 Year Book of the Academy of Applied Osteopathy*. See also *Ligamentous articular strain technique.*
  - *Combined method*. 1. A treatment strategy where the initial movements are indirect; as the technique is completed the movements change to direct forces. 2. A manipulative sequence involving two or more different osteopathic manipulative treatment systems (e.g. Spencer technique combined with muscle energy technique). 3. A concept described by Paul Kimberly.
  - *Counterstrain (CS)*. 1. A system of diagnosis and treatment that considers the dysfunction to be a continuing, inappropriate strain reflex, which is inhibited by applying a position of mild strain in the direction exactly opposite to that of the reflex; this is accomplished by specific directed positioning about the point of tenderness to achieve the desired therapeutic response. 2. Australian and French use: Jones technique (correction spontaneous by position), spontaneous release by position. 3. Developed by Lawrence Jones in 1955 (originally 'spontaneous release by positioning', later termed 'strain–counterstrain').
  - *Strain–counterstrain*. 1. An osteopathic system of diagnosis and indirect treatment in which the patient's somatic dysfunction, diagnosed by (an) associated myofascial tenderpoint(s), is treated by using a passive position, resulting in spontaneous tissue release and at least 70% decrease in tenderness. 2. Developed by Lawrence H. Jones in 1955. See Figure 14.5. See video link 4.
  - *Direct method (D/DIR)*. An osteopathic treatment strategy by which the restrictive barrier is engaged and a final activating force is applied to correct somatic dysfunction.
  - *Facilitated positional release (FPR)*. 1. A system of indirect myofascial release treatment. The component region of the body is placed into a neutral position, diminishing tissue and joint tension in all planes, and an activating force (compression or torsion) is added. 2. A technique developed by Stanley Schiowitz.
  - *Fascial unwinding*. A manual technique involving constant feedback to the osteopathic practitioner who is passively moving a portion of the patient's body in response to the sensation of movement. Its forces are localized using the sensations of ease and bind over wider regions.
  - *Functional method*. An indirect treatment approach that involves finding the dynamic balance point and one of the following: applying an indirect guiding force, holding the position or adding compression to exaggerate position and allow for spontaneous readjustment. The osteopathic practitioner guides the manipulative procedure while the dysfunctional area is being palpated in order to obtain a continuous feedback of the physiological response to induced motion. The osteopathic practitioner guides the dysfunctional part so as to create a decreasing sense of tissue resistance (increased compliance). See Figure 14.4. See video link 3.
  - *High-velocity/low-amplitude technique (HVLA)*. An osteopathic technique employing a rapid, therapeutic force of brief duration that travels a short distance within the anatomic range of motion of a joint, and that engages the restrictive barrier in one or more planes of motion to elicit release of restriction. Also known as thrust technique. See Figures 14.3 and 14.9. See video links 2 and 7a.
  - *Indirect method (I/IND)*. A manipulative technique where the restrictive barrier is disengaged and the dysfunctional body part is moved away from the restrictive barrier until tissue tension is equal in one or all planes and directions.
  - *Inhibitory pressure technique*. The application of steady pressure to soft tissues to reduce reflex activity and produce relaxation.
  - *Ligamentous articular strain technique (LAS)*. 1. A manipulative technique in which the goal of treatment is to balance the tension in opposing ligaments where

Continued

Box 14.3

Osteopathic terminology (ECOP 2009)—cont'd

there is abnormal tension present. 2. A set of myofascial release techniques described by Howard Lippincott and Rebecca Lippincott. 3. Title of reference work by Conrad Speece and William Thomas Crow.

- *Lymphatic pump*. 1. A term used to describe the impact of intrathoracic pressure changes on lymphatic flow. This was the name originally given to the thoracic pump technique before the more extensive physiologic effects of the technique were recognized. 2. A term coined by C. Earl Miller.
- *Muscle energy*. A form of osteopathic manipulative diagnosis and treatment in which the patient's muscles are actively used on request, from a precisely controlled position, in a specific direction and against a distinctly executed physician counterforce. First described in 1948 by Fred Mitchell Sr. See Figures 14.2, 14.6, 14.7 and 14.8. See video links 1 and 5.
- *Myofascial release (MFR)*. A system of diagnosis and treatment first described by Andrew Taylor Still and his early students, which engages continual palpatory feedback to achieve release of myofascial tissues.
- *Direct MFR*. A myofascial tissue-restrictive barrier is engaged for the myofascial tissues and the tissue is loaded with a constant force until tissue release occurs. See Figure 14.1.
- *Indirect MFR*. The dysfunctional tissues are guided along the path of least resistance until free movement is achieved.
- *Osteopathy in the cranial field (OCF)*. 1. A system of diagnosis and treatment by an osteopathic practitioner using the primary respiratory mechanism and balanced membranous tension. 2. Refers to the system of diagnosis and treatment first described by William Garner Sutherland.
- *Soft tissue technique*. A direct technique that usually involves lateral stretching, linear stretching, deep pressure, traction and/or separation of muscle origin and insertion while monitoring tissue response and motion changes by palpation. Also called myofascial treatment. See video link 6.
- *Thoracic pump*. 1. A technique that consists of intermittent compression of the thoracic cage. 2. Developed by C. Earl Miller.

immaturity and primarily cartilaginous structure of the young child's pelvis, imprecise aggressive treatment of these joints could disrupt cartilaginous portions of pelvic bones, induce membranous strains, and possibly result in fractures or deranged joint structures.

- Other adjustments to how much OMT to provide need to be made for the ill patient who often has limited energy reserves, weakness and pain.
- Soft tissue, articulatory procedures, such as joint springing, and thrust, or high-velocity/low-amplitude (HVLA), OMT, when performed gently and precisely are effective and well-tolerated in most patients; thrust (HVLA) for SIJ dysfunction and PGP has been used successfully during pregnancy (Daly et al. 1991). Counterstrain, myofascial release, balanced ligamentous tension, and cranial balanced membranous tension treatments are all helpful for patients of any age; they may be most often utilized in infants and young children (Hayes & Bezilla 2006) as well as elderly patients with advanced arthritis or other degenerative disease processes (Hruby 2008). Similar to chiropractic articulatory adjustments, osteopathic manipulations involving thrust are the techniques most likely to have contraindications (bony metastases, bony infections, osteoporosis, etc.), while soft tissue and non-thrust techniques are relatively safe when prudently performed by skilled practitioners (Kuchera et al. 2003).

Respiratory–circulatory model

Somatic dysfunction involves neurogenic inflammatory processes, decreased lymph and blood flow, and palpable congestion of the soft tissues (Pickar 2002, Howell & Willard 2005). A goal of manipulation is to relieve congestion (see Chapter 11).

- Osteopathic manual procedures to the thorax, thoracic inlet and diaphragm have been shown to improve cardiopulmonary function (O-Yurvati et al. 2005).
- Spontaneous breathing improves movement of lymph from the abdominal to the thoracic cavity (Lattuada & Hedenstierna 2006).
- External manual rhythmical abdominal pumping increasing lymph flow and flux in the thoracic duct (Hodge et al. 2007, Downey et al. 2008).

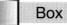

The respiratory–circulatory model views somatic dysfunction in relation to the influence on the ease of respiration and lymph and venous drainage, more than the view of neural entrapment or biomechanically altered function. Skeletal muscles and the thoracic and pelvic diaphragms are pumps of the low-pressure venous and lymphatic systems. Diaphragms and the body core maintain pressure differentials to facilitate flow of the low-pressure circulatory system. Inhalation and exhalation movements are coupled with this fluid flow mechanism (Knott et al. 2005, Lattuada 2006). Based on clinical experience, it is theorized that in order to maximize the potential of these physiological processes (and thoracic diaphragm function in particular) the pelvis, vertebral column and thorax must be functionally flexible and balanced, to maintain appropriate muscle tone. One therapeutic goal of osteopathic manipulation is enhancing pumping action of the musculoskeletal system to aid the return of venous and lymphatic flow to the heart and the reduction of the 'work' of breathing, by increasing the efficiency of each breath.

The balance and maintenance of negative pressures of the thorax and the pelvis depend on efficient and related functions of both the respiratory and pelvic diaphragms. Pelvic congestion, lower extremity oedema, pelvic inflammation and infection are relieved not only when mechanical obstructions are cleared, but also when the blood can deliver nutrition to tissues and, along with the lymph system, remove toxic products of metabolism. Exercise influences the pelvic diaphragm from below to stimulate pumping actions to move fluids (Hodges et al. 1997, Hodges & Richardson 1997) and therefore is an important component of the patient care plan.

Another, and primary, area to be treated in order to move body fluids to reduce inflammation and oedema is the thoracic inlet (Zink 1973, Hodges et al. 2003). By first relieving back pressure caused by fascial restrictions in the left and right supraclavicular fossae and around the left and right first ribs, referred to as 'opening' the thoracic inlet (the area of terminal lymphatic drainage), then relieving myofascial restrictions in the abdominal and pelvic diaphragms, it is theorized that fluid congestion in the pelvis is better able to drain. After addressing other restrictions – skeletal, arthrodial, ligamentous, fascial – a lymphatic pump would extend the benefit of continued fluid motion, augmented by respiration and posture (Nicholas & Oleski 2002, Knott et al. 2005).

Neurological model

The neurological model of osteopathic treatment strives to address autonomic imbalance, relieve peripheral and central sensitization and alleviate pain. Viscerosomatic reflexes, when successfully treated, reduce residual effects in somatic structures that have resulted from a visceral problem; or the viscus may be influenced as a result of stimulation of somatovisceral reflexes (Patterson & Howell 1992, Jänig 2008). Sympathetic nerve supply to pelvic organs is primarily from the thoracolumbar spine. Somatic dysfunction of this area could refer pain to the pelvis (Beal 1985, Patterson & Howell 1992). However, the parasympathetic supply to the pelvis is primarily through the pelvic nerves (S2–4). Somatic dysfunction of the sacrum theoretically could affect bladder (Weiss 2001, Arab et al. 2010) and bowel (Ng 2007) function, as well as influence dysmenorrhoea (Holtzman et al. 2008) and dyspareunia (Gentilcore-Saulnier et al. 2010) through somatovisceral reflexes (Patterson & Howell 1992, Jänig 2008). One purpose of treating the sacrum from the neurological perspective would be to rule out mechanical causes of the PGP. This is particularly useful when the pain is not relieved by OMT, forcing the astute clinician to consider organ dysfunction as a possible generator of pelvic pain through viscerosomatic reflexes (Patterson & Howell 1992) or through central sensitization (Winkelstein 2004, Howell & Willard 2005).

Additional manual approaches to PGP include deep inhibition of myofascial trigger points located on muscles and fascias on the pelvic floor, which are attached to bones of the pelvic girdle (Anderson et al. 2009) (see Chapters 14 and 15). Some of these trigger points may refer pain to other muscles in the pelvis. Relief of these myofascial trigger points through physical therapeutics may also decrease pain sensations related to bladder function, as in the case of patients with interstitial cystitis (Weiss 2001). The points may be located externally on the pelvis, or internally in the vagina. In addition to relieving PGP and chronic pelvic pain, urogenital function may also improve from specific myofascial manual therapy (FitzGerald et al. 2009).

Counterstrain tenderpoints, on the other hand, do not refer pain to other structures. These tenderpoints were empirically identified in the clinical practice of Lawrence Jones, in the 1950s. Dr. Jones found that certain points that were sensitive to digital provocation were relieved (by at least 70%) during sustained passive positioning (from up to 90–120 seconds) of the body in postures. Subsequent evaluation commonly notes reduced sensitivity and enhanced mobility and functionality of soft tissues and associated joints (Dardzinski et al. 2000, Lewis

& Flynn 2001, Speicher et al. 2004). There are also many hypotheses regarding the mechanisms that might explain how strain–counterstrain works. Most researchers consider that modified nociception, as well as the Golgi tendon organ, and alpha Ia afferent and gamma efferents are involved (Bailey & Dick 1992). The exact mechanism of action of the relationship between somatic tender, or trigger, points and somatic and visceral pain and function continues to be investigated (Patterson & Howell 1992, Meltzer & Standley 2007).

Metabolic energy model

The metabolic energy approach to treating pelvic pain addresses hormonal and biochemical factors that influence pelvic girdle pain. In patients with musculoskeletal complaints who only temporarily respond to manipulative treatment, in spite of correctly addressing somatic dysfunctions, it might be useful to consider, for example, investigating thyroid dysfunction, calcium levels, vitamin D levels, abnormal cortisol levels or diabetes (Goldman et al. 2008). Frequently these patients complain of muscle weakness or general fatigue. On palpatory evaluation, changes in tissue texture may lead one to consider laboratory evaluation of a metabolic problem influencing a structural problem (i.e. osteoporosis). In females, oestrogen and relaxin hormones may alter ligament function during and after the childbearing years. In such individuals, in addition to treating hormonal imbalances, nutritional counselling to obtain optimal weight for her age, a practitioner would also advise the patient about types of exercises for weight maintenance, structural stability and flexibility. The patient would also benefit from evaluation of her posture and gait to reduce musculoskeletal strains and injuries.

Consider also a patient with compromised cardiopulmonary function who has PGP and dysfunction that increases the effort of sitting and ambulating, thus taxing the energy economy of the entire musculoskeletal system while exerting excessive energy demand on the heart and lungs. The management plan needs to be modified for patients with cardiopulmonary intolerance to exercises and manual treatments that depend on patient force, such as muscle energy techniques. The practitioner should control the amount of counterforce provided by the patient depending on patient comfort and tolerance without compromising efficacy. Patient respiratory and ocular motion assists (synkinesis) can be utilized to facilitate energy conservation as needed in select patients (Lewit et al. 1997).

Behavioural model

The behavioural model of osteopathic care strives to identify mind–body issues affecting pelvic girdle pain. Thoughts and emotions related to pain are explored to discover a possible somatic component to the problem. Chronic pain is a factor in treating depression. Sleep becomes disrupted, causing increased fatigue and pain (Goldman et al. 2008, Tibbits 2008). Discussion about medical treatment including pain relief medication, hormone replacement therapy, antidepressants and anti-anxiety agents should also include concern about self- or over-medication. Recommendations for care might include counselling, supportive care and an exercise programme to keep active to tolerance (Tettambel 2007). Osteopathic treatment may relieve fascial strains to aid relaxation or reduce anxiety; it may not fully alleviate PGP. Behavioural changes of the patient may help the individual accept the complexity of the symptoms and possibly a long course of treatment.

The cause of low back pain in general is of unknown aetiology in 85% of patients (Deyo & Weinstein 2001) and is feared by 40% of sufferers to be a sign of a serious problem (Waddell 1998); thus, reassurance is one of the most important aspects of the management plan. Vleeming et al. (2007) address this directly in terms of psychosocial and emotional aspects of body–mind medicine. In lumbopelvic girdle pain, imbalance and dysfunction alter gait, posture, functional capacities and other essential tasks that can shift a person's outlook as well as presentation of ability to others.

A key component of the osteopathic examination of the patient with pelvic girdle pain is to make an accurate diagnosis and propose a rational management plan. Establishing a trusting doctor–patient relationship and assuring dedication to helping the patient alleviate pain is critical to successful management of the problem. Indeed, the patient's belief in the possibility of improvement (i.e. hope) has been demonstrated to be a predictor of clinical significance in women having PGP postpartum (Vøllestad & Stuge 2009).

Case study 14.1: Male

A 64-year-old male complains of low back pain and PGP for 5 days after he lifted a bag of groceries. He is unable to extend backwards due to lumbosacral pain, so he avoids it. He has left SIJ pain and urinary urgency sensations and intermittent tingling paraesthesias in his left foot involving his fifth toe and heel. He has had these symptoms off and on for 30 years. Lumbar MRI, urinalysis, cystoscopy and prostate examinations have been normal; the last battery of these tests was performed 2 years ago. Symptoms are intermittent and only appear when he has mechanical dysfunction of his sacroiliac and thoracolumbar spine. Lifting objects over 10 pounds (5 kg) causes a pulling sensation and pain in the right SIJ region. Lying supine or side lying helps relieve the discomfort. Medication does not help.

He has a long history of problems with his low back and pelvis. He was 8 when he was playing on a see-saw with a friend. While up high, his friend jumped off the low end and he suddenly fell to the ground onto his right sacrum and hip. He had disabling pain, but as a resilient child, that resolved in a few weeks. In his teenage life, he began having low back pain. An avid skier, he had no problem during skiing, until he grew older. In his twenties he attended professional school and began practising his trade by the time he was 30 years old. As he began his stressful career and began to raise a family, he developed incapacitating low back and pelvic pain to the extent that he could barely get out of bed.

Full medical workup has consistently been negative for organic disease except for testicular failure requiring testosterone replacement since last year. He has sought osteopathic manual treatments for 30 years to alleviate his pain and dysfunction. Osteopathic manipulative treatment to balance the muscles and mobilize the joints of the pelvis and low back has consistently enabled him to return to work pain-free. For decades he has had urinary frequency and urgency that waxes and wanes in amount relative to the degree of pelvic girdle dysfunction, but no pathology of his bladder, urethra or prostate has ever been found by his urologists. Sexual function was intact until 2 years ago. Testicular failure now causes testosterone deficiency and, without replacement, muscle wasting is noticeable throughout his body.

For 30 years, intermittent osteopathic manipulative care three or four times a year has helped him maintain his professional practice, raise his family and continue skiing. He spends an hour daily stretching his lower extremity, low back and neck muscles to remain supple and balanced. He has sinus allergies, for which he gets desensitization injections every 3–5 years, and occasional vertigo, which has responded to osteopathic manipulation of his cervical somatic dysfunction and the use of a rocker board for balance training. For the past 5 years he has had occasional palpitations for which a full cardiology workup was unable to discern a pathological condition; palpitations resolved following correction of his second left rib somatic dysfunction.

An osteopathic structural examination using a combination of visual, motion and palpatory tests for tenderness and tissue abnormalities (STAR) in the standing, seated, supine and prone positions revealed the following findings:

- Neurological examination is negative for eliciting any deficiencies in motor strength, sensation or coordination.
- In the standing postural assessment, his thoracic kyphosis is flattened and his head is held anterior to the lateral postural line of gravity. He has a right convex scoliosis at the thoracolumbar junction from T10–L2 with apex at T12.
- His gait appears normal and gross range of motion of the upper and lower extremities is full.
- Seated and supine active and passive straight leg raising tests are negative for shooting posterior leg pain at 70° bilaterally.
- There are no signs of a short leg.
- The right hamstring muscle group is more hypertonic than the left.
- His pelvic anatomic landmarks, including iliac crest levels, anterior posterior diameter between posterior superior iliac spines and anterior iliac spines are asymmetrical; his right hemipelvis is noticeably smaller than the left side.
- Motion restriction is present at the lumbosacral and SIJs and pubic symphysis. He has a lumbosacral torsion and an iliosacral shear.
- Muscle imbalances are present in the psoas, multifidi, erector spinae, quadratus lumborum, piriformis and gluteus medius muscles.
- On the seated examination, his L5 is found to be flexed, rotated left, sidebent left; the sacrum is rotated right on a left oblique axis; L4 is also rotated left; L3 is flexed, rotated right, sidebent right; T10–L2 is neutral, rotated right, sidebent left.

- The left piriformis and psoas muscles are tense and tender, and have decreased range of motion. The right inferior surface of the posterior superior iliac spine, right side of the L5 spinous process and the left iliolumbar ligament are tender to palpation.
- Backward bending in the prone position causes the sacrum to rotate more to the right and the lumbosacral posterior-anterior spring test is positive (resistant).
- The right thoracic diaphragm and right pelvic diaphragm excursions are restricted during exhalation.
- The left thoracic spine between T4 and T8 is neutral, rotated left, sidebent right. T2 is extended, rotated right, sidebent right. The right first rib is elevated, with hypertonic and tender middle scalene muscles. The cervical spine is restricted at C3–6 possibly due to the scalene muscle spasm. The atlantoaxial joint is rotated left and the occipitoatlas joint is extended, rotated right, sidebent left. The right posterior quadrant of the cranium has decreased compliance compared to the contralateral side.

There are biomechanical, neurological, respiratory–circulatory, metabolic and behavioural considerations in designing a management plan for his recurrent PGP problem. Viewing the clinical situation from the biomechanical perspective, he has an asymmetrical pelvis probably due to a traumatic incident during his formative years. The sacrum comprises five separate bones separated by compliant cartilage until age 25. It is plausible that the fall inhibited full growth of one side of his pelvis. It is also possible this is a congenital asymmetrical development. His pelvic dysfunction on the left side is compensated by the right rotation of the thoracolumbar junction, and the left rotation of the thoracic spine, then right rotation of the cervical spine. Previous attempts to just treat his sacroiliac and lumbosacral mechanics have failed to resolve his symptoms. Treating the entire neuromusculoskeletal system at each visit gives him lasting relief for weeks to months. After several weeks of work, he develops an imbalance of muscle tension throughout his body and symptoms recur. Manual procedures utilized to resolve somatic dysfunction to improve posture and motion included:

- Myofascial release to the thoracolumbar fascia (see Figure 14.1);
- Muscle energy techniques for the lumbosacral somatic dysfunction (see Figure 14.2 and video link 1);
- HVLA for the pelvic shear (see Figure 14.3 and video link 2);
- Functional technique for the lumbar spine dysfunction (see Figure 14.4 and video link 3);
- Strain–counterstrain for the piriformis tender points (see Figure 14.5 and video link 4);

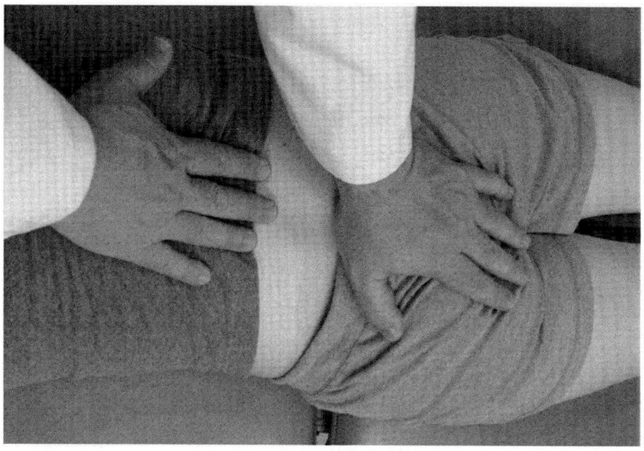

Figure 14.1 • Myofascial release to the thoracolumbar fascia

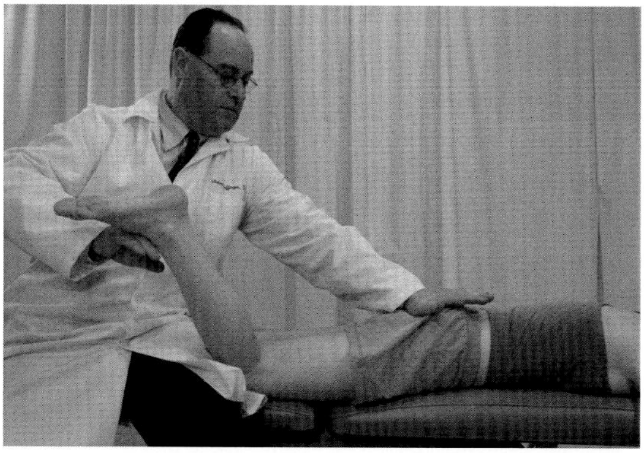

Figure 14.2 • Muscle energy techniques for lumbosacral somatic dysfunction

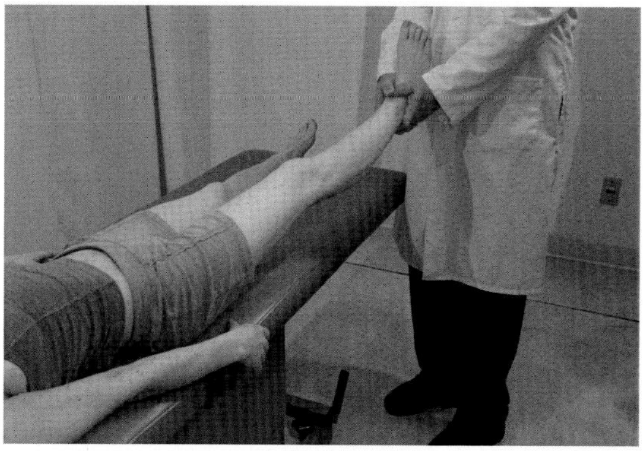

Figure 14.3 • HVLA for pelvic shear

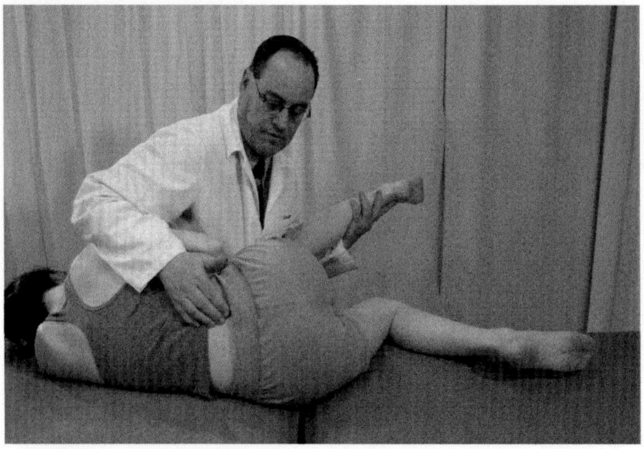

Figure 14.4 • Functional technique for lumbar spine dysfunction

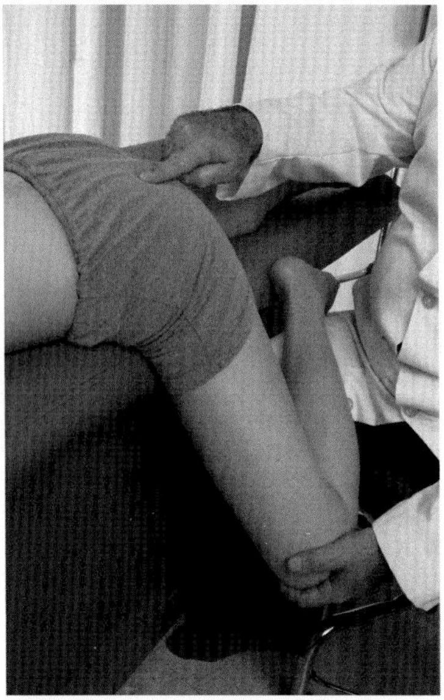

Figure 14.5 • Strain–counterstrain for piriformis tender points

- Muscle energy treatment to stretch the hypertonic psoas muscles (see Figure 14.6);
- Muscle energy for the pubic dysfunction (see Figure 14.7);
- Muscle energy for lumbar spine somatic dysfunction with the patient in the seated position was performed at times during his treatments, as depicted in Figure 14.8 and video link 5;
- HVLA for the lumbar spine somatic dysfunctions with the patient sidelying was used often as depicted in Figure 14.9 and video link 7a;
- Soft tissue massage for the thoracic and lumbar paraspinal muscle hypertonicity (see video link 6);

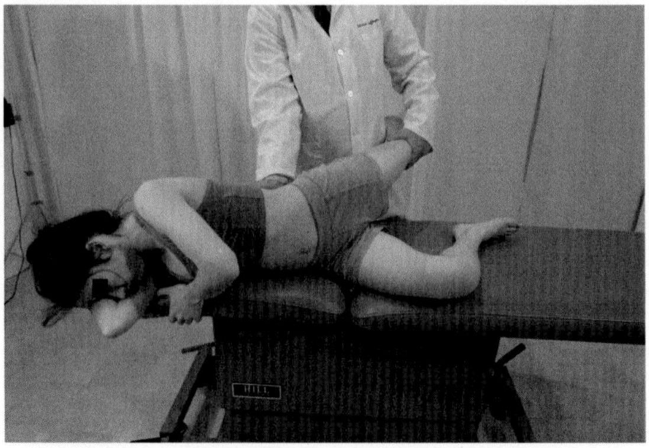

Figure 14.6 • Muscle energy treatment to stretch hypertonic psoas muscles

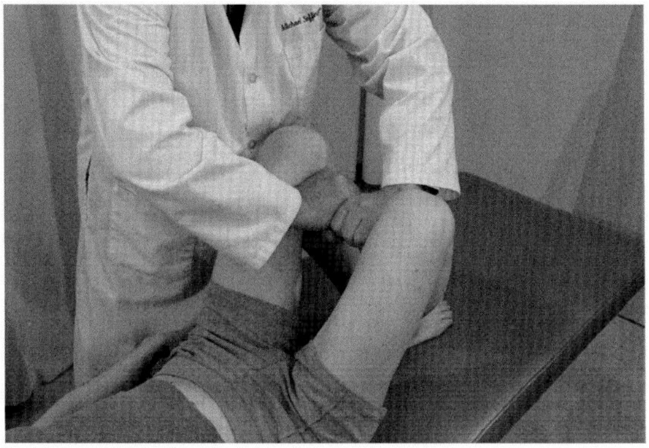

Figure 14.7 • Muscle energy for pubic dysfunction

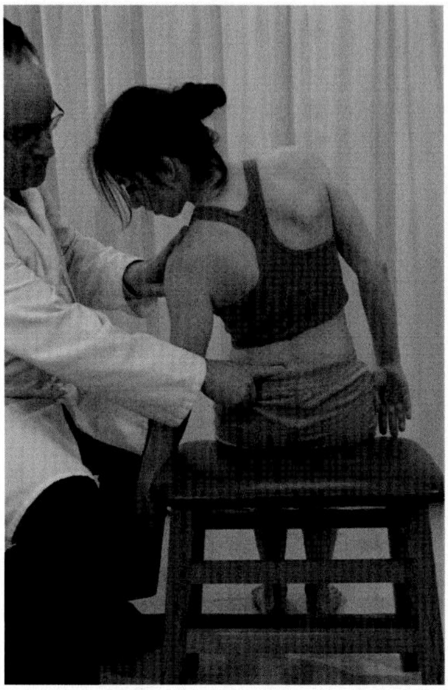

Figure 14.8 • Muscle energy for lumbar spine somatic dysfunction with the patient in the seated position

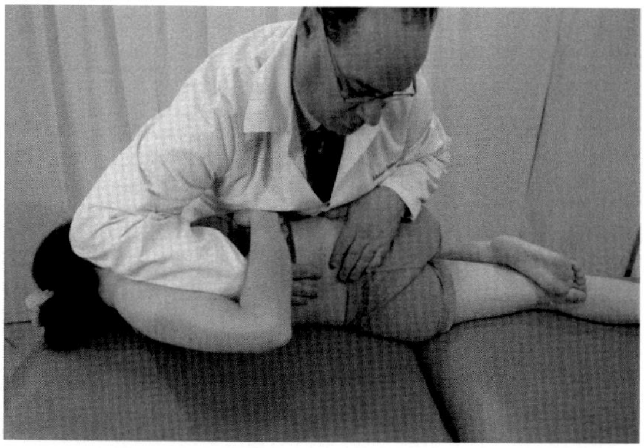

Figure 14.9 • HVLA for lumbar spine somatic dysfunctions with the patient sidelying

- HVLA for the cervical spine somatic dysfunction;
- Muscle energy for the costal cage dysfunctions;
- Balanced membranous tension for the cranium somatic dysfunctions.

From the neurological perspective, most commonly, PGP involving the SIJ is accompanied by pain radiating no further down the leg than the knee (Szadek et al. 2009). However, this patient had non-painful paraesthesias to the foot. This suggested that there was a neurological root being compromised at S1 or the sciatic nerve itself was irritated as it passes by, or through, the piriformis muscle (Boyajian-O'Neill et al. 2008). To decrease lumbosacral pain and peripheral sensitization, tenderness was reduced with strain–counterstrain techniques for the sacral and lumbar regions, including the piriformis muscle tender point. The urinary urgency sensation resolved a couple of days after the somatic dysfunctions resolved (somatovisceral reflex), possibly due to a decrease in afferent stimuli from the joint and soft tissue nociceptors in the spine and pelvis (Howell & Willard 2005).

For improvement in respiration–circulation, myofascial release was provided for the lumbodorsal fascia, the thoracic inlet, and thoracic and pelvic diaphragm somatic dysfunctions. Muscle energy was used to release the scalene spasm. Improved costal cage and diaphragm motion was restored to maximize respiratory function (see also Chapter 12).

Metabolic treatment with testosterone supplementation helped restore muscle wasting (Bassil et al. 2009), but since he had an asymmetry of muscle mass due to his scoliotic lumbosacral spine mechanics, he had an increase in his asymmetric paraspinal thoracolumbar muscle mass with increasing doses of testosterone, which made him uncomfortable and in more pain. OMT did not help decrease the hypertonicity or hypertrophy of the thoracolumbar muscle mass, but decreased doses of testosterone did. Subsequently, OMT was effective in relieving pain and improving muscle balance and lumbopelvic stability in posture and motion. Urinary urgency symptoms diminished as well.

From the behavioural viewpoint, he has had chronic pelvic pain for over 50 years, but has learned to live with it with daily exercises, medication, osteopathic manipulative treatment and surveillance for organic disorders. He does not smoke or drink alcohol. Other than skiing (he rarely falls unless someone crashes into him), he does not engage in risky behaviours.

Case study 14.2: Female

Throughout a woman's life, there are many instances where PGP can occur and be treated. Following is a discussion of osteopathic treatment of a female patient who has had various instances of PGP throughout her life. At age 16 she developed low back pain after sustaining a fall onto a balance beam in a gymnastics competition. Structural findings included shear of pubic symphysis, upslipped left innominate, left lumbosacral tenderness. X-rays confirmed a pars interarticularis fracture of the fifth lumbar vertebra. She responded well to balanced ligamentous tension and, later, to muscle energy treatment. Because she also has an increased lumbar lordosis, she tries to maintain an exercise programme to stabilize her low back and to avert spondylolisthesis.

At age 24, the patient was having severe menstrual discomfort, dyspareunia and inability to become pregnant after 3 years of marriage. She reported that exercise occasionally helped diminish her menstrual cramps. She also exercised to control her weight as she had gained about 20 pounds since the wedding. This extra weight also bothered her low back and hips. On gynaecological examination, posterior vaginal vault tenderness was elicited, and the uterus was fixed in retroversion. This examination was quite uncomfortable and the discomfort she experienced was similar to painful intercourse. A diagnosis of endometriosis and pelvic adhesions was confirmed with laparoscopy. Prior to surgery, osteopathic treatment to her sacral base to attempt to restore physiological motion and reduce menstrual discomfort was useful, but not entirely successful. Post-operatively, the patient experienced pelvic pain relief as adhesions from her pelvic organs to her pelvic floor were released. Increased mobility of the sacro-iliac joints was noted. The patient also reported that she could do more exercising for longer time periods. Her dyspareunia was also relieved as she became pregnant 3 months after surgery.

Her pregnancy aggravated her low back and hip pain due to postural changes, pre-existing lumbar lordosis with spondylolysis, anteriorly tipped pelvic bowl, and weight gain. Hormone influence of relaxin on all of her pelvic joints also increased her misery. She delivered her first baby, a breech presentation, by caesarian section at term. She did not experience a long labour, but stated that most of her contractions started in her back instead of anterior pelvis. She responded well to osteopathic treatment which focused on mobilizing her SIJs.

Three years later, she delivered her second child vaginally after a long labour and forceps-assisted delivery, with large episiotomy. During this pregnancy, she experienced tearing pains, most likely due to stretching of recurrent endometrial adhesions, as well as adhesions from previous surgical delivery. Postpartum pain was reported in the rectal area. Walking and using the toilet were extremely painful. X-ray confirmed a twisted coccyx. Osteopathic treatment to the muscles of the pelvic floor, the pubic symphysis, and the sacrococcygeal area provided relief. Family members also assisted with baby care so that the patient could get additional much-needed rest.

Shortly thereafter, during a 'well woman' gynaecology visit, the patient complained of low back and hip pain. She related it to lifting children and groceries and doing housework. No abnormalities were noted on her intrapelvic examination, but on her musculoskeletal structural examination, a bilateral posterior sacral base was found and treated with OMT. This resolved the back and hip pain. The dysfunction could have been related to her delivery that did not entirely resolve and was merely exacerbated by lifting.

At age 46, the patient had a hysterectomy with bilateral oophorectomy for adenomyosis and uterine fibroids. She reported that she was having painful and heavy menstrual flow. A large posterior uterine fibroid was putting pressure on her colon and pelvic floor. Venous congestion of her pelvis caused hip pain with walking or doing low back exercises. Surgery provided musculoskeletal relief and osteopathic manipulative treatment stabilized her pelvic girdle with related ligaments so that she could resume an exercise routine. She is menopausal and currently considering health management options for this phase of her life: hormone replacement therapy, dietary changes, re-evaluation of her exercise regimen to keep her musculoskeletal system flexible and stable, while protecting herself from osteoporosis and debilitating degenerative arthritis.

In summary, PGP has many opportunities to manifest throughout the life of a female patient. It may be the result of physical trauma in adolescence, pelvic organ dysfunction, hormone influences throughout pre- and post-reproductive years, childbirth, and menopause. Osteopathic care can modify potential physical and metabolic disabilities influencing PGP by addressing structural influences affecting a woman's body changes throughout her life.

Home exercise programme

Osteopathic manipulative treatment in-office effects are supported by providing an individualized exercise regimen for self-care between sessions. Regular exercise also helps to maintain the progress made during a series of treatment sessions. Exercise prescriptions are generated from four methodical steps:

- A detailed history;
- Physical examination including functional assessment;
- Treatment of kinetic chain dysfunctions;
- Reassessment as to goals (Liebenson 2003).

Goals of treatment are reassurance, reactivation and functional restoration. Together with OMT, exercise serves as a catalyst for recovery by promoting kinetic stability and reducing further dysfunction. At each office visit, functional re-assessment enables the practitioner and patient to determine degree of progress, re-establish goals and modify exercise prescriptions.

A detailed history should ascertain whether remote injuries, procedures or events might inform the current presentation in ways that impact function or expectation. Setting attainable short- and long-term goals and reviewing them periodically helps track and quantify clinical and personal success. Age, gender, chronicity and expectations are factors to consider when setting goals. Specific therapeutic measures may target distinct clinical presentations such as piriformis syndrome, trochanteric bursitis, iliopectineal bursitis, osteitis pubis, groin or thigh strains, and other pelvic girdle conditions (DePalma 2001).

Rehabilitation of pelvic girdle disorders includes consideration of the pelvic girdle, visceral contents and functions, adjacent structures (low back, abdominal core, SIJs, coccyx, hips) and kinetic chain biomechanics. Because structural assessment is related intrinsically to functional integrity, it is necessary to address the bones, joints, muscles, nerves, internal organs and connective tissues including fascia and skin.

Individualized exercise programme prescriptions can help people improve mobility, stretching and strengthening of the lumbopelvic region. When designing a programme, it is necessary to consider the structural components and their attachments while testing to determine functional compromise, imbalance or pain provocation guide exercise selection. It is helpful to consider the sequencing of exercises by introducing relaxed breathing first to promote functional releasing of regional tension (Vleeming et al. 2007). Stretching sequentially can facilitate mobilization; Sahrmann (2001) advocates addressing the hip flexors and anterior capsule, then piriformis, and then hamstrings, first in passive and then progressively independent active activation. Following Janda's guidelines (1977, 1986), Isaacs and Bookhout (2002) and Greenman (2003) propose that muscle groups that are commonly tight release well when agonist–antagonist groups are treated by alternate contract–release intervals, as in muscle energy technique (see Chapter 11 and elsewhere in this chapter).

The effect of exercise on women with postpartum PGP has been evaluated in two randomized controlled trials (Mens et al. 2000, Stuge et al. 2004a, 2004b). In 2006 Stuge and colleagues compared the studies to determine variant findings (Stuge et al. 2006). Overall, the studies demonstrated that the group of women that performed specific stabilizing exercises reported lower pain and disability ratings and higher quality of life for the duration of the study and for 1–2 years postpartum.

Stuge and colleagues (Stuge et al. 2004a, 2004b) chose Lee and Vleeming's integrated model (1998) of self-expansion, where components of form closure and force closure are augmented by motor control and an appreciation of emotions and awareness related to pelvic girdle stability. The pelvic girdle's structural elements comprise what Lee calls a Circle of Integrity. In the Stuge group's protocol, greater emphasis was placed on deep core local muscles and the larger torque-producing global muscle

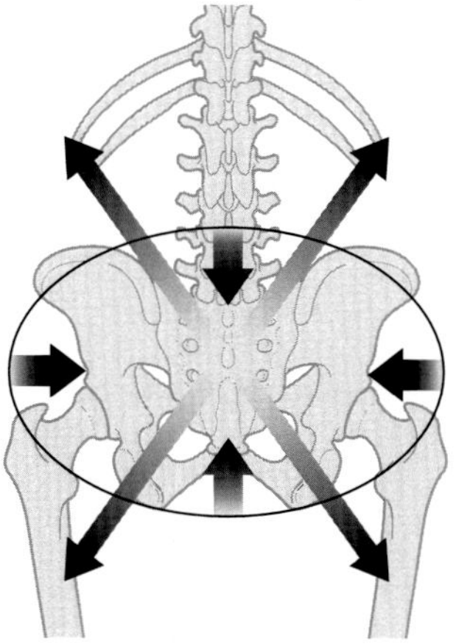

Figure 14.10 • An illustration of muscles with implication for lumbopelvic stability and control. Short arrows indicate deep local muscles (the transverse abdominals, the multifidus, diaphragm and the pelvic floor muscles). Long arrows indicate the posterior oblique muscle sling with latissimus dorsi, gluteus maximus and the intervening thoracolumbar fascia (Stuge et al. 2006)

systems in order to stabilize the spine as well as the pelvic girdle (Figure 14.10). Coordinated motor activation was emphasized and individualized during training to promote improved motor control of the deeper core muscles independent of superficial muscles (see Box 14.4). Asymmetric SIJ motion called for muscle energy mobilization by the individuals or by their therapist. Three sets of ten repetitions were performed by participants three times a week, and intensity was scaled to avoid lumbopelvic trembling or uncomfortable pain sensations during or after training. Preloading of superficial muscles before global muscle recruitment was encouraged to promote stability instead of rigidity.

> [W]e have learned how to teach others to achieve mobile stability through touch, imagery, and movement – a different way to exercise.
>
> (Diane Lee 2004)

Exercise regimens and therapeutic options

The pelvic girdle is a parabolic bowl capable of integrated load distribution through form closure, force closure and motor control. Hence, rehabilitation of the patient with PGP integrates functional and structural elements by manipulation, manual treatments

Box 14.4

The abdominal rectus sheath

The abdominal rectus sheath, also known as the 'six-pack' of buff bodybuilders, is the anterior superficial layer overlying the true core abdominal muscles: transversus abdominis internal and external obliques. These layers form a three-ply wrap of muscles from the lumbar spine and thoracolumbar fascia behind, to the pubic rami, thoracic costal outlet and linea alba in front, supported from below by the coordinated activity of the pelvic floor. The multifidus muscles at the base of the lumbosacral spine comprise 90% of the caudal sacral paraspinal musculature (Mitchell 2001).

---

and individualized exercise programmes. Progressive exercise programmes for dynamic lumbopelvic stabilization have been recommended by Lee (2004), Liebenson (2003, 2004, 2007, 2008, 2010), Creager (2001), Akuthota et al. (2008), Cusi (2010a) and many others. Cusi simplifies the regimen: After diagnosing the type, location, and extent of 'load transfer failure', a specific, targeted and progressive treatment programme consisting of exercise and other therapeutics is started. The exercise regimen he proposes has three steps:

1. *Isolation*. Engage the involved structures to restore deep core strength and reduce faulty global recruitment (Lee's 'downtraining') so that the person learns 'neutral' lumbopelvic positioning (slight lumbar lordosis, or 12 o'clock for the pelvic clock).
2. *Combination*. Improve endurance and coordination by progressive challenges such as adding limb movements while maintaining the core and breathing.
3. *Function*. Progress to functional activities of daily living, work and recreation. If structural integrity is not consistently maintained despite consistent effort and appropriate programme practice, direct stabilization of disrupted tissues may be attained by use of prolotherapy before resorting to surgery (Dagenais et al. 2007, Cusi et al. 2010b).

Exercise equipment such as balls, resistance bands and foam rolls may provide additional learning opportunities (Creager 1994, 1998, 2001, Leibenson 2010). Liebenson (2008) recommends stabilizing the entire lumbopelvic region by training in 'abdominal brace' methods of all-around co-activation. Pelvic belts might help certain individuals improve stability while regaining internal strength and stamina (or until postpartum) (Nillson-Wickmar et al. 2005).

Exercises for the pelvic girdle, lumbar spine and hips are best addressed as a unity comprising components (Lee 2004). After establishing which structures are involved (form control), determine faulty function (force control) and disproportional global and local muscle recruitment (motor control). Breath and relaxation training add the fourth element (emotions and awareness) to the integrated model (Lee 2004, Vleeming et al. 2007).

Certain principles are common to treatment programmes:

- Neutral spine mechanics;
- Progressive dynamic core stabilization;
- Functional integration.

The first step of the exercise regimen is learning neutral spine mechanics, a process of tilting the pelvis anteriorly and cephalad in a symmetrical and controlled manner. The desired small amount of lumbar lordosis is maintained while the person breathes; this position corresponds to 12 o'clock of a pelvic clock (a figurative clock on the person's belly facing forward) (Sahrmann 2001, Isaacs & Bookhout 2002, Greenman 2003). This is accomplished by co-contracting the transversus abdominis and multifidus muscles simultaneously; learning to do this is facilitated by in-session training and take-home exercises (Creager 2001, Lee 2004, Vleeming et al. 2007). Following Janda's lead, Liebenson (2007) advances the classic TrA-MF focus to performing circumferential contraction of the entire abdominal wall as an 'abdominal brace' that provides stability while a person is responding to postural perturbations. Kinesthetic awareness can be facilitated if the individual self-monitors smooth and even movement at the anterior superior iliac spines while moving from 12 to 6 o'clock, 3 (left) to 9 (right) o'clock, and then through clockwise and counterclockwise rotations while keeping the pelvis on the exercise surface instead of bridging (Isaacs & Bookhout 2002).

Once neutral spine and clock movements are coordinated with breathing, this kinesthetic awareness is applied to dynamic lumbopelvic core stabilization movements involving the limbs while the person is supine, prone, on all fours (quad position) or standing. Liebenson (2008) cites McGill (1995, 1998) who found that safe loading of the lumbopelvic region is accomplished with quad single leg raise, opposite arm/leg raise, side bridge on knees or on ankles, and curl-up positions. Good form is essential and should be the emphasis from the start rather than the number of repetitions. McGill (2007) recommends doing cat-cow in quad position 8–10 times to warm up, then doing three sets of a 'reverse pyramid' (15, 12, and then eight repetitions) of any manoeuvre. Liebenson (2007, 2008) outlines 'stability training variables' to promote satisfactory motor control and movement pattern re-education:

- Intensity: submaximal, less than 50% of single repetition maximum.
- Sets and repetitions: start with one set of approximately six repeats, then progress to 15 repeats, then McGill's reverse pyramid.
- Hold times: emphasize endurance by holding for 1–2 breaths (6–10 s).
- Form: movements should be performed slowly with appropriate form for motor control training and injury prevention.
- Frequency: daily or twice a day.
- Duration: improvement noted after consistent performance for at least 3 months.
- Goals: structural stability and functional improvement should reach individualized needs for performance capacities and activities of daily living.

Liebenson provides examples of several exercises to add: side-lying bridges, bird-dog quad elevation of opposite arm and leg, and dying bug supine activation of the limbs bent and extended (Liebenson 2008). Supine bridges can be performed with or without a ball between the knees or resistance band around them (Creager 1994, Liebenson 2007); pubic symphysis self-mobilization can be done from this position if the person exhales while contracting knees together into the ball or apart into the band. Creager (1994, 1998, 2001) and Lee (2004) provide many other progressive exercise routines using equipment such as balls and resistance bands. Liebenson (2010) implements foam roll exercises. A person is encouraged to progress to integrating dynamic core stabilization principles and practices into functional and occupational activities that can be performed as an independent home programme.

Elden et al. (2008a, 2008b) has found that both acupuncture and stabilizing exercises are safe treatments for pregnant women having PGP without increased fetal risk; with repeated clinical assessment, nearly all of the women in the study were found to be pain-free 12 weeks after giving birth. Schlinger (2006) finds that Feldenkrais, Alexander Technique and yoga body-awareness approaches are useful adjuncts to medical care.

Independent home exercise programmes must be done consistently at least 3 days per week, with additional activities or sports participation as tolerated. Granath et al. (2006) found that healthy pregnant women who participated in water aerobics once a week reported less back pain or absenteeism than those women doing land-based exercises once a week. DiFrancisco-Donoghue et al. (2007) conducted strength training in older adults (65–79 years old) and found that once or twice weekly produced similar levels of health and functional benefit. The adage 'you rest, you rust' has been confirmed by an animal model showing that exercise reduces joint stiffness after blunt trauma (Weaver & Haut 2005).

Conclusion

In conclusion, PGP is multifactorial. There are structural–mechanical, respiratory–circulatory, metabolic–immune–endocrine, neurological and behavioural components to the problem. Evaluation should be specific to the patient, giving credence to all of the related components and in consideration of the variety of circumstances that cause the painful symptom, thus enabling an accurate diagnosis of the underlying condition. Therapeutic options and regimens should be goal-specific and rational, and respectful of the abilities and preferences of the individual being treated. Osteopathic manipulative treatment is utilized to alleviate somatic dysfunction, decrease or alleviate pain and improve motion and function of the neuromuscular system. Improvement in posture and motion, circulation, respiration, metabolic processes, neurological balance/integration and behaviour are the ultimate goals of treatment. Individualized exercise programmes complement osteopathic medical management and manipulative treatment.

References

Akuthota, V., Ferreiro, A., Moore, T., et al., 2008. Core stability exercise principles. Curr. Sports Med. Rep. 7 (1), 39–44.

Anderson, R.U., Sawyer, T., Wise, D., Morey, A., et al., 2009. Painful myofascial trigger points and pain sites in men with chronic prostatitis/chronic pelvic pain syndrome. J. Urol. 182 (6), 2753–2758.

Arab, A.M., Abdollahi, I., Joghataei, M.T., et al., 2009. Inter and intra examiner reliability of single and composites of selected motion palpation and pain provocation tests for sacroiliac joint. Man. Ther. 14 (2), 213–221.

Arab, A.M., Behbahani, R.B., Lorestani, L., et al., 2010. Assessment of pelvic floor muscle function in women with and without low back pain using transabdominal ultrasound. Man. Ther. Jan 18[Epub ahead of print], 1–5.

Bahr, R., Andersen, S.O., Løken, S., et al., 2004. Low back pain among endurance athletes with and without specific back loading: a cross-sectional survey of cross-country skiers, rowers, orienteerers, and nonathletic controls. Spine 29 (4), 449–454.

Bailey, H.W., Beckwith, C.G., 1937. Short leg and spinal anomalies: their incidence and effects on spinal mechanics. In: Peterson, B. (Ed.), 1983. Postural balance and Imbalance. American Academy of Osteopathy, Indianapolis, pp. 63–70.

Bailey, M., Dick, L., 1992. Nociceptive considerations in treating with counterstrain. J. Am. Osteopath. Assoc. 92 (3), 334–341.

Barney, S.P., 2008. Pelvic masses. Med. Clin. North Am. 92 (5), 1143–1161.

Bassil, N., Alkaade, S., Morley, J.E., 2009. The benefits and risks of testosterone replacement therapy: a review. Ther. Clin. Risk Manage. 5 (3), 427–448.

Beales, D.J., O'Sullivan, P.B., Briffa, N.K., Spine 2009a. Motor control patterns during an active straight leg raise in pain-free subjects. Spine 34 (1), E1–E8.

Beales, D.J., O'sullivan, P.B., Briffa, N.K., Spine 2009b. Motor control patterns during an active straight leg raise in chronic pelvic girdle pain subjects. Spine 34 (9), 861–870.

Beal, M.C., 1982. The sacroiliac problem: Review of anatomy, mechanics, and diagnosis. J. Am. Osteopath. Assoc. 81, 667–679.

Beal, M.C., 1985. Viscerosomatic reflexes: A review. J. Am. Osteopath. Assoc. 85, 786–801.

Biering-Sorensen, F., 1984. Physical measurements as risk indicators for low-back trouble over a one-year period. Spine 9, 106–119.

Bo, K., Backe-Hansen, K., 2007. Do elite athletes experience low back, pelvic girdle and pelvic floor complaints during and after pregnancy? Scand. J. Med. Sci. Sports 17 (5), 480–487.

Boyajian-O'Neill, L., McClain, R., Coleman, M., et al., 2008. Diagnosis and management of piriformis syndrome: an osteopathic approach. J. Am. Osteopath. Assoc. 108, 657–664.

Boyle, K.J., 2008. Benign gynecologic conditions. Surg. Clin. North Am. 88 (2), 245–264.

Bronfort, G., Haas, M., Evans, R.L., et al., 2006. Efficacy of spinal manipulation and mobilization for low back pain and neck pain: A systematic review and best evidence synthesis. Spine J. 4, 335–356.

Browning, J.E., 1990. Mechanically induced pelvic pain and organic dysfunction in a patient without low back pain. J. Manipulative Physiol. Ther. 13 (7), 406–411.

Chen, C.H., Huang, M.H., Chen, T.W., et al., 2005. Relationship between ankle position and pelvic floor muscle activity in female stress urinary incontinence. Urology 66 (2), 288–292.

Creager, C.C., 1994. Therapeutic Exercises Using the Swiss Ball. Executive Physical Therapy, Inc, Berthoud, Colorado.

Creager, C.C., 1998. Therapeutic Exercises Using Resistive Bands. Executive Physical Therapy, Inc, Berthoud, Colorado.

Creager, C.C., 2001. Bounce Back Into Shape After Baby: The Ultimate Guide to aFun-Filled, Time and Energy Efficient Workout – With Your Baby. Executive Physical Therapy, Inc, Berthoud, CO.

Cusi, M.F., 2010a. Paradigm for assessment and treatment of SIJ mechanical dysfunction. J. Bodyw. Mov. Ther. 14 (2), 152–161.

Cusi, M., Saunders, J., Hungerford, B., et al., 2010b. The use of prolotherapy in the sacroiliac joint. Br. J. Sports Med. 44 (2), 100–104.

da Costa, B.R., Vieira, E.R., 2009. Risk factors for work-related musculoskeletal disorders: a systematic review of recent longitudinal studies. Am. J. Ind. Med. 14, 1–39.

Dagenais, S., Mayer, J., Wooley, J., et al., 2007. Safety and toxicity of prolotherapy for back pain. In: Vleeming, A., Mooney, V., Cusi, M. (Eds.), Sixth Interdisciplinary World Congress on Low Back & Pelvic Pain. Diagnosis and Treatment; the Balance Between Research and the Clinic. ECO, Barcelona, Spain.

Daly, J.M., Frame, P.S., Rapoza, P.A., 1991. Sacroiliac subluxation: a common, treatable cause of low-back pain in pregnancy. Fam. Pract. Res. J. 11 (2), 149–159.

Damen, L., Buyruk, H., Güler-Uysal, F., et al., 2001. Pelvic pain during pregnancy is associated with asymmetric laxity of the sacroiliac joints. Acta Obstet. Gynecol. Scand. 80 (11), 1019–1024.

Dardzinski, J.A., Ostrov, B.E., Hamann, L.S., 2000. Myofascial pain unresponsive to standard treatment: Successful use of a strain and counterstrain technique with physical therapy. J. Clin. Rheumatol. 6 (4), 169–174.

DeMann Jr., L.E., 1997. Sacroiliac dysfunction in dancers with low back pain. Man. Ther. 2 (1), 2–10.

DePalma, B., 2001. Rehabilitation of the groin, hip, and thigh. In: Prentice, W.E. (Ed.), Techniques in Musculoskeletal Rehabilitation. McGraw-Hill, New York, pp. 509–525.

Deyo, R.A., Weinstein, J.N., 2001. Low back pain. N. Engl. J. Med. 344 (5), 363–370.

DiFrancisco-Donoghue, J., Werner, W., Douris, P.C., 2007. Comparison of once-weekly and twice-weekly strength training in older adults. Br. J. Sports Med. 41 (1), 19–22.

Dinnar, U., Beal, M.C., Goodridge, J.P., et al., 1982. Description of fifty diagnostic tests used with osteopathic manipulation. J. Am. Osteopath. Assoc. 81, 314–321.

DonTigny, R.L., 2005a. Critical analysis of the functional dynamics of the sacroiliac joints as they pertain to normal gait. J. Orthopedic Med. 27, 3–10.

DonTigny, R.L., 2005b. Pathology of the sacroiliac joint and its effect on normal gait. J. Orthopedic Med. 27, 61–69.

Downey, H.F., Durgam, P., Williams Jr., A.G., et al., 2008. Lymph flow in the thoracic duct of conscious dogs during lymphatic pump treatment, exercise, and expansion of extracellular fluid volume. Lymphat. Res. Biol. 6 (1), 3–13.

Eberhard-Gran, M., Eskild, A., 2008. Diabetes mellitus and pelvic girdle syndrome in pregnancy. Is there an association? Acta Obstet. Gynecol. Scand. 87 (10), 1015–1019.

Educational Council on Osteopathic Principles (ECOP), 1987. Core Curriculum Outline. American Association of Colleges of Osteopathic Medicine, Washington, DC.

Educational Council on Osteopathic Principles (ECOP), 2009. Glossary of Osteopathic Terminology. American Association of Colleges of Osteopathic Medicine, Washington, DC.

Elden, H., Ostgaard, H.C., Fagevik-Olsen, M., et al., 2008a. Treatments of pelvic girdle pain in pregnant women: adverse effects of standard treatment, acupuncture and stabilizing exercises on the pregnancy, mother, delivery and the fetus/neonate. BMC Complement. Altern. Med. Jun 26:8, 34.

Elden, H., Hagberg, H., Olsen, M.F., et al., 2008b. Regression of pelvic girdle pain after delivery: follow-up of a randomized single blind controlled trial with different treatment modalities. Acta Obstet. Gynecol. Scand. 87 (2), 201–208.

Esquinazi, A., Mukul, T., 2008. Gait analysis: technology and clinical applications. In: Braddom, R.L. (Ed.), Physical medicine and rehabilitation. third ed. Saunders, Philadelphia, pp. 93–110.

Fall, M., Baranowski, A.P., Elneil, S., et al., 2010. Guidelines on Chronic Pelvic Pain. European Association of Urology. Eur. Urol. 57, 35–48.

Ferreira, M.L., Ferreira, P.H., Latimer, J., et al., 2003. Efficacy of spinal manipulative therapy for low back pain of less than three months' duration. J. Manipulative Physiol. Ther. 26, 593–601.

FitzGerald, M.P., Anderson, R.U., Potts, J., 2009. Randomized multicenter feasibility trial of myofascial physical therapy for the treatment of urological chronic pelvic pain syndromes. J. Urol. 182 (2), 570–580.

Fryer, G., Morris, T., Gibbons, P., 2004a. Relation between thoracic paraspinal tissues and pressure sensitivity measured by digital algometer. J. Osteopathic Med. 7 (2), 64–69.

Fryer, G., Morris, T., Gibbons, P., 2004b. Paraspinal muscles and intervertebral dysfunction: Part two. J. Manipulative Physiol. Ther. 27 (5), 348–357.

Fryer, G., Morris, T., Gibbons, P., 2005. The relationship between palpation of thoracic tissues and deep paraspinal muscle thickness. Int. J. Osteopathic Med. 8 (1), 22–28.

Fryer, G., Morse, C.M., Johnson, J.C., 2009. Spinal and sacroiliac assessment and treatment techniques used by osteopathic physicians in the United States. Osteopathic Med. Primary Care 3, 4.

Gabbe, S.G. (Ed.), 2007. Skeletal and Postural Changes. Williams' Obstetrics: Normal and Problem Pregnancies, fifth ed. Elsevier, Philadelphia (Chapter 3).

Gentilcore-Saulnier, E., McLean, L., Goldfinger, C., 2010. Pelvic floor muscle assessment outcomes in women with and without provoked vestibulodynia and the impact of a physical therapy program. J. Sex. Med. Jan 6 [Epub ahead of print].

Goldman, L., Ausiello, D. (Eds.), 2008. Cecil's Textbook of Internal Medicine, twenty-third ed. Elsevier, Philadelphia, pp. 1663, 1700–1708, 1761–1767, 1897–1906, 2078–2083.

Goodridge, J.P., 1981. Muscle energy technique: definition, explanation, methods of procedure. J. Am. Osteopath. Assoc. 81 (4), 249–253.

Granath, A.B., Hellgren, M.S., Gunnarsson, R.K., 2006. Water aerobics reduces sick leave due to low back pain during pregnancy. J. Obstet. Gynecol. Neonatal Nurs. 35 (4), 465–471.

Greenman, P.E., 1996. Syndromes of the lumbar spine, pelvis, and sacrum. Phys. Med. Rehabil. Clin. North Am. 7, 773–785.

Greenman, P.E., 2003. Principles of Manual Medicine, third ed. Lippincott, Williams & Wilkins, Philadelphia.

Gutke, A., Josefsson, A., Oberg, B., 2007. Pelvic girdle pain and lumbar pain in relation to postpartum depressive symptoms. Spine 32 (13), 1430–1436.

Gutke, A., Kjellby-Wendt, G., Oberg, B., 2009. The inter-rater reliability of a standardized classification system for pregnancy-related lumbopelvic pain. Man. Ther. Jul 24 [Epub ahead of print].

Hancock, M.J., Maher, C.G., Latimer, J., et al., 2007. Systematic review of tests to identify the disc, SIJ or facet joint as the source of low back pain. Eur. Spine J. 16, 1539–1550.

Haneline, M.T., Young, M., 2009. A review of intraexaminer and interexaminer reliability of static spinal palpation: a literature synthesis. J. Manipulative Physiol. Ther. 32 (5), 379–386.

Hayes, N.M., Bezilla, T.A., 2006. Incidence of iatrogenesis associated with osteopathic manipulative treatment of pediatric patients. J. Am. Osteopath. Assoc. 106 (10), 605–608.

Hestbaek, L., Leboeuf-Yde, C., 2000. Are chiropractic tests for the lumbo-pelvic spine reliable and valid? A systematic critical literature review. J. Manipulative Physiol. Ther. 23, 258–275.

Hincapié, C.A., Morton, E.J., Cassidy, J.D., 2008. Musculoskeletal injuries and pain in dancers: A systematic review. Arch. Phys. Med. Rehabil. 89 (9), 1819–1829.

Hodge, L.M., King, H.H., Williams Jr., A.G., et al., 2007. Abdominal lymphatic pump treatment increases leukocyte count and flux in thoracic duct lymph. Lymphat. Res. Biol. 5 (2), 127–133.

Hodges, P.W., Mosely, G.L., 2003. Pain and motor control of the lumbopelvic region: effect and possible mechanisms. J. Electromyogr. Kinesiol. 13, 361.

Hodges, P.W., Richardson, C.A., 1997. Contraction of the abdominal muscles associated with movement of the lower limb. Phys. Ther. 77, 132.

Hodges, P.W., Gandevia, S., Richardson, C.A., 1997. Contractions of specific abdominal muscles in postural tasks are affected by respiratory maneuvers. J. Appl. Physiol. 83 (3), 753.

Holtzman, D.A., Petrocco-Napuli, K.L., Burke, J.R., 2008. Prospective case series on the effects of lumbosacral manipulation on dysmenorrhea. J. Manipulative Physiol. Ther. 31 (3), 237–246.

Howell, J.N., Willard, F., 2005. Nociception: New understandings and their possible relation to somatic dysfunction and its treatment. Ohio Res. Clin. Rev. 15, 12–15.

Hruby, R.J., 1991. Pathophysiologic models: aids to the selection of manipulative techniques. Am. Acad. Osteopathy J. 1 (3), 8–10.

Hruby, R.J., 1992. Pathophysiologic models and the selection of osteopathic manipulative techniques. J. Osteopath. Med. 6 (4), 25–30.

Hruby, R.J., 2008. Osteopathic medicine and the geriatric patient. Am. Acad. Osteopathy J. 18 (3), 16–20.

Hu, H., Meijer, O.G., van Dieën, J.H., et al., 2010. Muscle activity during the active straight leg raise (ASLR), and the effects of a pelvic belt on the ASLR and on treadmill walking. J. Biomech. 43 (3), 532–539.

Hungerford, B., Gilleard, W., Lee, D., 2004. Altered patterns of pelvic bone motion determined in subjects with posterior pelvic pain using skin markers. Clin. Biomech. 19 (5), 456–464.

Isaacs, E.R., Bookhout, M.R., 2002. Bourdillon's Spinal Manipulation. sixth ed. Butterworth/Heinemann, Boston, pp. 283–314.

Janda, V., 1977. Muscles, central nervous motor regulation and back problems. In: Korr, I.M. (Ed.), The Neurobiologic Mechanisms in Manipulative Therapy. Plenum Press, New York, pp. 27–41.

Janda, V., 1986. Muscle weakness and inhibition (pseudoparesis) in back pain syndromes. In: Grieve, G.P. (Ed.), Modern Manual Therapy of the Vertebral Column. Churchill Livingstone, Edinburgh, pp. 197–201.

Jänig, W., 2008. Pain in the sympathetic nervous system: pathophysiological mechanisms. In: Mathias, C.J., Bannister, R. (Eds.), Autonomic Failure, fifth ed. Oxford University Press, New York.

Jordan, T.R., 2006. Conceptual and treatment models in osteopathy II: Sacroiliac mechanics revisited. Am. Acad. Osteopathy J. 16 (2), 11–17.

Juhl, J.H., Ippolito Cremin, T.M., Russell, G., 2004. Prevalence of frontal plane pelvic postural asymmetry – part 1. J. Am. Osteopath. Assoc. 104 (10), 411–421. Erratum in: J. Am. Osteopath. Assoc. 105 (1), 5.

Kerrigan, D., Della Croce, U., Carciello, M., et al., 2000. A revised view of the determinants of gait: significance of heel rise. Arch. Phys. Med. Rehabil. 81, 1077–1080.

Kerrigan, D., Riley, P., Lelas, J., et al., 2001. Quantification of pelvic rotation as a determinant of gait. Arch. Phys. Med. Rehabil. 82, 217–220.

Kimberly, P., 1976. Formulating a prescription for osteopathic manipulative treatment. J. Am. Osteopath. Assoc. 75, 486–499.

Knott, E.M., Tune, J.D., Stoll, S.T., et al., 2005. Increased lymphatic flow in the thoracic duct during manipulative intervention. J. Am. Osteopath. Assoc. 105 (10), 447–456.

Kristiansson, P., Svardsudd, K., 1996. Discriminatory power of tests applied in back pain during pregnancy. Spine 21 (20), 2337–2343, discussion 2343–2344.

Kuchera, M.L., DiGiovanna, E.L., Greenman, P.E., 2003. Efficacy and complications. In: Ward, R.C., et al. (Eds.), Foundations for Osteopathic Medicine, second ed. Lippincott, Williams & Wilkins, Philadelphia, pp. 1143–1152.

Laslett, M., Young, S.B., Aprill, C.N., et al., 2003. Diagnosing painful sacroiliac joints: a validity study of a McKenzie evaluation and sacroiliac joint provocation tests. Aust. J. Physiother. 49, 89–97.

Laslett, M., Aprill, C.N., McDonald, B., et al., 2005. Diagnosis of sacroiliac joint pain: validity of individual provocation tests and composites of tests. Man. Ther. 10, 207–218.

Latthe, P., 2006. Factors predisposing women to chronic pelvic pain: systematic review. Br. Med. J. 332 (7544), 749–755.

Lattuada, M., Hedenstierna, G., 2006. Abdominal lymph flow in an endotoxin sepsis model: influence of spontaneous breathing and mechanical ventilation. Crit. Care Med. 34 (11), 2792–2798.

Lee, D.G., 2004. The Pelvic Girdle, third ed. Elsevier Science, Edinburgh.

Lee, D.G., Vleeming, A., 1998. Impaired load transfer through the pelvic girdle – a new model of altered neutral zone function. In: Proceedings from the 3rd Interdisciplinary World Congress on Low Back and Pelvic Pain. Vienna, Austria.

Lee, D.G., Lee, L.J., McLaughlin, L., 2008. Stability, continence and breathing: The role of fascia following pregnancy and delivery. J. Bodyw. Mov. Ther. 12, 333–348.

Lesho, E.P., 1999. An overview of osteopathic medicine. Arch. Fam. Med. (6), 477–484.

Lewis, T., Flynn, C., 2001. Use of strain-counterstrain in treatment of patients with low back pain. J. Manual Manip. Ther. 9 (2), 92–98.

Lewit, K., Berger, M., Holzmüller, G., 1997. Breathing movements: The synkinesis of respiration with looking up and down. J. Musculoskeletal Pain 5 (4), 57–69.

Licciardone, J.C., Brimhall, A.K., King, L.N., 2005. Osteopathic manipulative treatment for low back pain: a systematic review and meta-analysis of randomized controlled trials. BMC Musculoskelet. Disord. Aug 4; 6, 43.

Licciardone, J.C., Buchanan, S., Hensel, K.L., et al., 2010. Osteopathic manipulative treatment of back pain and related symptoms during pregnancy: a randomized controlled trial. Am. J. Obstet. Gynecol. 202 (1), 43.e1–43.e8.

Liebenson, C., 2003. Functional training. Part 2: integrating functional training into clinical practice. J. Bodyw. Mov. Ther. 7 (1), 20–21.

Liebenson, C., 2004. Spinal stabilization an update. Part 2: functional assessment. J. Bodyw. Mov. Ther. 8 (2), 199–213.

Liebenson, C., 2007. Hip dysfunction and back pain. J. Bodyw. Mov. Ther. 11, 111–115.

Liebenson, C., 2008. A modern approach to abdominal training. Part III: Putting it together. J. Bodyw. Mov. Ther. 12, 31–36.

Liebenson, C., 2010. Self-management: patient section. Postural exercises on the foam roll. J. Bodyw. Mov. Ther. 14 (2), 203–205.

Lipton, J.A., Flowers-Johnson, J., Bunnell, M.T., et al., 2009. The use of heel lifts and custom orthotics in reducing self-reported chronic musculoskeletal pain scores. Am. Acad. Osteopathy J. (1), 15–17 19–20.

Marx, S., Cimniak, U., Beckert, R., et al., 2009. Chronic prostatitis/chronic pelvic pain syndrome. Influence of osteopathic treatment - a randomized controlled study [Article in German]. Urologe A 48 (11), 1339–1345.

McGill, S.M., 1995. The mechanics of torso flexion: sit-ups and standing dynamic flexion manouvres [sic]. Clin. Biomech. 10, 184–192.

McGill, S.M., 1998. Low back exercises: prescription for the healthy back and when recovering from injury. In: Resources Manual for Guidelines for Exercise Testing and Prescription. third ed. American College of Sports Medicine, Indianapolis, IN. Williams & Wilkins, Baltimore.

McGill, S.M., 2007. Low Back Disorders: Evidence Based Prevention and Rehabilitation, second ed. Human Kinetics Publishers, Champaign, IL.

Meleger, A.L., Krivickas, L.S., 2007. Neck and back pain: musculoskeletal disorders. Neurological Clinics 25 (2), 419–438.

Meltzer, K.R., Standley, P.R., 2007. Modeled repetitive motion strain and indirect osteopathic manipulative techniques in regulation of human fibroblast proliferation and interleukin secretion. J. Am. Osteopath. Assoc. 107 (12), 527–536.

Mens, J.M.A., Snijders, C.J., Stam, H.J., 2000. Diagonal trunk muscle exercises in peripartum pelvic pain: a randomized clinical trial. Phys. Ther. 80 (12), 1164–1173.

Mitchell Jr., F., 2001. The muscle energy manual – evaluation and treatment of the pelvis and sacrum. MET Press, East Lansing, Michigan.

Mitchell Sr., F.L., 1958. Structural pelvic function. Yearbook of the American Academy of Osteopathy, American Academy of Osteopathy, Carmel, CA (now Indianapolis), pp. 71–90.

Mottola, M.F., 2009. Exercise prescription for overweight and obese women: pregnancy and post-partum. Obstet. Clin. North Am. 36 (2), 301–316.

Nadler, S.F., Malanga, G.A., Bartoli, L.A., et al., 2002. Hip muscle imbalance and low back pain in athletes: influence of core strengthening. Med. Sci. Sports Exerc. 34 (1), 9–16.

Ng, C.L., 2007. Levator ani syndrome - a case study and literature review. Aust. Fam. Physician 36 (6), 449–452.

Nicholas, A., Oleski, S., 2002. Osteopathic manipulative treatment for postoperative pain. J. Am. Osteopath. Assoc. 102 (S3), S5–S8.

Nillson-Wikmar, L., Holm, K., Oijerstedt, R., et al., 2005. Effect of three different physical therapy treatments on pain and activity in pregnant women with pelvic girdle pain: a randomized clinical trial with 3, 6, and 12 months follow-up postpartum. Spine 30 (8), 850–856.

O'Connell, J., 2003. Bioelectric responsiveness of fascia: A model for understanding the effects of manipulation. Tech. Orthopaedics 18 (1), 67–73.

O'Sullivan, P.B., Beales, D.J., 2007. Diagnosis and classification of pelvic girdle pain disorders—Part 1: A mechanism based approach within a biopsychosocial framework. Man. Ther. 12 (2), 86–97.

O'Sullivan, P.B., Beales, D.J., Beetham, J.A., et al., 2002. Altered motor control strategies in subjects with sacroiliac joint pain during the active straight-leg-raise test. Spine 27 (1), E1–E8.

O-Yurvati, A.H., Carnes, M.S., Clearfield, M.B., et al., 2005. Hemodynamic effects of osteopathic manipulative treatment immediately after coronary artery bypass graft surgery. J. Am. Osteopath. Assoc. 105 (10), 475–481.

Patterson, M.M., Howell, J.N. (Eds.), 1992. The Central Connection: Somatovisceral/ Viscerosomatic Interaction. American Academy of Osteopathy, Indianapolis.

Pickar, J.G., 2002. Neurophysiological effects of spinal manipulation. Spine J. 2, 357–371.

Pool-Goudzwaard, A.L., ten Hove, M.C.P.H.S., Vierhout, M.E., 2005. Relations between pregnancy-related low back pain, pelvic floor activity and pelvic floor dysfunction. Int. Urogynecol. J. 16, 468–474.

Prather, H., 2007. Recognizing and treating pelvic pain and pelvic floor dysfunction. Phys. Med. Rehabil. Clin. North Am. 18 (3), 477–496.

Robinson, H.S., Brox, J.I., Robinson, R., et al., 2007. The reliability of selected motion and pain provocation tests for the sacroiliac joint. Man. Ther. 2 (1), 72–79.

Ronchetti, I., Vleeming, A., van Wingerden, J.P., 2008. Physical characteristics of women with severe pelvic girdle pain after pregnancy: A descriptive cohort study. Spine 33 (5), E145–E151.

Sahrmann, S., 2001. Diagnosis and Treatment of Movement Impaired Syndromes. Mosby, St. Louis.

Schlinger, M., 2006. Feldenkrais Method, Alexander Technique, and yoga--body awareness therapy in the performing arts. Phys. Med. Rehabil. Clin. N. Am. 17 (4), 865–875.

Seffinger, M.A., Najm, W.I., Mishra, S.I., et al., 2004. Reliability of spinal palpation for diagnosis of back and neck pain: a systematic review of the literature. Spine 29, E413–E425.

Selkow, N.M., Grindstaff, T.L., Cross, K.M., et al., 2009. Short-term effect of muscle energy technique on pain in individuals with non-specific lumbopelvic pain: a pilot study. J. Man. Manip. Ther. 17 (1), E14–E18.

Sembrano, J.N., Polly Jr., D.W., 2009. How often is low back pain not coming from the back? Spine 34 (1), E27–E32.

Speicher, T., et al., 2004. Effect of strain counterstrain on pain and strength in hip musculature. J. Man. Manip. Ther. 12 (4), 215–223.

Stochkendahl, M.J., Christensen, H.W., Hartvigsen, J., et al., 2006. Manual examination of the spine: a systematic critical literature review of reproducibility. J. Manipulative Physiol. Ther. 29 (6), 475–485.

Stuge, B., Laerum, E., Kirkesola, G., et al., 2004a. The efficacy of a treatment program focusing on specific stabilizing exercises for pelvic girdle pain after pregnancy. A randomized controlled trial. Spine 29 (4), 351–359.

Stuge, B., Veierød, M.B., Laerum, E., et al., 2004b. The efficacy of a treatment program focusing on specific stabilizing exercises for pelvic girdle pain after pregnancy. A two-year follow-up of a randomized clinical trial. Spine 29 (10), E197–E203.

Stuge, B., Holm, I., Vøllestad, N., 2006. To treat or not treat postpartum pelvic girdle pain with stabilising exercises? Man. Ther. 11, 337–343.

Szadek, K., van der Wurff, P., van Tulder, M., et al., 2009. Diagnostic validity of criteria for sacroiliac joint pain: a systematic review. J. Pain 10 (4), 354–368.

Tettambel, M.A., 2005. An osteopathic approach to treating women with chronic pelvic pain. J. Am. Osteopath. Assoc. 105 (9 Suppl. 4), S20–S22.

Tettambel, M.A., 2007. Using integrative therapies to treat women with chronic pelvic pain. J. Am. Osteopath. Assoc. 107 (10 Suppl. 6), ES 17–20.

Tibbits, G.M., 2008. Sleep disorders: causes, effects, solutions. Prim. Care 35 (4), 817–837.

Tong, H.C., Heyman, O.G., Lado, D.A., et al., 2006. Interexaminer reliability of three methods of combining test results to determine side of sacral restriction, sacral base position, and innominate bone position. J. Am. Osteopath. Assoc. 106, 464–468.

Van der Hulst, L.A., 2006. Bad experience, good birthing: Dutch low-risk pregnant women with a history of sexual abuse. J. Psychosom. Obstet. Gynaecol. 27 (1), 59–66.

Van der Wurff, P., Hagmeijer, R.H.M., Meyne, W., 2000a. Clinical tests of the sacroiliac joint. A systematic methodological review. Part 1: Reliability. Man. Ther. 5 (1), 30–36.

Van der Wurff, P., Hagmeijer, R.H.M., Meyne, W., 2000b. Clinical tests of the sacroiliac joint. A systematic methodological review. Part 2: Validity. Man. Ther. 5, 89–96.

Van der Wurff, P., Buijs, E.J., Groen, G.J., 2006. A multitest regimen of pain provocation tests as an aid to reduce unnecessary minimally invasive sacroiliac joint procedures. Arch. Phys. Med. Rehabil. 87, 10–14.

Van Wingerden, J.P., Vleeming, A., Buyruk, H.M., et al., 2004. Stabilization of the SIJ in vivo: verification of muscular contribution to force closure of the pelvis. Eur. Spine J. 13 (3), 199–205.

Van Wingerden, J.P., Vleeming, A., Ronchetti, I., 2008. Differences in standing and forward bending in women with chronic low back or pelvic girdle pain: indications for physical compensation strategies. Spine 33 (11), E334–E341.

Vleeming, A., Stoeckart, R., Volkers, A.C.W., et al., 1990a. Relation between form and function in the sacroiliac joint. 1: Clinical anatomical aspects. Spine 15, 130–132.

Vleeming, A., Volkers, A.C.W., Snijders, C.J., et al., 1990b. Relation between form and function in the sacroiliac joint. 2. Biomechanical aspects. Spine 15 (2), 133–136.

Vleeming, A., Mooney, V., Stoeckart, R., 2007. Movement, stability and lumbopelvic pain: Integration of research and therapy, second ed. Churchill Livingstone, Edinburgh.

Vleeming, A., Albert, H.B., Östgaard, H.C., et al., 2008. European guidelines for the diagnosis and treatment of pelvic girdle pain. Eur. Spine J. 17 (6), 794–819.

Vøllestad, N.K., Stuge, B., 2009. Prognostic factors for recovery from postpartum pelvic girdle pain. Eur. Spine J. 18 (5), 718–726.

Waddell, G., 1998. The Back Pain Revolution. Churchill Livingstone, New York.

Ward, R., Sprafka, S., 1981. Glossary of osteopathic terminology. J. Am. Osteopath. Assoc. 80 (8), 552–567.

Weaver, B.T., Haut, R.C., 2005. Enforced exercise after blunt trauma significantly affects biomechanical and histological changes in rabbit retro-patellar cartilage. J. Biomech. 38 (5), 1177–1183.

Weiss, J.M., 2001. Pelvic floor myofascial trigger points: manual therapy for interstitial cystitis and the urgency-frequency syndrome. J. Urol. 166 (6), 2226–2231.

Wilson, E., Payton, O., Donegan-Shoaf, L., et al., 2003. Muscle energy technique in patients with acute low back pain: A pilot clinical trial. J. Orthop. Sports Phys. Ther. 33, 502–512.

Winkelstein, B.A., 2004. Mechanisms of central sensitization, neuroimmunology & injury biomechanics in persistent pain: implications for musculoskeletal disorders. J. Electromyogr. Kinesiol. 14 (1), 87–93.

Wu, W.H., Meijer, O.G., Bruijn, S.M., et al., 2008. Gait in pregnancy-related pelvic girdle pain: amplitudes, timing, and coordination of horizontal trunk rotations. Eur. Spine J. 17 (9), 1160–1169; Epub 2008 Jul 26.

Wu, W., Meijer, O.G., Lamoth, C.J., et al., 2004. Gait coordination in pregnancy: transverse pelvic and thoracic rotations and their relative phase. Clin. Biomech. (Bristol, Avon) 19 (5), 480–488.

Zink, G.G., 1973. Applications of the osteopathic holistic approach to homeostasis. In: American Academy of Osteopathy Yearbook. American Academy of Osteopathy, Indianapolis, p. 37.

Intramuscular manual therapy: Dry needling

15

Jan Dommerholt Tracey Adler

CHAPTER CONTENTS

Introduction

Intramuscular manual therapy or dry needling, as it is more commonly known, is a relatively new intervention in the treatment of patients diagnosed with myofascial pain and myofascial trigger points. In the US, the American Physical Therapy Association has suggested that the term 'intramuscular manual therapy' is the preferred term to be used when physical therapists employ dry needling techniques, while physical therapists in Spain have recommended the term 'invasive physical therapy' (Mayoral del Moral 2005). Since dry needling is within the scope of practice of multiple disciplines, including medicine, physical therapy, chiropractic and acupuncture, the terminology used may vary between disciplines. It is important to note that dry needling is just a technique, which does not define or represent any particular profession or discipline. Comprehensive dry needling techniques are rarely covered in entry-level educational programmes and post-graduate training is generally indicated. In medical practice, the term trigger point needling is commonly used, but in many jurisdictions physicians appear to prefer trigger point injections (Peng & Castano 2005). A few States in the US, including Maryland, have ruled that dry needling is within the scope of chiropractic practice. Acupuncturists are qualified to use dry needling techniques but, as with other disciplines, acupuncture training programmes rarely include specific education about trigger point management (Dommerholt et al. 2006b).

Acupuncture

There is controversy about the possible correspondences between the location of acupuncture points and the location of trigger points. The traditional concept of acupuncture is based on a mixture of natural laws, metaphysical beliefs, and the practice of blood-letting, and the specific body points in Chinese medicine have similarities with points traditionally used in Ayurvedic and Arabic mediaeval medicine. The original 365 classical acupuncture points and meridians were based on the cosmological relationship between the number of points and the days of the year, and the sun's annual journey across the celestial sphere. Nevertheless, there are close resemblances between ancient acupuncture point maps and maps for blood-letting (Unschuld 1987, 1999, Pas, 1998, Whorton, 2004, Kavoussi 2009).

Throughout the centuries, the number of points used in the various schools and traditions of acupuncture has increased to over 2500, with all schools claiming therapeutic efficacy (Ma et al. 2005). Yet, the existence of acupuncture points and meridians has never been confirmed scientifically, in spite of numerous histological, biochemical, imaging, philosophical and electrical studies (Liu et al. 1975, Rabischong et al. 1975, Bossy 1984, Ramey 2000, Langevin & Yandow 2002, Dorsher 2009, Dorsher & Fleckenstein 2009). Mann, co-founder of the British Medical Acupuncture Society, concluded that acupuncture points simply do not exist. Instead of focusing on acupuncture points, he recommended to either needle anywhere on the body, needle in the dysfunctional quadrant, needle in a neighbouring dermatome, myotome or sclerotome, needle in a small circumscript area near the location of pain, or needle trigger points, in order of increasing specificity (Mann 2000).

With regard to trigger points, there is also no evidence or even any indication that they have defined anatomical locations. The locations of trigger points, initially reported by Travell, have been duplicated by many; however, Travell never suggested that trigger points would be limited to these locations or that these locations would somehow be absolute (Travell & Rinzler 1952, Travell & Simons 1992, Simons et al. 1999). Several authors have suggested that trigger points are comparable to so-called ashi points in traditional Chinese acupuncture or kori in Japanese acupuncture (Hong 2000, Audette & Blinder 2003, Cardinal 2004, Campbell 2006, Amaro 2007, Seem, 2007). Ashi points are defined as points where the patient expresses pain and discomfort in response to pressure. Kori is defined as a tight myofascial constriction that may or may not elicit discomfort with palpation, but which can be felt by the practitioner. In the acupuncture nomenclature, ashi points or kori are not located on the traditional meridians or channels. Others suggested that trigger point dry needling is similar to treating musculotendinous meridian points (Amaro 2007, Seem 2007). Even if topographical correspondences could be confirmed, considering the metaphysical origin of acupuncture points, and the lack of distinct anatomical locations of acupuncture points and trigger points, there is no reason to believe that such assumed correspondences would have any meaningful relevancy or alter the clinical management of patients with myofascial pain. Dry needling does not require any knowledge of traditional acupuncture theory or Chinese medicine (White 2009).

Trigger points

Trigger point therapy is particularly suited to improve abnormal pain processing (Dommerholt 2005, Dommerholt et al. 2006a). Individuals with myofascial trigger points were found to have abnormal central processing with enhanced brain activity in somatosensory and limbic regions, suppressed activity in the hippocampus, and hyperalgesia in response to electrical stimulation and compression of the trigger point (Niddam et al. 2007, 2008). There is increasing evidence that trigger points contribute to the development of central sensitization and as such may cause or contribute to various pain syndromes (Fernández de las Peñas et al. 2007, 2009, Giamberardino et al. 2007, Cuadrado et al. 2008). Muscle nociceptors are more effective at inducing neuroplastic changes in wide-dynamic-range dorsal horn neurons than cutaneous receptors (Wall & Woolf 1984).

Inactivating trigger points with a needle requires an excellent kinesthetic sense and awareness, based on training, experience and anatomical knowledge. The clinician must know the exact location of the tip of the needle to assure that needling procedures are safe. Experienced clinicians will be able to appreciate changes in structures and accurately identify skin, the subcutaneous connective tissue and fascial layers, the muscle, and ultimately the taut band and trigger point with a needle (Dommerholt et al. 2006b).

Invasive trigger point therapies can be divided into dry needling and injections. Dry needling can be divided into superficial and deep dry needling techniques (Dommerholt et al. 2006b). Superficial dry needling techniques are performed over a trigger point without aiming to elicit local twitch responses (Baldry 2002).

Injections are administered with a hypodermic syringe; dry needling is administered with a solid filament needle. Injections are performed with either an anaesthetic, such as procaine, lidocaine, mepivacaine, bupivacaine, levobupivacaine, or ropivacaine, botulinum toxin, or serotonin antagonists, including tropisetron (Travell et al. 1942, Müller & Stratz 2004, Göbel et al. 2006, Zaralidou et al. 2007, Garcia-Leiva et al. 2007). When using lidocaine, the recommendation is to use a 0.25% lidocaine solution, which was found to be more effective than stronger solutions (Iwama & Akama 2000, Iwama et al. 2001). Stronger concentrations of 0.5%, 1%, or even 2% solutions are frequently reported (Carlson et al. 1993, Hong 1994, Kamanli et al. 2005, Peng & Castano 2005). There is no evidence of any advantage of administering injections with vitamin B12, non-steroidal anti-inflammatories or steroids (Dommerholt & Gerwin 2010). Although there are no trigger point studies, there are some indications that injections with bee venom may be beneficial, as bee venom has an anti-nociceptive and anti-inflammatory effect through activation of brainstem catecholaminergic neurons and activation of the α_2-adrenergic and serotonergic pathways of the descending inhibitory system (Kwon et al. 2001a, 2001b, Kim et al. 2005).

Sham needling

It is very difficult, if not impossible, to perform studies with sham needling procedures and create meaningful control groups. Any needling will have a physiological effect, including a release of endorphins, a change in pain thresholds, or an expectancy of a positive outcome. Therefore, studies comparing needling with sham needling may actually compare active treatment regimens with little value for clinical practice (Pariente et al. 2005, Birch 2006, Lund & Lundeberg 2006, Wang et al. 2008, Lund et al. 2009, Lundeberg et al. 2009). In some studies, sham needling is attempted by tapping a von Frey monofilament on the skin. However, both needling and tapping induce specific but different brain responses. Needling procedures can trigger strong placebo responses (Wager et al. 2004, Bausell et al. 2005, Pariente et al. 2005, Kong et al. 2009). Even light touch of the skin can stimulate mechanoreceptors coupled to slow conducting unmyelinated C-fibre afferents, and activate the insular region (Olausson et al. 2002). White and Cummings suggested discontinuing the use of sham needling procedures, and instead to compare the clinical efficacy of invasive procedures with other interventions using standardized outcome measures (White & Cummings 2009).

Evidence of intramuscular manual therapy

Although recent meta-reviews of acupuncture, dry needling and trigger point injections in the management of myofascial trigger points showed only limited evidence (Garvey et al. 1989, Berman et al. 1999, Ezzo et al. 2000, Cummings & White, 2001, Scott et al. 2009, Tough et al. 2009), there are several studies that offer support for including dry needling in the treatment of individuals with low back and pelvic pain (Furlan et al. 2005). Meta-reviews often conclude that there is a lack of high-quality studies, and they tend to be limited in their scope and conclusions, partly because only double-blind randomized controlled studies are included even though in the context of evidence-based medicine multiple levels of evidence are recognized. An authoritative Cochrane meta-review concluded that dry needling is a potentially useful adjunct in the treatment of individuals with chronic low back pain, although the researchers agreed that more high-quality studies are needed (Furlan et al. 2005). Two studies compared trigger point injections with dry needling using hypodermic needles in both interventions and concluded that dry needling with a syringe caused more post-needling soreness (Hong 1994, Kamanli et al. 2005). A more recent study looked at trigger point injections in comparison with dry needling using a solid filament needle. This study showed that the effectiveness of trigger point injections is comparable to intramuscular manual therapy but the dry needling procedures had a longer-lasting effect (Ga et al. 2007).

Shah and colleagues observed that the abnormal concentrations of especially substance P and calcitonin gene-related peptide in the immediate region of active trigger points decreased significantly after eliciting a local twitch response with a needle, suggesting that the effects of trigger point dry needling are at least partially due to the reduction of nociceptive input into muscle receptors (Shah et al. 2005, 2008). The positive effects of dry needling are also related to the reduction of endplate noise (Chen et al. 2001), which is the summation of miniature endplate potentials found in myofascial trigger points (Hong & Simons 1998, Simons 2004). Eliciting local twitch responses by dry needling reduced the endplate noise associated with trigger points in rabbits (Chen et al. 2001). The prevalence of endplate noise in a trigger point region has been correlated with the pain intensity of that trigger point (Kuan et al. 2007).

As described in Chapters 9, 11, 12, 13 and 14, many studies, reviews and case reports have confirmed a correlation between trigger points and chronic pelvic pain. The European Association of Urology and the Society of Obstetricians and Gynaecologists of Canada recommended that trigger points be considered in the diagnosis of chronic pelvic pain (Jarrell et al. 2005, Fall et al. 2009). There is, however, no evidence for the often assumed pain–spasm–pain cycle, which suggests that pain would lead to muscle spasms, which in turn would increase pain. Quite the contrary, muscle pain is more likely to inhibit the contractile activity of muscles (Mense & Simons 2001).

Few studies have explored the effects of needling therapies in patients with these diagnoses. As a general rule, needling therapies increase the specificity of the stimulus. Several papers explored the use of acupuncture and electro-acupuncture for patients with endometriosis, vulvodynia, piriformis syndrome, prostatitis, urinary tract infections and constipation, among others (Aune et al. 1998, Powell & Wojnarowska 1999, Wang 2001, Chen & Nickel, 2004, Spiller 2007, Lee et al. 2008, Lundeberg & Lund 2008, Wayne et al. 2008, Han et al. 2009, Lee & Lee 2009). Abdominal trigger point injections were very effective in the treatment of myofascial pain (Kuan et al. 2006) and the efficacy of superficial dry needling was confirmed in a randomized study of subjects with chronic lumbar trigger points (Macdonald et al. 1983). Giamberardino and colleagues established that patients with visceral referred pain and hyperalgesia are likely to have clinically relevant abdominal trigger points (Giamberardino et al. 1999).

Nearly 90% of women with pelvic pain, interstitial cystitis or incontinence have painful trigger points in the pelvic floor muscles, abdominal and gluteal muscles (Weiss 2001, FitzGerald & Kotarinos 2003). The International Continence Society and European Association of Urology suggested that pelvic pain can be divided into pelvic pain of muscular origin and pelvic floor muscle pain syndrome (Abrams et al. 2003, Fall et al. 2009); however, trigger points in the abdominal, gluteal, obturator internus, piriformis, psoas, iliacus, quadratus lumborum and lumbar multifidi muscles frequently refer pain to the pelvic floor, perineum, vagina, labia, clitoris, scrotum and penis (Segura et al. 1979, King Baker 1993, Zermann et al. 1999, King & Goddard 1994, Doggweiler-Wiygul & Wiygul 2002, Prendergast & Weiss 2003, Doggweiler-Wiygul 2004). Empirical data suggest that pain and trigger points in the perineal or lower abdominal region can be treated successfully by inactivating the more remote trigger points which frequently is the first step in reducing pain levels. Inactivation of trigger points in the perineal muscles, such as the bulbospongiosus and ischiocavernosus muscles, is not commonly indicated after trigger points in the low back, gluteal and abdominal regions have been inactivated. Langford and colleagues described intravaginal trigger point injection techniques for the levator ani muscles using an Iowa trumpet pudendal needle guide (Langford et al. 2007). Thirty percent of the subjects were completely pain-free following the injection. Thirteen out of 18 subjects reported significant improvement (Langford et al. 2007).

It seems reasonable to consider dry needling studies in other regions of the body, but some caution is warranted in applying the findings of these studies to the pelvic area. Dry needling of trigger points in the infraspinatus muscle decreased the pain intensity of the shoulder, increased active and passive shoulder internal rotation, and increased the pressure pain threshold of myofascial trigger points in the ipsilateral anterior deltoid and extensor carpi radialis longus muscles (Hsieh et al. 2007). A recent study by Anderson and colleagues offers support for first treating muscles that refer pain and other paraesthesia into the pelvic area (Anderson et al. 2009), but fascial releases of the vaginal and perineal areas may still be indicated (FitzGerald & Kotarinos 2003). In reverse, it is also conceivable that treatment of trigger points in the perineal region may have an impact on trigger points outside the perineal region, which means that clinicians should not become too dogmatic in the order of treatment. Dry needling of trigger points in the extensor carpi radialis longus reduced the irritability of trigger points in the ipsilateral trapezius muscle, the overall pain intensity and improved range of motion (Tsai et al. 2009).

Trigger point dry needling and stretching restored normal muscle activation patterns in a study of the effects of latent trigger points on muscle activation patterns in the shoulder region (Lucas et al. 2004). After only four dry needling treatments of patients with shoulder pain following a cerebrovascular accident, patients reported significantly less frequent and less intense pain, had more restful sleep, decreased the use of analgesic medications, and increased compliance with the rehabilitation programme compared to patients who received the regular rehabilitation programme (Dilorenzo et al. 2004). Another randomized prospective study concluded that the combination of dry needling and stretching was more effective than stretching only or no treatment (Edwards & Knowles 2003). A multicentre study of the feasibility to conduct myofascial pain studies confirmed that trigger point therapy is effective in chronic pelvic pain syndromes (FitzGerald et al. 2009).

General guidelines

To reduce the risk of vasodepressive syncope, patients are lying down during any needling procedures. Anatomical landmarks must be identified before any needling procedures. After the needle is tapped into the skin, it is moved in and out of the region of the trigger point to elicit so-called local twitch responses (Hong 1994). Following needling procedures, haemostasis must be accomplished to prevent or minimize local bleeding, help restore and maintain range of motion, and facilitate a return to normal function. It is recommended to apply ice or heat following the treatment for patient comfort and to reduce the risk of haematoma.

Muscles included in the following section either cause or contribute to local pain or referred pain in the pelvic region. Please note that the skills needed to safely and accurately use dry needling can only be learned through attending hands-on courses offered by qualified and experienced tutors. Excellent anatomical knowledge is a prerequisite for all needling procedures. Reading this chapter does not constitute any qualification to use dry needling in clinical practice. Informed consent is assumed for all treatments. When treating patients in the pelvic region, specific consent to treatment may be advisable.

Low back and hip muscles

Quadratus lumborum muscle (Figure 15.1)

Needling technique

The patient is side lying, with the side to be treated superior, on a pillow at waist level to elongate the quadratus lumborum. The clinician, standing or sitting behind the patient, palpates the 12th rib, iliac crest and transverse process. Insert a 50-mm or 60-mm needle towards the transverse process.

Precautions

To avoid needling the kidney, which lies anterior to the quadratus lumborum, the muscle is needled preferably below the level of L2.

Iliocostalis thoracis muscle (Figure 15.2)

Needling technique

The patient is prone or side lying. The needle is directed in an inferior medial direction with the muscle between the index and middle fingers. The muscle is fixed over a rib, to avoid going between the ribs and into the lungs. A superficial technique may also be used.

Precautions

Avoid directing the needle between the ribs and into the lungs.

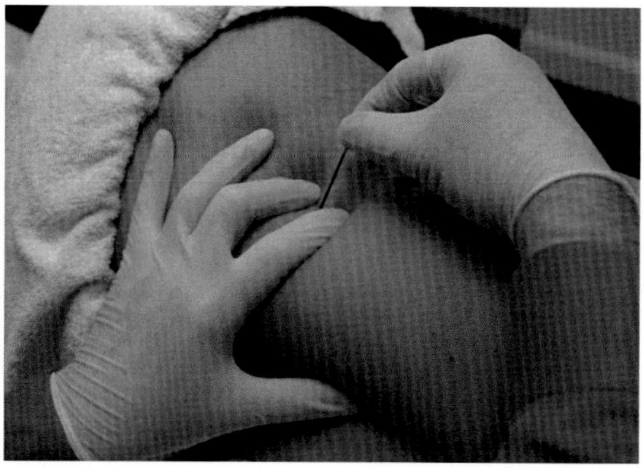

Figure 15.1 • Dry Needling of TrPs in the quadratus lumborum muscle

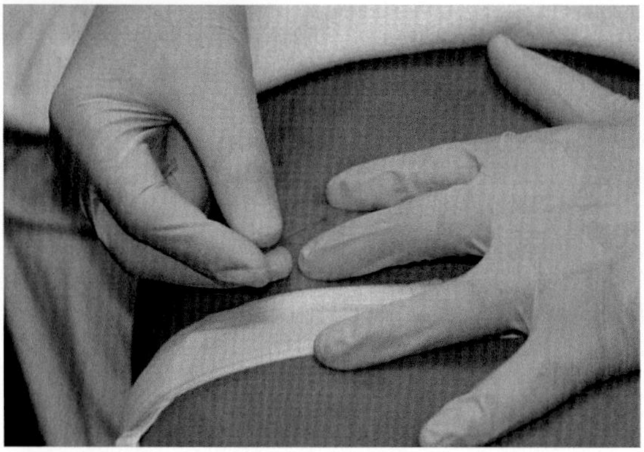

Figure 15.2 • Dry Needling of TrPs in the iliocostalis thoracis muscle

Iliocostalis lumborum muscle

Needling technique

Similar to method described above for iliocostalis thoracis.

Precautions

There are no precautions related to the lungs.

Semispinalis/multifidus/rotatory muscle (deep) (Figures 15.3 and 15.4)

Needling technique

The patient is in a prone position. The needle is directed caudally and medially, aiming toward the base (lamina) of the spinous process. Using a Japanese needle plunger can improve accuracy of needling.

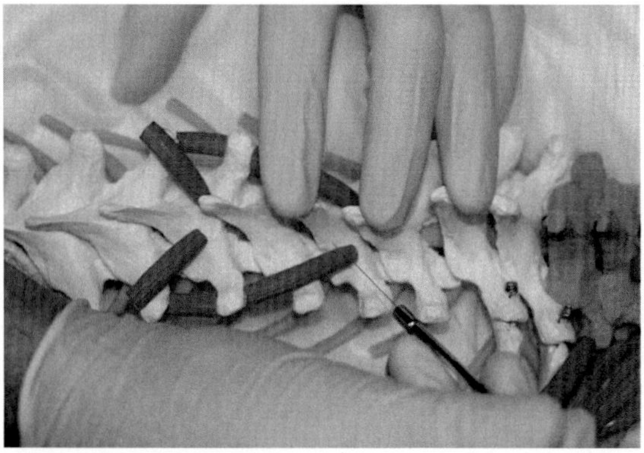

Figure 15.3 • Dry Needling of TrPs in the semispinalis – multifidus - rotatory muscles on a spinal model

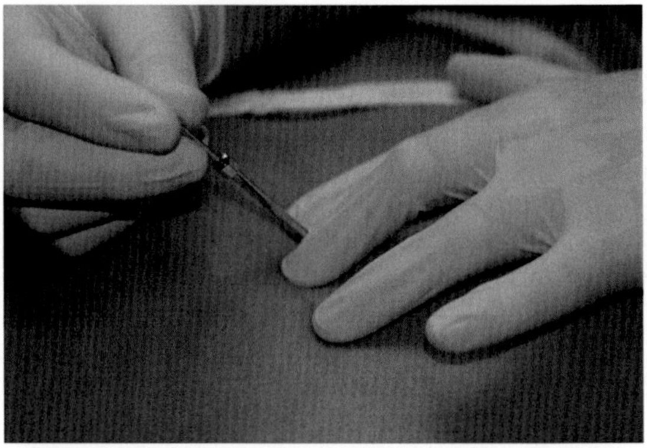

Figure 15.4 • Dry Needling of TrPs in the semispinalis – multifidus - rotatory muscles using a Japanese needle plunger

Precautions

Avoid needling in a cranial direction and possibly entering the epidural space.

Gluteus maximus muscle (Figure 15.5)

Needling technique

The patient is in prone or side lying with the side to be treated superior. Insert the needle into the trigger point. Due to the size of taut bands in this muscle, the twitch response may be quite strong.

Precautions

Avoid needling the sciatic nerve between the posterior superior iliac spine and the ischial tuberosity.

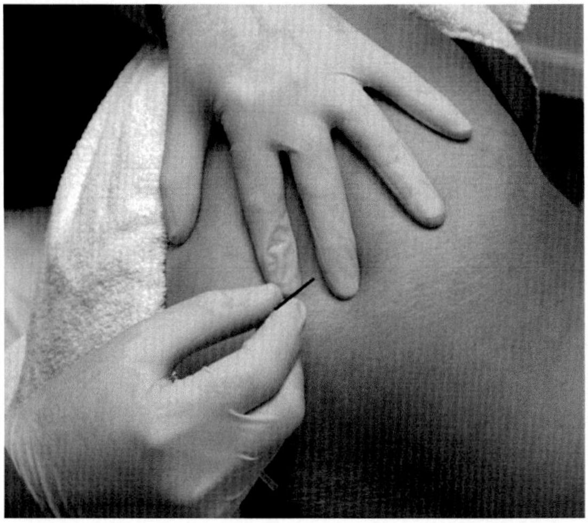

Figure 15.5 • Dry Needling of TrPs in the gluteus maximus muscle

Gluteus medius and minimus muscles (Figures 15.6 and 15.7)

Needling technique

The patient is positioned prone or side lying with the side to be treated superior. Insert needle into trigger point.

Precautions

Avoid needling the ischiotibial band.

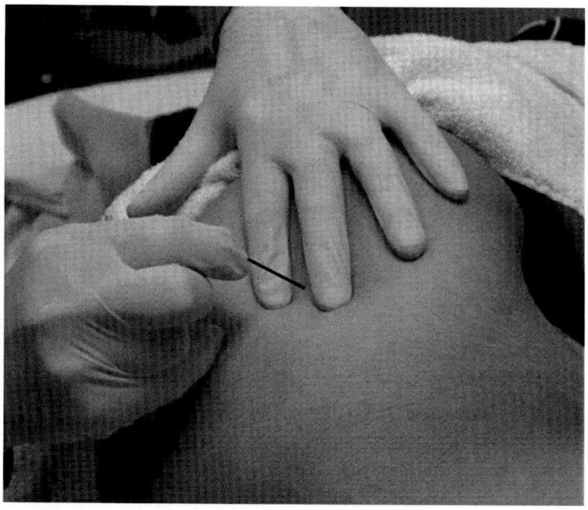

Figure 15.6 • Dry Needling of TrPs in the gluteus medius muscle

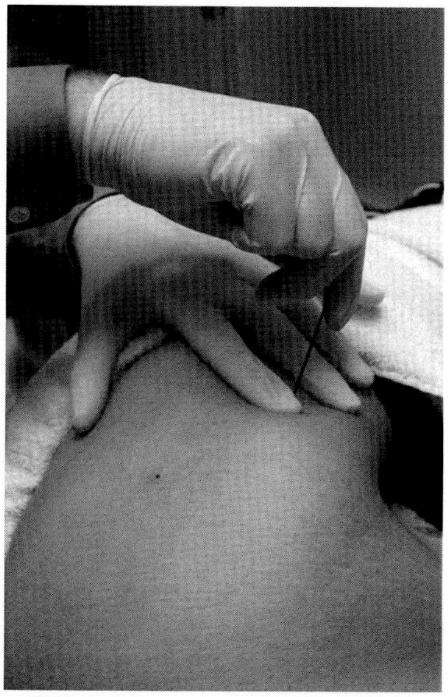

Figure 15.7 • Dry Needling of TrPs in the gluteus minimus muscle

Piriformis muscle (Figure 15.8)

Needling technique

The patient may be prone or side lying with the affected hip superior. Slightly flex the hip and knee, and support with a pillow between the legs. Palpate the superior aspect of the greater trochanter, identify the lateral aspect of the piriformis and the inferior angle of the sacrum for the proximal attachment. Insert the needle. When needling the middle third be cautious of the sciatic nerve.

Precautions

Sciatic nerve – middle third of the piriformis.

Note: The treatment of the gemelli superior and inferior and obturator internus and externus muscles is very similar to that for the piriformis muscle.

Obturator internus muscle (Figure 15.9)

Needling technique for the medial part

Position the patient in side lying with the affected side down and the knee flexed. Stand in front of the patient. With one hand palpate the medial aspect of the muscle. Depress the contralateral buttocks to improve access. Insert the needle into the muscle perpendicular to the table.

Precautions

Avoid needling the pudendal nerve.

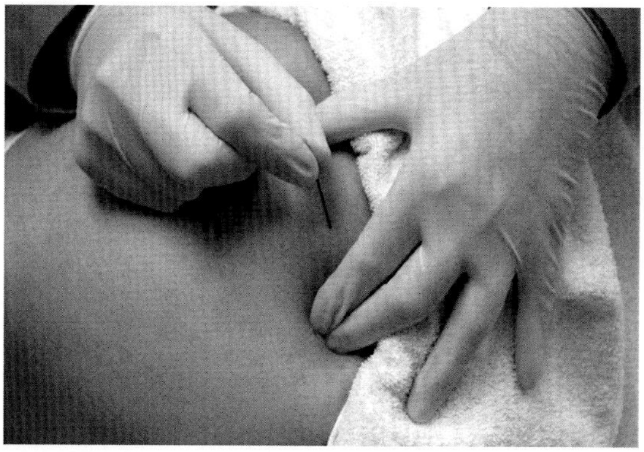

Figure 15.8 • Dry Needling of TrPs in the piriformis muscle

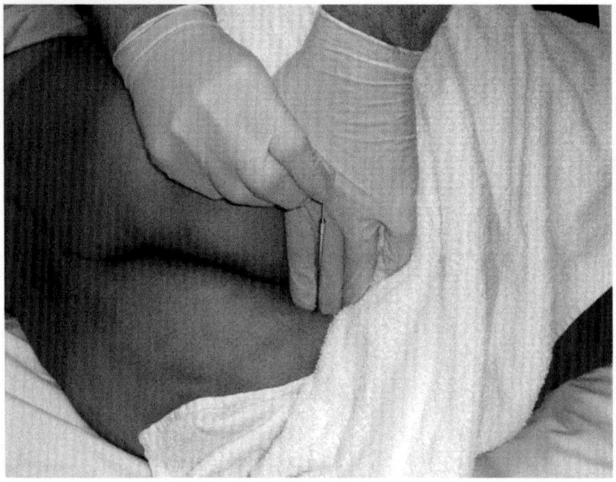

Figure 15.9 • Dry Needling of TrPs in the obturator internus muscle

Adductor muscles

Adductor longus/brevis muscle (Figure 15.10)

Needling technique

The patient is in the supine position. Flex the hip and knee. Identify the femoral triangle (inguinal ligament, medial border of the sartorius muscle and the lateral border of the adductor longus muscles) to avoid the femoral nerve, artery, and vein. Using a pincer grasp, insert the needle anterior/posterior.

Precautions

Intimate body location. Educate and inform the patient. Confirm consent.

Adductor magnus muscle (Figure 15.11)

Needling technique

The patient is in side lying or supine with the leg to be treated flexed at the hip and knee, externally rotated and abducted. Using flat palpation, insert the needle.

Precautions

Inform the patient and obtain consent when treating the proximal part of the muscle.

Pectineus muscle (Figure 15.12)

Needling technique

Position the patient supine with the lower extremity flexed and externally rotated. Palpate the femoral artery. Insert the needle at least 0.5 cm medially from the femoral artery.

Precautions

Femoral nerve, artery and vein laterally and the obturator nerve medially. Educate and inform the patient. Get consent to work in this personal area.

Abdominal muscles

External oblique, internal oblique, transverse abdominus, rectus abdominis muscles (Figure 15.13)

Needling technique

Insert the needle at a shallow angle, using a pincher grasp for the obliques.

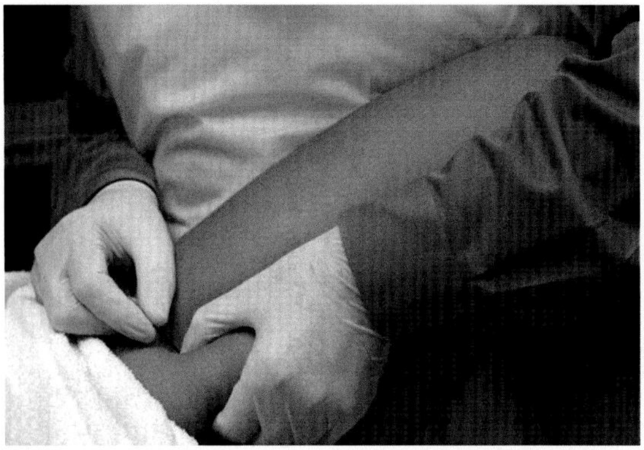

Figure 15.10 • Dry Needling of TrPs in the adductor longus/brevis muscles

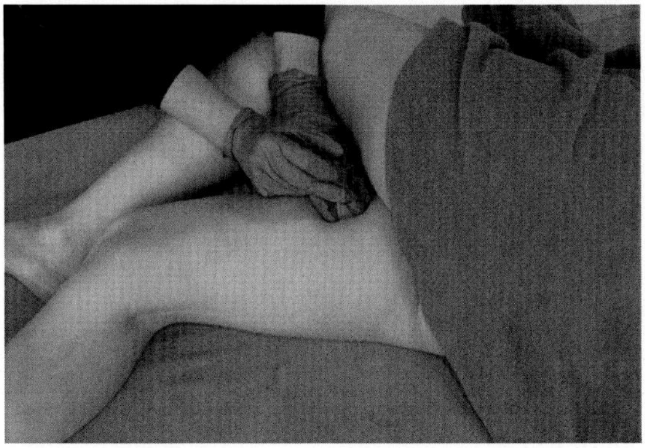

Figure 15.11 • Dry Needling of TrPs in the adductor magnus muscle

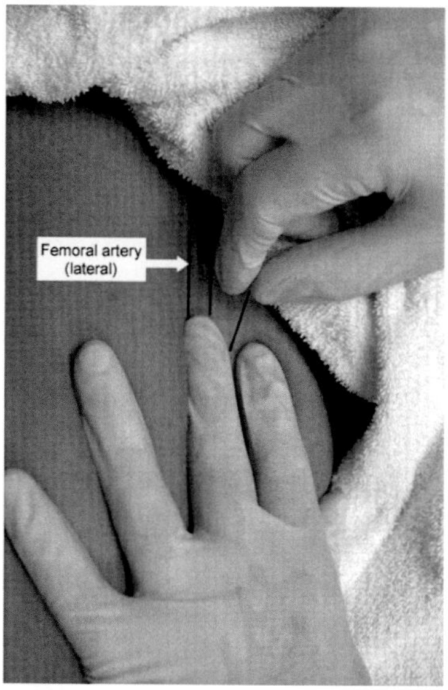

Figure 15.12 • Dry Needling of TrPs in the pectineus muscle

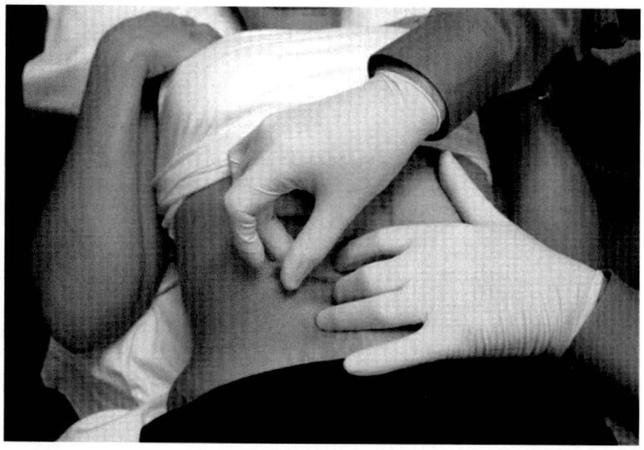

Figure 15.13 • Dry Needling of TrPs in the abdominal muscles

Precautions

Avoid perpendicular insertion of the needle to decrease risk of entering the abdominal cavity/viscera. Avoid the intercostal space and the lungs when needling the lateral abdominals.

Pyramidalis muscle (Figure 15.14)

Needling technique

The patient is supine and the needle is inserted at a shallow, tangential angle, towards the pubic ramus.

Precautions

Avoid perpendicular insertion of the needle to decrease risk of entering the abdominal cavity/viscera.

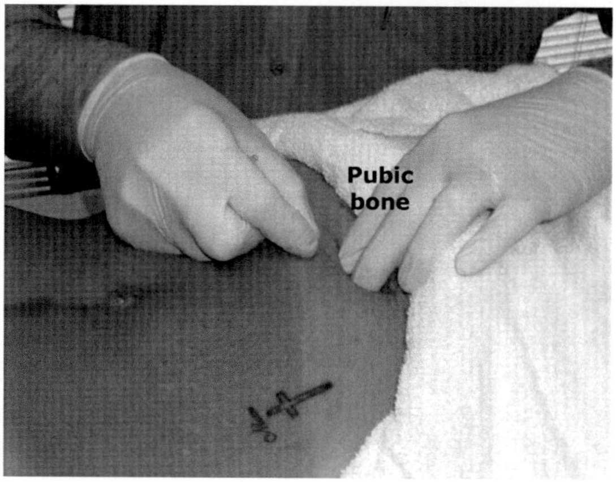

Figure 15.14 • Dry Needling of TrPs in the pyramidalis muscle

Hip flexors

Iliacus muscle (Figure 15.15)

Needling technique

The patient is positioned side lying on the opposite hip. Insert the needle toward the iliac crest away from the abdominal contents. Use a 50 mm needle.

Precautions

Avoid needling the abdominal contents.

Psoas major/minor muscle (Figure 15.16)

Needling technique

The patient is side lying. Palpate the transverse processes of L3–4 and L4–5 and the top of the iliac crest. Insert the needle just lateral to the paraspinals using a 75-mm needle. Direct the needle in an

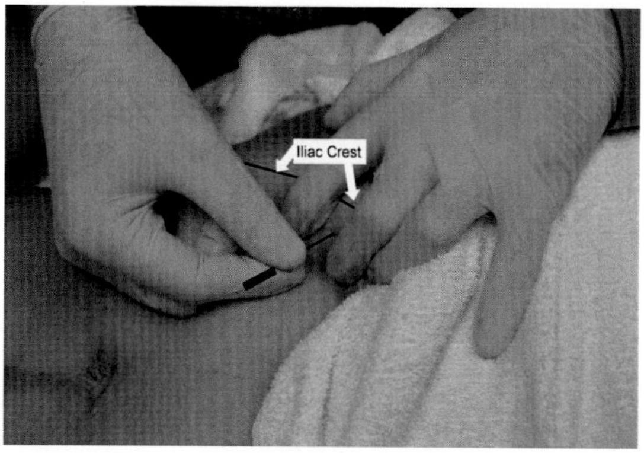

Figure 15.15 • Dry Needling of TrPs in the iliacus muscle

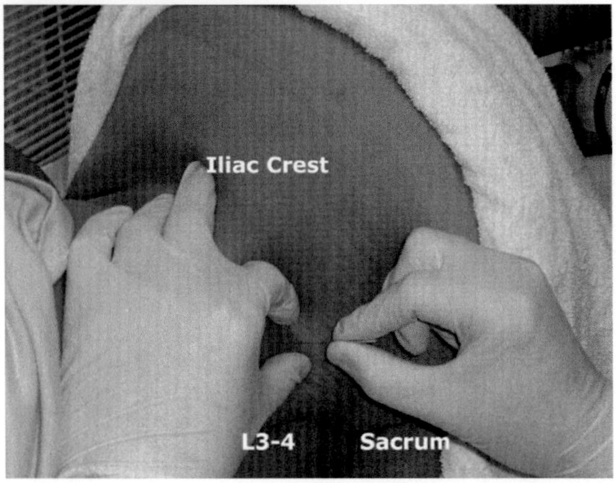

Figure 15.16 • Dry Needling of TrPs in the psoas major/minor muscles

anterior direction in between the transverse processes. The muscle belly lies immediately anterior to the transverse processes.

Precautions

To avoid needling the kidney, the psoas is needled only below the level of L2. Advance the needle slowly to avoid needling the lumbar nerve roots.

Pelvic floor (perineal) muscles

Bulbospongiosus muscle (Figure 15.17)

Needling technique: Female

Needle the muscle using a pincer palpation with the index finger inserted into the vagina. For male and female patients, the muscle can also be treated in a slightly tangential angle, which in women may be preferred in cases of hypersensitivity or when patients do not consent to vaginal insertion.

Precautions

Educate and inform the patient. Get consent to work in this personal area.

Ischiocavernosus muscle (Figure 15.18)

Needling technique

The muscle is needled in a slightly tangential angle.

Precaution

Educate and inform the patient. Get consent to work in this personal area.

Transverse perineal muscle

Needling technique

The transverse perineal muscle is treated in a similar fashion to the ischiocavernosus. The muscle is needled in a slightly tangential angle.

Precaution

Educate and inform the patient. Get consent to work in this personal area.

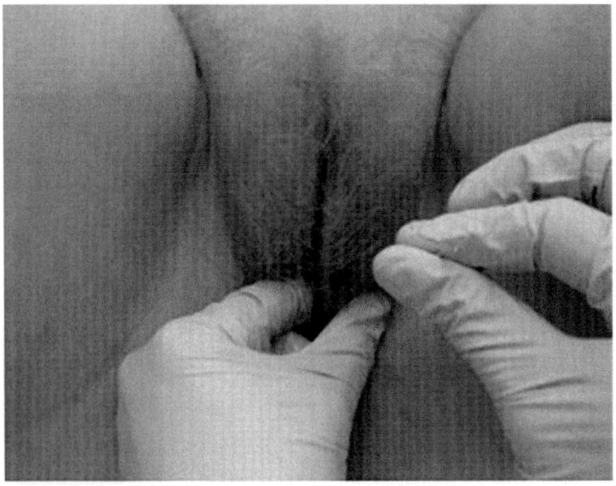

Figure 15.17 • Dry Needling of TrPs in the bulbospongiosus muscle

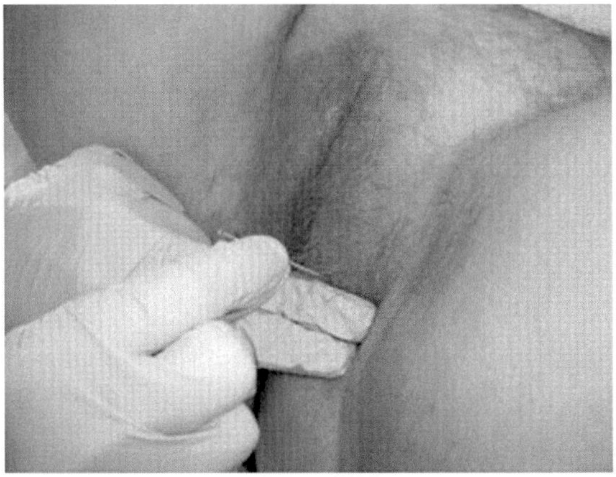

Figure 15.18 • Dry Needling of TrPs in the ischiocavernosus muscle

References

Abrams, P., Cardozo, L., Fall, M., Griffiths, D., Rosier, P., Ulmsten, U., et al., 2003. The standardisation of terminology in lower urinary tract function: report from the standardisation sub-committee of the International Continence Society. Urology 61, 37–49.

Amaro, J.A., 2007. When acupuncture becomes "dry needling". Acupuncture Today.

Anderson, R.U., Sawyer, T., Wise, D., Morey, A., Nathanson, B.H., 2009. Painful myofascial trigger points and pain sites in men with chronic prostatitis/chronic pelvic pain syndrome. J. Urol. 182, 2753–2758.

Audette, J.F., Blinder, R.A., 2003. Acupuncture in the management of myofascial pain and headache. Curr. Pain Headache Rep. 7, 395–401.

Aune, A., Alraek, T., Lihua, H., Baerheim, A., 1998. Acupuncture in the prophylaxis of recurrent lower urinary tract infection in adult women. Scand. J. Prim. Health Care 16, 37–39.

Baldry, P., 2002. Superficial versus deep dry needling. Acupunct. Med. 20, 78–81.

Bausell, R.B., Lao, L., Bergman, S., Lee, W.L., Berman, B.M., 2005. Is acupuncture analgesia an expectancy effect? Preliminary evidence based on participants' perceived assignments in two placebo-controlled trials. Eval. Health Prof. 28, 9–26.

Berman, B.M., Ezzo, J., Hadhazy, V., Swyers, J.P., 1999. Is acupuncture effective in the treatment of fibromyalgia? J. Fam. Pract. 48, 213–218.

Birch, S., 2006. A review and analysis of placebo treatments, placebo effects, and placebo controls in trials of medical procedures when sham is not inert. J. Altern. Complement. Med. 12, 303–310.

Bossy, J., 1984. Morphological data concerning the acupuncture points and channel network. Acupunct. Electrother. Res. 9, 79–106.

Campbell, A., 2006. Point specificity of acupuncture in the light of recent clinical and imaging studies. Acupunct. Med. 24, 118–122.

Cardinal, S., 2004. Points détente et acupuncture: approche neurophysiologique. Centre Collégial de Développement de Matériel Didactique, Montreal.

Carlson, C.R., Okeson, J.P., Falace, D.A., Nitz, A.J., Lindroth, J.E., 1993. Reduction of pain and EMG activity in the masseter region by trapezius trigger point injection. Pain 55, 397–400.

Chen, J.T., Chung, K.C., Hou, C.R., Kuan, T.S., Chen, S.M., Hong, C.Z., 2001. Inhibitory effect of dry needling on the spontaneous electrical activity recorded from myofascial trigger spots of rabbit skeletal muscle. Am. J. Phys. Med. Rehabil. 80, 729–735.

Chen, R.C., Nickel, J.C., 2004. Acupuncture for chronic prostatitis/chronic pelvic pain syndrome. Curr. Urol. Rep. 5, 305–308.

Cuadrado, M.L., Young, W.B., Fernandez-De-Las-Penas, C., Arias, J.A., Pareja, J.A., 2008. Migrainous corpalgia: body pain and allodynia associated with migraine attacks. Cephalalgia 28, 87–91.

Cummings, T.M., White, A.R., 2001. Needling therapies in the management of myofascial trigger point pain: a systematic review. Arch. Phys. Med. Rehabil. 82, 986–992.

Dilorenzo, L., Traballesi, M., Morelli, D., Pompa, A., Brunelli, S., Buzzi, M.G., et al., 2004. Hemiparetic shoulder pain syndrome treated with deep dry needling during early rehabilitation: a prospective, open-label, randomized investigation. J. Musculoskeletal Pain 12, 25–34.

Doggweiler-Wiygul, R., 2004. Urologic myofascial pain syndromes. Curr. Pain Headache Rep. 8, 445–451.

Doggweiler-Wiygul, R., Wiygul, J.P., 2002. Interstitial cystitis, pelvic pain, and the relationship to myofascial pain and dysfunction: a report on four patients. World J. Urol. 20, 310–314.

Dommerholt, J., 2005. Persistent myalgia following whiplash. Curr. Pain Headache Rep. 9, 326–330.

Dommerholt, J., Gerwin, R.D., 2010. Neurophysiological effects of trigger point needling therapies. In: Fernández De Las Peñas, C., Arendt-Nielsen, L., Gerwin, R.D. (Eds.), Diagnosis and management of tension type and cervicogenic headache. Jones & Bartlett, Boston.

Dommerholt, J., Bron, C., Franssen, J.L.M., 2006a. Myofascial trigger points; an evidence-informed review. J. Man. Manip. Ther. 14, 203–221.

Dommerholt, J., Mayoral, O., Gröbli, C., 2006b. Trigger point dry needling. J. Man. Manip. Ther. 14, E70–E87.

Dorsher, P.T., 2009. Myofascial referred-pain data provide physiologic evidence of acupuncture meridians. J. Pain 10, 723–731.

Dorsher, P.T., Fleckenstein, J., 2009. Trigger points and classical acupuncture points part 3: Relationships of myofascial referred pain patterns to acupuncture meridians. Dt. Ztschr. Akup. 52, 10–14.

Edwards, J., Knowles, N., 2003. Superficial dry needling and active stretching in the treatment of myofascial pain: a randomised controlled trial. Acupunct. Med. 21, 80–86.

Ezzo, J., Berman, B., Hadhazy, V.A., Jadad, A.R., Lao, L., Singh, B.B., 2000. Is acupuncture effective for the treatment of chronic pain? A systematic review. Pain 86, 217–225.

Fall, M., Baranowski, A.P., Elneil, S., Engeler, D., Hughes, J., Messelink, E.J., et al., 2009. EAU Guidelines on Chronic Pelvic Pain. Eur. Urol.

Fernández De Las Peñas, C., Cuadrado, M., Arendt-Nielsen, L., Simons, D., Pareja, J., 2007. Myofascial trigger points and sensitization: an updated pain model for tension-type headache. Cephalalgia 27, 383–393.

Fernández De Las Peñas, C., Galán Del Rio, F., Fernández Carnero, J., Pesquera, J., Arendt-Nielsen, L., Svensson, P., 2009. Bilateral widespread mechanical pain sensitivity in women with myofascial temporomandibular disorder: evidence of impairment in central nociceptive processing. J. Pain 10, 1170–1178.

Fitzgerald, M.P., Kotarinos, R., 2003. Rehabilitation of the short pelvic floor. II: Treatment of the patient with the short pelvic floor. Int. Urogynecol. J. Pelvic Floor Dysfunct. 14, 269–275, discussion 275.

Fitzgerald, M.P., Anderson, R.U., Potts, J., Payne, C.K., Peters, K.M., Clemens, J.Q., et al., 2009. Randomized multicenter feasibility trial of myofascial physical therapy for the treatment of urological chronic pelvic pain syndromes. J. Urol. 182, 570–580.

Furlan, A., Tulder, M., Cherkin, D., Tsukayama, H., Lao, L., Koes, B., et al., 2005. Acupuncture and dry-needling for low back pain: an updated systematic review within the framework of the Cochrane Collaboration. Spine 30, 944–963.

Ga, H., Koh, H.J., Choi, J.H., Kim, C.H., 2007. Intramuscular and nerve root stimulation vs lidocaine injection to trigger points in myofascial pain syndrome. J. Rehabil. Med. 39, 374–378.

Garcia-Leiva, J.M., Hidalgo, J., Rico-Villademoros, F., Moreno, V., Calandre, E.P., 2007. Effectiveness of ropivacaine trigger points inactivation in the prophylactic management of patients with severe migraine. Pain Med. 8, 65–70.

Garvey, T.A., Marks, M.R., Wiesel, S.W., 1989. A prospective, randomized, double-blind evaluation of trigger-point injection therapy for low-back pain. Spine 14, 962–964.

Giamberardino, M.A., Affaitati, G., Iezzi, S., Vecchiet, L., 1999. Referred muscle pain and hyperalgesia from viscera. J. Musculoskeletal Pain 7, 61–69.

Giamberardino, M.A., Tafuri, E., Savini, A., Fabrizio, A., Affaitati, G., Lerza, R., et al., 2007. Contribution of myofascial trigger points to migraine symptoms. J. Pain 8, 869–878.

Göbel, H., Heinze, A., Reichel, G., Hefter, H., Benecke, R., 2006. Efficacy and safety of a single botulinum type A toxin complex treatment (Dysport) for the relief of upper back myofascial pain syndrome: results from a randomized double-blind placebo-controlled multicentre study. Pain 125, 82–88.

Han, Y.F., Hou, L.H., Zhou, Y.J., Wu, X.K., 2009. A survey of TCM treatment for endometriosis. J. Tradit. Chin. Med. 29, 64–70.

Hong, C.Z., 1994. Lidocaine injection versus dry needling to myofascial trigger point. The importance of the local twitch response. Am. J. Phys. Med. Rehabil. 73, 256–263.

Hong, C.Z., 2000. Myofascial trigger points: pathophysiology and correlation with acupuncture points. Acupunct. Med. 18, 41–47.

Hong, C.Z., Simons, D.G., 1998. Pathophysiologic and electrophysiologic mechanisms of myofascial trigger points. Arch. Phys. Med. Rehabil. 79, 863–872.

Hsieh, Y.L., Kao, M.J., Kuan, T.S., Chen, S.M., Chen, J.T., Hong, C.Z., 2007. Dry needling to a key myofascial trigger point may reduce the irritability of satellite MTrPs. Am. J. Phys. Med. Rehabil. 86, 397–403.

Iwama, H., Akama, Y., 2000. The superiority of water-diluted 0.25% to near 1% lidocaine for trigger-point injections in myofascial pain syndrome: a prospective, randomized, double-blinded trial. Anesth. Analg. 91, 408–409.

Iwama, H., Ohmori, S., Kaneko, T., Watanabe, K., 2001. Water-diluted local anesthetic for trigger-point injection in chronic myofascial pain syndrome: evaluation of types of local anesthetic and concentrations in water. Reg. Anesth. Pain Med. 26, 333–336.

Jarrell, J.F., Vilos, G.A., Allaire, C., Burgess, S., Fortin, C., Gerwin, R., et al., 2005. Consensus guidelines for the management of chronic pelvic pain. J. Obstet. Gynaecol. Can. 27, 781–826.

Kamanli, A., Kaya, A., Ardicoglu, O., Ozgocmen, S., Zengin, F.O., Bayik, Y., 2005. Comparison of lidocaine injection, botulinum toxin injection, and dry needling to trigger points in myofascial pain syndrome. Rheumatol. Int. 25, 604–611.

Kavoussi, B., 2009. The untold story of acupuncture. Focus Altern. Compliment. Ther., in press.

Kim, H.W., Kwon, Y.B., Han, H.J., Yang, I.S., Beitz, A.J., Lee, J.H., 2005. Antinociceptive mechanisms associated with diluted bee venom acupuncture (apipuncture) in the rat formalin test: involvement of descending adrenergic and serotonergic pathways. Pharmacol. Res. 51, 183–188.

King Baker, P., 1993. Musculoskeletal origins of chronic pelvic pain; diagnosis and treatment. In: Contemporary Management of Chronic Pelvic Pain. W.B. Saunders Company, Philadelphia.

King, J.C., Goddard, M.J., 1994. Pain rehabilitation. 2. Chronic pain syndrome and myofascial pain. Arch. Phys. Med. Rehabil. 75, S9–S14.

Kong, J., Kaptchuk, T.J., Polich, G., Kirsch, I., Vangel, M., Zyloney, C., et al., 2009. An fMRI study on the interaction and dissociation between expectation of pain relief and acupuncture treatment. Neuroimage 47, 1066–1076.

Kuan, L.C., Li, Y.T., Chen, F.M., Tseng, C.J., Wu, S.F., Kuo, T.C., 2006. Efficacy of treating abdominal wall pain by local injection. Taiwan J. Obstet. Gynecol. 45, 239–243.

Kuan, T.S., Hsieh, Y.L., Chen, S.M., Chen, J.T., Yen, W.C., Hong, C.Z., 2007. The myofascial trigger point region: correlation between the degree of irritability and the prevalence of endplate noise. Am. J. Phys. Med. Rehabil. 86, 183–189.

Kwon, Y.B., Kim, J.H., Yoon, J.H., Lee, J.D., Han, H.J., Mar, W.C., et al., 2001a. The analgesic efficacy of bee venom acupuncture for knee osteoarthritis: a comparative study with needle acupuncture. Am. J. Chin. Med. 29, 187–199.

Kwon, Y.B., Lee, J.D., Lee, H.J., Han, H.J., Mar, W.C., Kang, S.K., et al., 2001b. Bee venom injection into an acupuncture point reduces arthritis associated edema and nociceptive responses. Pain 90, 271–280.

Langevin, H.M., Yandow, J.A., 2002. Relationship of acupuncture points and meridians to connective tissue planes. Anat. Rec. 269, 257–265.

Langford, C.F., Udvari Nagy, S., Ghoniem, G.M., 2007. Levator ani trigger point injections: An underutilized treatment for chronic pelvic pain. Neurourol. Urodyn. 26, 59–62.

Lee, S.H., Lee, B.C., 2009. Electroacupuncture relieves pain in men with chronic prostatitis/chronic pelvic pain syndrome: three-arm randomized trial. Urology 73, 1036–1041.

Lee, S.W., Liong, M.L., Yuen, K.H., Leong, W.S., Chee, C., Cheah, P.Y., et al., 2008. Acupuncture versus sham acupuncture for chronic prostatitis/chronic pelvic pain. Am. J. Med. 121 (79), e1–e7.

Liu, Y.K., Varela, M., Oswald, R., 1975. The correspondence between some motor points and acupuncture. Am. J. Chin. Med. 3, 347–358.

Lucas, K.R., Polus, B.I., Rich, P.S., 2004. Latent myofascial trigger points: their effect on muscle activation and movement efficiency. J. Bodyw. Mov. Ther. 8, 160–166.

Lund, I., Lundeberg, T., 2006. Are minimal, superficial or sham acupuncture procedures acceptable as inert placebo controls? Acupunct. Med. 24, 13–15.

Lund, I., Naslund, J., Lundeberg, T., 2009. Minimal acupuncture is not a valid placebo control in randomised controlled trials of acupuncture: a physiologist's perspective. Chin. Med. 4, 1.

Lundeberg, T., Lund, I., 2008. Is there a role for acupuncture in endometriosis pain, or 'endometrialgia'? Acupunct. Med. 26, 94–110.

Lundeberg, T., Lund, I., Sing, A., Naslund, J., 2009. Is placebo acupuncture what it is intended to be? Evidence Based Complement. Altern. Med.

Macdonald, A.J., Macrae, K.D., Master, B.R., Rubin, A.P., 1983. Superficial acupuncture in the relief of chronic low back pain. Ann. R. Coll. Surg. Engl. 65, 44–46.

Mann, F., 2000. Non-existent acupuncture points. In: Reinventing Acupuncture. second ed. Butterworth-Heinemann, Oxford.

Mayoral Del Moral, O., 2005. Fisioterapia invasiva del síndrome de dolor miofascial. Fisioterapia 27, 69–75.

Ma, Y.T., Ma, M., Cho, Z.H., 2005. Biomedical acupuncture for pain management; an integrative approach. Elsevier, St. Louis.

Mense, S., Simons, D.G., 2001. Muscle pain; understanding its nature, diagnosis, and treatment. Lippincott Williams & Wilkins, Philadephia.

Müller, W., Stratz, T., 2004. Local treatment of tendinopathies and myofascial pain syndromes with the 5-HT3 receptor antagonist tropisetron. Scand. J. Rheumatol. (Suppl.) 44–48.

Niddam, D.M., Chan, R.C., Lee, S.H., Yeh, T.C., Hsieh, J.C., 2007. Central modulation of pain evoked from myofascial trigger point. Clin. J. Pain 23, 440–448.

Niddam, D.M., Chan, R.C., Lee, S.H., Yeh, T.C., Hsieh, J.C., 2008. Central representation of hyperalgesia from myofascial trigger point. Neuroimage 39, 1299–1306.

Olausson, H., Lamarre, Y., Backlund, H., Morin, C., Wallin, B.G., Starck, G., et al., 2002. Unmyelinated tactile afferents signal touch and project to insular cortex. Nat. Neurosci. 5, 900–904.

Pariente, J., White, P., Frackowiak, R.S., Lewith, G., 2005. Expectancy and belief modulate the neuronal substrates of pain treated by acupuncture. Neuroimage 25, 1161–1167.

Pas, J.F., 1998. Historical dictionary of Taoism. Rowman & Littlefield Publishing Group, Lanham.

Peng, P.W., Castano, E.D., 2005. Survey of chronic pain practice by anesthesiologists in Canada. Can. J. Anaesth. 52, 383–389.

Powell, J., Wojnarowska, F., 1999. Acupuncture for vulvodynia. J. R. Soc. Med. 92, 579–581.

Prendergast, S.A., Weiss, J.M., 2003. Screening for musculoskeletal causes of pelvic pain. Clin. Obstet. Gynecol. 46, 773–782.

Rabischong, P., Niboyet, J.E., Terral, C., Senelar, R., Casez, R., 1975. Bases experimentales de l'analgesie acupuncturale. Nouv. Presse Med. 4, 2021–2026.

Ramey, D.W., 2000. A review of the evidence for the existence of acupuncture points and meridians. AAEP Proc. 46, 220–224.

Scott, N.A., Guo, B., Barton, P.M., Gerwin, R.D., 2009. Trigger point injections for chronic non-malignant musculoskeletal pain: a systematic review. Pain Med. 10, 54–69.

Seem, M., 2007. A new American acupuncture; acupuncture osteopathy. Blue Poppy Press, Boulder.

Segura, J.W., Opitz, J.L., Greene, L.F., 1979. Prostatosis, prostatitis or pelvic floor tension myalgia? J. Urol. 122, 168–169.

Shah, J.P., Phillips, T.M., Danoff, J.V., Gerber, L.H., 2005. An in-vivo microanalytical technique for measuring the local biochemical milieu of human skeletal muscle. J. Appl. Physiol. 99, 1977–1984.

Shah, J.P., Danoff, J.V., Desai, M.J., Parikh, S., Nakamura, L.Y., Phillips, T.M., et al., 2008. Biochemicals associated with pain and inflammation are elevated in sites near to and remote from active myofascial trigger points. Arch. Phys. Med. Rehabil. 89, 16–23.

Simons, D.G., 2004. Review of enigmatic MTrPs as a common cause of enigmatic musculoskeletal pain and dysfunction. J. Electromyogr. Kinesiol. 14, 95–107.

Simons, D.G., Travell, J.G., Simons, L.S., 1999. Travell and Simons' myofascial pain and dysfunction; the trigger point manual. Williams & Wilkins, Baltimore.

Spiller, J., 2007. Acupuncture, ketamine and piriformis syndrome: a case report from palliative care. Acupunct. Med. 25, 109–112.

Tough, E.A., White, A.R., Cummings, T.M., Richards, S.H., Campbell, J.L., 2009. Acupuncture and dry needling in the management of myofascial trigger point pain: A systematic review and meta-analysis of randomised controlled trials. Eur. J. Pain 13, 3–10.

Travell, J., Rinzler, S.H., 1952. The myofascial genesis of pain. Postgrad. Med. 11, 425–434.

Travell, J.G., Simons, D.G., 1992. Myofascial pain and dysfunction: the trigger point manual. Williams & Wilkins, Baltimore.

Travell, J., Rinzler, S.H., Herman, M., 1942. Pain and disability of the shoulder and arm: Treatment by intramuscular infiltration with procaine hydrochloride. J. Am. Med. Assoc. 120, 417–422.

Tsai, C.T., Hsieh, L.F., Kuan, T.S., Kao, M.J., Chou, L.W., Hong, C.Z., 2009. Remote effects of dry needling on the irritability of the myofascial trigger point in the upper trapezius muscle. Am. J. Phys. Med. Rehabil., in press.

Unschuld, P.U., 1987. Traditional Chinese medicine: some historical and epistemological reflections. Soc. Sci. Med. 24, 1023–1029.

Unschuld, P.U., 1999. The past 1000 years of Chinese medicine. Lancet 354 (Suppl.), SIV9.

Wager, T.D., Rilling, J.K., Smith, E.E., et al., 2004. Placebo-induced changes in FMRI in the anticipation and experience of pain. Science 303, 1162–1167.

Wall, P.D., Woolf, C.J., 1984. Muscle but not cutaneous C-afferent input produces prolonged increases in the excitability of the flexion reflex in the rat. J. Physiol. 356, 443–458.

Wang, S., 2001. Electroacupuncture treatment for constipation due to spasmodic syndrome of the pelvic floor: a report of 36 cases. J. Tradit. Chin. Med. 21, 205–206.

Wang, S.M., Kain, Z.N., White, P.F., 2008. Acupuncture analgesia: II. Clinical considerations. Anesth. Analg. 106, 611–621.

Wayne, P.M., Kerr, C.E., Schnyer, R.N., Legedza, A.T., Savetsky-German, J., Shields, M.H., et al., 2008. Japanese-style acupuncture for endometriosis-related pelvic pain in adolescents and young women: results of a randomized sham-controlled trial. J. Pediatr. Adolesc. Gynecol. 21, 247–257.

Weiss, J.M., 2001. Pelvic floor myofascial trigger points: manual therapy for interstitial cystitis and the urgency-frequency syndrome. J. Urol. 166, 2226–2231.

White, A., 2009. Western medical acupuncture: a definition. Acupunct. Med. 27, 33–35.

White, A., Cummings, M., 2009. Does acupuncture relieve pain? BMJ 338, a2760.

Whorton, J.C., 2004. Nature cures: the history of alternative medicine in America. Oxford University press, New York.

Zaralidou, A.T., Amaniti, E.N., Maidatsi, P.G., Gorgias, N.K., Vasilakos, D.F., 2007. Comparison between newer local anesthetics for myofascial pain syndrome management. Methods Find. Exp. Clin. Pharmacol. 29, 353–357.

Zermann, D.H., Ishigooka, M., Doggweiler, R., Schmidt, R.A., 1999. Chronic prostatitis: a myofascial pain syndrome? Infect. Urol. 12, 84–92.

Electrotherapy and hydrotherapy in chronic pelvic pain

16

Eric Blake

CHAPTER CONTENTS

Introduction

This chapter provides an overview of the role of electrotherapy and hydrotherapy modalities in the clinical management of chronic pelvic pain. These modalities are commonly applied for a wide variety of reasons such as musculoskeletal dysfunction, rehabilitation, pain management, infection or specific localized tissue effect. They may be utilized individually or in combination with one another depending upon therapeutic strategy and desired outcome. The hallmark of electrical hydrotherapy and electrotherapy modalities is that they elicit predictable physiological responses. Application of the modality and evaluation of the effect can have both therapeutic and diagnostic significance. The potential role of hydro-electrotherapy methods in CPP is extensive and supported by research. Each modality subsection has a synopsis of the research and a description of a relevant representative example.

Goals of hydrotherapy and electrotherapy treatment in chronic pelvic pain

Therapeutic goals include the reduction of pain, inflammation, oedema, muscular spasm, improved sexual function and improved urinary function. Therapeutic effect may include intrinsic antimicrobial activity of the modality, enhancement of endogenous antimicrobial activity of the body, improved muscular strength, resorption of scar tissue, increased circulation, enhanced quality of tissue repair, or a combination of these effects. Immediate symptom reduction may or may not be one of the goals of the therapy. The principles of treating the whole person and identifying and treating the cause of illness may require indirect strategies to achieve the goal of improved health and reduction of symptoms. Of course the ultimate goal of resolution of the patient's complaints is an important overarching outcome that, when possible to achieve, is the important end outcome. In conditions or situations when this is not possible or unlikely to occur, palliative techniques may be all that can be offered. Electrotherapy and hydrotherapy modalities can be useful in both resolution and palliation.

Modalities

For purposes of convenience, hydrotherapy and electrotherapy are discussed as separate entities. However, these modalities are commonly employed simultaneously, along with other interventions relevant to the management of associated causes of chronic pelvic pain. In the case of women with chronic pelvic pain, consideration of the endocrine changes associated with the menstrual cycle may be of significant importance to symptomatic improvement along with electotherapeutic and hydrotherapy interventions (Zharkin et al. 1991).

During the discussion of electrotherapy methods, the electrical aspects of neuromuscular junction depolarization should be considered. For example, research has demonstrated neuromuscular dysfunction in non-bacterial prostatitis (Hellstrom et al. 1987). It has also been demonstrated that baseline study and evaluation of sympathetic skin response of the lower abdomen to electrical stimulation of the dorsal nerve may be a useful means of evaluating response to treatment (Opsomer et al. 1996). The implications of this will become more apparent as individual modalities and their therapeutic effectiveness are examined.

Electrotherapy

Electrogalvanic and iontophoresis

Galvanism is a direct current with a low voltage and amperage. Galvanic current is one of the oldest forms of therapeutic electricity. The waveform is a continuous or pulsed flow of electrons. The flow of electrons in the direction of the negative pole results in electrochemical effects at each of the poles of the circuit. Eliciting physiological changes of the tissue based upon the effects of the current is referred to as *medical galvanism*. This effect is harnessed for driving ionic medication into tissues in the process of *iontophoresis*.

Mechanism of action and physiological effects

The galvanic current produces predictable electrochemical and physiological effects at the site of application (Jaskoviak 1993) (Table 16.1).

Table 16.1 The physiological and electrochemical effects of positive and negative poles

Positive pole (anode)	Negative pole (cathode)
Electrochemical effects	
Attracts acids	Attracts bases (alkaloids)
Attracts oxygen	Attracts hydrogen
Promotes oxidation	
Physiological effects	
Stops haemorrhage	Increases haemorrhage
Relieves acute inflammation	Relieves chronic inflammation
Dehydrates/hardens tissue	Congests/irritates tissue
Constricts arterioles	Dilates arterioles
Decreases nerve irritability	Increases nerve irritability

Safety and contraindications

The galvanic current is relatively safe. Caution should be observed for allergic sensitivity to ions applied. Electrode pads should not be applied over broken skin. Patients with electronic implants should not be treated with galvanism or there is risk of interference with the operation of the implant. Tissues that have impaired pain sensation should not have electrodes applied to them (Starkey 1999).

Galvanic treatment has demonstrated benefit in pelvic floor dyssynergia, levator syndrome, urinary incontinence and vaginal muscle stimulation for sexual dysfunction (Chiationi et al. 2004, Nicosia et al. 1985, Scott & Hsueh 1979, Hull et al. 1993). The therapeutic benefits of electrogalvanic treatment for these conditions of discordant muscular synchronization appear to be retained over time.

Galvanic current and levator ani syndrome

In one study 45 patients with levator syndrome were treated by negative high-voltage electrogalvanic stimulation of the levator ani with an intra-anal probe (150–400 volts, 80 cycles per second, 20-minute application every other day). An average of five treatments was needed for complete pain relief. Excellent results (total pain relief) were obtained in 36 patients, good results in five, fair results in two, and poor results (no relief) in two (Nicosia et al. 1985). Note that this method utilized high-voltage galvanic which has a high voltage and low amperage output.

Galvanic iontophoresis

Galvanic current can be utilized to drive charged ions, ionic medication, into the tissues. Like charges repel one another therefore positively charged medications will be delivered by the positive pole of the circuit and negative by the negative. The galvanic current penetrates only into the corium of the dermis, approximately 1 mm. The medication is then dispersed via capillary circulation to a larger amount of tissue.

Galvanic iontophoresis has demonstrated benefit in chronic prostatitis, adnexal inflammation, epididymitis and urethritis. Associated diagnosis of these conditions as underlying causes in chronic pelvic pain warrants consideration of their use. Iontophoretic medication for chronic pelvic pain may include potassium iodide, brine extract, therapeutic mud (esobel), shrishal concentrate (containing magnesium sulphate) and other drugs. The brine, mud and shirshal are naturally occurring substances containing antimicrobial and anti-inflammatory compounds (Iunda & Grinchuk 1980, Tikhonovskaia et al. 2000, Tikhonovskaia & Logvinov 1998, Leĭtes et al. 1990, Dikke & Ruzaeva 1993, Reshetov et al. 1996).

Additional naturopathic indications

Naturopathic physicians have historically described various methods of clinical application of medical galvanism and iontophoresis. Relative to chronic pelvic pain and associated diagnoses adjunctive galvanic treatment is recommended in dysmenorrhoea, amenorrhoea, adhesion resorption, colitis, endometritis, uterine and intestinal haemorrhage, pelvic inflammation, orchitis and salpingitis (Lust 1939, Scott 1990). This clinical documentation is consistent with the modern research listed above.

Low-voltage electrical stimulation

Low-voltage alternating current is a biphasic current produced with a low voltage and low amperage. There are a variety of biphasic waveforms such as rectangular, sawtooth and square. However, the sinusoidal current can be considered as representative. Unlike galvanic treatment the biphasic waveform does not produce any polarity effect (Starkey 1999).

Mechanism of action and physiological effects

The sinusoidal current is utilized to depolarize sensory and motor nerves. The depolarization of the sensory nerves is utilized in transcutaneous electrical nerve stimulation (TENS), which is discussed in detail later in this chapter, for pain control. Muscle stimulators employ the sinusoidal output. The sensory nerves are stimulated in a fashion that disrupts pain perception through gate control or opiate system mechanisms (Starkey, 1999). The stimulation of the motor nerves elicits muscular contractions.

The physiological effects of the sine wave encourage tissue healing by promoting increased tissue perfusion of arterial blood, increased venous return and increased lymphatic circulation. These effects can be utilized to mechanically reduce oedema. The sinusoidal current can also be used for muscular re-education, strengthening and relaxation of muscular spasm by causing muscular fatigue. The sinusoidal current is typically applied in a constant, surging or pulsed fashion (Jaskoviak 1993).

Safety and contraindications

Low-voltage current has a long history of use with a relatively high margin of safety. Implanted neurological devices and cardiac pacemakers or defibrillators should be considered contraindications. Diminished neurological sensation or motor capabilities should be approached with caution. Active contraction of muscular tissue in the vicinity of a thrombotic clot may precipitate emboli. Caution should be exercised in the event of vascular insufficiency (Starkey 1999).

Indications

Intravaginal low-volt alternating current (LVAC) application has demonstrated improved pelvic floor functioning and re-education in chronic pelvic pain with a reduction in pain (Skilling & Petros 2004, de Oliveira Bernardes et al. 2005). Levator ani spasm has also demonstrated improvement from intravaginal application (Fitzwater et al. 2003). LVAC has shown benefit in a variety of conditions that may be the underlying cause of chronic pelvic pain such as chronic prostatitis (Iunda et al. 1990, Pryima et al. 1996) and salpingitis (Evseeva et al. 2006). Fallopian tube postsurgical application has demonstrated improvement in fertility and pain reduction if applied early after surgery (Tereshin et al. 2008). Chronic prostatitis may benefit from improved non-surgical drainage via transurethral electrical stimulation (Gus'kov et al. 1997).

Intravaginal electrical stimulation in chronic pelvic pain

Twenty-four women with chronic pelvic pain with no identifiable cause underwent ten sessions of intravaginal electrical stimulation (8 Hz frequency, pulse train 1 msec, intensity to patient tolerance). Applications were administered 2–3 times weekly for 30 minutes. Visual analogue scale of pain was evaluated pre- and post-treatment and at the end of the treatment series. Follow-up pain evaluation was performed at 2 weeks, 4 weeks and 7 months. Pain reduction was statistically significant with fewer complaints of dyspareunia and benefit was retained at the 7-month evaluation (de Oliveira Bernardes et al. 2005).

The therapeutic re-education of muscular activity is largely the province of LVAC (Yamanishi & Yasuda 1998). In this regard conditions associated with chronic pelvic pain and disorders such as stress incontinence and sexual dysfunction such as dyspareunia and vaginismus have shown benefit from low-voltage sinusoidal treatment (Castro et al. 2004, Yamanishi & Yasuda 1998, Nappi et al. 2003, Castro et al. 2008, Lorenzo et al. 2008, Santos et al. 2009, Eyjólfsdóttir et al. 2009). Interestingly vaginal electrical stimulation may not actually cause pelvic muscle contraction directly suggesting other mechanisms of action may be present to explain the therapeutic effect (Bø & Maanum 1996). Biofeedback (see Chapter 13) along with intravaginal electrical stimulation has shown benefit in pelvic floor re-education and symptom reduction and may be a worthwhile direction to explore to understand these benefits (Bendaña et al. 2009).

Transcutaneous electrical nerve stimulation

TENS is an electrotherapy utilizing a biphasic sinusoidal waveform similar to LVAC. TENS is primarily a non-invasive alternative to pharmacological pain management. The therapy activates sensory nerves through electrical stimulation. The sensory stimulation interferes with pain transmission at the associated spinal level reflexogenically via gate control (proposed by Melzack & Wall 1965).

TENS is primarily indicated for pain management and has been validated for chronic prostatitis, interstitial cystitis and detrusor overactivity, and stress incontinence. Treatment is generally required for a considerable (3 months or longer) period of time and daily application is required. Units are typically prescribed for home use and are relatively simple, safe and cost-effective as the units are relatively inexpensive (Fall et al. 1980, Bristow et al. 1996, Everaert et al. 2001, Sikiru et al. 2008).

TENS in the symptomatic management of chronic pelvic pain

Twenty-four patients with chronic prostatitis/chronic pelvic pain were treated with analgesics, no treatment, or TENS treatment. All patients received concurrent antibiotic treatment. The TENS groups received treatment 5 days weekly for 4 weeks (60 Hz, 100 μsec, 25 mA, 20 minutes). Post-treatment pain level evaluation demonstrated a statistically significant benefit from the inclusion of TENS treatment (Sikiru et al. 2008).

Electroacupuncture

Electroacupuncture involves a combination of electrical stimulation device and TENS with insertion of thin trigger point needles. Electrodes are attached to inserted needles and electrical stimulation is applied to sensation or beyond to muscular contraction. The proposed mechanism of action is through modulation of ergoreceptors and somatic modulation of sympathetic nerve activity (Stener-Victorin et al. 2009).

Elcctroacupuncture has shown benefit in chronic prostatitis, prostodynia and chronic pelvic pain associated with those diagnoses. Electroacupuncture outperformed sham electroacupuncture and yielded improvement in pain scores as well as measurements of inflammatory substances in prostatic massage (Lee & Lee 2009). Cases that were refractory to medical treatment have also demonstrated significant response when treatment was directed to utilize the electroacupuncture in a local fashion to reduce prostatic congestion (Ikeuchi & Iguchi 1994).

Electroacupuncture has also demonstrated benefit via reduction of high muscle sympathetic nerve activity in polycystic ovary syndrome with associated symptomatic improvement (Stener-Victorin et al. 2009). Combined with moxabustion electroacupuncture has also shown benefit in chronic pelvic infection disease (Wang 1989). Both ear and body electroacupuncture have demonstrated benefit in dysmenorrhoea associated with endometriosis (Jin et al. 2009).

Electroacupuncture relieves pain in chronic prostatitis/chronic pelvic pain

Sixty-three participants were randomized to three treatment groups. Group 1 received advice and exercise prescription with electroacupuncture, Group 2 received the same with sham electroacupuncture, Group 3 received advice and exercise prescription. Six acupuncture points were chosen to stimulate the sacral plexus and piriformis muscle. Response was evaluated with the NIH Chronic Prostatitis Symptom Index, prostaglandin E_2 and beta-endorphin levels in postmassage urine samples. At 6 weeks Group 1 had statistically significant benefit as compared to Group 2 and 3 in pain perception and decreased prostaglandin level (Lee & Lee 2009).

Percutaneous tibial nerve stimulation

Percutaneous tibial nerve stimulation (PTNS) involves the insertion of a fine needle electrode immediately superior to the medial malleolus. A grounding electrode is applied to the same foot medial to the calcaneus. Electrical stimulation, galvanic or sinusoidal, is applied until flexion of the phalanges occurs. This electrode placement allows for stimulation of the sacral plexus.

The therapeutic rationale of PTNS is primarily for pain and symptom management, and is not directed at underlying conditions. For this reason the therapeutic response dissipates with discontinuation over time. The therapeutic response requires weekly treatment for up to 12 weeks and may also require periodic maintenance therapy (van der Pal et al. 2006, Zhao et al. 2008). The need for ongoing therapeutic impression has led to consideration of implantable devices (van Belken 2007). The current approach includes periodic maintenance treatment every 21 days to maintain the gains of the initial 12 week course (MacDiarmid et al. 2010).

Similar methods of reflex electrical stimulation for dysfunction not associated directly with the anatomic region are also applied in other conditions such as trigeminal neuralgia, occipital neuralgia, angina and peripheral ischaemia (Lou 2000). The therapeutic impression appears to be beyond the local reflex influence of the sacral plexus. Research into the physiological response to PTNS for overactive bladder has demonstrated changes in cortical somatosensory pathways (Finazzi-Agro et al. 2009).

PTNS has been found to be effective for chronic pelvic pain as well as a variety of associated diagnoses (van Balken et al. 2003, Finazzi-Agro et al. 2009) including chronic prostatitis, interstitial cystitis, urinary incontinence, faecal incontinence, various types of lower urinary dysfunction in children, overactive bladder and various types of neurogenic bladder pain (Capitanucci et al. 2009, Kabay et al. 2009). An important theoretical consideration is that the needle of PTNS is inserted at the site of the acupuncture point San Yin Jiao, Spleen 6. Spleen 6 is an important acupuncture point for abdominal and pelvic complaints. Perhaps PTNS is more accurately described as a specific electro-acupuncture protocol.

Posterior tibial nerve stimulation in chronic prostatitis/chronic pelvic pain

Eighty-nine patients with category IIIB chronic nonbacterial prostatitis/chronic pelvic pain that were therapy-resistant were randomized to receive either nerve stimulation or sham treatment. The NIH Chronic Prostatitis Symptom Index and VAS (visual analogue scale) were used to evaluate response at 12 weeks of treatment and showed statistically significant improvement (Kabay et al. 2009).

Magnetic and pulsed electromagnetic therapy

Magnet therapy is the application of static or pulsed magnetic fields to the patient. Magnetic application can be applied as a static or electromagnetic field of varying Gauss strength. Early ideas as to the mechanism of action focused upon blood microcirculation enhancement via magnetic field influence upon the iron in haemoglobin. However, the mechanism of action relative to microcirculation appears to be influenced through calcium ion channels (Okano & Ohkubo 2001, Skalak & Morris 2008). This influence may be through inflammation reduction via capillary constriction and may influence neurological signalling of pain (Gmitrov et al. 2002). There are several magnetotherapy units that also apply concurrent laser and electrical stimulation.

Indications

Magnetotherapy alone has shown benefit in urinary stress incontinence and chronic abacterial prostatitis, and some research has demonstrated benefit for chronic pelvic pain syndrome with others showing limited or no benefit (Kirschner-Hermanns & Jakse 2003, Leippold et al. 2005, Shaplygin et al. 2006, Neĭmark et al. 2009). Magnetotherapy combined with laser and electrical stimulation has also shown long-term remission in chronic prostatitis patients (Alekseev & Golubchikov 2002). Some reduction in uterine myoma has also been demonstrated in long-term follow-up after a series of magnetotherapy treatments when compared with controls (Kulishova et al. 2005).

Application has consistently demonstrated improvement in pelvic floor functioning when applied in incontinence (Takahashi & Kitamura 2003, Kirschner-Hermanns & Jakse 2007). Chronic salpingitis has also shown positive response to magnetotherapy, particularly with the addition of iodine-bromine balneotherapy, discussed later in this chapter (Iarustovskaia et al. 2005). Infectious prostatitis similarly demonstrates magnetotherapy response when combined with chymotrypsin galvanic electrophoresis (Churakov et al. 2007).

Magnetic therapy for stress incontinence

Twenty-seven patients were treated with magnetic stimulation with pulsating fields by sitting on a therapeutic chair for 20 minutes, twice a week, for 2 weeks. Females with grade I and II stress incontinence, who could not actively flex the pelvic floor musculature during physiotherapy treatment, and who had been previously unresponsive to anticholinergic therapy, demonstrated the best response.

Incontinence episodes were decreased 67%. Non-organically tangible pelvic pain syndrome did not benefit (Kirschner-Hermanns & Jakse 2003).

Diathermy and inductothermy

Diathermy literally means 'through heat'. The depth of penetration of the therapeutic heat is one of the deepest produced by physiotherapy modalities (Jaskoviak 1993). The heat is generated by the resistance of the tissues to the passage of the current. Inductothermy is another term for an inductance-type applicator of diathermy. For a period of time microwave diathermy units were produced but have demonstrated some deleterious health risk and their clinical use is uncommon today. Note: Shortwave diathermy is discussed in this section, whereas microwave diathermy is not (Prentice 1998, Starkey 1999).

Mechanism of action of shortwave diathermy

Shortwave diathermy produces an electromagnetic radio wave. The most common frequency is 27.12 MHz which produces an 11-metre wavelength. The waveform can be delivered in a constant or pulsed fashion at a variety of intensity settings. The absorption of the electromagnetic energy by the tissues in the treatment field results in increased kinetic energy and therefore heat. The high frequency of the diathermy wave (greater than 10 MHz) does not elicit muscular contraction or nerve depolarization (Starkey 1999). The absorption of energy, increased kinetic energy, and therefore heat increases cellular metabolism in the treatment field (Jaskoviak 1993).

Thermal effects

As the tissues resist the flow of current, the physiological effects of diathermy are mediated through high-frequency vibration of molecules in the treatment field. The result of the vibration is friction that creates a heating effect. The heating is to a depth of 2–5 cm depending upon type of application. The thermal effects increase tissue perfusion, increase capillary pressure and cell membrane permeability, relax muscles, increase transfer of metabolites across cell membranes, increase local metabolic rate, increase pain threshold, increase range of motion and decrease tension in collagenous tissues and enhance tissue recovery (Prentice 1998, Starkey 1999).

The degree of heat delivered to the tissue by shortwave units is not a quantified unit. Heating in tissue occurs as the equivalent of the current density squared multiplied by the resistance. Doses are measured by verbal communication from the patient as to the perceived intensity. Four levels are commonly utilized:

I: No perceived heat;
II: Mild heat;
III: Moderate heat – described by patients as a comfortable 'velvety warmth';
IV: Vigorous and barely tolerable heat.

Athermal effects

Pulsed diathermy allows a train of pulsed waveforms whose amplitude and frequency can be manipulated. The pulse train allows for a brief pause during which the kinetic energy can be dispersed and distributed by the target tissues. This theoretically creates an athermal treatment where the energy transferred does not appreciably absorb in the target tissues. The effect of the treatment is theorized to be a product of the primary field effect of the energy rather than the secondary effects of the heat produced (Jaskoviak 1993).

The pulsed shortwave diathermy proposes a field effect due to the influence of the electromagnetic field independent of thermal impressions. The proposed mechanism of action is via changes in cellular ion levels and cell membrane potential. The proposed mechanism of action is the influence of the wave on the cellular sodium pump that encourages normalization of the cell's ionic balance. This proposed mechanism has not yet been substantiated (Sanseverino 1980).

Observations of the clinical effect include (Cameron 1961, Goldin et al. 1981, Van den Bouwhuijsen et al. 1990):

1. Increased number of white cells, histocytes and fibroblasts in a wound;
2. Improved rate of oedema dispersion;
3. Enhanced fat activity;
4. Encourages canalization and absorption of haematoma;
5. Reduction of the inflammatory process;
6. Promotes a more rapid rate of fibrin fibre orientation and deposition of collagen;

7. Improves collagen formation;
8. Stimulation of osteogenesis;
9. Improved healing of the peripheral and central nervous systems.

Safety and contraindications

Diathermy has been utilized for decades with a relatively strong safety record (Prentice 1998). Most of the negative reported effects attributed to diathermy were associated with microwave diathermy, and not to short-wave diathermy (Prentice 1998, Starkey 1999). The recent evidence of beneficial tissue effects of pulsed diathermy is not only a validation of the relative safety of the electromagnetic wave field but is also evidence of a positive influence of the field (Nevropatol et al. 1995, Hill et al. 2002, Kerem & Yigiter 2002).

Diathermy should never be applied directly over any metal, as metal selectively heats and can burn the patient. Likewise diathermy should not be used over anything wet as the water is likely to turn to steam, potentially resulting in a burn. Sensible precautions should be taken to ensure that the area to be treated is dried so avoiding common clinical errors.

It is best to have patients remove jewellery in the area to be treated – most dental work is safe and no adverse response to use over fillings or other dental implants has been reported. A Danish study on abdominal diathermy in women with copper IUDs demonstrated no adverse effects and the researchers concluded that it is safe in commonly used dosages (Heick 1991).

Diathermy should not to be used if a patient has a pacemaker or implanted neurological device. Patients with a pacemaker or implanted neurological device should not be allowed within a 25-foot radius of an active diathermy unit. The waveform can interfere with the functions of these devices.

Diathermy is not used directly over the abdomen of pregnant patients, and generally avoided with pregnancy primarily because of its temperature-elevating ability. The balance of studies on pregnant physiotherapist diathermy operators has shown no consistent significant differences in pregnancy outcomes or newborn health when compared with controls (Taskinen 1990, Larsen 1991, Guberan et al. 1994, Lerman et al. 2001). Studies and case reports associated with negative outcome appear to involve the microwave forms of diathermy and the high volume of exposure for operators using diathermy (Oullett Helstrom & Stewart 1993). A study on the mutagenicity for short-wave radiofrequency has demonstrated no negative effect (Hamnerius 1985).

Diathermy should not be used over an active epiphysis and is generally not advised directly over malignant tissue (Starkey 1999). The latter may change with future research as local hyperthermia is being investigated in the treatment of malignancies (Laptev 2004, Hurwitz et al. 2005, Tilly et al. 2005).

Diathermy indications

Diathermy has been validated for infectious conditions that may be a part of the underlying cause in chronic pelvic pain. Adjunctive diathermy application is indicated in infections such as prostatitis, epididymitis, gonorrhoea, chronic urethritis, and pelvic inflammatory disease (Braitsev et al. 1978, Barabanov & Pyzhik 1989, Leĭtes et al. 1990, Stepanenko & Koliadenko 1990, Balogun & Okonofua 1988).

Relative to infection management a relevant historical passage from a 1975 electrotherapy manual states: 'The effective use of antibiotics has eliminated the need to treat infected body cavities with diathermy over lengthy periods' (Shriber 1975). While the advent of antibiotics may have contributed to the decline of the application of diathermy in infectious processes, with the modern rise of antibiotic resistance and the challenges of controlling tissue perfusion of medications diathermy may have a potentially much larger role to play again in the future.

Pulsed short-wave indications

Pulsed short wave has shown improvement in fibronectin synthesis with local and hepatic treatment has shown a positive influence in post-surgical healing times (Argiropol et al. 1992). Case reports and evaluation in dysmenorrhoea, endometriosis, dyspareunia, ovarian cyst and pelvic inflammatory disease (Trojel & Lebech 1969, Jorgensen et al. 1994). Chronic pelvic pain that involves vulval epithelial lesions has also shown a response (Grönroos et al. 1979).

Ultrasound

Ultrasound involves applying acoustic energy to living tissues in order to elicit a rise in tissue temperature. The acoustic energy of ultrasound can also be used to drive molecules into tissues; this method, phonophoresis, is analogous to the electrical iontophoresis of galvanism. However, phonophoresis does not utilize polarity effect and is a mechanical aspect of the acoustic energy waves (Starkey 1999).

Safety and contraindications

Care should be utilized in areas of tendon insertions and along the periosteum. Absorption of the energy produced by ultrasound is greatest in tissues with high collagen content. Treatment over the eye, implanted medical devices, a gravid uterus, malignancies, thrombophlebitis and the carotid sinus are generally contraindicated (Starkey 1999, Chaitow et al. 2008).

The effects of ultrasound include increased tissue extensibility, increased enzyme activity, increased skin and cell membrane permeability, increased mast cell degranulation, increased macrophage responsiveness, increased fibroblastic protein synthesis leading to increased collagen synthesis, and increased angiogenesis (Starkey 1999, Chaitow et al. 2008).

Indications

While the therapeutic application of ultrasound is widely known in physiotherapy, relative to chronic pelvic pain and associated diagnoses, ultrasound has primarily been evaluated and shown benefit in chronic prostatitis, plastic induration of the penis and associated sexual dysfunction of these conditions (Karpukhin & Nesterov 1975, Karpukhin et al. 1977, Papp & Csontay 1979).

Low-level laser therapy

LASER (light amplification by stimulating emission of radiation) light is a focused beam of light that emits photon energy. There are several different means by which laser light is generated including the gaseous helium-neon (HeNe) laser, the gallium-arsenide (GaAs), and the gallium-aluminium-arsenide (GaAlAs) semiconductor or diode lasers (Belanger 2002). Lasers used in physical medicine and rehabilitation are low power (1–20 mW) and athermal. As a result of this low-power intensity, this type of laser therapy is referred to as cold, low-power or low-level laser therapy (LLLT) (Shank & Randall 2002).

Laser light may be in light's visible spectrum (390–770 nm) or invisible spectrum (600–1200 nm). Similar to most other electrotherapy modalities laser may be applied in a continuous form or a non-continuous pulsed form with varying duty cycles intensity levels. Application is made via topical probes directly or at a distance from the surface of the body and typically while moving the probe over the area of application (Smith 1991).

Mechanism of action and physiological effects

Laser light therapy activates athermic photochemical reactions dependent upon specific wavelengths and frequencies. The type of reactions is dependent upon tissue chromophores within cell membranes and organelles (mitochondria). This mechanism of action is known as photobiomodulation.

Safety and contraindications

The main contraindications for laser therapy are direct exposure over the eye, over a pregnant uterus, malignancies, photosensitive patients or those taking photosensitizing medications (Chaitow et al. 2008).

Indications

Laser therapy for conditions associated with chronic pelvic pain has primarily been in proprietary combination devices that utilize low-voltage electrical, electromagnetic and laser therapy simultaneously. These devices have demonstrated benefit in interstitial cystitis and also for associated infectious causes of chronic pelvic pain including chronic bacterial and specifically chlamydial prostatitis (Tiktinskii et al. 1997, Alekseev & Golubchikov 2002, Kalinina et al. 2004, Shaplygin et al. 2004, Shaplygin et al. 2006, Pryima et al. 1996).

Hydrotherapy

The modern field of hydrotherapy is sometimes referred to as medical hydrology. Balneology or balneotherapy is a branch of the science that studies baths and their therapeutic uses. Crenology or crenotherapy is the science and use of waters from mineral springs (Boyle & Saine 1988). Today, we use the terms hydrotherapy and medical hydrology interchangeably, with medical hydrotherapy indicating all uses of water therapeutically (Bender 2006).

History of hydrotherapy

Medical hydrology has a rich history. Water was used for healing in biblical records and by the ancient Greeks and Romans. Hippocrates (460 BCE), the father of systematic medicine, applied water for healing, along with diet, exercise, manipulation and herbs. In his tract on the use of fluids he laid down rules for the treatment of acute and chronic diseases by water, which were followed by the hydropaths in the nineteenth century and which, together with subsequent developments, place hydrotherapy among orthodox and scientific methods of treatment. Galen (129 CE), Celsus (25 BCE) and Asclepiades (100 BCE) also used water therapeutically (Baruch 1892).

Selected clinical hydrotherapy research

Laboratory and clinical research on hydrotherapy has been ongoing for well over 150 years. Awareness of the current terminology for the terms hydrotherapy, balneotherapy and spa therapy are useful for proper interpretation of the literature.

- Hydrotherapy generally refers to plumbed water applied at various temperatures, aquatic therapy and therapeutic rehabilitation methods.
- Balneotherapy is the therapeutic use of bathing agents such as mineral and thermal waters, muds and gases.
- Spa therapy combines hydrotherapy, balneotherapy and drinking cures in an inpatient setting.

Balneotherapy and chronic pelvic pain

Chronic pelvic pain symptoms and their relationship to body temperature perception

- A Swedish study documented that ambient temperature that was perceived as cold by patients suffering from chronic pelvic pain tended to aggravate symptoms while heat tended to ameliorate symptoms. This would suggest that heating methods of hydrotherapy may warrant clinical trial in chronic pelvic pain if for no reason other than symptom management (Hedelin & Jonsson 2007).
- Comparison of every other day warm water (38°C) baths for 20 minutes and water containing alum, ten bathing sessions total, in 40 patients with pelvic inflammatory disease, demonstrated improvement of symptoms in both groups with the alum-containing waters statistically more effective. Neither group showed pathological change reduction (Zámbó et al. 2008).
- While radon-containing waters have widespread application for pain reduction in musculoskeletal disorders, evaluation of the endocrine system during treatment failed to demonstrate any changes that would attribute the improvements to endocrine effects (Nagy et al. 2009).
- Research into the evaluation of C-reactive protein, cholesterol and triglycerides show a marked reduction after a series of balneotherapy (Oláh et al. 2009).

Balneotherapy with antibiotics in the management of acute adnexitis and salpingitis

- Infectious conditions associated with chronic pelvic pain include adnexitis and salpingitis. Evaluation of the co-administration of antibiotic therapy with the addition of warm water balneotherapy was performed in infertile patients. Symptom reduction was improved by the addition of balneotherapy to a statistically significant effect. The reduction in tubal occlusion and adhesion was better in the balneotherapy arm compared to antibiotic administration alone, but not in a statistically significant manner (Jaworska-Karwowska 1980, Gerber et al. 1992).

Brine electrophoresis in acute inflammation of female genitalia

- A brine from Lake Karachi electrophoretically applied reduced inflammation of uterine appendages and sclerotic alterations of ovarian stroma, repair of intramural nerves, and correction of follicular atresia (Tikhonovskaia & Logvinov 1998).

- Ultraphonophoresis of a preparation of Eplir mud in an experimental model of uterine inflammation demonstrated a reduction in scar tissue formation, follicular atresia, exudation and haemodynamic disorders when applied in combination with antibiotic therapy (Tikhonovskaia et al. 1999).
- Russian researchers report on sacroabdominal electrophoresis with vaginal baths of brine acute salpingitis (Radionchenko & Tepliakova 1989).
- Research as to the positive effect of brine and mud phonophoresis suggests that normalization of vaginal microflora is likely the beneficial mechanism of action of this approach in chronic adnexitides, pelvic inflammation and pain (Abdrakhmanov et al. 2004).

Vaginal Irrigations with arsenical-ferruginous water in chronic vaginitis and vulvovaginal dystrophy

- Italian case-controlled research demonstrated a statistically significant symptom reduction and inflammation reduction with vaginal irrigation of arsenical-ferruginous water in chronic vaginitis and vulvovaginal dystrophy (Tikhonovskaia et al. 1999, Danesino 2001, Zámbó et al. 2008).

Spa therapy and pelvic inflammatory diseases

- Russian researchers report on cases treated at health resorts for pelvic inflammatory conditions interfering with pregnancy. Twelve-month post-treatment follow-up showed no recurrence of the condition and pregnancy rate improved by 2.5 times (Vorovskaia et al. 1994).
- Czech research showed improvement in a 12-month follow-up in chronic pelvic pain with 40% of female patients indicating improvement in sexual dysfunction (Urbánek et al. 1998).
- There are numerous European, Russian and Bulgarian reports and studies that demonstrate improvement in chronic adnexal inflammation, uterine myoma, salpingitis and sterility (Prokopiev and Nikolova 1971, Korenevskaia et al. 1982, Suchy & Cekański 1982, Burgudzhieva 1981, Lytkin 1982, Bero 1977, Burgudzhieva 1984, Burgudshieva & Slaveĭkova 1980, Maslarova 1984a, Esartiia et al. 1973, Borovskaia 1986, Burgudzhieva et al. 1981, Maslarova 1984b, Keshokova 1981) as well as case reports on balneotherapy and uterine retrodeviation (Sokolova 1981).

Case study 16.1

A 35-year-old woman presented to the naturopathic clinic with a primary complaint of abdominal pain radiating bilaterally through the inguinal region. She had previously been to her primary care physician, gynaecologist, as well as presenting to the emergency room for her current symptoms without relief of symptoms. Her gynaecological examination had been normal, normal blood counts, urinalysis, and abdominal CT negative. She had a recurring pattern of abdominal and inguinal pain for several years, since her last vaginal birth, at various levels of intensity. At the time of presentation her pain was very severe (8/10 VAS) and increasing. She had also suffered from low back pain for over 20 years and was a gymnast as a child and teenager. Her previous work-up led to no clear diagnosis or treatment recommendations. Her current pain pattern was a recurrent one that appeared several times annually.

A thorough abdominal examination was performed notable for diffuse tenderness to palpation, mostly around the umbilicus and in the region for McBurney's point. Right thigh flexion with passive internal rotation of the femur was provocative (obturator sign). Passive side lying extension was also provocative on the right (psoas sign). Based on these physical findings with a previous negative abdominal CT scan a working diagnosis of chronic sub-acute inflammation of the appendix was made. The patient was educated about referral for laparascopic management and appendiceal removal and the option for conservative non-surgical management with the purpose of reducing inflammation. Conservative approach was agreed upon and it was understood that worsening of symptoms could necessitate emergent referral.

At that visit a hydro-electrotherapy treatment was performed. The treatment goal was reduction of abdominal pain and appendiceal inflammation. Contrast hydrotherapy to the chest and abdomen was first administered using the constitutional hydrotherapy method.

Constitutional hydrotherapy method

The patient was supine, undressed from the waist up, covered with a vellux blanket.

1. Two turkish towels, each folded in half to allow for four layers of towelling, very well wrung from hot water (130–140°F) were applied covering chest and abdomen – from clavicle to ASIS, laterally the towels reached the anterior axillary line. The patient was covered with a vellux or wool blanket.
2. At the 5-minute mark one turkish towel, folded in half, very well wrung from hot water, replaced the two turkish towels previously applied.
3. The hot towel was then quickly replaced with one turkish towel well wrung from cold water (40–55°F) and folded in half, allowing for two layers of toweling. The application covered the same area as the hot towels, from clavicle to anterior superior iliac spine, anterior axillary line to anterior axillary line. Again the patient was covered with a blanket. The cold towel remains in place for 10 minutes and will be observed to rewarm to body temperature (Chaitow et al. 2008).

After the anterior application of contrast hydrotherapy in the constitutional hydrotherapy method, high frequency was applied to the right lower abdomen for 8 minutes by means of a topical electrode. High-frequency current has anti-inflammatory, sedative and analgesic properties (Chaitow et al. 2008). Throughout the anterior treatment a trigger point needle was placed 3 inches below the acupuncture location for Stomach 36 on the right lower leg. This corresponds to the 'extra point' for appendicitis (the term 'extra point' refers to an acupuncture point not identified as a specific point on one of the primary acupuncture meridian channels and is typically associated with specific therapeutic effect).

After the application of the anterior contrast hydrotherapy according to the constitutional hydrotherapy method, high frequency to the right lower abdominal quadrant, and trigger point treatment, the patient positioned herself in a prone position and the contrast hydrotherapy treatment was applied to the back of the torso in a similar fashion:

1. Two turkish towels (the same as previously used), freshly well wrung from hot water, each folded in half for a total of four layers, were applied to the patient's back. The towels covered from the superior edge of the scapula to the posterior superior iliac spine laterally to the posterior axillary line.
2. At the 5-minute mark, the two towels are replaced with one fresh towel wrung from hot water. This towel was quickly replaced with a towel well wrung from cold water.
3. At the 10-minute mark the patient had warmed the towel to body temperature. Finish with a dry friction rub to the back.
4. A fresh dry towel was used to give a 20–30-second dry friction rub to the patient's back.

At the end of treatment (45 minutes) her pain on the VAS was 1/10, a reduction from 8 of 10 at the start of the procedure.

The following day the patient returned to the clinic reporting that the umbilical pain was much improved, however the inguinal pain had returned and the low back pain was still present. On physical examination the tenderness at McBurney's point was diminished and the challenge to the obturator muscle and psoas muscle were negative suggesting reduction in the presumed appendiceal inflammation. The previous day's treatment was repeated with the inclusion of LVAC at the end of the procedure series. The LVAC was applied in the following fashion: one 4″ × 4″ electrode pad placed on the sole of each foot. Constant tetanizing current was applied to patient tolerance for 5 minutes (this was felt by the patient as a gentle tingling and very minor contraction of the muscles of the lower leg). The therapeutic strategy was to relax muscle spasm in the pelvic girdle musculature indirectly through exhaustion of muscular spasm. A third treatment was administered 3 days later at which point the patient was not experiencing significant abdominal discomfort and the low back pain had improved. She was leaving for a 1-week holiday.

Upon return from holiday she reported that all abdominal symptoms had abated, she was able to lie on her side during sleep for the first time in a year, and she was left with only a minimal low back pain on the left side, though it did continue to radiate through the groin in a typical discogenic fashion.

Physical examination also revealed significant tenderness at the sacroiliac joints and iliolumbar ligaments bilaterally. Upon inquiry the patient revealed that her chronic low back pain followed a pattern of worsening of symptoms always in the later part of the day. Hackett identifed this pattern as one suggesting laxity of the sacroiliac and lumbar ligaments (Hackett 1958, 1991). Treatment recommended for ligament laxity is the injection of dextrose into the ligamentous tissue to provoke fibroblast formation and soft tissue production (prolotherapy) (Hackett 1991, Yelland et al. 2004).

It was now possible to perform a more thorough abdominal examination. Tenderness at the right pubis with superior pressure and iliac crest with posterior palpation was elicited corresponding to the diagnostic reflexes of kidney ptosis according to Failor (1979). Inquiry based on physical findings revealed frequent urge to pass urine but only passing small amounts of urine.

A combination of therapeutic interventions were applied over a period of 3 weeks:

1. Neuromuscular treatment according to Lief to the spine and abdomen (Chaitow 1988) and abdominal manipulation according to Ralph Failor (Failor 1979). The goal of treatment was reduction of trigger point and recurrent muscular spasm to the areas treated. This method was applied once weekly.
2. Contrast hydrotherapy according to the constitutional hydrotherapy method anterior and posterior applications with the inclusion of LVAC to the feet and high frequency to the abdomen as previously described. Therapeutic goal was to reduce pain, muscular spasm and inflammation and to improve circulation. Trigger point needling at Large Intestine 4, Liver 3, and Bai Hui was also administered (Takahashi 2011, Dorsher 2011). Therapeutic goal was to reduce pain through reflex mechanisms. This method was applied twice weekly, once in combination with the soft tissue manipulation and once independently.

The patient responded well to this combination of treatment and indicated a significant decrease in back pain and improved functions with urination. Her pubic and iliac tenderness to palpation resolved. Treatment was administered twice weekly for 3 weeks.

At the end of 3 weeks of hydroelectrotherapy treatment, injection therapy according to Hackett (prolotherapy) to the iliolumbar and sacroiliac ligament was administered and was well tolerated (Yelland et al. 2004).

During this treatment phase the patient admitted that she had also suffered since her last childbirth (6 years) significant dyspareunia at the midpoint of penile penetration which on many occasions prevented intercourse. Diluted Cactus Grandiflorus, Citrullus Colocynthis and Delphinium Staphisagria was administered orally, ten drops once daily for 3 weeks to reduce the genital pain. The hydroelectrotherapy treatment was continued once weekly according to the previous description for 4 weeks (Marzouk et al. 2010a, 2010b, Diaz et al. 2008).

At the end of 2 months of therapy her low back pain symptoms, inguinal pains, abdominal pains, urinary frequency and urgency, and dyspareunia symptoms were all fully resolved. She became pregnant 6 months later and successfully had a vaginal childbirth. At 3-year follow-up her symptoms have not returned.

References

Abdrakhmanov, A.R., Kartashova, O.L., Kirgizova, S.B., 2004. Characteristics of microflora isolated in chronic adnexitides and effects of balneotherapy on biological properties of microorganisms in experimental and clinical conditions. Vopr. Kurortol. Fizioter. Lech. Fiz. Kult. (4), 21–24.

Alekseev, M.I.a., Golubchikov, V.A., 2002. Comparative analysis of long-term results of treating chronic prostatis with the use of the Andro-Gin device. Urologiia (1), 14–17.

Argiropol, M., et al., 1992. The stimulation of fibronectin synthesis by high peak power electromagnetic energy (Diapulse). Rev. Roum. Physiol. 29 (3–4), 77–81.

Balogun, J.A., Okonofua, F.E., 1988. Management of chronic pelvic inflammatory disease with shortwave diathermy. A case report. Phys. Ther. 68 (10), 1541–1545.

Barabanov, L.G., Pyzhik, I.M., 1989. Ethymisole and inductothermy in the treatment of patients with chronic gonorrhea. Vestn. Dermatol. Venerol. (2), 69–72.

Baruch, S., 1892. The Uses of Water in Modern Medicine. George S. Davis, Detroit, MI, pp. 2–22.

Belanger, A., 2002. Evidence-Based Guide to Therapeutic Physical Agents. Lippincott Williams & Wilkens, p. 191.

Bendaña, E.E., Belarmino, J.M., Dinh, J.H., et al., 2009. Efficacy of transvaginal biofeedback and electrical stimulation in women with urinary urgency and frequency and associated pelvic floor muscle spasm. Urol. Nurs. 29 (3), 171–176.

Bender T, 2006 International Society of Medical Hydrology and Climatology, www.ismh-direct.net.

Bero, L.I., 1977. Berdiansk mud therapy of inflammatory processes of the female genitalia at the subacute stage. Akush. Ginekol. (Mosk) (4), 26–29.

Bø, K., Maanum, M., 1996. Does vaginal electrical stimulation cause pelvic floor muscle contraction? A pilot study. Scand. J. Urol. Nephrol. Suppl. 179, 39–45.

Borovskaia, V.D., 1986. Results of health resort treatment of women with chronic inflammation of the adnexae and uterine myoma. Vopr. Kurortol. Fizioter. Lech. Fiz. Kult. (1), 44–46.

Boyle, W., Saine, A., 1988. Lectures in Naturopathic Hydrotherapy. Buckeye Naturopathic Press, East Palestine, Ohio.

Braitsev, A.V., Grachev, I.u.I., Ovchinnikov, V.I., Kul'kov, V.I.u., Zastenker, F.S., 1978. Therapeutic effectiveness of inductothermy in treating prostatitis. Vestn. Dermatol. Venerol. (8), 66–69.

Bristow, S.E., Hasan, S.T., Neal, D.E., 1996. TENS: a treatment option for bladder dysfunction. Int. Urogynecol. J. Pelvic Floor Dysfunct. 7 (4), 185–190.

Burgudzhieva, T., 1981. Hemodynamics of the pelvic organs in women with chronic salpingo-oophoritis resulting from ambulatory treatment using Varna Gulf mud. Akush. Ginekol. (Sofiia) 20 (4), 320–324.

Burgudzhieva, T., 1984. Mud therapy of inflammatory gynecologic diseases and sterility of inflammatory etiology in Bulgaria. Akush. Ginekol. (Sofiia) 23 (4), 341–344.

Burgudshieva, T., Slaveĭkova, O., 1980. Comparative hemodynamic changes in the organs of the lesser pelvis of women with inflammatory gynecologic diseases and sterility following treatment with Baikal peat and sulfide mineral waters. Akush. Ginekol. (Sofiia) 19 (5–6), 518–521.

Burgudzhieva, T., Marovski, S., Tabakova, P., 1981. Effect of peat treatment at the Kyustendil health resort on cortisol and androgen secretion in inflammatory gynecologic diseases and female sterility. Akush. Ginekol. (Sofiia) 20 (6), 463–466.

Cameron, B.M., 1961. Experimental acceleration of wound healing. Am. J. Orthop. 3, 336–343.

Capitanucci, M.L., Camanni, D., Demelas, F., 2009. Long-term efficacy of percutaneous tibial nerve stimulation for different types of lower urinary tract dysfunction in children. J. Urol. 182 (4 Suppl.), 2056–2061.

Castro, R.A., et al., 2004. Does electrical stimulation of the pelvic floor make any change in urodynamic parameters? When to expect a cure and improvement in women with stress urinary incontinence? Clin. Exp. Obstet. Gynecol. 31 (4), 274–278.

Castro, R.A., Arruda, R.M., Zanetti, M.R., et al., 2008. Single-blind, randomized, controlled trial of pelvic floor muscle training, electrical stimulation, vaginal cones, and no active treatment in the management of stress urinary incontinence. Clinics (Sao Paulo) 63 (4), 465–472.

Chaitow, L., 1988. Soft Tissue Manipulation. Healing Arts Press.

Chaitow, L., et al., 2008. Naturopathic Physical Medicine. Elsevier.

Chiationi, G., Chistolin, F., Menegotti, M., et al., 2004. One year follow up study on the effects of electrogalvanic stimulation in chronic idiopathic constipation with pelvic floor dyssynergia. Dis. Colon Rectum 47 (3), 346–353.

Churakov, A.A., Popkov, V.M., Zemskov, S.P., Glybochko, P.V., Bliumberg, B.I., 2007. Combined physiotherapy of chronic infectious prostatitis. Urologiia (1), 61–65.

Danesino, V., 2001. Balneotherapy with arsenical-ferruginous water in chronic cervico-vaginitis. A case-control study. Minerva Ginecol. 53 (1), 63–69.

de Oliveira Bernardes, N., Bahamondes, L., 2005. Intravaginal electrical stimulation for the treatment of chronic pelvic pain. J. Reprod. Med. 50 (4), 267–272.

Diaz, J., Carmona, A., de Paz, P., 2008. Acylated flavonol glycosides from Delphinium staphisagria Phytochemistry Letters, 1 (2):125.

Dikke, G.B., Ruzaeva, I.u.F., 1993. The use of the Shirsal concentrate in treating chronic inflammatory diseases of the uterine adnexa. Vopr. Kurortol. Fizioter. Lech. Fiz. Kult. (6), 30–33.

Dorsher, P., 2011. Acupuncture for chronic pain Techniques in Regional Anesthesia and Pain Management, 15(2):55–63.

Esartiia, T.P., Loriia, E.K., Bochorishvili, L.G., 1973. Treatment of chronic inflammatory diseases of the female sex organs using Gagry mineral water. Vopr. Kurortol. Fizioter. Lech. Fiz. Kult. 38 (3), 237–239.

Everaert, K., Devulder, J., De Muynck, M., et al., 2001. The pain cycle: implications for the diagnosis and treatment of pelvic pain syndromes. Int. Urogynecol. J. Pelvic Floor Dysfunct. 12 (1), 9–14.

Evseeva, M.M., Serov, V.N., Tkachenko, N.M., 2006. Chronic salpingo-oophoritis: clinical and physiological rationale for therapeutic application of impulse low-frequency electrostatic field. Vopr. Kurortol. Fizioter. Lech. Fiz. Kult. (1), 21–24.

Eyjólfsdóttir, H., Ragnarsdóttir, M., Geirsson, G., 2009. Pelvic floor muscle training with and without functional electrical stimulation as treatment for stress urinary incontinence. Laeknabladid 95 (9), 575–580 quiz 581.

Failor, R.M., 1979. New Era Chiropractor. Failor, Palm Desert, CA.

Fall, M., Carlsson, C.A., Erlandson, B.E., 1980. Electrical stimulation in interstitial cystitis. J. Urol. 123 (2), 192–195.

Finazzi-Agro, E., Rocchi, C., Pachatz, C., et al., 2009. Percutaneous tibial nerve stimulation produces effects on brain activity: study on the modifications of the long latency somatosensory evoked potentials. Neurourol. Orodyn. 28 (4), 320–324.

Fitzwater, J.B., Kuehl, T.J., Schrier, J.J., 2003. Electrical stimulation in the treatment of pelvic pain due to levator ani spasm. J. Reprod. Med. 48 (8), 573–577.

Gerber, B., Wilken, H., Zacharias, K., Barten, G., Splitt, G., 1992. Treatment of acute salpingitis with tetracycline/metronidazole with or without additional balneotherapy, Augmentin or ciprofloxacin/ metronidazole: a second-look laparoscopy study. Geburtshilfe Frauenheilkd. 52 (3), 165–170.

Gmitrov, J., Ohkubo, C., Okano, H., 2002. Effect of 0.25 T static magnetic field on microcirculation in rabbits. Bioelectromagnetics 23 (3), 224–229.

Goldin, J., et al., 1981. The effects of Diapulse on the healing of wounds a double blind randomised controlled trial in man. Br. J. Plast. Surg. 34, 267–270.

Grönroos, M., Liukko, P., Rauramo, L., Punnonen, R., 1979. Treatment of vulval epithelial lesions by pulsed high-frequency therapy. Acta Obstet. Gynecol. Scand. 58 (2), 187–189.

Guberan, E., Campana, et al., 1994. Gender ratio of offspring and exposure to shortwave radiation among female physiotherapists. Scand. J. Work Environ. Health 20 (5), 345–348.

Gus'kov, A.R., Vasil'ev, A.I., Bogacheva, I.D., Kulinich, A.I.u., Abrazheev, V.G., 1997. Transurethral drainage of the prostate in chronic prostatitis by means of the Intraton-4 electrostimulator-aspirator. Urol. Nefrol. (Mosk) (1), 34–37.

Hackett, G.S., 1958. Ligament and Tendon Relaxation Treated by Prolotherapy.

Hamnerius, Y., 1985. Biological effects of high-frequency electromagnetic fields on *Salmonella typhimurium* and *Drosophila melanogaster*. Bioelectromagnetics 6 (4), 405–414.

Hellstrom, W.J., Schmidt, R.A., Lue, T.F., Tanagho, E.A., 1987. Neuromuscular dysfunction in nonbacterial prostatitis. Urology 30 (2), 183–188.

Hedelin, H., Jonsson, K., 2007. Chronic prostatitis/chronic pelvic pain syndrome: symptoms are aggravated by cold and become less distressing with age and time. Scand. J. Urol. Nephrol. 41 (6), 516–520.

Heick, E., 1991. Is diathermy safe in women with copper-bearing IUDs? Acta Obstet. Gynecol. Scand. 70 (2), 153–155.

Hill, L., et al., 2002. Pulsed short-wave diathermy effects on human fibroblast proliferation. Arch. Phys. Med. Rehabil. 83 (6), 832–836.

Hull, T.L., Milsom, J.W., Church, J., 1993. Electrogalvanic stimulation for levator syndrome: how effective is it in the long-term? Dis. Colon Rectum 36 (8), 731–733.

Hurwitz, et al., 2005. Hyperthermia combined with radiation in treatment of locally advanced prostate cancer is associated with a favourable toxicity profile. Int. J. Hyperthermia 21 (7), 649–656.

Iarustovskaia, O.V., Rodina, E.V., Orekhova, E.M., Markina, L.P., 2005. Amplipulse-magnetotherapy and iodine-bromine waters in combined treatment of patients with chronic nonspecific salpingo-oophoritis. Vopr. Kurortol. Fizioter. Lech. Fiz. Kult. (5), 14–16.

Ikeuchi, T., Iguchi, H., 1994. Clinical studies on chronic prostatitis and prostatitis-like syndrome (7). Electric acupuncture therapy for intractable cases of chronic prostatitis-like syndrome. Hinyokika Kiyo 40 (7), 587–591.

Iunda, I.F., Grinchuk, V.A., 1980. Comparative effectiveness of rectal electrophoresis with sinusoidal modulated currents and other methods of treating chronic nonspecific prostatitis with a pain syndrome. Vopr. Kurortol. Fizioter. Lech. Fiz. Kult. (2), 58–61.

Iunda, I.F., Gorpinchenko, I.I., Israilov, S.R., Boĭko, N.I., 1990. Urethral electrothermal stimulation in treating patients with chronic non-gonococcal urethro-prostatitis. Vrach Delo. (3), 21–22.

Jaskoviak, P.A., 1993. Applied Physiotherapy: Practical Clinical Applications with Emphasis on the Management of Pain and Related Syndrome. The American Chiropractic Association, Arlington, VA.

Jaworska-Karwowska, J., 1980. Evaluation of the results of treatment of acute adnexitis with sulfonamides and antibiotics in the course of balneotherapy. Ginekol. Pol. 51 (6), 539–543.

Jin, Y.B., Sun, Z.L., Jin, H.F., 2009. Randomized controlled study on ear-electroacupuncture treatment of endometriosis-induced dysmenorrhea in patients. Zhen Ci Yan Jiu 34 (3), 188–192.

Jorgensen, W.A., Frome, B.M., Wallach, C., 1994. Electrochemical therapy of pelvic pain: effects of pulsed electromagnetic fields (PEMF) on tissue trauma. Eur. J. Surg. Suppl. (574), 83–86.

Kabay, S., Kabay, S.C., Yucel, M., Ozden, H., 2009. Efficiency of posterior tibial nerve stimulation in category IIIB chronic prostatitis/chronic pelvic pain: a sham-controlled comparative study. Urol. Int. 83 (1), 33–38 Epub 2009 Jul 27.

Kalinina, S.N., Molchanov, A.V., Rutskaia, N.S., 2004. Combined therapy of interstitial cystitis using the "Aeltis-Synchro-02-Iarilo" device. Urologiia (2), 20–22.

Karpukhin, V.T., Nesterov, N.I., Roman, D.L., 1977. Ultrasonic therapy of chronic prostatitis. Vopr. Kurortol. Fizioter. Lech. Fiz. Kult. (3), 75–77.

Karpukhin, V.T., Nesterov, N.I., 1975. Treatment of chronic nonspecific prostatitis by rectally administered ultrasound. Nov. Med. Tekh. (2), 104–105.

Kerem, M., Yigiter, K., 2002. Effects of continuous and pulsed short-wave diathermy in low back pain. Pain Clinic 14 (1), 55–59 (5).

Keshokova, M.P., 1981. Changes in the cervical factor and isolation of pathogenic microbes from the genital organs of women with chronic salpingo-oophoritis and infertility undergoing treatment at the Nalchik health resort. Vopr. Kurortol. Fizioter. Lech. Fiz. Kult. (6), 55–57.

Kirschner-Hermanns, R., Jakse, G., 2003. Magnet stimulation therapy: a simple solution for the treatment of stress and urge incontinence? Urologe A 42 (6), 819–822 Epub 2003 Jan 17.

Kirschner-Hermanns, R., Jakse, G., 2007. Magnetic stimulation of the pelvic floor in older patients. Results of a prospective analysis. Urologe A 46 (4), 377–378 380–381.

Korenevskaia, E.E., Markina, L.P., Perfil'eva, I.F., 1982. Comparative evaluation of the effect of nitrogen-containing and fresh water on hemodynamics of organs of the small pelvis in patients with chronic salpingo-oophoritis. Vopr. Kurortol. Fizioter. Lech. Fiz. Kult. (1), 52–54.

Kulishova, T.V., Tabashnikova, N.A., Akker, L.V., 2005. Efficacy of general magnetotherapy in conservative therapy of uterine myoma in women of reproductive age. Vopr. Kurortol. Fizioter. Lech. Fiz. Kult. (1), 26–28.

Larsen, A.I., 1991. Congenital malformations and exposure to high-frequency electromagnetic radiation among Danish physiotherapists. Scand. J. Work Environ. Health 17 (5), 318–323.

Laptev, P.I., 2004. Use of local UHF hyperthermia and CO(2) laser in treatment of cancer of the lip, lingual mucosa, and bottom of the oral cavity. Stomatologiia (Mosk) 83 (1), 30–32.

Lee, S.H., Lee, B.C., 2009. Electroacupuncture relieves pain in men with chronic prostatitis/chronic pelvic pain syndrome: three-arm randomized trial. Urology 73 (5), 1036–1041.

Leippold, T., Strebel, R.T., Huwyler, M., et al., 2005. Sacral magnetic stimulation in non-inflammatory chronic pelvic pain syndrome. BJU Int. 95 (6), 838–841.

Leĭtes, V.G., Pavlov, V.N., Mozzhukhin, P.A., 1990. Experience with the use of physiotherapy in treating epididymitis. Vestn. Dermatol. Venerol. (9), 55–58.

Lerman, et al., 2001. Pregnancy outcome following exposure to shortwaves among female physiotherapists in Israel. Am. J. Ind. Med. 39 (5), 499–504.

Lorenzo Gómez, M.F., Silva Abuín, J.M., García Criado, F.J., Geanini Yagüez, A., Urrutia Avisrror, M., 2008. Treatment of stress urinary incontinence with perineal biofeedback by using superficial electrodes. Actas Urol. Esp. 32 (6), 629–636.

Lou, L., 2000. Uncommon areas of electrical stimulation for pain relief. Curr. Rev. Pain. 4 (5), 407–412.

Lytkin, V.V., 1982. Substantiation of the duration of radon vaginal irrigations in patients with uterine myoma. Vopr. Kurortol. Fizioter. Lech. Fiz. Kult. (1), 54–55.

MacDiarmid, S.A., Peters, K.M., Shobeiri, A., et al., 2010. Long-term durability of percutaneous tibial nerve stimulation for the treatment of overactive bladder. J. Urol. 183, 234–240.

Marzouk, B., Marzouk, Z., Décor, R., 2010a. Antibacterial and antifungal activities of several populations of Tunisian Citrullus colocynthis Schrad immature fruits and seeds. Journal of Medical Mycology 20 (3), 179–184.

Marzouk, B., Marzouk, Z., Haloui, E., et al., 2010b. Screening of analgesic and anti-inflammatory activities of Citrullus colocynthis from southern Tunisia. Journal of Ethnopharmacology, 128(1):15–19.

Maslarova, Z., 1984a. Comparative results of balneotherapy with mineral water from the Vlasa and Chepino springs in Velingrad in women with nonspecific inflammatory gynecologic diseases and sterility. Akush. Ginekol (Sofiia) 23 (2), 151–154.

Maslarova, Z., 1984b. Efficacy of using mineral water from "Chepino" spring, Velingrad, alone and in combination with vibration therapy in the treatment of chronic nonspecific inflammatory gynecologic diseases and sterility in women. Akush. Ginekol. (Sofiia) 23 (3), 245–248.

Melzack, R., Wall, P.D., 1965. Pain mechanisms: a new theory. Science 150 (699), 971–979.

Nagy, K., Berhés, I., Kovács, T., et al., 2009. Does balneotherapy with low radon concentration in water influence the endocrine system? A controlled non-randomized pilot study. Radiat. Environ. Biophys. 48 (3), 311–315.

Nappi, R.E., Ferdeghini, F., Abbiati, I., et al., 2003. Electrical stimulation (ES) in the management of sexual pain disorders. J. Sex Marital Ther. 29 (Suppl. 1), 103–110.

Neĭmark, A.I., Aliev, R.T., Klepikova, I.I., et al., 2009. Efficacy of vibrothermomagnetic impact on the perineum from the device Avim-1 in the treatment of chronic abacterial prostatitis patients with chronic pelvic pain syndrome. Urologiia (4), 40–44.

Nevropatol, Zh., Psikhiatr, Im., Korsakova, S.S., 1995. The use of pulsed and continuous UHF electrical fields in the rehabilitation of patients with the Guillain-Barre syndrome and other peripheral myelinopathies 95 (5), 22–26.

Nicosia, J.F., Abcarian, H., 1985. Levator syndrome A treatment that works. Dis. Colon Rectum 28 (6), 406–408.

Oláh, M., Koncz, A., Fehér, J., et al., 2009. The effect of balneotherapy on C-reactive protein, serum cholesterol, triglyceride, total antioxidant status and HSP-60 levels. Int. J. Biometeorol.

Okano, H., Ohkubo, C., 2001. Modulatory effects of static magnetic fields on blood pressure in rabbits. Bioelectromagnetics 22 (6), 408–418.

Opsomer, R.J., Boccasena, P., Traversa, R., Rossini, P.M., 1996. Sympathetic skin responses from the limbs and the genitalia: normative study and contribution to the evaluation of neurological disorders. Electroenceph. Clin. Neurophysiol. 101 (1), 25–31.

Oullet Hellstrom, R., Stewart, W.F., 1993. Miscarriages among female physical therapists who report using radio- and microwave-frequency electromagnetic radiation. Am. J. Epidemiol. 138 (10), 775–786. Comment in: Am. J. Epidemiol. 141 (3), 273–274 (1995).

Papp, G., Csontay, A., 1979. Therapeutic use of ultrasound in urology. Acta Chir. Acad. Sci. Hung. 20 (2–3), 275–279.

Post-Graduate Study of Naturotherapy, 1939. Naturopath and Herald of Health. Benedict Lust Publications, NY, NY.

Prentice, W., 1998. Therapeutic Modalities for the Allied Health Professionals. McGraw Hill.

Prokopiev, V., Nikolova, L., 1971. The treatment of inflammatory diseases of the female genitalia with mineral baths of Kiustendil, ozokerite application and exercise therapy. Akush. Ginekol. (Sofiia) 10 (1), 63–67.

Pryĭma, O.B., Lysyk, O.S., Pidlisets'ka, M.M., et al., 1996. The use of laser and electrical physiotherapy in the combined treatment of patients with chronic prostatitis. Lik. Sprava (7–9), 128–131.

Radionchenko, A.A., Tepliakova, M.V., 1989. Combined treatment using brine in acute inflammatory diseases of the internal female genitalia. Vopr. Kurortol. Fizioter. Lech. Fiz. Kult. (2), 47–51.

Reshetov, P.P., Sedov, O.N., Reshetova, N.V., 1996. The treatment results in inflammatory diseases of the adnexa uteri with different methods of using sinusoidal modulated currents. Vopr. Kurortol. Fizioter. Lech. Fiz. Kult. (6), 27–28.

Sanseverino EG, 1980. Membrane phenomena and cellular processes under the action of pulsating magnetic fields. Presented at the 2nd International Congress of Magneto Medicine. Rome, Italy, 1980.

Santos, P.F., Oliveira, E., Zanetti, M.R., et al., 2009. Electrical stimulation of the pelvic floor versus vaginal cone therapy for the treatment of stress urinary incontinence. Rev. Bras. Ginecol. Obstet. 31 (9), 447–452.

Scott, L., 1990. Clinical Hydrotherapy. Leo Scott, Spokane, WA.

Scott, R.S., Hsueh, G.S., 1979. A clinical study of the effects of galvanic vaginal muscle stimulation in urinary stress incontinence and sexual dysfunction. Am. J. Obstet. Gynecol. 135 (5), 663–665.

Shank, K., Randall, K., 2002. Therapeutic Physical Modalities. Hanley & Befus, Inc., pp. 84–86.

Shaplygin, L.V., Begaev, A.I., V'iushina, V.V., 2006. Use of

Intramag devices with Intraterm and LAST-02 attachments in complex therapy of chronic prostatitis. Urologiia (4), 49–54.

Shaplygin, L.V., Koval', A.M., Pavlenko, A.V., Kazachenko, A.I.u., 2004. Apparatus Aeltis-Synchro-02-"Yarilo" and vacuum laser therapeutic urologic massager AMVL 01-"Yarovit" in the treatment of chronic prostatitis complicated with copulation dysfunction. Urologiia (5), 34–36.

Shriber, W., 1975. A Manual of Electrotherapy. Lea and Febiger, Philadelphia, PA, p. 219.

Sikiru, L., Shmaila, H., Muhammed, S.A., 2008. Transcutaneous electrical nerve stimulation (TENS) in the symptomatic management of chronic prostatitis/chronic pelvic pain syndrome: a placebo-control randomized trial. Int. Braz. J. Urol. 34 (6), 708–713, discussion 714.

Skalak, T.C., Morris, C.E., 2008. Acute exposure to a moderate strength static magnetic field reduces edema formation in rats. Am. J. Physiol. Heart Circ. Physiol. 294 (1), H50–H57.

Skilling, P.M., Petros, P., 2004. Synergistic non-surgical management of pelvic floor dysfunction: second report. Int. Urogynecol. J. Pelvic Floor Dysfunct. 15 (2), 106–110, discussion 110.

Smith, K., 1991. The photobiological basis of low-level laser radiation therapy. Laser Therapy 3, 19–24.

Sokolova, A.S., 1981. Balneotherapy of patients with retrodeviation of the uterus. Vopr. Kurortol. Fizioter. Lech. Fiz. Kult. (6), 44–46.

Starkey, C., 1999. Therapeutic Modalities, second ed. FA Davis.

Stener-Victorin, E., Jedel, E., Janson, P.O., Sverrisdottir, Y.B., 2009. Low-frequency electroacupuncture and physical exercise decrease high muscle sympathetic nerve activity in polycystic ovary syndrome. Am. J. Physiol. Regul. Integr. Comp. Physiol. 297 (2), R387–R395.

Stepanenko, V.I., Koliadenko, V.G., 1990. Experience in treating chronic urethritis in men by iontophoresis and inductothermy. Vestn. Dermatol. Venerol. (6), 55–59.

Suchy, H., Cekański, A., 1982. Treatment and sanatorium rehabilitation in chronic adnexitis and postinflammatory conditions of the adnexa uteri with regard to specific action of brine baths. Ginekol. Pol. 53 (9), 619–624.

Takahashi, T., 2011. Mechanism of Acupuncture on Neuromodulation in the Gut-A Review Neuromodulation: Technology at the Neural Interface, 14 (1):8–12.

Takahashi, S., Kitamura, T., 2003. Overactive bladder: magnetic versus electrical stimulation. Curr. Opin. Obstet. Gynecol. 15 (5), 429–433.

Taskinen, H., 1990. Effects of ultrasound, shortwaves, and physical exertion on pregnancy outcome in physiotherapists. J. Epidemiol. Commun. Health 44 (3), 196–201.

Tereshin, A.T., Vinogrdkiĭ, A.M., Avlastimov, I.a.I., Popov, S.A., 2008. Electropulse therapy in the early postoperative rehabilitation period after reconstructive and plastic surgery on fallopian tubes. Vopr. Kurortol. Fizioter. Lech. Fiz. Kult. (4), 26–28.

Tikhonovskaia, O.A., Evtushenko, I.D., Logvinov, S.V., 2000. An experimental and clinical validation of a method for treating acute inflammatory diseases of the adnexa uteri by using the electrophoresis of a therapeutic mud preparation. Vopr. Kurortol. Fizioter. Lech. Fiz. Kult. (4), 31–34.

Tikhonovskaia, O.A., Logvinov, S.V., 1998. The effect of the brine and mud extract from Lake Karachi on the morphofunctional status of the adnexa uteri in experimental inflammation. Vopr. Kurortol. Fizioter. Lech. Fiz. Kult. (5), 33–35.

Tikhonovskaia, O.A., Petrova, M.S., Logvinov, S.V., Shustov, L.P., Titkova, I.N., 1999. An experimental validation of the use of the ultraphonophoresis of the mud preparation Eplir in inflammation of the uterine adnexa. Vopr. Kurortol. Fizioter. Lech. Fiz. Kult. (4), 32–34.

Tiktinskiĭ, O.L., Kalinina, S.N., Novikova, L.I., Mishanin, E.A., Tiktinskiĭ, N.O., 1997. Electrolaser therapy on the Iarilo device in patients with chronic chlamydial prostatitis. Urol. Nefrol. (Mosk) (4), 25–29.

Tilly, et al., 2005. Regional hyperthermia in conjunction with definitive radiotherapy against recurrent or locally advanced prostate cancer T3 pN0 M0. Strahlenther. Onkol. 181 (1), 35–41.

Trojel, H., Lebech, P.E., 1969. Intermittent short waves (Diapulse) in the therapy of inflammatory pelvic disease. Nord. Med. 81 (10), 307–310.

Urbánek, V., Raboch, J., Raboch Jr., J., Sindlár, M., Boudník, V., 1998. Treatment of gynecologic inflammations in Frantiskových Lázních Health Spa. Ceska. Gynekol. 63 (5), 400–402.

van Balken, M.R., 2007. Percutaneous tibial nerve stimulation: the Urgent PC device. Expert Rev. Med. Devices 4 (5), 693–698.

van Balken, M.R., Vandoninck, V., Messelink, B.J., et al., 2003. Percutaneous tibial nerve stimulation as neuromodulative treatment of chronic pelvic pain. Eur. Urol. 43 (2), 158–163, discussion 163.

Van den Bouwhuijsen, F., et al., 1990. Pulsed and Continuous Short Wave Therapy. B.V. Enhaf-Nonius, Delft, Holland, p. 17.

van der Pal, F., van Balken, M.R., Heesakkers, J.P., Debruyne, F.M., Bemelmans, B.L., 2006. Percutaneous tibial nerve stimulation in the treatment of refractory overactive bladder syndrome: is maintenance treatment necessary? BJU Int. 97 (3), 547–550.

Vorovskaia, V.D., Dzhaginian, A.I., Til'ba, I.P., Ziuban, A.L., Khabinson, V.K.h., 1994. Possible approaches to improvement of the efficacy of health resort treatment of women with pelvic inflammatory diseases. Akush. Ginekol. (Mosk) (1), 47–51.

Wang, X.M., 1989. On the therapeutic efficacy of electric acupuncture with moxibustion in 95 cases of chronic pelvic infectious disease (PID). J. Tradit. Chin. Med. 9 (1), 21–24.

Yamanishi, T., Yasuda, K., 1998. Electrical stimulation for stress incontinence. Int. Urogynecol. J. Pelvic Floor Dysfunct. 9 (5), 281–290.

Yelland, M.J., Glasziou, P.P., Bogduk, N., et al., 2004. Prolotherapy injections, saline injections, and exercises for chronic low-back pain: a randomized trial. Spine 29 (1), 9–16.

Zámbó, L., Dékány, M., Bender, T., 2008. The efficacy of alum-containing ferrous thermal water in the management of chronic inflammatory gynaecological disorders: a randomized controlled study. Eur. J. Obstet. Gynecol. Reprod. Biol. 140 (2), 252–257.

Zhao, J., Bai, J., Zhou, Y., Qi, G., Du, L., 2008. Posterior tibial nerve stimulation twice a week in patients with interstitial cystitis. Urology 71 (6), 1080–1084.

Zharkin, A.F., Strugatsku, V.M., Kamara, K.M., 1991. Rationale for using physiotherapeutic procedures adapted to the phases of menstrual cycle in women of reproductive age. Akush. Ginekol. (Mosk) (1), 37–40.

Appendix: Clinical outcome measurement tools

Dee Hartman Ruth Lovegrove Jones Leon Chaitow

There are numerous validated outcome tools used as measures of rehabilitation changes in 'normal' dysfunction (e.g. stroke). However, when dealing with chronic pelvic pain (CPP) and its nuances, it becomes difficult to find an appropriate tool(s) that effectively addresses all the issues involved. When treating CCP, practitioners must consider the many overlapping co-morbid disorders that occur and which, when left untreated, may contribute to the dysfunction and interfere with full recovery. As a result, it is typical to use more than one outcome measurement (OM) tool to address more than one problem.

Below are brief summaries of suggested available OM tools, most of which are available online for clinical use. However, it is important to remember that these OM tools were in the most part developed for research purposes, and normative data are unavailable to assist in the interpretation of scores in individual cases. Nonetheless, for those practitioners dealing with pelvic pain who may not have considered urinary or sexual dysfunction co-morbidity, they may provide a useful resource of enquiry as well as a tool to monitor the effects of treatment over time.

1. The International Pelvic Pain Society (IPPS; see p. 397) has developed the Pelvic Pain Assessment Form for women. This is a complete questionnaire that incorporates extensive medical history (including sexual and abuse issues (Leserman et al. 1995)), VASs pain mapping, bowel/bladder/dietary habits, and a portion of the short-form McGill pain questionnaire (SF-MPQ). The final three pages are dedicated to physical assessment.
2. The Pelvic Pain and Urgency/Frequency questionnaire is an eight-question survey that inquires about bladder habits associated with pain, urgency, frequency and sexual activity. Its numerical scoring system differentiates between symptoms and bother created by the symptoms. It is included within the IPPS assessment form (see p. 402).
3. The original McGill questionnaire (MPQ; see p. 404, top box) was designed with questions about three areas of pain: how it feels, how it changes with time and how strong it is. It includes lists of word descriptors that are scored, with a greater total score representing greater pain. A shorter version was created (SF-MPQ) that includes 15 descriptors (11 sensory and four affective) and added measures using the Present Pain Intensity (PPI) index and a VAS (Melzak 1987). The SF-MPQ is found within the pelvic pain assessment form from the IPPS. There is no total score determined; rather a comparison of change over time is used.
4. The VAS and numeric pain rating (NRS) have both shown validity over time, are quick, easy and inexpensive to use, and are user-friendly. Patients are asked to rate their symptoms on a scale of 0 to 10 with 0 being 'no pain at all' and 10 as 'the worst pain you've ever experienced' (e.g. 5/10). Results can be recorded as a number or as a slash mark on a 10-cm line that denotes '0' on one end and '10' on the other. Statistically significant change is viewed as a change in two points, either up or down. A version of a VAS is to be found within the Stanford Pelvic Pain Symptom Score (PPSS) for men (see p. 408).

5. The Stanford Pelvic Pain Symptom Score (PPSS) (for men) has three domains: a pain location and severity (including a separate ten-point pain VAS a seven-item urinary symptom score similar to the IPPS described above; and a five-item sexual dysfunction score. It was modified from the survey initially developed at the University of Washington and reported in the *Journal of Urology* (2006). The PPSS (see p. 408) was not validated and it predates the availability of the NIH-CPSI (Anderson et al. 2005).
6. The National Institutes of Health developed the Chronic Prostatitis Symptom Index (NIH-CPSI; see p. 409) which has recently been adapted for use in female patients (see p. 411) with the female homologue of each male anatomical term used (Female Questionnaire) (Marszalek et al. 2009). It consists of nine questions that gather information on pain, urinary symptoms and quality of life issues. It has definitive scoring, 0–43, with the total score suggestive of mild (0–9), moderate (10–18) or severe (19–31) disease.
7. The Female Sexual Function Index (FSFI; see p. 413) is a 19-question self-administered survey including questions on six sexual domains, including desire, subjective arousal, lubrication, orgasm, satisfaction, and pain. Total and single domain numeric scores demonstrate change. A total score ≤ 26 suggests risk for sexual dysfunction. It has been validated for use in women with vulvodynia who, in the validation study, had an average total score of 15.5. The FSFI deals with self-perceived emotional and functional issues.
8. The Female Sexual Distress Scale (FSDS; see p. 420) is a 20-item questionnaire designed to measure female sex-related personal distress. A revised form (FSDS-R) has only 12 questions and has been validated in women with hypoactive sexual desire disorder. There are no ranges of normal to abnormal scoring (Derogatis et al. 2002).
9. The Vulvar Pain Functional Questionnaire (V-Q) is an 11-item questionnaire that deals with functional aspects of CPP as well as vulvar pain. There is a scoring system with improvement suggested by a decrease in overall scoring over time (see p. 423).
10. The Nijmegen questionnaire (see p. 425) assesses 16 symptoms associated with abnormal breathing on a five-point scale. A total symptom score of, or greater than, 23 has been reported as showing a sensitivity of 91% and a specificity of 95% as a screening instrument in patients with diagnosed hyperventilation syndrome (Van Dixhoorn & Duivenvoorden 1985).
11. The Self-Evaluation of Breathing Questionnaire (SEBQ; see p. 426) is a tool for measuring dysfunctional breathing symptoms and self-perception of breathing behaviours. It is most valuable for evaluating patients before and after treatment. The items of the SEBQ are based on research and clinical reports of breathing complaints and breathing behaviours associated with dysfunctional breathing. It has not been validated as a diagnostic instrument and cut-off scores for normal and abnormal have not been established; however, clinical experience suggests that normal individuals tend to score below 11. The SEBQ contains phrases that differentiate qualities of dyspnoea known to arise from different pathological mechanisms. The items 'I feel I cannot take a deep or satisfying breath' and 'My breathing feels stuck or restricted' are phrases typical of the quality of dyspnoea often referred to as unsatisfied respiration, which is often associated with poor neuromechanical coupling in breathing. Items such as 'I feel short of breath talking or reading', 'I can't catch my breath', 'the air feels stuffy' and other items that use the words breathless are more likely to be influenced by feedback from chemoreceptors and other cortical influences on dyspnoea (Courtney & Greenwood 2009).
12. A summary of descriptions of eight standard pelvic girdle pain provocation tests (see p. 427), derived from the European guidelines for the diagnosis and treatment of pelvic girdle pain (Vleeming et al. 2008).

THE INTERNATIONAL **PELVIC PAIN** SOCIETY

Pelvic Pain Assessment Form

Physician:________________________

Initial History and Physical Examination

*Date:*_______________

This assessment form is intended to assist the clinician with the initial patient assessment and is not meant to be a diagnostic tool.

Contact Information

Name:________________________ Birth Date:__________________ Chart Number:______________

Phone: Work:______________________ Home:_____________________ Cell:____________________

Referring Provider's Name and Address:____

Information About Your Pain

Please describe your pain problem (use a separate sheet of paper if needed):____________________

____

____

____

____

____

What do you think is causing your pain?____

Is there an event that you associate with the onset of your pain? ❑ Yes ❑ No If so, what?_______

How long have you had this pain? _____years _____months

For each of the symptoms listed below, please "bubble in" your level of pain over the last month using a 10-point scale:

0 – no pain 10 – the worst pain imaginable

How would you rate your pain?	0	1	2	3	4	5	6	7	8	9	10
Pain at ovulation (mid-cycle)	O	O	O	O	O	O	O	O	O	O	O
Pain just before period	O	O	O	O	O	O	O	O	O	O	O
Pain (not cramps) before period	O	O	O	O	O	O	O	O	O	O	O
Deep pain with intercourse	O	O	O	O	O	O	O	O	O	O	O
Pain in groin when lifting	O	O	O	O	O	O	O	O	O	O	O
Pelvic pain lasting hours or days after intercourse	O	O	O	O	O	O	O	O	O	O	O
Pain when bladder is full	O	O	O	O	O	O	O	O	O	O	O
Muscle/joint pain	O	O	O	O	O	O	O	O	O	O	O
Level of cramps with period	O	O	O	O	O	O	O	O	O	O	O
Pain after period is over	O	O	O	O	O	O	O	O	O	O	O
Burning vaginal pain after sex	O	O	O	O	O	O	O	O	O	O	O
Pain with urination	O	O	O	O	O	O	O	O	O	O	O
Backache	O	O	O	O	O	O	O	O	O	O	O
Migraine headache	O	O	O	O	O	O	O	O	O	O	O
Pain with sitting	O	O	O	O	O	O	O	O	O	O	O

Provider Comments

____

____

____

____

____

Information About Your Pain

What types of treatments/providers have you tried in the past for your pain? **Please check all that apply.**

❑ Acupuncture
❑ Anesthesiologist
❑ Anti-seizure medications
❑ Antidepressants
❑ Biofeedback
❑ Botox injection
❑ Contraceptive pills / patch / ring
❑ Danazol (Danocrine)
❑ Depo-provera
❑ Gastroenterologist
❑ Gynecologist
❑ Family practitioner
❑ Herbal medicine
❑ Homeopathic medicine
❑ Lupron, Synarel, Zoladex
❑ Massage
❑ Meditation
❑ Narcotics
❑ Naturopathic medication
❑ Nerve blocks
❑ Neurosurgeon
❑ Nonprescription medicine
❑ Nutrition / diet
❑ Physical therapy
❑ Psychotherapy
❑ Psychiatrist
❑ Rheumatologist
❑ Skin magnets
❑ Surgery
❑ TENS unit
❑ Trigger point injections
❑ Urologist
❑ Other________________

Pain Maps

Please shade areas of pain and write a number from 1 to 10 at the site(s) of pain. (10 = most severe pain imaginable)

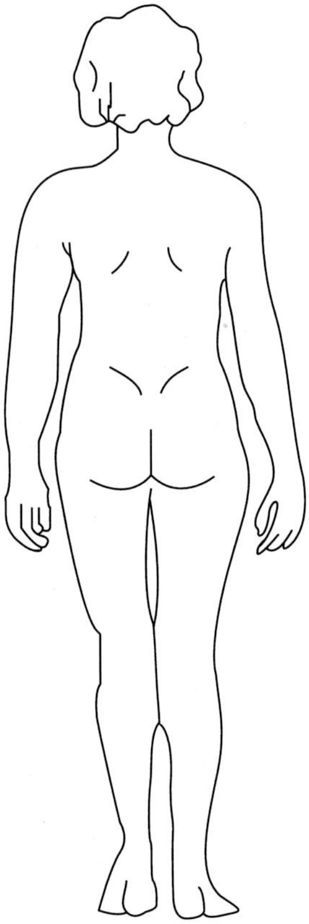

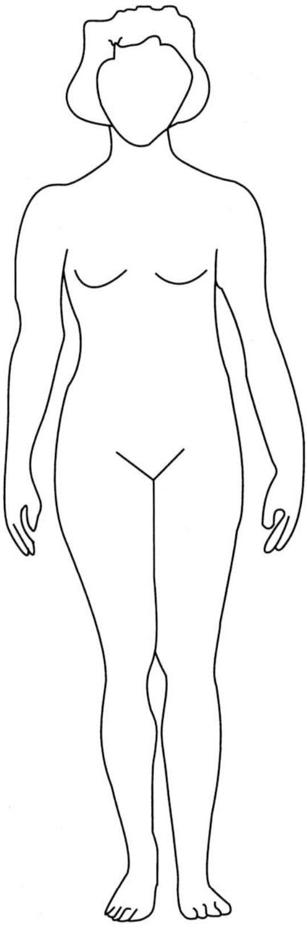

Left Right Right Left

Vulvar / Perineal Pain
(pain outside and around the vagina and anus)

If you have vulvar pain, shade the painful areas and write a number from 1 to 10 at the painful sites (10 = most severe pain imaginable)

Is your pain relieved by sitting on a commode seat? ❑ Yes ❑ No

Right Left

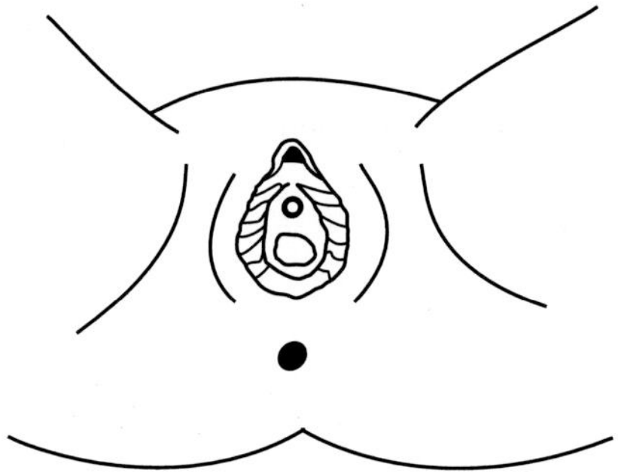

What physicians or health care providers have evaluated or treated you for **chronic pelvic pain**?

Physician / Provider	***Specialty***	***City, State, Phone***

Demographic Information

Are you (check all that apply):

❑ Married ❑ Widowed ❑ Separated ❑ Committed relationship

❑ Single ❑ Remarried ❑ Divorced

Who do you live with?________________________________

Education: ❑ Less than 12 years ❑ High School graduate

❑ College degree ❑ Postgraduate degree

What type of work are you trained for? ________________________________

What type of work are you doing?________________________________

Surgical History

Please list all surgical procedures you have had **related to this pain:**

Year	Procedure	Surgeon	Findings

Please list all **other** surgical procedures:

Year	Procedure

Year	Procedure

Provider Comments

____

____

____

____

Medications

Please list **pain medication** you have taken for your pain condition in the past 6 months, and the providers who prescribed them (use a separate page if needed):

Medication / dose	Provider	Did it help?
		❑ Yes ❑ No ❑ Currently taking
		❑ Yes ❑ No ❑ Currently taking
		❑ Yes ❑ No ❑ Currently taking
		❑ Yes ❑ No ❑ Currently taking
		❑ Yes ❑ No ❑ Currently taking
		❑ Yes ❑ No ❑ Currently taking
		❑ Yes ❑ No ❑ Currently taking
		❑ Yes ❑ No ❑ Currently taking

Please list all **other medications** you are presently taking, the condition, and the provider who prescribed them (use a separate page if needed):

Medication / dose	Provider	Medical condition

Obstetrical History

How many pregnancies have you had?_________

Resulting in (#): ______ Full 9 months ______ Premature ______ Miscarriage / Abortion ______ Living children

Where there any complications during pregnancy, labor, delivery, or post partum?

❑ 4° Episiotomy ❑ C-Section ❑ Vacuum ❑ Post-partum hemorrhaging

❑ Vaginal laceration ❑ Forceps ❑ Medication for bleeding ❑ Other______________

Family History

Has anyone in your family had: ❑ Fibromyalgia ❑ Chronic pelvic pain ❑ Irritable bowel syndrome

❑ Depression ❑ Interstitial cystitis ❑ Other chronic condition ________

❑ Endometriosis ❑ Cancer, type(s)________________________________

Medical History

Please list any medical problems / diagnoses ________________________________

____

____

Allergies (including latex allergy) ________________________________

Who is your primary care provider? ________________________________

Have you ever been hospitalized for anything besides childbirth? ❑ Yes ❑ No ❑ If yes, please explain________

____

Have you had major accidents such as falls or a back injury? ❑ Yes ❑ No

Have you ever been treated for depression? ❑ Yes ❑ No Treatments: ❑ Medication ❑ Hospitalization ❑ Psychotherapy

Birth control method: ❑ Nothing ❑ Pill ❑ Vasectomy ❑ Vaginal ring ❑ Depo provera

❑ Condom ❑ IUD ❑ Hysterectomy ❑ Diaphragm ❑ Tubal sterilization

❑ Other____________

Menstrual History
How old were you when your menses started? ___________
Are you still having menstrual periods? ❑ Yes ❑ No

Answer the following only if you are still having menstrual periods.
Periods are: ❑ Light ❑ Moderate ❑ Heavy ❑ Bleed through protection
How many days between your periods? ___________
How many days of menstrual flow? ___________
Date of first day of last menstrual period ___________
Do you have any pain with your periods? ❑ Yes ❑ No
Does pain start the day flow starts? ❑ Yes ❑ No Pain starts _______ days before flow
Are periods regular? ❑ Yes ❑ No
Do you pass clots in menstrual flow? ❑ Yes ❑ No

Gastrointestinal Eating
Do you have nausea? ❑ No ❑ With pain ❑ Taking medications ❑ With eating ❑ Other
Do you have vomiting? ❑ No ❑ With pain ❑ Taking medications ❑ With eating ❑ Other
Have you ever had an eating disorder such as anorexia or bulimia? ❑ Yes ❑ No
Are you experiencing rectal bleeding or blood in your stool? ❑ Yes ❑ No
Do you have increased pain with bowel movements? ❑ Yes ❑ No

The following questions help to diagnose irritable bowel syndrome, a gastrointestinal condition, which may be a cause of pelvic pain.
Do you have pain or discomfort that is associated with the following:

Change in frequency of bowel movement? ❑ Yes ❑ No
Change in appearance of stool or bowel movement? ❑ Yes ❑ No
Does your pain improve after completing a bowel movement? ❑ Yes ❑ No

Health Habits
How often do you exercise? ❑ Rarely ❑ 1-2 times weekly ❑ 3-5 times weekly ❑ Daily
What is your caffeine intake (number cups per day, include coffee, tea, soft drinks, etc)? ❑ 0 ❑ 1-3 ❑ 4-6 ❑ >6
How many cigarettes do you smoke per day? ___________ For how many years? ___________
Do you drink alcohol? ❑ Yes ❑ No
Number of drinks per week ___________
Have you ever received treatment for substance abuse? ❑ Yes ❑ No
What is your use of recreational drugs? ❑ Never used ❑ Used in the past, but not now ❑ Presently using ❑ No answer
❑ Heroin ❑ Amphetamines ❑ Marijuana ❑ Barbiturates ❑ Cocaine ❑ Other ___________
How would you describe your diet? (check all that apply) ❑ Well balanced ❑ Vegan ❑ Vegetarian ❑ Fried food
❑ Special diet ___________ ❑ Other ___________

Urinary Symptoms

Do you experience any of the following?

Loss of urine when coughing, sneezing, or laughing?	❑ Yes	❑ No
Difficulty passing urine?	❑ Yes	❑ No
Frequent bladder infections?	❑ Yes	❑ No
Blood in the urine?	❑ Yes	❑ No
Still feeling full after urination?	❑ Yes	❑ No
Having to void again within minutes of voiding?	❑ Yes	❑ No

The following questions help to diagnose painful bladder syndrome, which may cause pelvic pain

Please circle the answer that best describes your bladder function and symptoms.

	0	1	2	3	4
1. How many times do you go to the bathroom **DURING THE DAY** (to void or empty your bladder)?	3-6	7-10	11-14	15-19	20 or more
2. How many times do you go to the bathroom **AT NIGHT** (to void or empty your bladder)?	0	1	2	3	4 or more
3. If you get up at night to void or empty your bladder does it bother you?	Never	Mildly	Moderately	Severely	
4. Are you sexually active? ❑ Yes ❑ No					
5. If you are sexually active, do you now or have you ever had pain or symptoms during or after sexual intercourse?	Never	Occasionally	Usually	Always	
6. If you have pain with intercourse, does it make you avoid sexual intercourse?	Never	Occasionally	Usually	Always	
7. Do you have pain associated with your bladder or in your pelvis (lower abdomen, labia, vagina, urethra, perineum)?	Never	Occasionally	Usually	Always	
8. Do you have urgency after voiding?	Never	Occasionally	Usually	Always	
9. If you have pain, is it usually	Never	Mild	Moderate	Severe	
10. Does your pain bother you?	Never	Occasionally	Usually	Always	
11. If you have urgency, is it usually		Mild	Moderate	Severe	
12. Does your urgency bother you?	Never	Occasionally	Usually	Always	

KCI _____ *Not Indicated* _____ *Positive* _____ *Negative*

Coping Mechanisms

Who are the people you talk to concerning your pain, or during stressful times?

❑ Spouse / Partner ❑ Relative ❑ Support group ❑ Clergy
❑ Doctor /Nurse ❑ Friend ❑ Mental health provider ❑ I take care of myself

How does your partner deal with your pain?

❑ Doesn't notice when I'm in pain ❑ Takes care of me ❑ Not applicable
❑ Withdraws ❑ Feels helpless
❑ Distracts me with activities ❑ Gets angry

What helps your pain? ❑ Meditation ❑ Relaxation ❑ Lying down ❑ Music
❑ Massage ❑ Ice ❑ Heating pad ❑ Hot bath
❑ Pain medication ❑ Laxatives/enema ❑ Injection ❑ TENS unit
❑ Bowel movement ❑ Emptying bladder ❑ Nothing
❑ Other ___________________

What makes your pain worse? ❑ Intercourse ❑ Orgasm ❑ Stress ❑ Full meal
❑ Bowel movement ❑ Full bladder ❑ Urination ❑ Standing
❑ Walking ❑ Exercise ❑ Time of day ❑ Weather
❑ Contact with clothing ❑ Coughing/sneezing ❑ Not related to anything
❑ Other ___________________

Of all the problems or stresses of your life, how does your pain compare in importance?

❑ The most important problem ❑ Just one of many problems

Sexual and Physical Abuse History

Have you ever been the victim of emotional abuse? This can include being humiliated or insulted ❑ Yes ❑ No ❑ No answer

Check an answer for both as a child and as an adult	As a child (13 and younger)		As an adult (14 and over)	
1a. Has anyone ever exposed the sex organs of their body to you when you did not want it?	❑ Yes	❑ No	❑ Yes	❑ No
1b. Has anyone ever threatened to have sex with you when you did not want it?	❑ Yes	❑ No	❑ Yes	❑ No
1c. Has anyone ever touched the sex organs of your body when you did not want this?	❑ Yes	❑ No	❑ Yes	❑ No
1d. Has anyone ever made you touch the sex organs of their body when you did not want this?	❑ Yes	❑ No	❑ Yes	❑ No
1e. Has anyone forced you to have sex when you did not want this?	❑ Yes	❑ No	❑ Yes	❑ No
1f. Have you had any other unwanted sexual experiences not mentioned above?	❑ Yes	❑ No	❑ Yes	❑ No

If yes, please specify ____

2. When you were a child (13 or younger), did an older person do the following?

a. Hit, kick, or beat you?	❑ Never	❑ Seldom	❑ Occasionally	❑ Often
b. Seriously threaten your life?	❑ Never	❑ Seldom	❑ Occasionally	❑ Often

3. Now that you are an adult (14 or older), has any other adult done the following?

a. Hit, kick, or beat you?	❑ Never	❑ Seldom	❑ Occasionally	❑ Often
b. Seriously threaten your life?	❑ Never	❑ Seldom	❑ Occasionally	❑ Often

Leserman, J, Drossman D, Li Z. The reliability and validity of a sexual and physical abuse history questionnaire in female patients with gastrointestinal disorders. Behavioral Medicine 1995:21:141-148.

Short-Form McGill

The words below describe average pain. Place a check mark (✓) in the column which represents the degree to which you feel that type of pain. Please limit yourself to a description of the pain in your pelvic area only.

What does your pain feel like?

Type	***None (0)***	***Mild (1)***	***Moderate (2)***	***Severe (3)***
Throbbing	_______	_______	_______	_______
Shooting	_______	_______	_______	_______
Stabbing	_______	_______	_______	_______
Sharp	_______	_______	_______	_______
Cramping	_______	_______	_______	_______
Gnawing	_______	_______	_______	_______
Hot-Burning	_______	_______	_______	_______
Aching	_______	_______	_______	_______
Heavy	_______	_______	_______	_______
Tender	_______	_______	_______	_______
Splitting	_______	_______	_______	_______
Tiring-Exhausting	_______	_______	_______	_______
Sickening	_______	_______	_______	_______
Fearful	_______	_______	_______	_______
Punishing-Cruel	_______	_______	_______	_______

Melzak R. The Short-form McGill Pain Questionnaire. Pain 1987:30:191-197.

Pelvic Varicosity Pain Syndrome Questions

Is your pelvic pain aggravated by prolonged physical activity?	❑ Yes	❑ No
Does your pelvic pain improve when you lie down?	❑ Yes	❑ No
Do you have pain that is deep in the vagina or pelvis *during* sex?	❑ Yes	❑ No
Do you have pelvic throbbing or aching *after* sex?	❑ Yes	❑ No
Do you have pelvic pain that moves from side to side?	❑ Yes	❑ No
Do you have sudden episodes of severe pelvic pain that come and go?	❑ Yes	❑ No

Physical Examination – For Physician Use Only

Name:______________________________ Chart Number:______________________________

Date of Exam:________________ Height:________ Weight:________ BMI:________

BP:______ HR:______ Temp:______ Resp:______ LMP: ______

ROS, PFSH Reviewed: ❑ Yes ❑ No Physician Signature:______________________________

General Appearance: ❑ Well-appearing ❑ Ill-appearing ❑ Tearful ❑ Depressed
❑ Normal weight ❑ Underweight ❑ Overweight ❑ Abnormal Gait

NOTE: Mark "Not Examined" as N/E

HEENT ❑ WNL ❑ Other _____ ***Lungs*** ❑ WNL ❑ Other _____ ***Heart*** ❑ WNL ❑ Other _____ ***Breasts*** ❑ WNL ❑ Other___

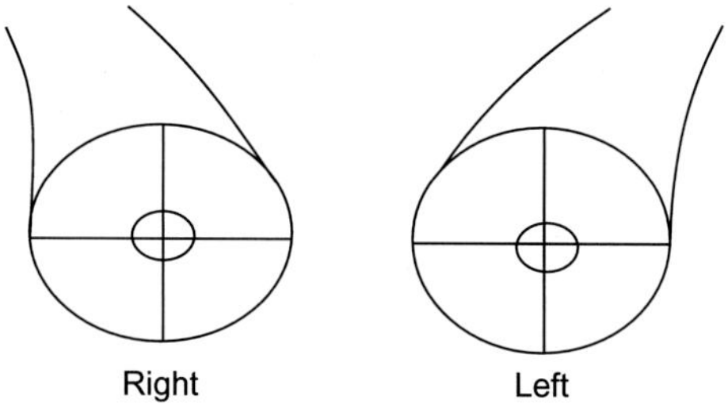

Abdomen

❑ Non-tender ❑ Tender ❑ Incisions ❑ Trigger Points
❑ Inguinal Tenderness ❑ Inguinal Bulge ❑ Suprapubic Tenderness ❑ Ovarian Point Tenderness
❑ Mass ❑ Guarding ❑ Rebound ❑ Distention
❑ Other ____

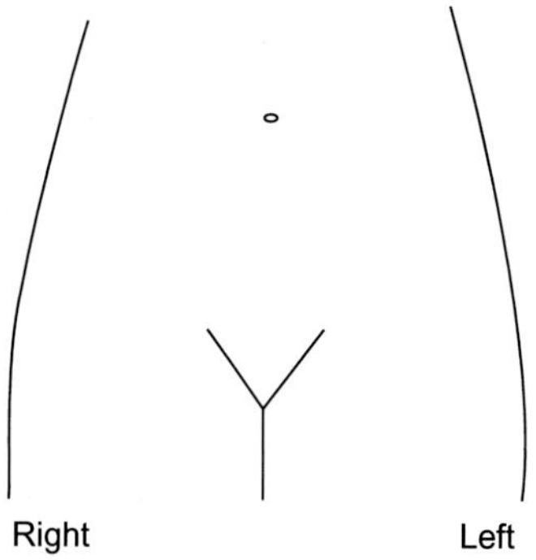

Trigger Points

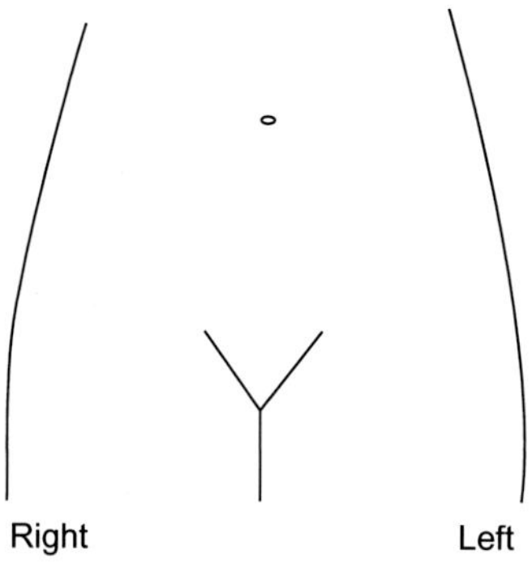

Surgical Scars

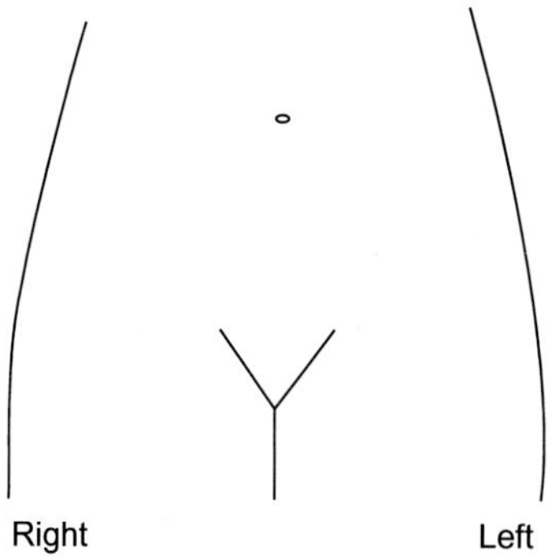

Other Findings

Back

❑ Non-tender ❑ Tender ❑ Alteration in posture ❑ SI joint rotation ________

Lower Extremities

❑ WNL ❑ Edema ❑ Varicosities ❑ Neuropathy ❑ Length Discrepancy ______

Neuropathy

❑ Iliohypogastric ❑ Ilioinguinal ❑ Genitofemoral ❑ Pudendal ❑ Altered Sensation

Fibromyalgia / Back / Buttock

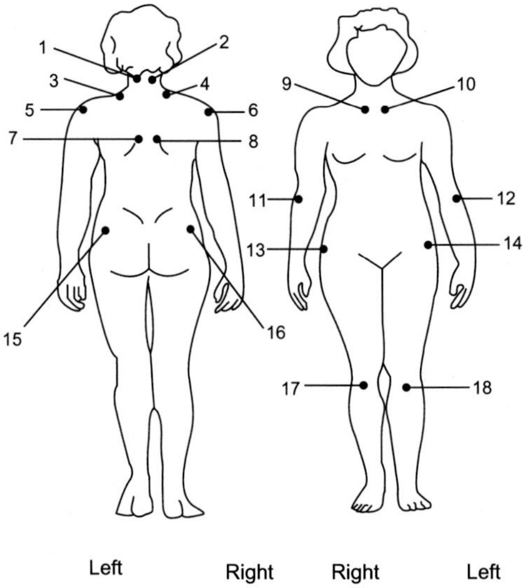

External Genitalia

❑ WNL ❑ Erythema ❑ Discharge ❑ Q-tip test (show on diagram) ❑ Tenderness (show on diagram)

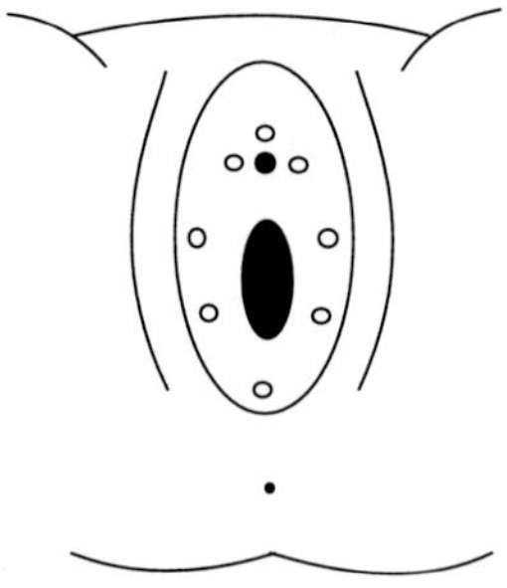

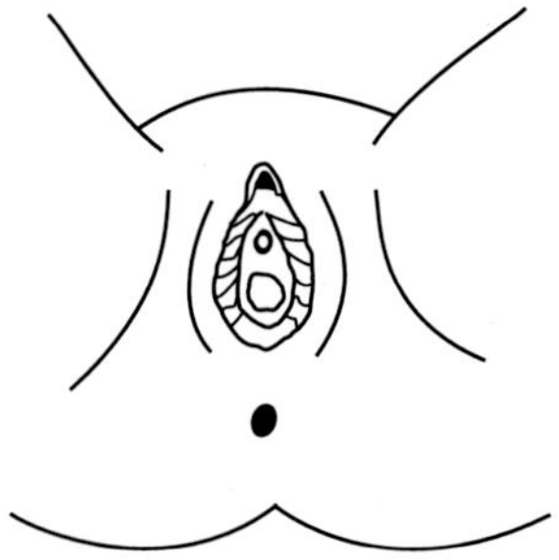

Q-tip Test (score each circle 0-4) **Total Score** ______ **Other Findings**______________________

Vagina

❑ WML ❑ Wet prep:____

❑ Local tenderness________________ Vaginal mucosa________________ Discharge______________

Cultures: ❑ GC ❑ Chlamydia ❑ Fungal ❑ Herpes

❑ Vaginal Apex Tenderness (post hysterectomy – show on diagram)

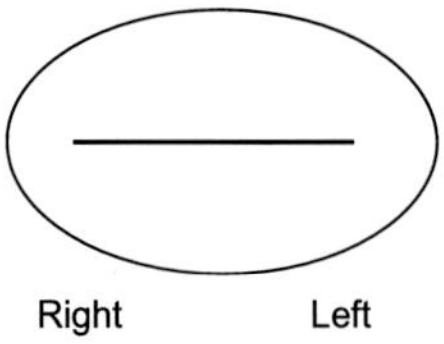

Transverse apex closure

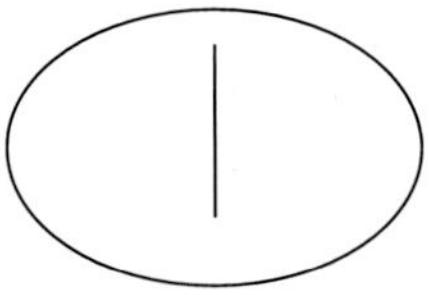

Vertical apex closure

Unimanual Exam

- ❑ WNL
- ❑ Introitus
- ❑ Uterine-cervical junction
- ❑ Urethra
- ❑ Bladder
- ❑ R ureter
- ❑ R inguinal
- ❑ Muscle awareness
- ❑ Cervix
- ❑ Cervical motion
- ❑ Parametrium
- ❑ Vaginal cuff
- ❑ Cul-de-sac
- ❑ L ureter
- ❑ L inguinal
- ❑ Clitoral tenderness

Rank muscle tenderness on 0-4 scale

- ❑ R obturator ____________________
- ❑ R piriformis ____________________
- ❑ R pubococcygeus ________________
- ❑ Total pelvic floor score ___________
- ❑ L obturator ________________
- ❑ L pyriformis ________________
- ❑ L pubococcygeus ____________
- ❑ Anal sphincter _____________

Bimanual Exam

Uterus:	❑ Tender	❑ Non-tender	❑ Absent
Position:	❑ Anterior	❑ Posterior	❑ Midplane
Size:	❑ Normal	❑ Other ______________________	
Contour:	❑ Regular	❑ Irregular	❑ Other
Consistency:	❑ Firm	❑ Soft	❑ Hard
Mobility:	❑ Mobile	❑ Hypermobile	❑ Fixed
Support:	❑ Well supported	❑ Prolapse	

Adnexal Exam

Right:

- ❑ Absent
- ❑ WNL
- ❑ Tender
- ❑ Fixed
- ❑ Enlarged _________ cm

Left:

- ❑ Absent
- ❑ WNL
- ❑ Tender
- ❑ Fixed
- ❑ Enlarged _________ cm

Rectovaginal Exam

- ❑ WNL
- ❑ Tenderness
- ❑ Nodules
- ❑ Mucosal pathology
- ❑ Guaiac positive
- ❑ Not examined

Assessment: ____

____

____

____

____

Diagnostic Plan: ____

____

____

Therapeutic Plan: ____

____

____

The Stanford Pelvic Pain Symptom Score (PPSS) for men (Stanford)

Appendix PPSS for men

Over the past month or so, including today, how much were you bothered by the following	Not at All	A Little Bit	Moderately	Quite a Bit	Extremely
Pain in the lower back	0	1	2	3	4
Pain in the lower abdomen or pubic area	0	1	2	3	4
Pain during urination	0	1	2	3	4
Pain with bowel movement	0	1	2	3	4
Pain in the rectum	0	1	2	3	4
Pain in the prostate gland	0	1	2	3	4
Pain in the testicles	0	1	2	3	4
Pain in the penis	0	1	2	3	4
Number of days pain experienced in the last month*	0	6	15	24	30
How bad is the pain on average? Put an X on the line from 0 to 10†	0				10
	No pain				Most painful
			Total Pain Score ________		
Difficulty postponing urination, hard to hold urgency	0	1	2	3	4
Need to urinate again less than 2 hours after urinating frequency	0	1	2	3	4
Number of times urinating at night	0	1	2	3	4
Bladder does not feel completely right after urinating	0	1	2	3	4
Stopping and starting several times while urinating intermittence	0	1	2	3	4
Weak urinary stream	0	1	2	3	4
Having to push or strain to begin urination	0	1	2	3	4
			Total Urinary Score ________		
Lack of interest in sexual activity	0	1	2	3	4
Difficulty getting an erection	0	1	2	3	4
Difficulty maintaining an erection	0	1	2	3	4
Difficulty reaching an ejaculation	0	1	2	3	4
Pain with ejaculation	0	1	2	3	4
			Total Sexual Score ________		

*The approximate number of days pain was experienced is scored in increments and is associated with a severity category for scoring; e.g. 10 days of pains represents moderate severity and is served as it.

†The 10 puzzle visual and scale score was used cloness the pain VAS, best the score was also incrementally included in the Total Pain Score. That is, the X mark on the line was scored as i of the 5 categoreis Not at All through Proximity based on position on the line. The maximum local pain score is 40, maximum total urinary score is 28, and maximum sexual score is 28, and maximum sexual score is 20.

NIH-Chronic Prostatitis Symptom Index (NIH-CPSI)

Pain or Discomfort

1. In the last week, have you experienced any pain or discomfort in the following areas?

	Yes	No
a. Area between rectum and testicles (perineum)	❑1	❑0
b. Testicles	❑1	❑0
c. Tip of the penis (not related to urination)	❑1	❑0
d. Below your waist, in your pubic or bladder area	❑1	❑0

2. In the last week, have you experienced:

	Yes	No
a. Pain or burning during urination?	❑1	❑0
b. Pain or discomfort during or after sexual climax (ejaculation)?	❑1	❑0

3. How often have you had pain or discomfort in any of these areas over the last week?

❑0 Never
❑1 Rarely
❑2 Sometimes
❑3 Often
❑4 Usually
❑5 Always

4. Which number best describes your AVERAGE pain or discomfort on the days that you had it, over the last week?

❑	❑	❑	❑	❑	❑	❑	❑	❑	❑	❑
0 NO PAIN	1	2	3	4	5	6	7	8	9	10 PAIN AS BAD AS YOU CAN IMAGINE

Urination

5. How often have you had a sensation of not emptying your bladder completely after you finished urinating, over the last week?

❑0 Not at all
❑1 Less than 1 time in 5
❑2 Less than half the time
❑3 About half the time
❑4 More than half the time
❑5 Almost always

6. How often have you had to urinate again less than two hours after you finished urinating, over the last week?

❑0 Not at all
❑1 Less than 1 time in 5
❑2 Less than half the time
❑3 About half the time
❑4 More than half the time
❑5 Almost always

Impact of Symptoms

7. How much have your symptoms kept you from doing the kinds of things you would usually do, over the last week?

❑0 None
❑1 Only a little
❑2 Some
❑3 A lot

8. How much did you think about your symptoms, over the last week?

❑0 None
❑1 Only a little
❑2 Some
❑3 A lot

Quality of Life

9. If you were to spend the rest of your life with your symptoms just the way they have been during the last week, how would you feel about that?

❑0 Delighted
❑1 Pleased
❑2 Mostly satisfied
❑3 Mixed (about equally satisfied and dissatisfied)
❑4 Mostly dissatisfied
❑5 Unhappy
❑6 Terrible

Scoring the NIH-Chronic Prostatitis Symptom Index Domains

Pain: Total of items 1a, 1b, 1c, 1d, 2a, 2b, 3, and 4 = ____________

Urinary Symptoms: Total of items 5 and 6 = ____________

Quality of Life Impact: Total of items 7, 8, and 9 = ____________

Female questionnaire

1. In the last week, have you experienced any pain or discomfort in the following areas?

a. Entrance to vagina	❑$_1$ Yes	❑$_0$ No
b. Vagina	❑$_1$ Yes	❑$_0$ No
c. Urethra	❑$_1$ Yes	❑$_0$ No
d. Below your waist, in your pubic or bladder area	❑$_1$ Yes	❑$_0$ No

2. In the last week, have you experienced:

a. Pain or burning during urination?	❑$_1$ Yes	❑$_0$ No
b. Pain or discomfort during or after sexual intercourse?	❑$_1$ Yes	❑$_0$ No
c. Pain or discomfort as your bladder fills?	❑$_1$ Yes	❑$_0$ No
d. Pain or discomfort relieved by voiding?	❑$_1$ Yes	❑$_0$ No

3. How often have you had pain or discomfort in any of these areas over the last week?

❑$_0$ Never ❑$_1$ Rarely ❑$_2$ Sometimes ❑$_3$ Often ❑$_4$ Usually ❑$_5$ Always

4. Which number best describes your AVERAGE pain or discomfort on the days you had it, over the last week?

❑	❑	❑	❑	❑	❑	❑	❑	❑	❑	❑
0 No pain	1	2	3	4	5	6	7	8	9	10 Pain as bad as you can imagine

5. How often have you had a sensation of not emptying your bladder completely after you finished urinating, over the last week?

❑$_0$ Not at all ❑$_1$ Less than 1 time in 5 ❑$_2$ Less than half the time ❑$_3$ About half the time ❑$_4$ More than half the time ❑$_5$ Almost always

6. How often have you had to urinate again less than two hours after you finished urinating, over the last week?

❑$_0$ Not at all ❑$_1$ Less than 1 time in 5 ❑$_2$ Less than half the time ❑$_3$ About half the time ❑$_4$ More than half the time ❑$_5$ Almost always

7. How much have your symptoms kept you from doing the kinds of things you would usually do, over the last week?

❑$_0$ None ❑$_1$ Only a little ❑$_2$ Some ❑$_4$ A lot

8. How much did you think about your symptoms, over the last week?

❑$_0$ None ❑$_1$ Only a little ❑$_2$ Some ❑$_4$ A lot

9. If you were to spend the rest of your life with your symptoms just the way they have been during the last week, how would you feel about that?

❑$_0$ Delighted
❑$_1$ Pleased
❑$_2$ Mostly satisfied
❑$_3$ Mixed (about equally satisfied and dissatisfied)
❑$_4$ Mostly dissatisfied
❑$_5$ Unhappy
❑$_6$ Terrible

Scoring

Pain subscale: Total of items 1a, 1b, 1c, 1d, 2a, 2b, 2c, 2d, 3, and 4	=_______	(range 0–23)
Urinary subscale: Total of items 5 and 6	=_______	(range 0–10)
QOL impact: Total of items 7, 8, and 9	=_______	(range 0–12)
Total score: Sum of subscale scores	=_______	(range 0–45)

Female Sexual Function Index (FSFI)©

Subject Identifier______________________ Date____________

INSTRUCTIONS: These questions ask about your sexual feelings and responses during the past 4 weeks. Please answer the following questions as honestly and clearly as possible. Your responses will be kept completely confidential. In answering these questions the following definitions apply:

Sexual activity can include caressing, foreplay, masturbation and vaginal intercourse.

Sexual intercourse is defined as penile penetration (entry) of the vagina.

Sexual stimulation includes situations like foreplay with a partner, self-stimulation (masturbation) or sexual fantasy.

CHECK ONLY ONE BOX PER QUESTION.

Sexual desire or interest is a feeling that includes wanting to have a sexual experience, feeling receptive to a partner's sexual initiation, and thinking or fantasizing about having sex.

1. Over the past 4 weeks, how **often** did you feel sexual desire or interest?
- Almost always or always
- Most times (more than half the time)
- Sometimes (about half the time)
- A few times (less than half the time)
- Almost never or never

2. Over the past 4 weeks, how would you rate your **level** (degree) of sexual desire or interest?
- Very high
- High
- Moderate
- Low
- Very low or none at all

Sexual arousal is a feeling that includes both physical and mental aspects of sexual excitement. It may include feelings of warmth or tingling in the genitals, lubrication (wetness), or muscle contractions.

3. Over the past 4 weeks, how **often** did you feel sexually aroused ("turn on") during sexual activity or intercourse?
- No sexual activity
- Almost always or always
- Most times (more than half the time)
- Sometimes (about half the time)
- A few times (less than half the time)
- Almost never or never

4. Over the past 4 weeks, how would you rate your **level** of sexual arousal ("turn on") during sexual activity or intercourse?
- No sexual activity
- Very high
- High
- Moderate
- Low
- Very low or none at all

5. Over the past 4 weeks, how **confident** were you about becoming sexually aroused during sexual activity or intercourse?
- No sexual activity
- Very high confidence
- High confidence
- Moderate confidence
- Low confidence
- Very low or no confidence

6. Over the past 4 weeks, how **often** have you been satisfied with your arousal (excitement) during sexual activity or intercourse?
- No sexual activity
- Almost always or always
- Most times (more than half the time)
- Sometimes (about half the time)
- A few times (less than half the time)
- Almost never or never

7. Over the past 4 weeks, how **often** did you become lubricated ("wet") during sexual activity or intercourse?
- No sexual activity
- Almost always or always
- Most times (more than half the time)
- Sometimes (about half the time)
- A few times (less than half the time)
- Almost never or never

8. Over the past 4 weeks, how **difficult** was it to become lubricated ("wet") during sexual activity or intercourse?
- No sexual activity
- Extremely difficult or impossible
- Very difficult
- Difficult
- Slightly difficult
- Not difficult

9. Over the past 4 weeks, how often did you **maintain** your lubrication ("wetness") until completion of sexual activity or intercourse?
- No sexual activity
- Almost always or always
- Most times (more than half the time)
- Sometimes (about half the time)
- A few times (less than half the time)
- Almost never or never

10. Over the past 4 weeks, how **difficult** was it to maintain your lubrication ("wetness") until completion of sexual activity or intercourse?
- No sexual activity
- Extremely difficult or impossible
- Very difficult
- Difficult

- Slightly difficult
- Not difficult

11. Over the past 4 weeks, when you had sexual stimulation or intercourse, how **often** did you reach orgasm (climax)?
- No sexual activity
- Almost always or always
- Most times (more than half the time)
- Sometimes (about half the time)
- A few times (less than half the time)
- Almost never or never

12. Over the past 4 weeks, when you had sexual stimulation or intercourse, how **difficult** was it for you to reach orgasm (climax)?
- No sexual activity
- Extremely difficult or impossible
- Very difficult
- Difficult
- Slightly difficult
- Not difficult

13. Over the past 4 weeks, how **satisfied** were you with your ability to reach orgasm (climax) during sexual activity or intercourse?
- No sexual activity
- Very satisfied
- Moderately satisfied
- About equally satisfied and dissatisfied
- Moderately dissatisfied
- Very dissatisfied

14. Over the past 4 weeks, how **satisfied** have you been with the amount of emotional closeness during sexual activity between you and your partner?
- No sexual activity
- Very satisfied
- Moderately satisfied
- About equally satisfied and dissatisfied
- Moderately dissatisfied
- Very dissatisfied

15. Over the past 4 weeks, how **satisfied** have you been with your sexual relationship with your partner?
- Very satisfied
- Moderately satisfied
- About equally satisfied and dissatisfied
- Moderately dissatisfied
- Very dissatisfied

16. Over the past 4 weeks, how **satisfied** have you been with your overall sexual life?
- Very satisfied
- Moderately satisfied
- About equally satisfied and dissatisfied
- Moderately dissatisfied
- Very dissatisfied

17. Over the past 4 weeks, how **often** did you experience discomfort or pain during vaginal penetration?

- Did not attempt intercourse
- Almost always or always
- Most times (more than half the time)
- Sometimes (about half the time)
- A few times (less than half the time)
- Almost never or never

18. Over the past 4 weeks, how **often** did you experience discomfort or pain following vaginal penetration?

- Did not attempt intercourse
- Almost always or always
- Most times (more than half the time)
- Sometimes (about half the time)
- A few times (less than half the time)
- Almost never or never

19. Over the past 4 weeks, how would you rate your **level** (degree) of discomfort or pain during or following vaginal penetration?

- Did not attempt intercourse
- Very high
- High
- Moderate
- Low
- Very low or none at all

Thank you for completing this questionnaire.

FSFI scoring appendix

Question	Response options
1. Over the past 4 weeks, how often did you feel sexual desire or interest?	5 = Almost always or always 4 = Most times (more than half the time) 3 = Sometimes (about half the time) 2 = A few times (less than half the time) 1 = Almost never or never
2. Over the past 4 weeks, how would you rate your level (degree) of sexual desire or interest?	5 = Very high 4 = High 3 = Moderate 2 = Low 1 = Very low or none at all
3. Over the past 4 weeks, how often did you feel sexually aroused ("turn on") during sexual activity or intercourse?	0 = No sexual activity 5 = Almost always or always 4 = Most times (more than half the time) 3 = Sometimes (about half the time) 2 = A few times (less than half the time) 1 = Almost never or never

4. Over the past 4 weeks, how would you rate your level of sexual arousal ("turn on") during sexual activity or intercourse?

0 = No sexual activity
5 = Very high
4 = High
3 = Moderate
2 = Low
1 = Very low or none at all

5. Over the past 4 weeks, how confident were you about becoming sexually aroused during sexual activity or intercourse?

0 = No sexual activity
5 = Very high confidence
4 = High confidence
3 = Moderate confidence
2 = Low confidence
1 = Very low or no confidence

6. Over the past 4 weeks, how often have you been satisfied with your arousal (excitement) during sexual activity or intercourse?

0 = No sexual activity
5 = Almost always or always
4 = Most times (more than half the time)
3 = Sometimes (about half the time)
2 = A few times (less than half the time)
1 = Almost never or never

7. Over the past 4 weeks, how often did you become lubricated ("wet") during sexual activity or intercourse?

0 = No sexual activity
5 = Almost always or always
4 = Most times (more than half the time)
3 = Sometimes (about half the time)
2 = A few times (less than half the time)
1 = Almost never or never

8. Over the past 4 weeks, how difficult was it to become lubricated ("wet") during sexual activity or intercourse?

0 = No sexual activity
1 = Extremely difficult or impossible
2 = Very difficult
3 = Difficult
4 = Slightly difficult
5 = Not difficult

9. Over the past 4 weeks, how often did you maintain your lubrication ("wetness") until completion of sexual activity or intercourse?

0 = No sexual activity
5 = Almost always or always
4 = Most times (more than half the time)
3 = Sometimes (about half the time)
2 = A few times (less than half the time)
1 = Almost never or never

10. Over the past 4 weeks, how difficult was it to maintain your lubrication ("wetness") until completion of sexual activity or intercourse?

0 = No sexual activity
1 = Extremely difficult or impossible
2 = Very difficult
3 = Difficult
4 = Slightly difficult
5 = Not difficult

11. Over the past 4 weeks, when you had sexual stimulation or intercourse, how often did you reach orgasm (climax)?	0 = No sexual activity 5 = Almost always or always 4 = Most times (more than half the time) 3 = Sometimes (about half the time) 2 = A few times (less than half the time) 1 = Almost never or never
12. Over the past 4 weeks, when you had sexual stimulation or intercourse, how difficult was it for you to reach orgasm (climax)?	0 = No sexual activity 1 = Extremely difficult or impossible 2 = Very difficult 3 = Difficult 4 = Slightly difficult 5 = Not difficult
13. Over the past 4 weeks, how satisfied were you with your ability to reach orgasm (climax) during sexual activity or intercourse?	0 = No sexual activity 5 = Very satisfied 4 = Moderately satisfied 3 = About equally satisfied and dissatisfied 2 = Moderately dissatisfied 1 = Very dissatisfied
14. Over the past 4 weeks, how satisfied have you been with the amount of emotional closeness during sexual activity between you and your partner?	0 = No sexual activity 5 = Very satisfied 4 = Moderately satisfied 3 = About equally satisfied and dissatisfied 2 = Moderately dissatisfied 1 = Very dissatisfied
15. Over the past 4 weeks, how satisfied have you been with your sexual relationship with your partner?	5 = Very satisfied 4 = Moderately satisfied 3 = About equally satisfied and dissatisfied 2 = Moderately dissatisfied 1 = Very dissatisfied
16. Over the past 4 weeks, how satisfied have you been with your overall sexual life?	5 = Very satisfied 4 = Moderately satisfied 3 = About equally satisfied and dissatisfied 2 = Moderately dissatisfied 1 = Very dissatisfied
17. Over the past 4 weeks, how often did you experience discomfort or pain during vaginal penetration?	0 = Did not attempt intercourse 1 = Almost always or always 2 = Most times (more than half the time) 3 = Sometimes (about half the time) 4 = A few times (less than half the time) 5 = Almost never or never

18. Over the past 4 weeks, how often did you experience discomfort or pain following vaginal penetration?

0 = Did not attempt intercourse
1 = Almost always or always
2 = Most times (more than half the time)
3 = Sometimes (about half the time)
4 = A few times (less than half the time)
5 = Almost never or never

19. Over the past 4 weeks, how would you rate your level (degree) of discomfort or pain during or following vaginal penetration?

0 = Did not attempt intercourse
1 = Very high
2 = High
3 = Moderate
4 = Low
5 = Very low or none at all

FSFI domain scores and full scale score

The individual domain scores and full scale (overall) score of the FSFI can be derived from the computational formula outlined in the table below. For individual domain scores, add the scores of the individual items that comprise the domain and multiply the sum by the domain factor (see below). Add the six domain scores to obtain the full scale score. It should be noted that, within the individual domains, a domain score of zero indicates that the subject reported having no sexual activity during the past month. Subject scores can be entered in the right-hand column.

Domain	Questions	Score Range	Factor	Minimum Score	Maximum Score	Score
Desire	1,2	1–5	0.6	1.2	6.0	
Arousal	3,4,5,6	0–5	0.3	0	6.0	
Lubrication	7,8,9,10	0–5	0.3	0	6.0	
Orgasm	11,12,13	0–5	0.4	0	6.0	
Satisfaction	14,15,16	0 (or 1)–5	0.4	0.8	6.0	
Pain	17,18,19	0–5	0.4	0	6.0	
Full Scale Score Range				2.0	36.0	

Female Sexual Distress Scale

Please fill in the following biographical information:

Name________________________ Type of treatment received________________

Date treatment was received (M/D/Y): _____/_____/_____

Below is a list of feelings and problems that women sometimes have concerning their sexuality. Please read each item carefully, and check the box that best describes how often that problem has bothered you or caused distress both before and after treatment. Please check only one box for each item, and take care not to skip ANY items. If you change your mind, erase your markings carefully. Read the example before beginning, and if you have any questions, please about them.

Example:

1. How often did you feel personal responsibility for your sexual problems?

	Pre-Treatment	Post-Treatment
NEVER	[ ]	[ ]
RARELY	[ ]	[ ]
OCCASIONALLY	[ ]	[ ]
FREQUENTLY	[ ]	[ ]
ALWAYS	[ ]	[ ]

2. How often did you feel unhappy about your sexual relationship?

	Pre-Treatment	Post-Treatment
NEVER	[ ]	[ ]
RARELY	[ ]	[ ]
OCCASIONALLY	[ ]	[ ]
FREQUENTLY	[ ]	[ ]
ALWAYS	[ ]	[ ]

3. How often did you feel guilty about your sexual difficulties?

	Pre-Treatment	Post-Treatment
NEVER	[ ]	[ ]
RARELY	[ ]	[ ]
OCCASIONALLY	[ ]	[ ]
FREQUENTLY	[ ]	[ ]
ALWAYS	[ ]	[ ]

4. How often did you feel frustrated by your sexual problems?

	Pre-Treatment	Post-Treatment
NEVER	[ ]	[ ]
RARELY	[ ]	[ ]
OCCASIONALLY	[ ]	[ ]
FREQUENTLY	[ ]	[ ]
ALWAYS	[ ]	[ ]

5. How often did you feel stressed about sex?

	Pre-Treatment	Post-Treatment
NEVER	[ ]	[ ]
RARELY	[ ]	[ ]
OCCASIONALLY	[ ]	[ ]
FREQUENTLY	[ ]	[ ]
ALWAYS	[ ]	[ ]

6. How often did you feel inferior because of sexual problems?

	Pre-Treatment	Post-Treatment
NEVER	[ ]	[ ]
RARELY	[ ]	[ ]
OCCASIONALLY	[ ]	[ ]
FREQUENTLY	[ ]	[ ]
ALWAYS	[ ]	[ ]

7. How often did you feel worried about sex?

	Pre-Treatment	Post-Treatment
NEVER	[ ]	[ ]
RARELY	[ ]	[ ]
OCCASIONALLY	[ ]	[ ]
FREQUENTLY	[ ]	[ ]
ALWAYS	[ ]	[ ]

8. How often did you feel sexually inadequate?

	Pre-Treatment	Post-Treatment
NEVER	[ ]	[ ]
RARELY	[ ]	[ ]
OCCASIONALLY	[ ]	[ ]
FREQUENTLY	[ ]	[ ]
ALWAYS	[ ]	[ ]

9. How often did you feel regrets about your sexuality?

	Pre-Treatment	Post-Treatment
NEVER	[ ]	[ ]
RARELY	[ ]	[ ]
OCCASIONALLY	[ ]	[ ]
FREQUENTLY	[ ]	[ ]
ALWAYS	[ ]	[ ]

10. How often did you feel embarrassed about your sexual problems?

	Pre-Treatment	Post-Treatment
NEVER	[ ]	[ ]
RARELY	[ ]	[ ]
OCCASIONALLY	[ ]	[ ]
FREQUENTLY	[ ]	[ ]
ALWAYS	[ ]	[ ]

11. How often did you feel dissatisfied with your sex life?

	Pre-Treatment	Post-Treatment
NEVER	[ ]	[ ]
RARELY	[ ]	[ ]
OCCASIONALLY	[ ]	[ ]
FREQUENTLY	[ ]	[ ]
ALWAYS	[ ]	[ ]

12. How often did you feel angry about your sex life?

	Pre-Treatment	Post-Treatment
NEVER	[ ]	[ ]
RARELY	[ ]	[ ]
OCCASIONALLY	[ ]	[ ]
FREQUENTLY	[ ]	[ ]
ALWAYS	[ ]	[ ]

Vulvar pain functional questionnaire (V-Q)

These are statements about how your pelvic pain affects your everyday life. Please check one box for each item below, choosing the one that best describes your situation. Some of the statements deal with personal subjects. These statements are included because they will help your health care provider design the best treatment for you and measure your progress during treatment. Your responses will be kept completely confidential at all times.

1. Because of my pelvic pain
- ❑ 3 I can't wear tight-fitting clothing like pantyhose that puts any pressure over my painful area.
- ❑ 2 I can wear closer fitting clothing as long as it only puts a little bit of pressure over my painful area.
- ❑ 1 I can wear whatever I like most of the time, but every now and then I feel pelvic pain caused by pressure from my clothing.
- ❑ 0 I can wear whatever I like; I never have pelvic pain because of clothing.

2. My pelvic pain
- ❑ 3 Gets worse when I walk, so I can only walk far enough to move around in my house, no further.
- ❑ 2 Gets worse when I walk. I can walk a short distance outside the house, but it is very painful to walk far enough to get a full load of groceries in a grocery store.
- ❑ 1 Gets a little worse when I walk. I can walk far enough to do my errands, like grocery shopping, but it would be very painful to walk longer distances for fun or exercise.
- ❑ 0 My pain does not get worse with walking; I can walk as far as I want to.
- ❑ 0 I have a hard time walking because of another medical problem, but pelvic pain doesn't make it hard to walk.

3. My pelvic pain
- ❑ 3 Gets worse when I sit, so it hurts too much to sit any longer than 30 minutes at a time.
- ❑ 2 Gets worse when I sit. I can sit for longer than 30 minutes at a time, but it is so painful that it is difficult to do my job or sit long enough to watch a movie.
- ❑ 1 Occasionally gets worse when I sit, but most of the time sitting is comfortable.
- ❑ 0 My pain does not get worse with sitting, I can sit as long as I want to.
- ❑ 0 I have trouble sitting for very long because of another medical problem, but pelvic pain doesn't make it hard to sit.

4. Because of pain pills I take for my pelvic pain
- ❑ 3 I am sleepy and I have trouble concentrating at work or while I do housework.
- ❑ 2 I can concentrate just enough to do my work, but I can't do more, like go out in the evenings.
- ❑ 1 I can do all of my work, and go out in the evening if I want, but I feel out of sorts.
- ❑ 0 I don't have any problems with the pills that I take for pelvic pain.
- ❑ 0 I don't take pain pills for my pelvic pain.

5. Because of my pelvic pain
- ❑ 3 I have very bad pain when I try to have a bowel movement, and it keeps hurting for at least 5 minutes after I am finished.
- ❑ 2 It hurts when I try to have a bowel movement, but the pain goes away when I am finished.
- ❑ 1 Most of the time it does not hurt when I have a bowel movement, but every now and then it does.
- ❑ 0 It never hurts from my pelvic pain when I have a bowel movement.

6. Because of my pelvic pain

- ❑ 3 I don't get together with my friends or go out to parties or events.
- ❑ 2 I only get together with my friends or go out to parties or events every now and then.
- ❑ 1 I usually will go out with friends or to events if I want to, but every now and then I don't because of the pain.
- ❑ 0 I get together with friends or go to events whenever I want, pelvic pain does not get in the way

7. Because of my pelvic pain

- ❑ 3 I can't stand for the doctor to insert the speculum when I go to the gynecologist.
- ❑ 2 I can stand it when the doctor inserts the speculum if they are very careful, but most of the time it really hurts.
- ❑ 1 It usually doesn't hurt when the doctor inserts the speculum, but every now and then it does hurt.
- ❑ 0 It never hurts for the doctor to insert the speculum when I go to the gynecologist.

8. Because of my pelvic pain

- ❑ 3 I cannot use tampons at all, because they make my pain much worse.
- ❑ 2 I can only use tampons if I put them in very carefully.
- ❑ 1 It usually doesn't hurt to use tampons, but occasionally it does hurt.
- ❑ 0 It never hurts to use tampons.
- ❑ 0 This question doesn't apply to me, because I don't need to use tampons, or I wouldn't choose to use them whether they hurt or not.

9. Because of my pelvic pain

- ❑ 3 I can't let my partner put a finger or penis in my vagina during sex at all.
- ❑ 2 My partner can put a finger or penis in my vagina very carefully, but it still hurts.
- ❑ 1 It usually doesn't hurt if my partner puts a finger or penis in my vagina, but every now and then it does hurt.
- ❑ 0 It doesn't hurt to have my partner put a finger or penis in my vagina at all.
- ❑ 0 This question does not apply to me because I don't have a sexual partner.
- ❑ 0 Specifically, I won't get involved with a partner because I worry about pelvic pain during sex.

10. Because of my pelvic pain

- ❑ 3 It hurts too much for my partner to touch me sexually even if the touching doesn't go in my vagina.
- ❑ 2 My partner can touch me sexually outside the vagina if we are very careful.
- ❑ 1 It doesn't usually hurt for my partner to touch me sexually outside the vagina, but every now and then it does hurt
- ❑ 0 It never hurts for my partner to touch me sexually outside the vagina.
- ❑ 0 This question does not apply to me because I don't have a sexual partner.
- ❑ 0 Specifically, I won't get involved with a partner because I worry about pelvic pain during sex.

11. Because of my pelvic pain

- ❑ 3 It is too painful to touch myself for sexual pleasure.
- ❑ 2 I can touch myself for sexual pleasure if I am very careful.
- ❑ 1 It usually doesn't hurt to touch myself for sexual pleasure, but every now and then it does hurt.
- ❑ 0 It never hurts to touch myself for sexual pleasure.
- ❑ 0 I don't touch myself for sexual pleasure, but that is by choice, not because of pelvic pain.

Nijmegen questionnaire

Please mark the score that best describes the frequency with which you experience the symptoms listed.

	Never 0	Rare 1	Sometimes 2	Often 3	Very often 4
Chest pain					
Feeling tense					
Blurred vision					
Dizzy spells					
Feeling confused					
Faster & deeper breathing					
Short of breath					
Tight feelings in chest					
Bloated feeling in stomach					
Tingling fingers					
Unable to breathe deeply					
Stiff fingers or arms					
Tight feelings round mouth					
Cold hands or feet					
Palpitations					
Feelings of anxiety					

Name:

Age: Male/Female

Medication: Main complaints:

The self-evaluation of breathing questionnaire

Scoring this questionnaire: *(0) never/not true at all; (1) occasionally/a bit true; (2) frequently/mostly true; and (3) very frequently/very true*

1. I get easily breathless out of proportion to my fitness	0	1	2	3
2. I notice myself breathing shallowly	0	1	2	3
3. I get short of breath reading and talking	0	1	2	3
4. I notice myself sighing	0	1	2	3
5. I notice myself yawning	0	1	2	3
6. I feel I cannot take a deep or satisfying breath	0	1	2	3
7. I notice that I am breathing irregularly	0	1	2	3
8. My breathing feels stuck or restricted	0	1	2	3
9. My ribcage feels tight and can't expand	0	1	2	3
10. I notice myself breathing quickly	0	1	2	3
11. I get breathless when I'm anxious	0	1	2	3
12. I find myself holding my breath	0	1	2	3
13. I feel breathless in association with other physical symptoms	0	1	2	3
14. I have trouble coordinating my breathing when speaking	0	1	2	3
15. I can't catch my breath	0	1	2	3
16. I feel that the air is stuffy, as if not enough air in the room	0	1	2	3
17. I get breathless even when resting	0	1	2	3
18. My breath feels like it does not go in all the way	0	1	2	3
19. My breath feels like it does not go out all the way	0	1	2	3
20. My breathing is heavy	0	1	2	3
21. I feel that I am breathing more	0	1	2	3
22. My breathing requires work	0	1	2	3
23. My breathing require effort	0	1	2	3
24. I breath through my mouth during the day	0	1	2	3
25. I breathe through my mouth at night while I sleep	0	1	2	3

Description of pelvic girdle pain tests (Vleeming et al. 2008)

Active straight leg raise test

The patient lies supine with straight legs and the feet 20 cm apart. The test is performed after the instruction: 'Try to raise your legs, one after the other, above the couch for 20 cm without bending the knee'. The patient is asked to score any feeling of impairment (on both sides separately) on a six-point scale: not difficult at all = 0; minimally difficult = 1; somewhat difficult = 2; fairly difficult = 3; very difficult = 4; unable to do = 5. The scores on both sides are added so that the sum score can range from 0 to 10 (Mens et al. 2001).

Gaenslen's test

The patient, lying supine, flexes the hip/knee and draws it towards the chest by clasping the flexed knee with both hands. The patient is then shifted to the side of the examination table so that the opposite leg extends over the edge while the other leg remains flexed. The examiner uses this manoeuvre to gently stress both sacroiliac joints simultaneously.

The test is positive if the patient experiences pain (either local or referred) on the provoked side (Gaenslen 1927).

Long dorsal sacroiliac ligament (LDL) test

The LDL test in postpartum women

The patient lies prone and is tested for tenderness on bilateral palpation of the LDL directly under the caudal part of the posterior superior iliac spine. A skilled examiner scores the pain as positive or negative on a 4-point scale: no pain = 0; mild = 1; moderate = 2; unbearable = 3.

The scores on both sides are added so that the sum score can range from 0 to 6 (Vleeming et al. 2002).

The LDL test in pregnant women

The patient lies on her side with slight flexion in both hip and knee joints. If the palpation causes pain that persists for more than 5 seconds after removal of the examiner's hand it is recorded as pain. If the pain disappears within 5 seconds it is recorded as tenderness (Albert et al. 2000).

Pain provocation of the symphysis by modified Trendelenburg's test

The patient stands on one leg and flexes the hip and knee at 90°. If pain is experienced in the symphysis the test is considered positive (Albert et al. 2000).

Patrick's Faber test

The patient lies supine: one leg is flexed, abducted and externally rotated so that the heel rests on the opposite knee. The examiner presses gently on the superior aspect of the tested knee joint. If pain is felt in the sacroiliac joints or in the symphysis the test is considered positive (Albert et al. 2000, Broadhurst & Bond 1998, Wormslev et al. 1994).

Posterior pelvic pain provocation test

The test is performed supine and the patient's hip flexed to an angle of 90° on the side to be examined. Light manual pressure is applied to the patient's flexed knee along the longitudinal axis of the femur while the pelvis is stabilized by the examiner's other hand resting on the patient's contralateral superior anterior iliac spine.

The test is positive when the patient feels a familiar well-localized pain deep in the gluteal area on the provoked side (Ostgaard 1994).

A similar test is described as the posterior shear or 'thigh thrust' test (Laslett & Williams 1994).

Symphysis pain palpation test

The patient lies supine. The entire front side of the pubic symphysis is palpated gently. If the palpation causes pain that persists more than 5 seconds after removal of the examiner's hand, it is recorded as pain. If the pain disappears within 5 seconds it is recorded as tenderness (Albert et al. 2000).

References

Clinical outcome measurement tools

Anderson, R., Wise, D., Sawyer, T., Chan, C., 2005. Integration of myofascial trigger point release and paradoxical relaxation training treatment of chronic pelvic pain in men. J. Urol. 174, 155–160.

Courtney, R., Greenwood, K.M., 2009. Preliminary investigation of a measure of dysfunctional breathing symptoms: the Self Evaluation of Breathing Questionnaire (SEBQ). Int. J. Osteopathic Med. 12, 121–127.

Derogatis, L.R., Rosen, R., Leiblum, S., Burnett, A., Heiman, J., 2002. The Female Sexual Distress Scale (FSDS): initial validation of a standardized scale for assessment of sexually related personal distress in women. J. Sex Marital Ther. 28 (4), 317–330.

Leserman, J., Drossman, D., Li, Z., 1995. The reliability and validity of a sexual and physical abuse history questionnaire in female patients with gastrointestinal disorders. Behav. Med. 21, 141–148.

Marszalek, M., Wehrberger, C., Temml, C., et al., 2009. Chronic pelvic pain and lower urinary tract symptoms in both sexes: analysis of 2749 participants of an urban health screening project. Eur. Urol. 55, 499–1408.

Melzack, R., 1987. The Short-form McGill Pain Questionnaire. Pain 30, 191–197.

Van Dixhoorn, Duivenvoorden, H.J., 1985. Efficacy of Nijmegen questionnaire in recognition of the hyperventilation syndrome. J. Psychosom. Res. 29, 199–206.

Description of pelvic girdle pain tests

Albert, H., Godskesen, M., Westergaard, J., 2000. Evaluation of clinical tests used in classification procedures in pregnancy related pelvic joint pain. Eur. Spine J. 9, 161–166.

Broadhurst, N.A., Bond, M.J., 1998. Pain provocation tests for the assessment of sacroiliac joint dysfunction. J. Spinal Disord. 11, 341–345.

Gaenslen, F.J., 1927. Sacro-iliac arthrodesis. J. Am. Med. Assoc. 89, 2031–2035.

Laslett, M., Williams, M., 1994. The reliability of selected pain provocation tests for sacroiliac joint pathology. Spine 19, 1243–1249.

Mens, J.M., Vleeming, A., Snijders, C.J., Koes, B.W., Stam, H.J., 2001. Reliability and validity of the active straight leg raise test in posterior pelvic pain since pregnancy. Spine 26, 1167–1171.

Ostgaard, H.C., Zetherström, G., Roos-Hansen, E., Svanberg, G., 1994. The posterior pelvic pain provocation test I pregnant women. Eur. Spine J. 3, 258–260.

Vleeming, A., de Vries, H.J., Mens, J.M., van Wingerden, J.P., 2002. Possible role of the long dorsal sacroiliac ligament in women with peripartum pelvic pain. Acta Obstet. Gynecol. Scand. 81, 430–436.

Vleeming, A., Albert, H.B., Ostgaard, H.C., Sturesson, B., Stuge, B., 2008. European guidelines for the diagnosis and treatment of pelvic girdle pain. [Review] [155 refs]. Eur. Spine J. 17 (6), 794–819.

Wormslev, M., Juul, A.M., Marques, B., et al., 1994. Clinical examination of pelvic Insufficiency during pregnancy. Scand. J. Rheumatol. 23, 96–102.

Index

Note: Page numbers followed by *b* indicate boxes, *f* indicate figures and *t* indicate tables.

A

B

C

D

E

F

J

K

L

M

N

O

P

Q

R

T

W

X

Printed in the United States
By Bookmasters